San Diego Christian College
Library
Santee, CA

San Diego Christian College
Library
Santee

Spatial Disorientation in Aviation

153.752
S732d

Spatial Disorientation in Aviation

Edited by

Fred H. Previc
Northrop Grumman Information Technology
San Antonio, Texas
William R. Ercoline
General Dynamics Advanced Information Systems
San Antonio, Texas

Volume 203
PROGRESS IN
ASTRONAUTICS AND AERONAUTICS

Paul Zarchan, Editor-in-Chief
MIT Lincoln Laboratory
Lexington, Massachusetts

Published by the
American Institute of Aeronautics and Astronautics, Inc.
1801 Alexander Bell Drive, Reston, Virginia 20191-4344

American Institute of Aeronautics and Astronautics, Inc., Reston, Virginia

1   2   3   4   5

Copyright © 2004 by the American Institute of Aeronautics and Astronautics, Inc. This work was created in the performance of a Cooperative Research and Development Agreement with the Department of the Air Force. The Government of the United States has certain rights to use this work. Printed in the United States of America. Reproduction or translation of any part of this work beyond that permitted by Sections 107 and 108 of the U.S. Copyright Law without the permission of the copyright owner is unlawful. The code following this statement indicates the copyright owner's consent that copies of articles in this volume may be made for personal or internal use, on condition that the copier pay the per-copy fee ($2.00) plus the per-page fee ($0.50) through the Copyright Clearance Center, Inc., 222 Rosewood Drive, Danvers, Massachusetts 01923. This consent does not extend to other kinds of copying, for which permission requests should be addressed to the publisher. Users should employ the following code when reporting copying from this volume to the Copyright Clearance Center:

1-56347-654-1 $2.00 + .50

Data and information appearing in this book are for informational purposes only. AIAA is not responsible for any injury or damage resulting from use or reliance, nor does AIAA warrant that use or reliance will be free from privately owned rights.

ISBN 1-56347-654-1

Progress in Astronautics and Aeronautics

Editor-in-Chief
Paul Zarchan
MIT Lincoln Laboratory

Editorial Board

David A. Bearden
The Aerospace Corporation

Richard C. Lind
University of Florida

John D. Binder

Richard M. Lloyd
Raytheon Electronics Company

Steven A. Brandt
U.S. Air Force Academy

Frank K. Lu
University of Texas at Arlington

Fred R. DeJarnette
North Carolina State University

Ahmed K. Noor
NASA Langley Research Center

L. S. "Skip" Fletcher
NASA Ames Research Center

Albert C. Piccirillo
Institute for Defense Analyses

Philip D. Hattis
Charles Stark Draper Laboratory

Ben T. Zinn
Georgia Institute of Technology

Foreword

To date there has never been an entire book written about the subject of spatial disorientation (SD) in aviation. Reasons may vary but most likely it is because our understanding has only recently matured to a level that enables a sufficient number of researchers to investigate and write about the different aspects of this known aircrew killer. Although the consequences of SD have been known for a long time, only within about the past ten years have most researchers reached agreement on a common definition, which has allowed the science to flourish. Our understanding of SD can be compared to our understanding produced from cancer research of a few decades ago. Much was being learned, yet a vast amount of knowledge remained to be discovered. And just as that cancer research produced an enormous amount of information about causes and methods of prevention, investigation into SD countermeasures is now following the same course.

SD is a many-faceted problem. Oddly enough, in one situation it may rapidly impair one's ability to fly an aircraft, yet in another under the same set of circumstances, it may not. Moreover, causes are numerous. The more commonly understood causes consist of visual illusions, vestibular and postural perceptions, and erroneous cognitive interpretations—some are well understood, while explanations for others are just beginning to unfold. Therein lies the real challenge of solving the SD problem and the need for a book dedicated to the subject of SD in aviation.

This broad-faced book begins with a historical overview of the early discovery of SD (referred to at the time as pilot vertigo). It continues into the neurological, physiological, and psychological mechanisms of spatial orientation and how normally functioning body systems produce misperceptions of the aircraft's position, motion, and attitude. The seriousness of the problem is explained in detail with a review of both civil and military SD-related accidents. Following this explanation is a chapter dealing with ground and flight training philosophy, including descriptions of devices used to optimize training practices. This chapter is followed by two others describing the means by which flight information is presented to the pilot via the flight instruments in an effort to enable the pilot to avoid any unrecognized SD through the use of a vigilant instrument cross-check. In these two chapters the relationship between aircraft movement and the flight instruments used to recognize aircraft movement is explained. Also, suggestions are made for using the more common research techniques of quantifying SD. The last chapter describes forward-thinking ideas that should prove useful for future research and development.

The authors—a selection of experts who have both research skills in the subject and extensive flight time—tell of their own experiences, their lessons learned, and their research findings. They have assembled a large amount of information pertinent to the causes and countermeasures of SD. There are other theories and ideas still emerging, as mentioned throughout the book, but most of the more thoroughly understood reasons of SD are explained. Notably, the authors have included information relevant to both fixed- and rotary-wing aircraft, while addressing military, general, and commercial aviation needs.

Within these pages is something for anyone interested in SD countermeasures, whether they are pilots, aeromedical specialists, avionics developers, or researchers. As compared earlier to the incremental progress in the continued search for a cure for cancer, this work is but a step in the right direction. You might not find all your answers about SD in this book—not all answers are known (as mentioned at the onset)—but you will find numerous answers to a puzzling problem confronting anyone who pilots an aircraft or decides to research the topic of SD. A book of this nature is long overdue. I suspect there will be more to come.

James W. Brinkley, SES
Director
Human Effectiveness Directorate
U.S. Air Force Research Laboratory

Table of Contents

Preface .... **xiii**

**Chapter 1. Spatial Disorientation in Aviation: Historical
Background, Concepts, and Terminology** **1**

Fred H. Previc, *Northrop Grumman Information Technology, San Antonio,
Texas*; and William R. Ercoline, *General Dynamics Advanced Information
Systems, San Antonio, Texas*

I.	Definition	1
II.	Historical Background	4
III.	Types of SD	20
IV.	Aircraft Motions in Flight	22
V.	Summary	32
	References	32

Chapter 2. Nonvisual Spatial Orientation Mechanisms **37**

Bob Cheung, *Defence Research and Development Canada, Toronto, Canada*

I.	Introduction	37
II.	Overview of Spatial Orientation Mechanisms in Flight	38
III.	Vestibular Input to Orientation	39
IV.	Vestibular Contribution to Gaze Stability	56
V.	Interactions Between the Semicircular Canals and Otoliths	62
VI.	Visual-Vestibular Interaction	63
VII.	Vestibular Influence on Cardiovascular Control	65
VIII.	Vestibular Habituation	67
IX.	Alignment with the Gravitational Vertical	68
X.	Vestibulospinal vs Corticospinal Motor Mechanisms	70
XI.	Somatosensory Input to Orientation	72
XII.	Auditory Input to Orientation	78
XIII.	Cortical Input to Spatial Orientation	80
XIV.	Summary	82
	References	82

Chapter 3. Visual Orientation Mechanisms **95**

Fred H. Previc, *Northrop Grumman Information Technology,
San Antonio, Texas*

I.	Introduction	95
II.	Nature of Three-Dimensional Space	97
III.	Function of Ambient Vision	99
IV.	Ambient Visual Mechanisms	102

V. Neurophysiology of Ambient Vision 127
VI. Summary 132
    References 133

Chapter 4. Psychological Factors 145
Valerie Gawron, *General Dynamics Advanced Information Systems,*
Buffalo, New York

I. Personality and Other Traits 145
II. Mental and Physical State 148
III. Experience 170
IV. Task 173
V. Environment 176
VI. SD Phenomena Related to Psychological Factors 179
VII. Summary 185
    References 185

Chapter 5. Spatial Disorientation Mishap Classification, Data,
and Investigation 197
Stephen J. H. Véronneau, *FAA Civil Aerospace Medical Institute, Oklahoma*
City, Oklahoma; and Richard H. Evans, *General Dynamics Advanced*
Information Systems, San Antonio, Texas

I. Introduction 197
II. Human Factors Modeling 199
III. Spatial Disorientation Mishap Classification Issues 203
IV. Mishap Statistics 207
V. Investigation Concerns and Techniques 227
VI. Summary 237
    References 239

Chapter 6. Nonvisual Illusions in Flight 243
Bob Cheung, *Defence Research and Development Canada,*
Toronto, Canada

I. Introduction 243
II. Illusions Primarily Involving the Semicircular Canals 244
III. Illusions Primarily Involving the Otoliths 251
IV. Illusions Involving Semicircular Canals and Otoliths 260
V. Visual and Audio Correlates of Somatic Illusions 264
VI. Illusions Contributed by the Somatosensory System 265
VII. Incapacitating Illusions 265
VIII. Inner-Ear Problems Contributing to SD 268
IX. Summary 271
Appendix A: Assortment of Practical Recommendations for
              Flight Surgeons 272
    References 275

Chapter 7. Visual Illusions in Flight **283**
Fred H. Previc, *Northrop Grumman Information Technology,*
San Antonio, Texas

   I.   Introduction 283
   II. Specific Visual Illusions of Flight 286
   III. Optical-Device Distortions and Illusions 310
   IV. Summary 317
       References 317

Chapter 8. Spatial Disorientation Instruction, Demonstration,
and Training **323**
Malcolm G. Braithwaite, *British Army, Hampshire, United Kingdom*; William
R. Ercoline, *General Dynamics Advanced Information Systems, San*
Antonio, Texas; and Lex Brown, *U.S. Air Force School of Aerospace*
Medicine, Brooks City-Base, Texas

   I.   Introduction 323
   II. Didactic Instruction 327
   III. Ground-Based Devices 336
   IV. In-Flight Demonstration and Training 348
   V. Efficacy of Demonstration and Training 354
   VI. Improvements in SD Education 359
   VII. Summary 360
   Appendix A: Didactic Syllabus of the SD Mechanisms 361
   Appendix B: Example of Disseminated Advice on Managing SD 364
   Appendix C: Use of Flight Simulators for SD Training 365
   Appendix D: Rotary Wing In-Flight SD Demonstration 368
   Appendix E: Fixed Wing In-Flight SD Demonstration 369
   Appendix F: Training Objective for Recovery from
                Unusual Attitudes 372
       References 372

Chapter 9. Flight Displays I: Head-Down Display Topics for
Spatial Orientation **379**
William R. Ercoline, *General Dynamics Advanced Information Systems, San*
Antonio, Texas; Carita A. DeVilbiss, *Army Research Laboratory, Ft. Sam*
Houston, Texas; and Richard H. Evans, *General Dynamics Advanced*
Information Systems, San Antonio, Texas

   I.   Introduction 379
   II. Piloting Topics 382
   III. Design Topics 401
   IV. Conclusion 438
   V. Summary 439
   Appendix A: Perceiving Horizon Position and Movement 440
   Appendix B: Visibility Definitions 442

Appendix C: Performance Standards 443
References 444

Chapter 10.   Flight Displays II: Head-Up and Helmet-Mounted Displays 451

Richard L. Newman, *Crew Systems, San Marcos, Texas*; and Loran A. Haworth, *Federal Aviation Administration, Seattle, Washington*

I.   Introduction 451
II.   Basic Characteristics of HUDs and HMDs 452
III. HUD Symbology and Spatial Disorientation 457
IV.   HMD Symbology and Spatial Disorientation 463
V.   Development of HUDs and HMDs and Their Standards 467
VI.   Spatial Disorientation Research Related to HUDs and HMDs 473
VII. Unusual-Attitude-Recovery Techniques 477
VIII. Conclusions and Recommendations 485
Appendix A: Flight-Test Techniques 486
References 500

Chapter 11.   Spatial Disorientation Countermeasures—Advanced Problems and Concepts 509

Willem Bles, *TNO Human Factors, Soesterberg, The Netherlands*

I.   Introduction 509
II.   Modeling Spatial Orientation for Advanced Technologies 511
III. Supermaneuverability 513
IV.   Future Cockpit 519
V.   Unmanned Aerial Vehicles 533
VI.   Summary 534
References 535

Glossary 541

Index 557

Series Listing 565

Preface

The concept for this book dates back to March 2000, when Lt. Col. Karl Friedl and Maj. Jim Ness of the U.S. Army Medical Research and Materiel Command—acting on behalf of the Armed Services Biomedical Research Evaluation and Management (ASBREM) Committee—visited our research facilities at Brooks AFB, Texas, and asked us what could be done to improve the state of knowledge concerning spatial disorientation in the aviation environment. We responded that no comprehensive reference text had ever been published on this expansive subject, although several excellent chapters on the topic were available, and that such a text would be quite useful to aviation operations, medicine, and research.

It was decided after this meeting that the U.S. Army would fund a workshop of leading experts in spatial disorientation countermeasures research from around the world, and that the event would be followed by the publication of a book solely devoted to the topic of spatial disorientation in the aerial environment. The U.S. Air Force Research Laboratory later joined forces with the Army Medical Research and Materiel Command in funding both efforts. The resulting conference, entitled "Recent Trends in Spatial Disorientation Research," was held in San Antonio, Texas, in November 2000 and consisted of 29 presenters and over 80 attendees. Shortly afterwards, the authors—most of whom were among the presenters at the conference—began writing this book.

Although titled *Spatial Disorientation in Aviation*, this book presents a comprehensive treatment of the various topics related to both spatial orientation (SO) and spatial disorientation (SD) as they relate to flying. After an introductory chapter, the text is divided into three major sections dealing with SO mechanisms, SD in flight, and SD countermeasures, respectively. While in other sources the topic of motion sickness has been included in some general chapters related to spatial orientation (e.g. Gillingham and Previc, 1996)—mainly because many of the same visual and vestibular mechanisms mediate both phenomena—the topic of motion sickness is mentioned only briefly in this text.

The three SO mechanisms chapters deal with nonvisual, visual, and cognitive mechanisms. Chapter 2 reviews the structure and function of the vestibular organs—the semicircular canals and otolith organs—as well as the somatosensory/proprioceptive and motor systems involved in the maintenance of spatial orientation. This chapter also highlights the functional limitations of our nonvisual orientation systems in the aerial environment. Chapter 3 describes the fundamental "ambient" visual mechanisms involved in perceiving self-motion and self-position in space and presents a general model of how humans interact in three-dimensional space, as well a discussion of the neurophysiology of ambient vision. Cognitive and attentional aspects of spatial orientation are reviewed in Chapter 4, which also addresses the relationship between situational awareness and spatial orientation and the contribution of specific psychological impairments and phenomena to SD.

The three chapters that speak to the problem of spatial disorientation in flight deal with SD accident statistics, nonvisual illusions of flight, and visual illusions of flight. Chapter 5 focuses on SD accident statistics across the various flying communities, principally general aviation, commercial aviation, and military aviation. It presents case studies of SD mishaps and also describes the processes involved in investigating and recreating an SD mishap. Chapter 6 reviews the specific SD illusions of flight that can primarily be attributed to ambiguous or erroneous vestibular signals (and, in some cases, abnormal somatosensory and motor processing). This chapter also contains some practical advice to flight surgeons and aircrew concerning medical or physiological conditions that affect functioning of the nonvisual orientation systems during flight. SD illusions of flight that primarily are of a visual nature are reviewed in Chapter 7, which also addresses the specific illusions caused by various displays and viewing devices.

The final section of the book deals with SD countermeasures and includes chapters on SD training, flight displays, and advanced countermeasures technologies. Chapter 8 reviews the various SD training methodologies, ranging from didactic instruction and ground-based SD demonstrations to in-flight SD demonstration sorties and instrument training practices. Chapter 9 presents general flight display concepts, with an emphasis on presentations of attitude and other primary flight information included on head-down displays. Chapter 10 discusses specific SD and information-processing issues pertaining to head-up displays and helmet-mounted displays (including night-vision devices). Finally, Chapter 11 presents a glimpse of both current and future technologies that may be fielded to either substantially reduce or even eliminate SD in the future. These technologies range from three-dimensional audio and tactile situational awareness systems to automated warning systems and even automated flight systems that maneuver the aircraft out of danger. This final chapter also discusses how future aircraft capabilities, such as agile flight, may generate new SD problems that will need to be counteracted.

The intent of producing this book is not only to present a review of the current knowledge on major SD topics but also to provide practical advice to aircrew, aeromedical professionals, and researchers and developers concerning SD. The ultimate goal is for readers to learn about the seriousness of the SD problem in flight and to then use that knowledge to reduce or eliminate the number of accidents caused by SD.

We are indebted to many individuals for their help in bringing this text to fruition. In addition to Karl Friedl and Jim Ness, Lt. Col. Todd Heinle of the U.S. Air Force Research Laboratory's Joint Cockpit Office was instrumental in funding and planning both the conference and book, and Dr. Robert Foster of the Department of Defense Research and Engineering Directorate provided supplemental funds for the project. Bruce Stuck and Dr. Wes Baumgardner helped manage the contractual effort for the U.S. Army and U.S. Air Force, respectively. Kathy Hitt and Christy Graham of General Dynamics not only helped produce the conference, but also provided invaluable technical editing support throughout the course of this writing and ultimately prepared the text for publication. Julie Larcher provided extra graphical and technical support for Chapter 5. The following experts helped review specific chapters: Dr. Jim Lackner (Chapter 2), Dr. Jeremy Beer (Chapter 3), Dr. Chuck Antonio (Chapter 7), and Kevin Greeley (Chapter 10). Finally, Dr. Alan Benson provided a critical review of all but one chapter prior to final revisions being made.

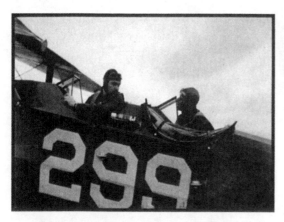

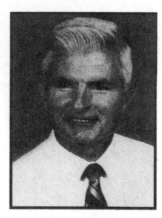

Lt. Carl Crane and Maj. William Ocker, c. 1930. (*Photo courtesy of Pam Crane*).   Dr. Kent Gillingham, c. 1990

We dedicate this textbook to the important SD researchers who preceded us at Brooks Air Force Base, Texas (formerly Brooks Field—and now Brooks City-Base). Three of these individuals, shown in the photos above, deserve special mention: William Ocker, Carl Crane, and Kent Gillingham. While stationed at Brooks Field as military officers in the late 1920s and early 1930s, Ocker and Crane performed experiments that demonstrated how flying with instruments countered spatial disorientation, developed the first instrument training programs, and co-authored a seminal textbook entitled *Blind Flight in Theory and Practice.* Carl Crane further inspired many to enhance flight safety through improving flight instrumentation and training, and he was a personal friend of one us (Bill Ercoline).

Dr. Kent Gillingham arrived at Brooks AFB in the mid–1960s as a young military flight surgeon and later headed the U.S. Air Force Spatial Disorientation Countermeasures Program as a civil servant. As a physician, physiologist, and private pilot, he became one of the world's leading experts in spatial disorientation and wrote several influential chapters on this topic. In the late 1980s, Dr. Gillingham hired both of us to assist him in SD countermeasures research and mentored us until his untimely death in 1993. He was posthumously honored with the first Kent K. Gillingham Award for Spatial Disorientation Research bestowed by the Aerospace Medical Association.

As we have been inspired toward continuing the effort to eradicate spatial disorientation in aviation by these undaunted advocates of SD countermeasures training and research, we hope the readers of this book are similarly motivated.

Fred Previc
Bill Ercoline
October 2003

Spatial Disorientation in Aviation: Historical Background, Concepts, and Terminology

Fred H. Previc*

Northrop Grumman Information Technology, San Antonio, Texas

William R. Ercoline[†]

General Dynamics Advanced Information Systems, San Antonio, Texas

I. Definition

S PATIAL orientation (SO) is arguably the most fundamental of all behaviors that humans engage in, and it involves a large number of different sensory and motor systems and brain regions. Spatial disorientation (SD) represents a failure to maintain SO, which in the flight environment all too frequently proves catastrophic. Indeed, SD, as broadly defined, constitutes over 25% of all fatal mishaps in military aviation and an even larger percentage of mishaps specifically related to pilot factors.[1]

Spatial orientation and disorientation are commonly used terms in neurology and neuropsychology as well as aviation, and they mean different things to different professions. Someone who suffers from brain damage and is spatially disoriented, for example, might have an inability to tell right from left, or might have trouble finding his or her way around unfamiliar surroundings. This is not what spatial disorientation refers to in the aviation environment, however. In the aviation world spatial orientation mainly refers not to our lack of awareness of our position and motion relative to particular places on Earth but in relation to *Earth-fixed space in general*. According to its most widely used definition, one that has been accepted by a large number of countries, SD refers to the pilot's: "... [failure] to sense correctly the position, motion or attitude of his aircraft or of him/herself within the fixed coordinate system provided by the surface of the earth and the gravitational vertical" (Ref. 2, p. 419). Added to this standard definition is the

This material is declared a work of the U.S. Government and is not subject to copyright protection in the United States.

*Senior Human Factors Specialist.

[†]Senior Scientist.

caveat that" . . . errors in perception by the pilots of their position, motion or attitude with respect to his aircraft, or their own aircraft relative to other aircraft, may also be embraced within a broader definition of spatial disorientation in flight" (Ref. 2, p. 419).

What the preceding definition implies is that the inability to maintain one's orientation with respect to particular objects or places on the ground— for example, landing at the wrong airport or other types of "getting lost,"— does not fall within the preceding definition of SD. Rather, such incidents would fall under the general category of *geographical disorientation*. Another way to view the distinction between spatial and geographical disorientation relates to the functions of the three major types of primary flight instruments, as described in Chapter 1 of the United States Air Force Manual 11-217, Volume 1, *Instrument Flight Procedures*[3]: control (attitude and engine power/thrust displays), performance (altitude, airspeed, heading, vertical velocity, acceleration, angle of attack, and turn-and-slip indicators), and navigation instruments (bearing-and-course indicators, range indicators, and glide-slope indicators). Spatial orientation is maintained by means of the control and performance instruments, whereas geographical orientation is mostly maintained with reference to the navigational instruments (Ref. 4, see Chapter 9, Sec. II.B). Although some definitions of SD do not include an erroneous perception of altitude,[5] misperception of altitude is clearly SD by the standard definition because it involves an erroneous sense of "position . . . within the fixed coordinate system provided by the surface of the earth and the gravitational vertical."

The second part of the definition goes beyond the problem of orienting in relation to Earth-fixed space to include the perception of the pilot's relationship to his or her own aircraft—as in the "break off" and related phenomena in which the pilot might feel detached and flying from outside the aircraft (Chapter 4, Sec. VI), as well as parameters such as separation distance and closure rate relative to other aircraft. Misperception of these latter elements might or might not occur in association with other manifestations of SD, and by no means should all midair collisions be listed as SD mishaps. However, some midair accidents can occur because the pilot is unaware of his or her own aircraft's velocity or trajectory in space, that is, a manifestation of SD. How such SD-related midair accidents might occur is illustrated by the crash of two U.S. Air Force (USAF) C-141 aircraft in the early 1990s. The prelude to this mishap occurred when the second C-141 aircraft in the formation of four engaged in a slow, evidently undetected roll away from the lead aircraft. This undetected change in bank attitude might have led to a visual illusion of the lead aircraft dropping in altitude that resulted in the pilot of the rejoining aircraft to push the control column forward, that is, nose down, thereby lowering his aircraft into the lead aircraft. As might be expected, broadening the category of SD mishaps to include disorientation relative to other aircraft results in a large increase in the SD mishap rate.

What is termed SD today was not always referred as such. Until the 1970s, SD was also referred to as aviator's vertigo or pilot vertigo, while spatial orientation was often referred to as aerial equilibrium. The term spatial orientation appeared in a classic early text on instrument flight,[6] and the term spatial disorientation was used shortly thereafter.[7] Although SD was a commonly used term by the 1950s, "vertigo" was still included in place of SD in aerospace medical textbooks until 1971 (Ref. 8) and in USAF mishap forms until 1989. Today, vertigo is recognized as a distinct set of symptoms that can accompany SD—usually referring to dizziness, light-headedness ("giddiness" in the older literature), visual-field instability, or other physical or emotional sensations produced by the motions of flight—whereas SD is recognized as a phenomenon that can occur with or without such sensations. Indeed, all too many pilots have gone to their death never feeling or suspecting that anything was amiss with their aircraft's altitude or trajectory. What might be experienced during one type of SD might be very different than what is experienced during a different type, as will be discussed further in Sec. III.

Another related term that became widely used in the 1980s and 1990s is *loss of situational awareness* (LSA) (see Chapter 4, Sec. II.F). This term, which dates back to World War II, was the subject of little research interest until the 1980s. It is a more general term than SD, as it refers to the loss of a pilot's "perception of the elements in the [aviation] environment within a volume of time and space, the comprehension of their meaning, and the projection of their status in the near future."[9] Because spatial orientation is undoubtedly a "key element in the aviation environment," spatial orientation is generally considered to be a subset of situational awareness (SA).[10,11] Thus, any pilot suffering from SD also has LSA, although the reverse is not always true. For example, a pilot can lose his or her navigational sense and suffer from geographical disorientation (and, by definition, LSA) without losing spatial orientation. Nevertheless, non-SD components of LSA, especially attention-management deficiencies, often precipitate SD. Any cognitive state or process that results in losing SA (fatigue, distraction, task saturation, etc.), or the task itself of regaining lost SA, can divert the pilot's attentional resources and lead to a failure to properly crosscheck the flight instruments. The relationship between spatial orientation and situational awareness is shown in Fig. 1.

A final term that has been used in conjunction with SD is controlled flight into terrain (CFIT).[12,13] According to Wiener,[13] CFIT can be defined as "... [those accidents] in which an aircraft, under the control of the crew, is flown into terrain (or water) with no prior awareness on the part of the crew of the impending disaster" (Ref. 13, p. 171). This definition implies that the crew must be flying the plane (engine failure or physiological incapacitation is excluded) and that no evidence exists that the pilot initiated a control action prior to the point at which the collision could not be averted. For example, an accident in which a futile last-second effort to alter the aircraft's flight path occurred could still qualify

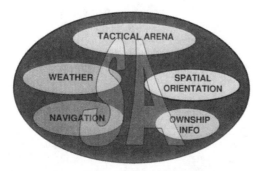

Fig. 1 Illustration of the relationship between spatial orientation and situational awareness. In this scheme spatial orientation is a subset of situational awareness. (Adapted from Ref. 11.)

as CFIT. Although the vast majority of CFIT accidents involve a misjudgment of altitude and therefore should be classified as SD, some CFIT mishaps might also result from geographical disorientation. If, for example, a pilot maintains adequate terrain clearance for a particular set of geographical coordinates that mistakenly differ from those the aircraft is actually flying over, the pilot might not be aware of impending mountains, power lines, etc.[14] Also, CFIT accidents typically occur during only one particular type of SD (Type I), in which the pilot is unaware of his or her misjudgment of terrain clearance (see Sec. III), whereas in many SD situations the pilot might be fighting a perceptual mismatch between perceived and actual altitude to maintain control of the aircraft before impacting the ground (Types II and III SD). [Another term that has recently been used by the U.S. National Transportation Safety Board (NTSB) to categorize mishaps involving human errors is "aircraft control not maintained." This term is synonymous with neither CFIT nor SD, but the number of SD-labeled mishaps declined considerably after the NTSB introduced this term in 1987 (see Chapter 5, Sec. IV.B).]

II. Historical Background

Virtually from the moment humans began to fly in maneuverable aircraft, they experienced SD. This is because our nonvisual and visual sensory systems were designed over tens of millions of years of mammalian evolution to maintain spatial orientation in a terrestrial environment. Conversely, our sensory systems turn out to be poorly suited to the abnormal acceleratory environment of flight, which can include prolonged turning and linear accelerations not typically encountered on Earth (except in vehicles). As stated by Gillingham and Previc (Ref. 4, pp. 339, 340), SD occurs because of the following:

> The evolution of humans saw us develop over millions of years as an aquatic, terrestrial, and even arboreal creature, but never an aerial one. In this development, we subjected ourselves to and were subjected to many different varieties of transient motions, but not to the relatively sustained linear and angular accelerations commonly experienced in aviation. As a result, humans acquired sensory systems well suited for maneuvering under our own power on the surface of the earth but poorly suited for flying. Even the birds, whose primary mode of locomotion is flying, are unable to maintain spatial orientation and fly safely when deprived of vision by fog and clouds. Only bats seem to have developed the ability to fly without vision, and then only by replacing vision with auditory echolocation. Considering our phylogenetic heritage, it should come as no surprise that our sudden entry into the aerial environment resulted in a mismatch between the orientational demands of the new environment and our innate ability to orient. The manifestation of this mismatch is spatial disorientation.

The recognition that SD is a serious problem in aviation did not come immediately, but rather occurred mostly during and just after World War I. Even prior to then, however, many of the common SD illusions were already known from research performed in the terrestrial environment, principally by Ernst Mach.

A. Pre-1919 SD Research

The credit for much of our early understanding of SD goes to the great physicist Ernst Mach.[15] Mach's fundamental contributions to fluid mechanics led him to the study of the vestibular system and its mechanisms. He became interested in the vestibular system and its role in motion detection during a train ride, in which he first encountered what was later to become known as the somatogravic illusion:

> "I myself became interested in consideration of movement sensation during a research project on fluids containing suspended particles, which one of my students carried out at my suggestion. . . . My view at that time was that the whole body contributed to movement sensation. The supposition of a special organ for movement sensation was far away at that time. . . . A chance happening led me back to the study of motion sensation. I noticed the tilting of houses and trees while I was traveling around a curve in a railroad. This is easily explained if one directly senses the resultant inertial acceleration. Although the physiological side of this subject was still very foreign to me even on reconsideration . . . this observation was nevertheless sufficient to stimulate my thoughts in their current direction" (Mach, *Fundamentals of the Theory of Motion Perception*, 1875, pps. 2, 3; cited in Ref. 15, p. 140). [Interestingly, Mach perceived something that is infrequently observed—the movement of the external visual world in response to a shift of the gravitoinertial vector, which normally only occurs for gravitoinertial shifts >15 deg and in subjects who are above average in field-dependence (see Chapter 3, Sec. III).]

Mach went on to study in his laboratory many prominent vestibular SD illusions using a rotating chair and a primitive centrifuge. He discovered or reproduced the somatogyral, somatogravic, oculogravic, oculogyral, and Coriolis illusions (see Chapters 6 and 7), although they were not known as such at the time. He also understood the key vestibular mechanism involved in angular motion sensation, namely, the torque or pressure of the endolymph on what was later determined to be the cupula, and the confusions generated between our inability to distinguish inertial forces from gravity, the basis of the somatogravic illusion.[15] Mach also studied visual-vestibular interactions using measurements of subject-fixed target displacements during whole-body movements and by adding a striped cylinder to his rotating chair. He is generally credited with first studying the phenomena of angular and linear vection (see Chapter 3, Sec. IV.A.1) and with first recognizing the importance of peripheral vision to it, as he described in 1875:

> The observer sits inside a hollow, turning, lined cylinder. When this drum alone is kept turning for minutes one quickly notices himself turning in the direction opposite to the drum along with all those things which are not hidden by the drum. . . . After several repetitions of this experiment it seems to be as though the peripheral part of the visual field appeared to be placed in motion most easily. . . . Various forms of this illusion are recognized, when one stands on a bridge over running water or observes moving trains from a still railroad car, whereby different parts of the visual field take on different movements" (Mach, *Fundamentals of the Theory of Movement Perception*, 1875, pp. 85, 86; cited in Ref. 15, p. 143).

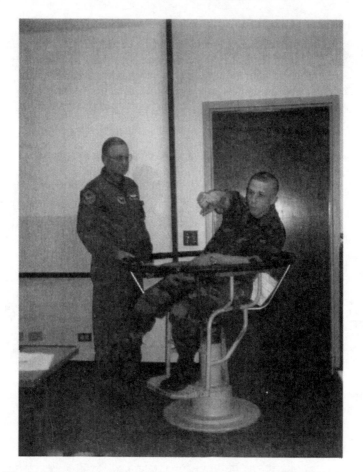

Fig. 2   **Barany chair developed in 1906 by the Nobel Prize-winning Austrian otologist Robert Barany that is still in use in most spatial disorientation countermeasures training curricula to demonstrate susceptibility to vestibular illusion. (Photo reproduced with permission of Lt. Col. Carlton, 12th ADS/SGGT, Randolph Air Force Base, Texas.)**

Mach did not conduct his studies in isolation, and many famous European scientists conducted similar work during this period, including Purkinje and Ewald. One vestibular scientist who requires special mention during the early part of the 20th century is Robert Barany, who developed many commonly used vestibular screening tests (caloric nystagmus, positional nystagmus) and investigated the brain pathways involved in the vestibular-ocular reflexes. Besides being awarded the Nobel Prize for medicine and physiology in 1913, his major contribution to countering SD lies in the reduced-friction chair that bears his name—the Barany chair (Fig. 2), which to this day remains a mainstay of ground-based SD training curricula (see Chapter 8, Sec. III).

B. SD Research from 1919–1945

This period was marked by the emergence of a clear understanding of the threat posed by SD in the aerial environment, as well as the beginnings of SD countermeasures efforts. Despite the many SD illusions that had been discovered in the laboratory prior to this time, how a pilot could overcome such illusions in the aerial environment by means of training and flight instrumentation remained a perplexing and contentious issue throughout most of this period.

The flying experiences during World War I led many flight surgeons and scientists around the world to the conclusion that vestibular processing was problematic in the aerial environment. Indeed, over 100 papers on the topic of the vestibular system in the aerial environment were published between World Wars I and II in a dozen languages.[16] Initially, the emphasis was on vestibular screening, and several countries started using various devices and tests before sending their pilot candidates into the air. The list of countries included England, where the neurologist Henry Head studied aviation-related vestibular problems,[17] as well as Italy, France, and the United States.[18] In the United States Capt. David Myers tested many pilots on a variation of the Barany chair known as the Jones–Barany chair. Another device used in the United States—the Ruggles Orientator—was a three-axis, interactive device that proved less effective as a screening device than as the progenitor of a long line of flight-simulators (see Fig. 3). [Indeed, a modified version of this device became the first patented flight simulator, whose rights were later acquired by Edwin Link of Link Aviation (later Singer–Link) fame.] Postural and other equilibrium tests were used as the chief criteria for accepting or rejecting pilots, along with the length of the postrotatory nystagmus interval following the cessation of a prolonged turn. The use of postrotatory nystagmus, which is an oculomotor measure of the inertial lag of the endolymph in the semicircular canals (see Chapter 2), was somewhat arbitrary and was found not to be predictive of which pilots would later succumb to SD. For example, the United States Army Air Services (later to become the U.S. Army Air Corps and eventually the USAF) required the postrotatory nystagmus to be between 16 and 36 s, which led to the rejection of many pilot candidates who then joined other air forces and became excellent aviators.[19]

Given the predictive failure of the burgeoning vestibular screening programs, it was clear that something more was needed to deal with SD in flight. The Dutch flight surgeon van Wulfften Palthe[19] provided a good account of many SD problems encountered during flight, including the somatogyral and somatogravic illusions and the effects of pressure vertigo. He attempted to distinguish between those caused mainly by the vestibular system and those involving the pressure sense (referred to as deeper sensibilities). One illusion that van Wulfften Palthe described in detail was the somatogravic illusion in bank, which occurs when the centrifugal force emanating from the center of a turn combines with the force of gravity and thereby leads the aviator to feel level when his or her aircraft might have actually assumed a large bank angle. From his studies, van Wulfften Palthe[19] concluded that, even for the most proficient aviator, spatial orientation requires vision:

> It is very difficult to imagine, when one sees an aeroplane in the air, standing almost vertically on its side, instead of in a horizontal position and making rather rapid

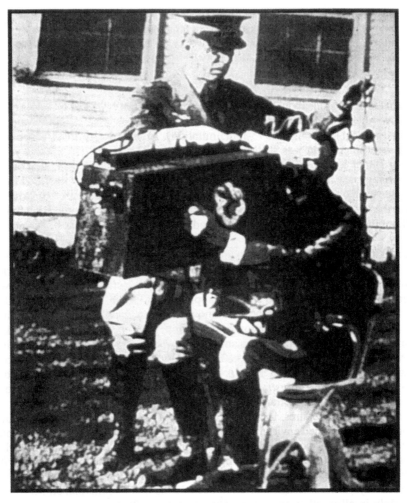

Fig. 4 Photo of Col. William Ocker (standing) and pilot trainee with the Ocker box attached to a Jones–Barany chair. (Photo reproduced with permission of Pam Crane.)

even birds could not fly by their own sensations when they were deprived of an outside reference (Carl Crane, personal communication, June 1975).

In the meantime Sperry would team up with a group of pilots and scientists in the United States to design the first instrument suite that allowed for total instrument flying, in a project funded by the Guggenheim Fund and carried out at Mitchel Field in Long Island, New York. This team would be led by a recent Ph.D. in aeronautics from the Massachusetts Institute of Technology by the name of Lt. (later Gen.) James Doolittle.[22] Besides the turn and airspeed indicators already in existence, the Guggenheim-funded effort produced an advanced radio altimeter and the first artificial horizon, which showed an airplane against a line aligned with the real horizon. The development of the advanced instrument display

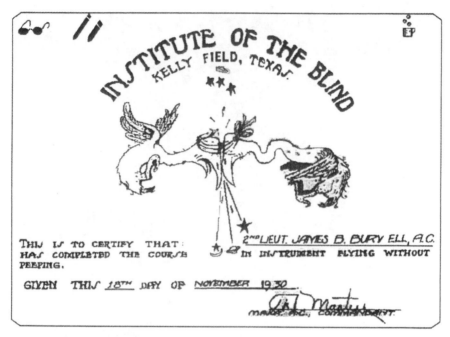

Fig. 5 Certificate from one of the first instrument flying courses in the United States, known as the Institute of the Blind. [Reproduced with permission of Maj. Gen. (Ret.) James Burwell.]

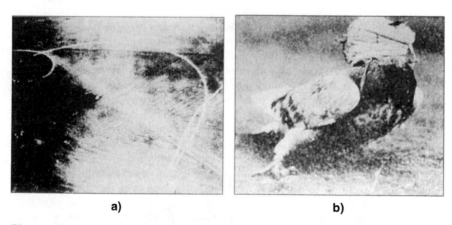

a) b)

Fig. 6 Photos from two of Col. Ocker's and Lt. Crane's demonstrations during the 1920s: a) the spiraling tendency during blindfolded locomotion in humans and b) the refusal to fly by blindfolded pigeons when released at altitude. (They elected to harmlessly glide to ground.) (Photo reproduced with permission of Pam Crane.)

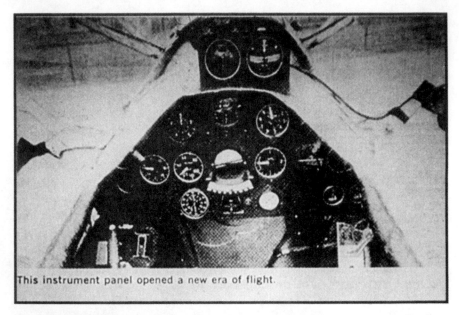

This instrument panel opened a new era of flight.

Fig. 7   Photo of the Guggenheim-funded experimental cockpit flown by Lt. Doolittle in 1929 during the first blind-flight sortie. (Photo reproduced with permission of USAF Instrument Flight Center, Randolph Air Force Base, Texas.)

suite (Fig. 7) allowed for a series of blind flights that included takeoffs and landings in 1929 (the first by Lt. Doolittle with a safety observer onboard) and the first solo blind flight by Capt. Albert Hegenberger in 1932.[6,22]

The year 1932 marked another important milestone in the history of instrument flight—the publication of the first major text on instrument flight, *Blind Flight in Theory and Practice* by Maj. Ocker and Lt. Crane.[6] This text, written while Ocker and Crane were teamed at Brooks Field in San Antonio, Texas, described the history of instrument flight, the major instruments available at that time, and procedures for instrument flight training and operations. It included an illustration of a novel integrated, pictorial flight display (Fig. 8) and a concept for grouping instruments according to their function in one of the first descriptions of the basic T arrangement (Ref. 6, pp. 115–120). It also distinguished between the instruments for maintaining spatial orientation vs those for navigation (which they termed "avigation"). Finally, Ocker and Crane offered a seminal definition of spatial orientation in flight as "an adjustment of position or change in position with respect to the three principal axes [including gravity]" (Ref. 6, p. 25) that is close to the standard definition used today (see Sec. I in this chapter). [Unfortunately, Maj. (later Col.) Ocker was independent minded and was eventually court martialed on two occasions. During his second trial, in which he was acquitted, Ocker called some of the most famous aviators in history to testify in his defense. One of these—Orville Wright of Wright Brothers fame—stated in a deposition that "[Ocker's] campaign of education has had more influence in bringing about the use of instruments than that of any other person."[23]]

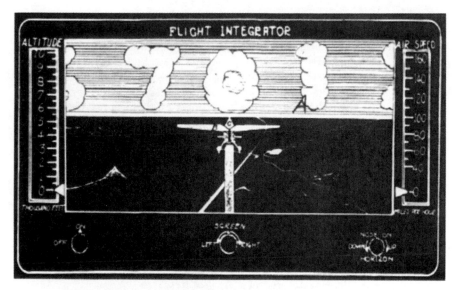

Fig. 8 Illustration of the pictorial flight integrator display (from Ref. 6). One of the first attempts at grouping information according to function, that is, control and performance information on one display.

By 1937, over 300 papers had been written on the topic of blind flight.[24] The development of instrument flight as a countermeasure to SD was not without its controversies and pitfalls, however. One major controversy that developed in the 1930s concerned the motion of the artificial horizon (attitude) display. The Sperry artificial horizon that was designed and flown by Doolittle and others during the early blind flights consisted of a line that moved in synchrony with the movement of the outside horizon, much as if the latter were viewed through a periscope from inside the aircraft; hence, it became known as an "inside-out" attitude format. Ocker and Crane's integrated flight display concept, on the other hand, showed a miniature aircraft changing its bank and pitch relative to a stable horizon, as if the aircraft were viewed from behind; hence, it became known as an "outside-in" attitude format. Sperry's artificial horizon that integrated both bank-and-pitch information became a standard early on, as the engineering prototype of Ocker and Crane's display was not built until after World War II. The supposed advantages of the inside-out concept were touted in an influential paper by Poppen,[25] although no formal comparisons between the two attitude concepts had been conducted at this stage. It became clear during World War II that flying with an inside-out attitude display could be very confusing to pilots, and the controversy has remained to this day[26] (see Chapter 9, Sec. III.A.1). A more serious problem facing aviation between the world wars involved instrument training. Instrument flying manuals were poorly written and confusing,[8] and instrument training was only sporadically adopted by most air services. This pitfall became especially apparent in the United States during the early days of World War II, when pilots were rushed into service and as many as 50 noncombat crashes a day occurred.

Colonel Joseph Duckworth recognized the problem and recommended the creation of an instrument flight school that would train all instructor pilots on the use of instruments. His recommendation led to the establishment of the U.S. Army Air Force's first Instrument Pilot Instructor School at Bryan Field, Texas, in 1943, as well as a dramatic decrease in the number of U.S. pilots lost to noncombat-related accidents during the latter course of the war. Graduates from this program would receive a "green card" that certified their instrument rating. (A USAF award for contributions to instrument flight was later named for Joseph Duckworth, which the authors of this chapter were honored to receive in 1995, as members of the U.S. Air Force Research Laboratory's SD Countermeasures team.)

C. SD Research from 1945–1970

The beginnings of formal SD research occurred during this era and were concentrated in four main areas: SD mechanisms research, SD mishap and incidence studies, primary flight displays, and SD training research.

The person most associated with the beginnings of postwar SD mechanisms research was Dr. Ashton Graybiel, who for several decades headed the SD research program at the Naval Aerospace Medical Research Laboratory (NAMRL) in Pensacola, Florida (Fig. 9a). Although the somatogyral and somatogravic illusions were known since the time of Mach, Graybiel and colleagues formally investigated their in-flight occurrence[27] as well as their ocular counterparts (the oculogyral and oculogravic counterparts) in terms of threshold, time course, types of visual cues, and many other factors.[28–30] The reference to the oculogyral and oculogravic illusions by Graybiel and colleagues actually preceded the use of the terms somatogyral and somatogravic by Drs. Alan Benson and Fred Guedry, who distinguished between the illusory effects on the bodily (somato) vs the visually manifested (ocular) effects (see Chapter 6). Dr. Graybiel assembled a very large and distinguished team of NAMRL scientists, including Dr. Fred Guedry (Fig. 9b) and began a long collaboration with NASA in the 1960s dealing with the visuomotor and perceptual effects of weightlessness. The NASA research effort in the area of SD would eventually bring in prominent academic teams led by Dr. James Lackner of Brandeis University and Dr. Larry Young of the Massachusetts Institute of Technology (MIT). Dr. James Lackner would later marry Dr. Ann Graybiel, the daughter of Capt. Graybiel and a prominent neurophysiologist in her own right, and would conduct most of his research at the Ashton Graybiel Spatial Orientation Laboratory at Brandeis University. Another historical note is that the first two living recipients of the Aerospace Medical Association's Gillingham Award for spatial disorientation research were Dr. Alan Benson and Dr. Fred Guedry, in 2000 and 2001, respectively.

By the end of this era, several other teams of SD researchers would surface around the world. One of these would be at the USAF School of Aerospace Medicine (USAFSAM) at Brooks Air Force Base, Texas, under the direction of Dr. Robert Cramer, where a young USAF captain by the name of Kent Gillingham would begin his career and later inherit and expand this SD research effort to include the authors of this chapter. Other SD research was conducted in civilian agencies such as the Federal Aviation Administration's Civil Aeromedical Institute (now known as the Civil Aerospace Institute), under the direction of Dr. William

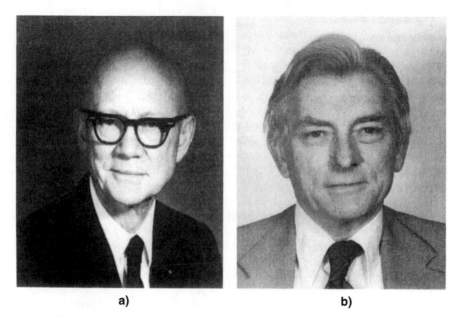

a)   b)

Fig. 9a   Captain Ashton Graybiel, head of the SD program at the U.S. Navy Aeromedical Research Laboratory and the leading SD researcher during the 1960s and 1970s. Fig. 9b   Dr. Fred Guedry, a noted SD researcher and colleague of Graybiel's at NAMRL since the 1970s and winner of the Aerospace Medical Association's Gillingham Award for SD research. (Photos reproduced with permission of Dr. Fred Guedry.)

Collins, and NASA's Ames Research Center, under the direction of Dr. Malcolm Cohen. Basic and applied SD research also flourished in different parts of the world, with Dr. Alan Benson heading a group at the Institute of Aviation Medicine in England, Dr. Vladimir Ponomarenko leading a team of researchers at the Russian Institute of Aviation and Space Medicine, and Dr. Geoffrey Melvill-Jones played a leading role in the Canadian SD program. One person who is not usually mentioned in conjunction with SD research was Dr. James Gibson, who in the early 1950s translated his experience as a researcher in the Army Air Corps in World War II into influential ecologically based theories of how humans visually orient in three-dimensional space, including the aviation environment.[31]

The first formal SD surveys and mishap analyses also began after World War II. Vinacke[32] published a survey dealing with what was termed aviator's vertigo as early as 1948, and another vertigo survey was published in 1957 by Clark and Graybiel.[33] The first formal SD mishap survey appears to be that of Nuttall and Sanford,[34] and this was followed by two other USAF studies based on mishap data from the 1950s and 1960s.[35,36] Interestingly, the percentage of total mishaps attributed to SD in each of these studies ranged from 4–9%, which is about half the 15% or more found in recent military aviation studies.[1,8,10,37] This difference is best explained by 1) the higher percentage of logistical (e.g., engine failure) mishaps that occurred in the early days of high-performance flying and 2) the concept of SD as synonymous with vertigo, which would exclude most Type I SD (see Sec. III of this chapter).

The first systematic research into primary flight displays and their role in pre-venting and recovering from SD began just after World War II by Dr. Paul Fitts and colleagues at Wright-Patterson Air Force Base, Ohio.[38] Based on an analysis of almost 500 incidents of pilot error,[39] it became clear that pilots were struggling to read and maneuver the flight instruments. One particular problem that occurred about 7% of the time was the pilot's perception of the wrong roll direction (bank angle) on the attitude display, which thereby contributed to a roll-reversal error (see Chapter 9, Sec. III.A.1). As noted by Fitts and Jones, "The proper directions of motion of flight instruments for maximum ease of sensing has been under dis-cussion since instrument flying was inaugurated.... However, after 20 years, the results of the present investigation indicate clearly that the problem has not been solved satisfactorily...." (Ref. 39, p. 22).

The U.S. Army Air Corps soon undertook an effort to investigate many aspects of primary flight displays,[40] and a great many studies were conducted in the ensuing 25 or so years dealing with the proper way to depict attitude and other primary flight parameters. One of the leading display researchers during this time was Dr. Stanley Roscoe, who collaborated with both industry and government agencies in studying a variety of primary flight displays, including inside-out, outside-in, frequency-separated, predictive, and periscopic ones. By the early 1970s, however, few truly novel concepts had been adopted by flying communities around the world, and the cockpits of the early 1960s looked much like the pre-war ones except that they contained many more gauges, novel flight-director displays, and, in some cases, color-coded attitude displays. Toward the end of this era, however, one important development was to take place—the development of the head-up display, first for targeting purposes and then as a platform for primary flight information (see Chapter 10).

The final major advance during this era occurred in the area of SD training devices.[41] For over 40 years the Barany chair was the mainstay of SD training, and it continues to be even today in many flying communities. By the 1960s, simulated cockpits were added to rotating platforms in an attempt to add realism to the basic turning illusions.[42] The first of the SD trainers with planetary motion capable of generating $> +1$ G of force was developed in 1964 at the USAFSAM; this device was known as the spatial disorientation demonstrator (Fig. 10). In 1967, the first planetary device that allowed pilots to actually fly into such illusions as the somatogravic pitch and graveyard spiral with a true-reading attitude instrument was also developed at USAFSAM; this device, known as the spatial orientation trainer (Fig. 10), was the forerunner of the modern advanced disorientation training devices.

D.   SD Research from 1970 to the Present

The pace of SD research quickened considerably during the last part of the 20th century. Over half of all SD studies were conducted in the 1990s alone, whereas little change occurred between the amount of SD research conducted in the 1970s and 1980s (Fig. 11). One of the more significant developments that occurred in this era was the accumulation of the knowledge in various areas (e.g., mechanisms, flight displays, training) into comprehensive SD chapters in leading aviation med-ical textbooks. Indeed, the term spatial disorientation replaced aviator's vertigo as

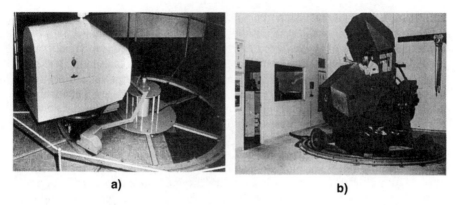

Fig. 10 Two of the first planetary SD countermeasures training devices developed at the USAF School of Aerospace Medicine during the 1960s: a) the spatial disorientation demonstrator and b) the spatial orientation trainer.

an aeromedical topic in leading textbooks only beginning with Benson.[44] Two of the more notable SD chapter authors during this period were Dr. Alan Benson[2,45–47] and Dr. Kent Gillingham.[4,48]

In terms of SD mechanisms, scientific verification of various in-flight illusions, including the g excess,[49] inversion,[50] and postroll illusions,[51] continued. An even greater advance occurred during this period in our understanding of the mechanisms of visual orientation. Although Mach had recognized the important

SD Research Trends

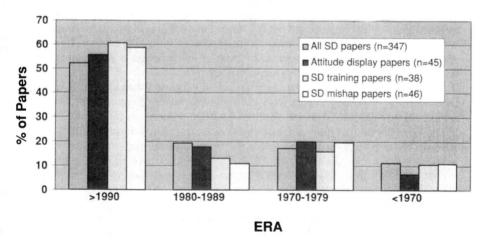

Fig. 11 Graph showing the trend in the overall number of SD publications and the trends in the number of attitude display, SD training, and SD mishap papers from 1940–2000.[43]

contribution of peripheral vision to spatial orientation, this concept resurfaced in an influential review of visual-vestibular interactions by Dichgans and Brandt, published in the *Handbook of Sensory Physiology* in 1978.[52] The distinction between focal and ambient vision—the system contributing to spatial orientation and most visual-vestibular interactions and dominated by the peripheral visual field—was first applied to the aviation and vehicular worlds by Leibowitz and Dichgans[76] in 1980 and later included as part of an expanded model of human visual interactions in three-dimensional space[53] (see Chapter 3, Sec. II).

The number of SD mishap studies also greatly increased after 1970, and the first analyses of civilian[54] and rotary-winged SD mishaps[55] were published in the open literature. Interestingly, the number of civilian SD mishaps turned out to be less than reported for military aviation—only 2.5% in Kirkham et al.'s study,[54] although SD mishaps constituted approximately 10% of the *fatal* mishaps in general aviation. In contrast, the rotary-winged SD percentage turned out to be higher (21% in Vrnwy-Jones' study[55]) than in fixed-wing aircraft. A slew of mishap analyses and SD surveys from around the world were published in the 1990s, as the implementation of electronic mishap databases made such analyses easier to perform, and the first analysis of SD mishap trends across decades was performed.[56]

The advent of the head-up display (HUD) and later on night-vision devices and other helmet-mounted displays (HMD) created additional SD "traps" for pilots, for numerous reasons: nonintuitive primary flight symbology, small fields of view, excessive clutter, etc. (see Chapter 10). One of the major milestones in SD countermeasures research was an attitude awareness workshop held at Wright-Patterson Air Force Base in 1985.[57] Many of the problems of the newer flight displays were discussed, and out of this meeting came an impetus for more intuitive, ambient primary flight displays and for greater standardization of flight-instrument symbology. Two working groups which coordinated several experiments designed to improve and standardize HUD symbology were later formed in the United States.[58,59] Progress also was made in the development of peripheral attitude displays, including the peripheral vision horizon display,[60] and electronic flight displays known as multifunction displays began to appear in the cockpits of aircraft around the world. Synthetic visual displays such as the highway in the sky were designed to present both navigational and spatial orientation information in a more intuitive manner than in the past[61,62] (see Chapters 9 and 10).

In the training arena the first formal studies of ground-based training effectiveness in the early 1970s gave way to the development of sophisticated hybrid systems involving both SD demonstrators and flight simulators by the mid-1990s. In addition, initial attempts at in-flight SD countermeasures training in the 1970s were followed by more comprehensive and systematic in-flight training regimes by the late 1990s.[63] In the 1970s and 1980s Dr. Alan Benson (see Fig. 12) cohosted two AGARD symposia dealing with SD countermeasures training issues[64,65] and authored an AGARD training report entitled *Orientation/Disorientation Training of Flying Personnel.*"[66]

Despite much debate as to the value of ground-based SD demonstrations, advances in computer capability eventually facilitated the development of an SD countermeasures training device known as the Gyrolab 2000 by the Environmental Tectonics Corporation. This device, delivered to three nations (United States, Germany, and Japan) in the early 1990s, included a wide field-of-view (FOV) computer scene, a reconfigurable head-down and HUD instrument suite, computerized

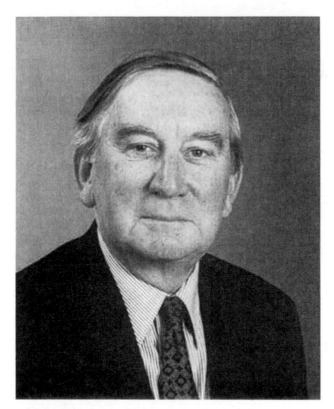

Fig. 12   Dr. Alan Benson, head of the SD research program at the United Kingdom's Institute of Aviation Medicine, a leading SD researcher in the 1970s–1990s, and winner of the Aerospace Medical Association's Gillingham Award for SD research. (Photo reproduced with permission of Dr. Alan Benson.)

motion in four axes (pitch, roll, yaw, and planetary), and three degree-of-freedom flight simulation (see Chapter 8). By the end of the century, an even more imposing SD countermeasures training device was being developed for the Royal Netherlands Air Force by AMST. This device, known as the Desdemona, is designed to have a fully computerized, nontraditional, six-degree-of-freedom motion base (see Chapter 8, Sec. III.D).

Despite the important gains in SD awareness and knowledge during the past three decades, the SD problem has not gone away. Indeed, one recent mishap study suggests that SD, as broadly defined, might actually have risen during the second half of the 1990s. The failure to eliminate SD prompted the U.S. Congress to fund a five-year effort aimed at reducing the number of CFIT/SD mishaps, which, in turn, led to the funding of an International SD conference in San Antonio, Texas (see Preface), the development of an SD Web site,* and the funding of this first comprehensive SD textbook.

---

*Data available online at http://www.spatiald.wpafb.af.mil [cited 27 Oct. 2003].

III. Types of SD

Spatial disorientation can take on various forms, depending on the flight situation and the pilot's reaction to it. Most researchers distinguish between two SD types—Type I (unrecognized) and Type II (recognized)—although many researchers also add a third category (Type III, or incapacitating).

In Type I SD the pilot does not consciously perceive any of the manifestations of SD, that is, the pilot experiences no disparity between natural and synthetic (instrument-derived) orientation percepts, has no suspicion that a flight instrument (e.g., attitude indicator) has malfunctioned, and feels that the aircraft is responding well to his or her control inputs. Basically, the pilot is oblivious to the SD episode and controls the aircraft in accordance with a false orientational percept. This type of SD, which has in the past been termed misorientation by some aeromedical professionals, is what occurs during most CFIT mishaps, in which the pilot does not appear to make any control movement to avoid an impact with the ground.

It can be assumed that most Type I SD incidents occur because the pilot is not maintaining concentration on the primary flight instruments, because of distractions that cause either prolonged fixation on other cockpit information (e.g., warning lights or audio messages) or prolonged fixation on targets outside of the cockpit. By some accounts it is also the type that is most likely to result in SD mishaps.[10] A recent USAF mishap study[8] showed that 100% (13 of 13) of SD mishaps between 1989–1991 were Type I, and a recent Canadian Air Force study[67] showed 12 of 14 SD mishaps to be of the Type I variety. In contrast, a U.S. Navy study[37] found most fighter aircraft SD mishaps to be of the Type II variety. However, Bellenkes et al.,[37] as well as a later U.S. Army helicopter survey,[68] found the largest percentage of rotary-winged SD mishaps to be of the Type I variety.

In Type II SD the pilot consciously perceives *some* manifestation of SD. Pilots might experience a conflict between what they feel the aircraft is doing and what the flight instruments show that it is doing or between their perception of aircraft orientation and what their out-the-window view tells them. Sometimes this occurs after a long period of glancing away from the instruments or after breaking out of a cloud in an unusual position, as first described by van Wulften Palthe.[19] Often, the first reaction of pilots during Type II SD is either to not believe the instruments or to misconstrue the position of the horizon or other out-the-window terrain features. An example of the former situation involved a C-5 aircraft over the Indian Ocean in a near-fatal SD incident. Just prior to the aircraft's entering a stall, the copilot was heard to say "What's up with the inertial nav[igation system]?" when the electronic attitude indicator showed the aircraft was climbing into a stall rather than flying level (which it was essentially doing relative to the experienced gravitoinertial force vector). The fact that primitive orientation sensations triumph over the information provided by flight instruments (whose failure rate in current aircraft is extremely rare) or a cognitive knowledge that true horizons do not "tilt" in space is a testament to the powerful influence exerted by our preconscious orientational systems.

It is important to stress that pilots might not realize that they are disoriented during Type II SD but only that there is a discrepancy between what their natural orientation senses convey vs what their synthetic orientation systems can glean from their flight instruments or other consciously processed information. Sometimes, the conflict is barely noticed and the pilot quickly resolves the discrepancy, but on other occasions the pilot might suffer from the physiological and emotional symptoms that are generally referred to as vertigo (see Sec. I of this chapter). The pilot can still control the aircraft in Type II SD but might not "feel right" as he or she attempts to fight off the discrepant, primitive orientation sensation. One common description of Type II SD by pilots is of a leaning percept in a level aircraft (i.e., the "leans") (see Chapter 6, Sec. IV.A). Another common occurrence is when pilots report that they "had a bad case of vertigo on final approach."[4,10]

Although only a minority of SD mishaps are attributable to Type II SD, it is likely that at least some Type I mishaps might actually be Type II situations in which pilots might recognize the conflict between the synthetic and natural orientation information but might misinterpret their instruments or might not have sufficient time to react. In one such instance, an F-15E pilot rolled into an overbank in poor weather over water, but he could not discern his aircraft's attitude initially from the HUD pitch ladder and subsequently from the head-down electronic attitude indicator. Had the pilot not ejected in time, his lack of control input would have been attributed to Type I SD, although we know from his later testimony that he refrained from corrective action because be was unable to determine which way to move the stick. Another example of this is an F-16 pilot who again ejected just prior to impact with his aircraft heading nose down into the ground. Later testimony indicated that the pilot thought he was in a much shallower bank and pulling a climb maneuver to evade a lead aircraft, but in reality was actually in an inverted bank and pulling the nose down. The pilot realized his aircraft was not responding as it should have to his stick pull, but he did not have sufficient time to realize what was causing the failure to climb. Even though the pilot was clearly experiencing Type II SD, had he not lived to tell about his experience the mishap would have probably been labeled as Type I SD because he did not make any action to reduce the overbank in the final seconds.

If Type II SD transitions into a more dangerous level of disorientation stress, some researchers argue that a third type of SD results, namely, Type III or inca-pacitating SD.[4,10] There are many reasons why pilots can become psychologically incapacitated during SD, such as an inability to control the aircraft manually, an inability to read the flight instruments, and/or concomitant psychological aberra-tions resulting in distorted time perception, heightened anxiety, and dissociative sensations involving loss of connectedness with the aircraft. In the "giant-hand" phenomenon,[69,70] for example, pilots can be psychologically incapable of mov-ing the control stick in the direction necessary to level the aircraft because of the intrusion of preconscious orientational inputs to the vestibulospinal motor system that controls their arm (see Chapter 4, Sec. VI.D and Chapter 6, Sec.VII.A). The inability to read the flight instruments can be a consequence of uncontrollable vestibulo-ocular nystagmus (known as vestibulo-ocular disorganization), as can frequently occur during aerodynamic spins[71] and in cases of pressure-induced vertigo (see Chapter 6, Sec.VII.B and VIII.A). Psychological aberrations that can affect the pilot's confidence in his or her ability to fly the aircraft occur in many forms (see Chapter 4, Sec.VI), but perhaps the most dramatic of these is the break-off phenomenon in which the pilot feels physically detached (i.e., lying outside) the airplane.[72]

Researchers have debated whether disorientation stress should be classified as a separate SD type. Some researchers[10,67] have lumped the SD situations just described above into a Type III category, partly because the procedures involved in recovering from this type of SD can be somewhat different than when control of the aircraft is not in jeopardy. For example, one procedure for overcoming the giant-hand phenomenon is to remove one's hand from the control stick and reapply stick control by means of the thumb and forefinger, which bypasses the vestibulospinal reflexes; however, this procedure would not necessarily be of value in overcoming Type II SD. One the other hand, Benson[2,47] has argued that Type II SD and Type III SD are too similar from a perceptual standpoint to justify a separate category and that the difficulty of overcoming the SD should not be a paramount consideration in classifying SD episodes. The debate over whether a separate Type III SD category should exist or not is not merely an academic concern, as some flying communities (e.g., the U.S. and Canadian Air Forces) use the Type III SD designation in classifying mishaps, whereas others (e.g., the U.S. Navy and United Kingdom's Royal Air Force) currently do not.

A general sequence of events can be described that often leads from Type I to Type III SD. Initially, the pilot can fly without awareness of being oriented differently than intended (Type I SD), for anywhere from a brief moment to an extended period of time lasting tens of seconds or even longer. In the vast majority of instances, a recognition by the pilot that the aircraft is not in the appropriate or perceived orientation in space occurs (Type II SD), which usually precipitates an effort to reestablish proper control of the aircraft's motion. If the conflict between the natural and synthetic orientation percepts is too great or the pilot becomes otherwise incapable of maintaining proper spatial orientation, extreme disorientation stress (synonymous with Type III SD) ensues with a resulting disintegration of skilled flying and, in rare cases, a failure to recover the aircraft. Usually, however, the pilot is able to reestablish control over the aircraft, although it might take a considerable time to reduce the disorientation stress to a manageable level. An illustration of the progression from Type I SD to disorientation stress (Type III SD) is shown in Fig. 13. It must be emphasized that not all instances of Type II or Type III SD progress through an earlier stage. For example, one might immediately recognize an SD situation and experience its conflict, thereby avoiding Type I SD, or one might experience Type III SD in the form of a giant hand without having previously experienced a Type II conflict (see Chapter 4, Sec. VI.D).

IV. Aircraft Motions in Flight

To understand and describe SD phenomena properly, it is important to understand the fundamental principles of motion and the nomenclature used to describe aircraft motions. Because some of the motion terminologies will be used repeatedly throughout this book, a review of them will be provided in this introductory chapter. An even more detailed discussion of aircraft motions is contained in Gillingham and Previc.[4]

A. Basic Motion Terminology

There are two types of physical motion: linear motion (translation) and angular motion (rotation). Linear motion can be further categorized as rectilinear (i.e., motion in a straight line) or curvilinear (i.e., motion in a curved path). Each

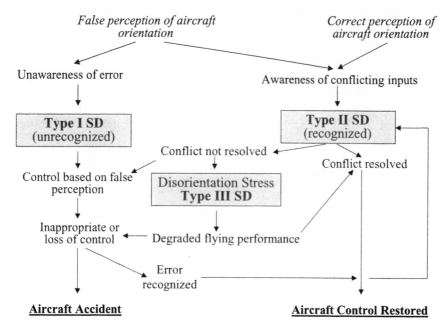

Fig. 13   Illustration of the progression from Type I to Type III SD. Adapted and modified from Benson.[2,47]

of the preceding motions can be further described in terms of various parameters, the most basic of which are displacement, velocity, acceleration, and jerk. Table 1 classifies the major linear and angular motion parameters that are used by SD researchers and other professionals, along with their symbols and units.

1. Linear Motion

The basic parameter of linear motion is *linear displacement*. The other three major parameters—velocity, acceleration, jerk—are derived from the concept of

Table 1   Linear and angular motion symbols and units

Motion parameter	Linear		Angular	
	Symbols	Units	Symbols	Units
Displacement	x	m 1 n mile (kn = 1852 m)	θ	degree rad = $360/2\pi$ (deg)
Velocity	v	m/s kn ($\approx$0.514 m/s)	ω	deg/s rad/s
Acceleration	a	m/s^2 g ($\approx$9.81 m/s^2)	α	deg/s^2 rad/s^2
Jerk	j	m/s^3 g/s	Υ	deg/s^3 rad/s^3

displacement over time. Linear displacement x is the distance and direction of the object under consideration from some reference point; as such, it is a vector quantity, having both magnitude and direction. Displacement in the flight environment can be described in a number of units, including feet (usually in reference to feet above ground), meters (m), kilometers (km), statute miles (1 mi = 1609 m), and nautical miles (1 n mile = 1.15 statute mi, or 1852 m). In this book all linear displacement and motion will be described in meters, which are the units used in the Systeme Internationale d'Unites (S.I.), but also in feet in reference to altitude above ground and changes thereof.

Linear velocity v occurs when linear displacement is changed during a period of time and is a vector with both a direction and magnitude. The formula for calculating the magnitude of the linear velocity, that is, the mean linear velocity v during a time interval Δt is as follows:

$$v = \frac{x_2 - x_1}{\Delta t} \tag{1}$$

where x_1 is the initial linear displacement, x_2 is the final linear displacement, and Δt is the elapsed time. Linear velocity of the aircraft is described in terms of meters per second or kilometers per hour and in nonmetric terms such as knots (1 kn = 0.51 m/s or 1.85 km/h) and ft/min (in reference to climb or descent rate). Linear velocity can also be described at a particular instant in time, that is, as Δt approaches zero. In this situation the *instantaneous linear velocity* can be defined as the first derivative of displacement with respect to time dx/dt.

When the linear velocity of an object changes over time, the difference in velocity divided by the elapsed time is referred as the mean *linear acceleration a*. The formula for acceleration is

$$a = \frac{v_2 - v_1}{\Delta t} \tag{2}$$

where v_1 is the initial velocity, v_2 is the final velocity, and Δt is the elapsed time. Linear acceleration is described in terms of meters per second squared. For example, an aircraft that accelerates from a dead stop to a velocity of 100 m/s in 5 s has a mean linear acceleration of 20 m/s^2. The *instantaneous linear acceleration* is the second derivative of displacement (d^2x/dt^2) or the first derivative of velocity (v or dv/dt) with respect to time. A very useful unit of acceleration is g_0, which is equal to the amount of acceleration exhibited by a free-falling body near the surface of the Earth, 9.81 m/s^2. To convert values of linear acceleration given in meters per second squared into g units, simply divide by 9.81. In the preceding example the aircraft's mean acceleration 20 m/s^2 can be expressed in g units as 2.04 g.

A final, less widely used linear motion parameter is *jerk j*, which refers to the rate of change of acceleration over time. Mean linear jerk is calculated using the formula:

$$j = \frac{a_2 - a_1}{\Delta t} \tag{3}$$

where a_1 is the initial acceleration, a_2 is the final acceleration, and Δt is the elapsed time. It has been argued by some researchers that neurons receiving inputs from the otolith organs of the vestibular system respond to jerk,[73] although most respond to linear acceleration and tilt (see Chapter 2). Although the metric unit for jerk is meters per cubic second, it is more customary to speak of jerk in terms of g-onset rate, measured in gs per second.

2. Angular Motion

The derivation of the parameters of angular motion parallels the scheme used to derive the parameters of linear motion. As with linear motion, angular displacement, velocity, and acceleration are all vectors with a specific direction and magnitude. The basic parameter of angular motion is angular displacement relative to a reference direction. *Angular displacement*, symbolized by θ, is generally measured in degrees, revolutions (1 rev = 360 deg), or radians (1 rad = 1 rev/2π, or approximately 57.3 deg). The radian is the angle subtended by a circular arc of the same length as the radius of the circle and is the S.I. unit for angular displacement. [The radian is a particularly convenient unit to use when dealing with circular motion (e.g., the motion of an SD demonstrator) because it is necessary only to multiply the angular displacement in radians by the length of the radius to find the value of the linear displacement along the circular path.]

Angular velocity ω is the rate of change of angular displacement. The mean angular velocity occurring in a time interval Δt is calculated as follows:

$$\omega = \frac{\theta_2 - \theta_1}{\Delta t} \tag{4}$$

where θ_1 is the initial angular displacement and θ_2 is the final angular displacement. *Instantaneous angular velocity* is $\partial\theta/\partial t$. An aircraft following a standard rate turn of 3 deg/s travels 180 deg in one minute, which can also be described as 0.5 rpm or as 0.052 rad/s.

The rate of change of angular velocity is termed *angular acceleration* α. The mean angular acceleration is calculated as follows:

$$\alpha = \frac{\omega_2 - \omega_1}{\Delta t} \tag{5}$$

where ω_1 is the initial angular velocity, ω_2 is the final angular velocity, and Δt is the time interval over which the angular velocity changes. If a figure skater spinning at 3 rev/s (1080 deg/s, or 18.9 rad/s) decelerates to a complete stop (0 rad/s) in 2 s, the mean angular acceleration α is –9.5 rad/s^2. *Instantaneous angular acceleration* is symbolized either as the second derivative of angular displacement ($d^2\theta/dt^2$) or as the first derivative of angular velocity ($d\omega/dt$) with respect to time.[10]

Although not commonly used by SD researchers, the final major parameter derived from angular displacement is *angular jerk*, the rate of change of angular acceleration. Its description is completely analogous to that for linear jerk, with the exception that angular rather than linear symbols and units are used.

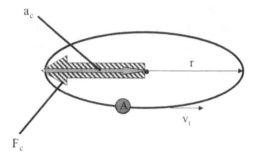

Fig. 14   Illustration of the concept of centripetal (radial) acceleration and centrifugal force. An object A moving in a circular path has a tangential velocity v_t equal to the object's angular velocity in radians/second ω multiplied by the radius of the path r, a centripetal acceleration a_c equal to v_t^2/r, and a centrifugal force F_c equal to the object's mass $m \times a_c$.

A special type of angular motion—*radial* or *centripetal acceleration a_c*—results in curvilinear (usually circular) motion and produces a similar physiological reaction to that of linear acceleration. Radial acceleration acts along the line represented by the radius of the curve and is directed toward the center of curvature (Fig. 14). Radial acceleration occurs as a result of a continuous redirection of an object's tangential velocity v_t. The occurrence of radial/centripetal acceleration in an aeromedical context is exemplified when an aircraft pulls out of a dive or when the gondola of an SD demonstrator moves about its center-post in planetary rotation (see Chapter 8, Sec. III). The value of the centripetal acceleration a_c can be calculated given the tangential velocity v_t and the radius r of the curved path according to the following formula:

$$a_c = \frac{v_t^2}{r} \tag{6}$$

For example, the centripetal acceleration of an aircraft traveling at 300 m/s (approximately 600 kn) with a turning radius of 1500 m generates a centripetal acceleration of (300 m/s)^2/1500) or 60 m/s^2 (6.12 g). Centripetal acceleration a_c can also be calculated directly from the angular velocity of the planetary body ω and its radius r from the center of rotation using the formula

$$a_c = \omega^2 r \tag{7}$$

where ω is the angular velocity in rad/s. One can convert readily to the formula for centripetal acceleration based on tangential velocity [see Eq. (6)], given the following equivalence:

$$v_t = \omega r \tag{8}$$

For example, to calculate the centripetal acceleration generated by an SD demonstrator having a 2.4-m arm and engaging in planetary rotation at 30 rpm, Eq. (7)

is used after first converting 30 rpm to rad/s (i.e., 3.14 rad/s). Squaring the angular velocity and multiplying by the 2.4-m radius, a centripetal acceleration of $3.14^2 \times 2.4$ m/s^2, that is, 23.66 m/s^2 or 2.4 g, is obtained.

B. Gravitoinertial Force Environment

Linear and angular parameters are important for describing the motion of the aircraft, but they are less important from a physiological standpoint than are the forces and torques that result from linear and angular velocities and accelerations. In this section the concepts of force and torque will be discussed and applied to SD phenomena.

1. Force, Torque, and Inertia

Force is an influence that can produce linear acceleration, that is, changes in linear motion. By contrast, a *torque* produces angular motion or changes thereof. Torque has dimensions of both force and length because the torque is applied as a force at a certain distance from a center of rotation. The S.I. unit of force is the Newton, which is the force required to accelerate a mass of 1 kg at 1 m/s^2. The S.I. unit of torque is the Newton-meter. Force is sensed by the otolith organs of the vestibular system and by pressure sensors in our skin, whereas torque is sensed primarily by the semicircular canals of the vestibular system (see Chapter 2).

According to Newton's second Law of Motion,

$$F = ma \qquad (9)$$

where F is the unbalanced force applied to an object, m is the mass of the object, and a is linear acceleration. [For the case of the apparent force (termed centrifugal) resulting from radial or centripetal acceleration, $F_c = ma_c$.] To describe the analogous situation pertaining to angular motion, the following equation is used:

$$M = J\alpha \qquad (10)$$

where M is the unbalanced torque (or moment) applied to the rotating object, J is the rotational inertia (moment of inertia) of the object, and α is angular acceleration.

Another concept related to force is *momentum*. The product of mass and linear velocity ($m \times v$) is known as linear momentum. Momentum can only be changed when a force is applied over time: $F\Delta t = mv_2 - mv_1$. This also holds true for angular momentum, which is the product of moment of inertia and angular velocity ($J \times \omega$).

Thus, the mass of an object is the ratio of the force acting upon the object to the acceleration resulting from that force. Mass, therefore, is a measure of the *inertia* of an object, that is, its resistance to being accelerated. Similarly, rotational inertia is the ratio of the torque acting upon an object to the angular acceleration resulting from that torque—again, a measure of resistance to acceleration. The concept of inertial force is inherent in Newton's third Law of Motion, which states that for every force applied to an object there is an equal and opposite reactive force exerted by that object. Thus, inertial force is an apparent force opposite in direction to an accelerating force and equal to the mass of the object times its acceleration. For example, a forward-accelerating aircraft exerts an inertial force that is equal to the product of the pilot's mass and the aircraft's acceleration and is expressed as seat pressure on the pilot's back (See Chapter 2, Sec. XI).

2. Gravitoinertial Forces

Physicists since Mach have recognized that gravitational and inertial forces cannot be distinguished; hence, a pilot in a maneuvering aircraft is almost continuously exposed to a *gravitoinertial force environment*. The combination of inertial force and gravity yields a resultant gravitoinertial force vector whose magnitude and direction are calculated as a vectorial sum of the two forces. As a result of the outward centripetal force generated during a coordinated turn in combination with gravity, for example, the pilot of the inwardly banked aircraft normally experiences a resultant gravitoinertial force vector that is oriented downward through the aircraft. This force also exerts downward pressure on the pilot's blood flow (thereby increasing the risk of loss of consciousness) as well as pressure on the pilot against the bottom of the seat (see Chapter 2).

As with the individual forces themselves, the resultant gravitoinertial force vector is described in terms of G units. Strictly speaking, G is a measure of relative weight:

$$G = \frac{w}{w_0} \tag{11}$$

where w is the weight observed in the environment under consideration and w_0 is the normal weight on the surface of the Earth. Weight, like force, is the product of the object's mass m and its acceleration a, such that

$$w = ma \tag{12}$$

When only Earth's gravity is present, the magnitude of the force vector is equal to the object's mass times the acceleration caused by gravity, namely, 9.81 m/s^2 (or 9.81 N for a 1-kg object). The calculation of G can be further simplified as the ratio between the existing acceleratory field a and the acceleration caused by gravity g_0:

$$G = \frac{w}{w_0} = \frac{ma}{mg_0} = \frac{a}{g_0} \tag{13}$$

Thus, whereas g is used as a unit of acceleration referenced to the acceleration associated with gravity (e.g., $a_c = 8\ g$), G is reserved for describing the resultant gravitoinertial force vector produced by that acceleration referenced to the gravitational force (e.g., $F = 8$ G, an 8-G load, or pulling 8 Gs). For example, when a 1-G forward acceleration (thrust) is applied to an aircraft that is flying level, the pilot experiences both an opposite (backward) 1 G inertial force as well as the downward 1-G force of gravity, which sum to a resultant gravitoinertial vector of 1.414 G, which is tilted backward from the gravitational vertical at an angle of 45 deg (see Fig. 15). In contrast, a pilot leveling off from a climb experiences the

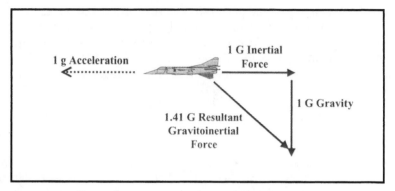

Fig. 15 Illustration of how an inertial force combines with gravity to produce a resultant gravitoinertial vector that represents the sum of the two individual vectors.

centrifugal force in an opposite direction to gravity, so that the resultant gravitoinertial vector is less than 1 G (perhaps even negative). A confusion of the direction of the gravitoinertial vector with the direction of the gravitational vertical is the source of many SD illusions in flight (see Chapter 6).

C. Description of Aircraft Motions

Linear and angular motions of the aircraft in space are typically described in reference to three principal Cartesian axes (see Fig. 16). The three linear axes are the longitudinal (fore-aft), lateral (right-left), and vertical (up-down) axes. Angular motion about the longitudinal, lateral, and vertical axes of the aircraft is termed roll, pitch, and yaw, respectively. Hence, the longitudinal axis is referred to as the

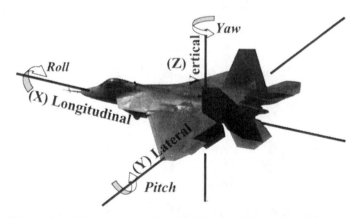

Fig. 16 Illustration of the system used to describe aircraft linear and angular motion (in italics) in reference to all three Cartesian axes.

roll axis, the lateral axis as the pitch axis, and the vertical axis as the yaw axis. By contrast, angular position or direction is referenced to the Earth, with bank referring to the lateral tilt relative to the horizon, elevation (and more commonly pitch) referring to the vertical tilt relative to the horizon, and heading referring to the angle (0–360 deg) about an Earth-vertical axis in relationship to the direction of true north. Although terms like roll and bank are often interchanged, they are often quite different. When the aircraft is in a 90-deg vertical climb, for example, roll motion about the longitudinal axis would not lead to any change in bank. All of these aircraft parameters are discussed further in Chapter 9 in reference to the aircraft instruments.

Most linear accelerations in aircraft occur along the longitudinal axis (where thrust usually occurs) or the vertical axis (where lift develops) or some combination thereof. Most angular accelerations in fixed-wing aircraft occur in the roll-and-pitch planes, although yaw motion is common in rotary-wing aircraft as well as fixed-wing aircraft performing spins and other aerobatic maneuvers. Vectored-thrust ("agile") aircraft that have only recently been tested and fielded operate with still greater freedom of linear and angular motion than do traditional fixed-wing aircraft (see Chapter 11, Sec. III).

A practical system for describing linear and angular aircraft accelerations and forces (torques) is shown in Fig. 17. This widely used nomenclature[74] refers to the longitudinal, lateral, and vertical axes as the x, y, and z axes, respectively. Linear and angular accelerations are labeled a and α, respectively, and their inertial reactions are referred to as G and R, respectively. The positive directions for accelerations are forward $(+a_x)$, upward $(+a_z)$, and rightward $(+a_y)$, whereas the positive inertial reactions are reversed (i.e., backward is $+G_x$, downward is $+G_z$),

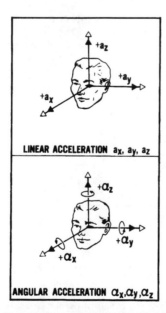
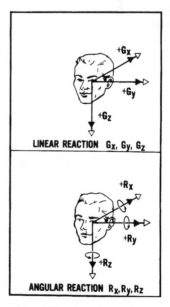

Fig. 17 Nomenclature for labeling the direction of linear and angular accelerations and inertial reactions (forces/torques).

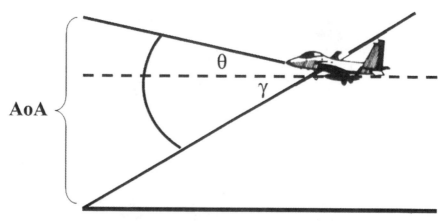

Fig. 18 The distinction between the pitch attitude of the aircraft (θ) and its velocity-vector (γ) during landing relative to a line that projects to the horizon (dashed line). The sum of θ and γ is angle-of-attack (AoA).

except in the case of the lateral axis (where rightward force is termed $+G_y$). Radial acceleration is similarly described, such that the acceleration directed toward the center of an aircraft turn is, in a banked aircraft, mostly $+a_{cz}$, and the resulting centrifugal force is mostly $+G_{cz}$ or G_z for short that is, head to foot. The direction of angular motions can also be named according to this convention, in that positive roll acceleration ($+\alpha_x$) is clockwise to the right, positive pitch acceleration ($+\alpha_y$) is downward, and positive yaw acceleration ($+\alpha_z$) is to the left (see Fig. 17). However, although these motions are shown relative to the head, as is appropriate for laboratory experiments, the vertical angle of the head is not always aligned with the vertical axis of the aircraft during flight.[75] Hence, SD researchers must be careful in specifying the reference system used to describe motions as they impact the pilot.

Although the preceding terminology is adequate for describing the direction of aircraft motion relative to a starting position of the aircraft, it is not adequate for completely describing the motion of the aircraft in space. Hence, researchers use an additional term to describe the motion/trajectory of the aircraft relative to Earth-fixed space, namely, its *velocity-vector*. The velocity-vector, or γ, usually approximates the orientation and acceleration of the aircraft, for example, rolling and yawing the aircraft to the right results in a turning of the aircraft in that same direction. The velocity-vector can deviate quite substantially from the orientation of the aircraft during landing, however. This is because the reduction in airspeed on approach results in reduced lift and a loss of altitude, despite the nose-high attitude of the plane when it flares (see Fig. 18). The difference between the aircraft's pitch and velocity vectors is known as the *angle of attack* (AoA). (Angle of attack also is typically denoted by the symbol α, but in this text α will refer exclusively to angular acceleration.) In most aircraft AoA can only reach a few degrees before a stall results, but vectored-thrust and other advanced high-performance aircraft can maneuver with AoAs equal to 20 deg or more. Whether to display orientation information in terms of aircraft attitude or velocity vector is a complex issue that will be discussed further in Chapter 9.

V. Summary

Spatial disorientation is a relatively mature research field that has steadily developed over the past century. Although laboratory discoveries by Mach and others provided some of the initial insights into the causes of SD illusions, research into the causes and prevention of SD in the aviation environment began in earnest only after World War I. In the 1920s and 1930s, the development of flight instrument displays and flight instrument training made it possible for pilots to fly safely in all kinds of weather. A steady expansion of the body of SD knowledge occurred after World War II, and the amount of SD research accelerated rapidly in the 1990s. The first efforts to treat spatial disorientation in flight as a comprehensive discipline began in the 1960s and 1970s and ultimately led to the creation of this first comprehensive textbook on SD.

As the SD research field matured, so did many of the concepts, definitions, and other terminologies used by SD researchers. Some of the terminology related to the types and axes of motion have gained near-universal acceptance, and a standard definition and usage of even more general conceptual terms such as controlled flight into terrain; loss of situational awareness; Types I, II, and III SD; etc. have been embraced by at least the majority of SD researchers. To ensure that SD research continues to progress and mature as a discipline, future researchers will hopefully review the hundreds of papers that currently form the core body of the knowledge in this area—the vast majority of which are cited in this textbook—and adhere to the commonly accepted SD terminology.

References

[1]Neubauer, J. C., "Classifying Spatial Disorientation Mishaps Using Different Definitions," *IEEE Engineering in Medicine and Biology,* Vol. 19, No. 2, 2000, pp. 28–34.

[2]Benson, A. J., "Spatial Disorientation—General Aspects," *Aviation Medicine*, 3rd ed., edited by J. Ernsting, A. N. Nicholson, and D. J. Rainford, Butterworth Heinemann, Oxford, England, U.K., 1999, pp. 419–436.

[3]*Instrument flight procedures*, Vol. 1, Air Force Manual 11–217, U.S. Air Force, Washington, D.C., 2000.

[4]Gillingham, K. K., and Previc, F. H., "Spatial Orientation in Flight," *Fundamentals of Aerospace Medicine*, 2nd ed., edited by R. L. DeHart, Williams and Wilkins, Baltimore, MD, 1996, pp. 309–397.

[5]Navathe, P. D., and Singh, B., "An Operational Definition for Spatial Disorientation," *Aviation, Space, and Environmental Medicine,* Vol. 65, 1994, pp. 1153–1155.

[6]Ocker, W. C., and Crane, C. J., *Blind Flight in Theory and Practice*, Naylor, San Antonio, TX, 1932.

[7]Macurdy, J. T., "Disorientation and Vertigo, with Special Reference to Aviation," *British Journal of Psychology,* Vol. 25, 1934, pp. 42–54.

[8]Lyons, T. J., Ercoline, W. R., Freeman, J. E., and Gillingham, K. K., "Classification Problems of U.S. Air Force Spatial Disorientation Accidents, 1989–91," *Aviation, Space, and Environmental Medicine,* Vol. 65, 1994, pp. 147–152.

[9]Endsley, M. R., "Toward a Theory of Situation Awareness in Dynamic Systems," *Human Factors,* Vol. 37, 1995, pp. 32–64.

[10]Gillingham, K. K., "The Spatial Disorientation Problem in the United States Air Force," *Journal of Vestibular Research,* Vol. 2, 1992, pp. 297–306.

[11]Previc, F. H., Yauch, D. W., DeVilbiss, C. A., Ercoline, W. R., and Sipes, W. E., "In Defense of Traditional Views of Spatial Disorientation and Loss of Situation Awareness: A Reply to Navathe and Singh's 'An Operational Definition of Spatial Disorientation,'" *Aviation, Space, and Environmental Medicine,* Vol. 66, 1995, pp. 1103–1106.

[12]Scott, W. B., "New Research Identifies Causes of CFIT," *Aviation Week and Space Technology,* Vol. 144, No. 25, 1994, pp. 70, 71.

[13]Wiener, E. L., "Controlled Flight into Terrain Accidents: System-Induced Errors," *Human Factors,* Vol. 19, 1977, pp. 171–181.

[14]Corwin, W. H., (1995) "Controlled Flight into Terrain Avoidance: Why the Ground Proximity Warning is Too Little, Too Late," *Proceedings of the 21st Conference of the European Association for Aviation Psychology,* Avebury Aviation, Brookfield, VT, 1995, pp. 155–160.

[15]Henn, V., and Young, L. R., "*Ernst Mach* on the Vestibular Organ 100 Years Ago," *ORL,* Vol. 37, 1975, pp. 138–148.

[16]Hoff, E. C., and Fulton, J. F., *A Bibliography of Aviation Medicine,* C. C. Thomas, Springfield, IL, 1942.

[17]Head, H., "The Sense of Stability and Balance in the Air," *The Medical Problems of High Flying,* His Majesty's Stationery Office, London, 1920, pp. 214–256.

[18]Koonce, J. M., "A Brief History of Aviation Psychology," *Human Factors,* Vol. 26, 1984, pp. 499–508.

[19]van Wulfften Palthe, P. M., "Function of the Deeper Sensibility and of the Vestibular Organs in Flying," *Acta Otolaryngologica,* Vol. 4, 1922, pp. 415–448.

[20]Macready, J. A., (1924). "The Non-Stop Flight Across America," *National Geographic Magazine,* Vol. 441, No. 1, 1924, pp. 1–83.

[21]Schaeffer, A. A., "Spiral Movement in Man," *Journal of Morphology and Physiology,* Vol. 45, 1928, pp. 293–398.

[22]Doolittle, J. H., "Early Experiments in Instrument Flying," *Annual Report of the Smithsonian Institution,* Smithsonian Publication No. 4478, 1961, pp. 337–355.

[23]Stokes, R. L., "First 'Blind' Flyer Reaches Goal," *Washington Star,* 13 July 1941.

[24]*Bibliography of Aeronautics (Part 21),* U.S. Works Progress Administration, Washington, D.C., 1937.

[25]Poppen, J. R., "Equilibratory Functions in Instrument Flying," *Journal of Aviation Medicine,* Vol. 7, 1936, pp. 148–160.

[26]Previc, F. H., and Ercoline, W. R., "The 'Outside-In' Attitude Display Concept Revisited," *International Journal of Aviation Psychology,* Vol. 9, 1999, pp. 377–401.

[27]Clark, B., and Graybiel, A., "Linear Acceleration and Deceleration as Factors Influencing Non-Visual Orientation During Flight," *Journal of Aviation Medicine,* Vol. 20, 1949, pp. 92–101.

[28]Graybiel, A., " Oculogravic Illusion," *A.M.A. Archives of Ophthalmology,* Vol. 48, 1952, pp. 605–615.

[29]Graybiel, A., and Hupp, D. I., "The Oculo-Gyral Illusion: A Form of Apparent Motion Which May Be Observed Following Stimulation of the Semicircular Canals," *Journal of Aviation Medicine,* Vol. 17, 1946, pp. 3–27.

[30]Graybiel, A., and Patterson, J. L., Jr., "Thresholds of Stimulation of the Otolith Organs as Indicated by the Oculogravic Illusion," *Journal of Applied Physiology,* Vol. 7, 1955, pp. 666–670.

[31]Gibson, J. J., *The Perception of the Visual World,* Houghton Mifflin, Boston, 1950.

[32]Vinacke, W. E., "Aviator's Vertigo," *Journal of Aviation Medicine,* Vol. 19, 1948, pp. 158–170.

[33]Clark, B., and Graybiel, A., "Vertigo as a Cause of Pilot Error in Jet Aircraft," *Journal of Aviation Medicine,* Vol. 28, 1957, pp. 469–478.

[34]Nuttall, J. B., and Sanford, W. G., *"Spatial Disorientation in Operational Flying,"* USAF Directorate of Flight Safety Research, Publication M-27-56, Norton AFB, CA, 1956.

[35]Barnum, F., and Bonner, R. H., "Epidemiology of USAF Spatial Disorientation Aircraft Accidents, 1 Jan 1958–31 Dec 1968," *Aerospace Medicine,* Vol. 42, 1971, pp. 896–898.

[36]Moser, R., Jr., "Spatial Disorientation as a Factor in Accidents in an Operational Command," *Aerospace Medicine,* Vol. 40, 1969, pp. 174–176.

[37]Bellenkes, A., Bason, R., and Yacavone, D. O., "Spatial Disorientation in Naval Aviation Mishaps: A Review of Class A Incidents from 1980 Through 1989," *Aviation, Space, and Environmental Medicine,* Vol. 63, 1992, pp. 128–131.

[38]Johnson, S. L., and Roscoe, S. N., "What Moves, the Airplane or the World?" *Human Factors,* Vol. 14, 1972, pp. 107–129.

[39]Fitts, P. M., and Jones, R. E., *"Psychological Aspects of Instrument Display: 1. Analysis of 270 'Pilot-Error' Experiences in Reading and Interpreting Aircraft Instruments,"* Air Materiel Command, Memorandum Rep. TSEAA-694-12A, Wright-Patterson Air Force Base, OH, 1947.

[40]Fitts, P. (ed.), *Psychological Research on Equipment Design,* Army Air Forces Aviation Psychology Research Report No. 19, U.S. Government Printing Office, Washington, D.C., 1947.

[41]Previc, F. H., and Ercoline, W. R., "Ground-Based Spatial Disorientation Training in the United States Air Force: Past and Current Devices," *Proceedings of the Eighth International Symposium on Aviation Psychology*, edited by R. A. Jensen and L. Rakovan, Ohio State University, Columbus, OH, 1995, pp. 1318–1322.

[42]Collins, W. E., *"Effective Approaches to Disorientation Familiarization for Aviation Personnel,"* Federal Aviation Administration, AM-7017, Oklahoma City, OK, 1970.

[43]Previc, F. H., and Ercoline, W. R., "Trends in Spatial Disorientation Research," *Aviation, Space, and Environmental Medicine,* Vol. 72, 2001, pp. 1048–1050.

[44]Benson, A. J., (1965). "Spatial Disorientation in Flight," *A Textbook of Aviation Physiology,* edited by J.A. Gilles, Pergamon, Oxford, England, U.K., pp. 1086–1132.

[45]Benson, A. J., "Spatial Disorientation—General Aspects," (Eds.), *Aviation Medicine: Physiology and Human Factors,* Vol. I, edited by G. Dhenin and J. Ernsting, Tri-Med, London, 1978, pp. 405–433

[46]Benson, A. J., "Spatial Disorientation—Common Illusions," *Aviation Medicine,* 2nd ed., edited by J. Ernsting and P. King, Butterworths, London, 1988, pp. 297–317.

[47]Benson, A. J., "Spatial Disorientation—General Aspects," *Aviation Medicine,* 3rd ed., edited by J. Ernsting, A. N. Nicholson and D.J. Rainford, Butterworth Heinemann, Oxford, England, U.K., 1999, pp. 419–436.

[48]Gillingham, K. K., and Wolfe, J. W., "Spatial Orientation in Flight," *Fundamentals of Aerospace Medicine*, 1st ed., edited by R. L. DeHart, Lea and Febiger, Philadelphia, PA, 1986, pp. 299–381.

[49]Gilson, R. D., Guedry, F. E., Jr., Hixson, W. C., and Niven, J. I., "Observations on Perceived Changes in Aircraft Attitude Attending Head Movements Made in a 2-g Bank and Turn," *Aviation, Space, and Environmental Medicine,* Vol. 44, 1973, pp. 90–92.

[50]McCarthy, G. W., and Stott, J. R. R., (1994). "In Flight Verification of the Inversion Illusion," *Aviation, Space, and Environmental Medicine,* Vol. 65, 1994, pp. 341–344.

[51]Ercoline, W. R., DeVilbiss, C. A., Yauch, D. W., and Brown, D. L., "Post-Roll Effects on Attitude Perception: The Gillingham Illusion," *Aviation, Space, and Environmental Medicine,* Vol. 71, 2000, pp. 489–495.

[52]Dichgans, J., and Brandt, T., "Visual-Vestibular Interaction: Effects on Self-Motion Perception and Postural Control," *Handbook of Sensory Physiology*, Vol. 8: *Perception*, edited by R. Held, H. Leibowitz, and H.-L. Teuber, Springer-Verlag, New York, 1978, pp. 755–804.

[53]Previc, F. H., (1998). "The Neuropsychology of 3-D Space," *Psychological Bulletin*, Vol. 124, 1998, pp. 123–164.

[54]Kirkham, W. R., Collins, W. E., Grape, P. M., Simpson, J. M., and Wallace, T. F., "Spatial Disorientation in General Aviation Accidents," *Aviation, Space, and Environmental Medicine*, Vol. 49, 1998, pp. 1080–1086.

[55]Vyrnwy-Jones, P., "A Review of Army Air Corps Helicopter Accidents, 1971–1982," *Aviation, Space, and Environmental Medicine*, Vol. 56, 1985, pp. 403–409.

[56]Ercoline, W., DeVilbiss, C. A., and Lyons, T. J., (1994). "Trends in USAF Spatial Orientation Accidents—1958–1992," edited by R. J. Lewandowski, W. Stephens, and L. A. Haworth, *Helmet and Head-Mounted Displays and Symbology Design Requirements Conference*, Vol. 2218, Society of Photo-Optical Instrumentation Engineers, Bellingham, WA, 1994.

[57]McNaughton, G., *Proceedings of the Aircraft Attitude Awareness Workshop*, Air Force Flight Dynamics Lab. Wright-Patterson AFB, OH, 1987.

[58]Newman, R. L., Haworth, L. A., Kessler, G. K., Eksuzian, D. J., Ercoline, W. R., Evans, R. H., Hughes, T. C., and Weinstein, L. F., "*TRISTAR I: Evaluation Methods for Testing Head-Up Display (HUD) Flight Symbology*," NASA TM 4665, 1994.

[59]Weinstein, L. F., Gillingham, K. K., and Ercoline, W. R., "United States Air Force Head-up Display Control and Performance Symbology Evaluations," *Aviation, Space, and Environmental Medicine*, Vol. 65, 1994, pp. A20–A30.

[60]Malcolm, R., "Pilot Disorientation and the Use of a Peripheral Vision Display," *Aviation, Space, and Environmental Medicine*, Vol. 55, 1984, pp. 231–238.

[61]Reising, J. M., Liggett, K. K., Solz, T. J., and Hartsock, D. C. "Comparison of Two Head Up Display Formats Used to Fly Curved Instrument Approaches," *Proceedings of the 39th Annual Meeting of the Human Factors and Ergonomics Society*, Human Factors and Ergonomics Society, Santa Monica, CA, 1995, pp. 1–5.

[62]Watler, J., and Logan, W., "The Maneuvering Flight Path Display—A Flight Trajectory Solution Display Concept," *Proceedings of the National Aerospace and Electronics Conference*, Inst. of Electrical and Electronics Engineers, New York, 1981, pp. 1254–1260.

[63]Braithwaite, M. G., Hudgens, J. J., Estrada, A., and Alvarez, E. A., "An Evaluation of the British Army Spatial Disorientation Sortie in U.S. Army Aviation," *Aviation, Space, and Environmental Medicine*, Vol. 69, 1998, pp. 727–732.

[64]Benson, A. J. (ed.), "The Disorientation Incident," AGARD-CP-95-Pt.1, AGARD, Neuilly sur Seine, France, 1971.

[65]Perdriel, G., and Benson, A. J. (eds.), "*Spatial Disorientation in Flight: Current Problems*," AGARD CP-287, AGARD, Neuilly-sur-Seine, France, 1980.

[66]Benson, A. J. (ed.), "Orientation/Disorientation Training of Flying Personnel: A Working Group Report, AGARD-R-625, AGARD, Neuilly sur Seine, France, 1974.

[67]Cheung, B., Money, K., Wright, H., and Bateman, W., "Spatial Disorientation-Implicated Accidents in Canadian Forces, 1982–1992," *Aviation, Space, and Environmental Medicine*, Vol. 66, 1995, pp. 579–585.

[68]Braithwaite, M. G., Durnford, S. J., Crowley, J. S., Rosado, N. R., and Albano, J. P., "Spatial Disorientation in U.S. Army Rotary-Wing Operations," *Aviation, Space, and Environmental Medicine*, Vol. 69, 1998, pp. 1031–1037.

[69]King, P. A. H., "A Report of an Incident of Extreme Spatial Disorientation in Flight," *Aeromedical Reports*, Vol. 1, Inst. of Aviation Medicine, Royal Canadian Air Force, Toronto, Canada, 1962, pp. 22–28.

[70]Lyons, T. J., and Simpson, C. G., "The Giant Hand Phenomenon," *Aviation, Space, and Environmental Medicine,* Vol. 60, 1989, pp. 64–66.

[71]Melvill Jones, G., "Disturbance of Oculomotor Control in Flight," *Aerospace Medicine,* Vol. 36, 1965, 461–465.

[72]Clark, B., and Graybiel, A., "The Break-Off Phenomenon: A Feeling of Separation from the Earth Experienced by Pilots at High Altitude," *Journal of Aviation Medicine,* Vol. 28, 1957, pp. 121–126.

[73]Angelaki, D. E., Bush, G. A., and Perachio, A. A., "Two-Dimensional Spatiotemporal Coding of Linear Acceleration in Vestibular Nuclei Neurons," *Journal of Neuroscience,* Vol. 13, 1993, pp. 1403–1417.

[74]Hixson, W. C., Niven, J. I., and Correia, M. J., *"Kinematics Nomenclature for Physiological Accelerations: With Special Reference to Vestibular Applications,"* Naval Aerospace Medical Institute, Monograph 14, Pensacola, FL, 1966.

[75]Patterson, F. R., Cacioppo, A. J., Gallimore, J. J., Hinman, G. E., and Nalepka, J. P., "Aviation Spatial Orientation in Relationship to Head Position and Attitude Interpretation," *Aviation, Space, and Environmental Medicine,* Vol. 68, 1997, pp. 463–471.

[76]Leibowitz, H. W., and Dichgans, J. "The Ambient Visual System and Spatial Orientation," *Spatial Disorientation in Flight: Current Problems*, AGARD-CP-287, AGARD, Neuilly sur Seine, France, 1980, pp. B4-1–B4-4.

Chapter 2

Nonvisual Spatial Orientation Mechanisms

Bob Cheung*

Defence Research and Development Canada, Toronto, Canada

I. Introduction

I NFORMATION about the attitude, heading, and velocity of the body, with respect to the fixed frame of reference provided by the gravitational vertical and the surface of the earth, is necessary for head stabilization, postural control, orientation, and locomotion. Posture maintenance and self-motion perception is based on simultaneous stimulation of the visual, vestibular, and somatosensory systems. To a lesser extent, the auditory system also provides information on orientation. Within this multiloop control system the individual components are mutually interactive and partially redundant because their functional ranges overlap. To the extent that their functional ranges do not overlap, the individual components compensate for each other's deficiencies. For example, if visual function is normal and external visual cues are unambiguous, low-frequency (<1–2 Hz) visual signals provide reliable sensory information from which orientation can be perceived correctly. However, under instrument meteorological conditions (IMC), where the pilot has meager, if any, visual information outside of the instrument display, and at higher motion frequencies, vestibular information plays a significant role. In the latter case observed targets move with the head as suppression of unwanted eye movements relies on a visual pursuit mechanism that can fail at frequencies as low as 0.5 Hz.[1]

Our perception of correct orientation based on these sensory systems is developed under a normal G environment. The relative contribution of the various sensory systems is significantly altered when exposed to unusual gravitoinertial environments such as in the air, in space, or underwater. For example, once we are airborne and subjected to abnormal or unusual accelerative forces the information provided by different sensory modalities, particularly the vestibular apparatus and proprioceptors, might be interpreted incorrectly with potentially dangerous

This material is declared a work of the U.S. Government and is not subject to copyright protection in the United States.

*Senior Defense Scientist.

consequences. The effective muscular response is redirected to maintain control of the aircraft rather than the maintenance of posture and equilibrium. Under continuous variation in both the magnitude and direction of the apparent gravitational field and prolonged rotational movements, the central nervous system (CNS) has the added responsibility of determining which sensory information is valid and which is not. When presented with reduced and or conflicting sensory information, it is normal to experience episodes of spatial disorientation (SD).

Disorientation is not limited to the aerial environment. During a prolonged space flight and until some level of adaptation is attained, astronauts often experience unstable vision, motor-control disturbances, reduced eye–hand coordination, illusory self- and/or scene-motion, and space-motion sickness.[2] Preflight and postflight data suggest that adaptation in orbit and readaptation upon return to Earth involve a change in the sensorimotor integration of vestibular signals, most likely from the otolith organs. Specifically, while the otoliths detect head tilt and translation on the ground, no changes in otolith signals are associated with head tilt in prolonged weightlessness; hence, the brain reinterprets all otolith signals as indicating linear translation and corresponding eye movement reflexes and self-motion perception are also altered accordingly.[3] Following return from orbit, the interpretation of otolith signals as linear motion persists until readaptation to 1 G occurs.

When a person is submerged underwater in an accident, such as helicopter ditching, somatosensory cues are markedly reduced, because the muscles that are normally responsible for posture and balance are neutrally buoyant and not subjected to the normal effect of gravity. The otoliths of the vestibular system normally respond to tangential shearing forces and detect changes relative to gravity but become ineffective beyond 90 deg from vertical. They do not recognize whether the body is upright or inverted. Finally, the visual frame of reference underwater can be lost as a result of a reduction of ambient light, being obscured by bubbles and debris, or confusion caused by the underwater magnification effect.

Therefore, SD occurs when subjects lose the ability to sense accurately their position, motion, or attitude within the fixed frame of reference, regardless of whether they are in flight, in space, or underwater. When SD occurs on the ground, it is usually attributed to some underlying pathology of the inner ear or the CNS. In the air, however, SD must be regarded as an extension of a normal physiological response, in the absence of any pathology, which implies that it cannot be entirely prevented. This chapter reviews nonvisual mechanisms of orientation; the visual mechanisms of orientation are dealt with in Chapter 3. An overview of spatial orientation mechanisms in flight is followed by a description of the anatomical and physiological function of the vestibular system, its influence on cardiovascular control, its habituation, and its contribution to gaze stability and alignment to vertical. Vestibulospinal motor mechanisms and somatosensory, auditory, and cortical input to orientation will also be discussed.

II.   Overview of Spatial Orientation Mechanisms in Flight

A schematic diagram showing the various sensory organs and components of perception that are involved in spatial orientation in flight is illustrated in Fig. 1. Sensory information available for orientation can be divided into two levels: the conscious and subconscious. At the conscious level auditory cues provide for

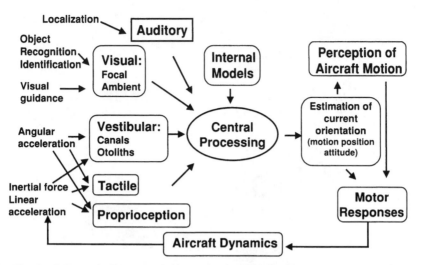

Fig. 1   Schematic diagram of the mechanisms of spatial orientation in flight.

sound localization, and focal vision is for object recognition and identification of flight instrument displays and symbolic data (see Chapter 3, Sec. IV.D.2). Conscious processing requires interpretation and intellectual construction from available information. At the subconscious level ambient vision is employed for visual guidance in positioning and orienting. Also, subconscious vestibular cues are used for detection of angular and linear acceleration, including gravity. The tactile and nonvestibular proprioceptive cues are for inertial force and linear acceleration detection. Neural processing in the CNS includes integration and interpretation of these sensory inputs and their comparison with internal models. These internal models are formulated based on past experience and training, which, in turn, generate expectations concerning estimation of the current motion, position, and attitude of the aircraft. Finally, the execution of the intended motor command occurs in response to current perception of aircraft motion.

III.   Vestibular Input to Orientation

A.   Labyrinth

Both the organ of hearing and the organ of balance are housed in the inner ear or labyrinth. The labyrinth is made up of the bony labyrinth, a series of channels embedded in the petrous portion of the temporal bone on each side of the head. Inside these channels, surrounded by a fluid called perilymph—high in sodium Na^+ and low in potassium K^+ concentration—is the membranous labyrinth, which more or less duplicates the shape of the bony channels and is constrained within the bony labyrinth by strands of connective tissue. The membranous labyrinth is filled with endolymph (high in K^+ and low in Na^+ concentration) and is composed of two different anatomical structures that subserve two distinct functions: the cochlea (organ of hearing) and the vestibular apparatus (organ of balance).

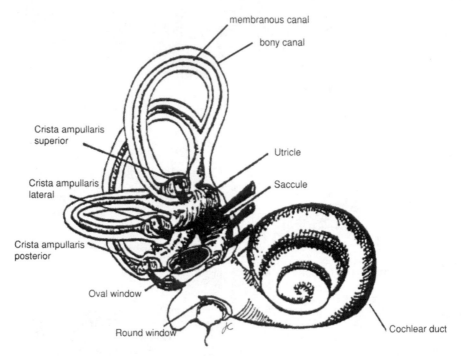

Fig. 2   Gross anatomy of the inner ear. A schematic illustration of relations among the semicircular canals, the utricle, and the saccule. The membranous semicircular canals are shown within their surrounding bony structure.

B.   Vestibular System

The vestibular sense does not have the conscious prominence of other orientation systems, such as vision, hearing, and touch. Normally, we are not aware of any vestibular dimension in our sensory experience. Only with clinical malfunction or provocative stimulation of the vestibular system—with resulting dizziness, nausea, vomiting, and other symptoms—does the function of the vestibular mechanism attain prominence. As mentioned before, the membranous portion of the vestibular apparatus is embedded within the bony labyrinth on each side of the skull and consists of three semicircular canals, a utricle, and a saccule. A schematic illustration of the anatomical relationship among the semicircular canals, the utricle, the saccule, and the cochlear duct is depicted in Fig. 2.

The vestibular apparatus, as a whole, functions in some respects like an inertial guidance system. It is an extremely sensitive device that provides information concerning movements of the head in space and its orientation to gravity. Our knowledge of the vestibular function is most complete for the primary canal and otolithic afferents. Relatively little progress has been made in understanding receptor mechanisms and the functional importance of the efferent vestibular system. At a frequency range between 0.1 and 5.0 Hz, which corresponds to that normally generated during natural movements such as locomotion, stepping, and jumping, the activity of the first-order afferent signals from the semicircular canals is close to being in phase with velocity.[4] At a lower or higher stimulus frequencies the afferent signal shifts toward acceleration. Angular velocity of head movements during normal locomotor activities seldom extends beyond a periodic time of 10 s, and shaking the head at frequencies higher than 5 Hz is quite uncomfortable. For linear translation the otolith afferent response, at a frequency range between 0.2 and 1.0 Hz, has the characteristic of a position response with a relative constant gain and a phase near zero across the frequency band.[5]

A considerable amount of knowledge has been accumulated regarding central vestibular reflex mechanisms. The major vestibular reflex systems include an ascending vestibulo-ocular reflex (VOR) that stabilizes gaze and ensures clear vision during head movements, particularly those that occur during locomotion. The otolith-ocular reflex becomes important when head translations cause image slip upon the retina, especially when viewing a near object. Naturally occurring head motion has both rotational and translational components so that both the otoliths and the semicircular canals contribute to the generation of compensatory slow-phase eye movements. The implications of the VOR for spatial orientation are discussed in Sec. V of this chapter.

The vestibular system also senses changes in posture for cardiovascular and other homeostatic control systems because significant changes in the orientation of the body (e.g., from supine to standing upright) result in stimulating the vestibular system at the time of movement. Therefore, the vestibular system could potentially anticipate the special demands of these regulatory systems during postural changes, allowing for rapid compensation for the altered posture. A descending vestibulospinal system is involved in head, limb, and postural control, and it provides input to the antigravity extensor muscle during quiet stance and locomotion.

As indicated in Sec. II, the mechanism of spatial orientation is "multimodal," that is, information from the vestibular receptors is actively integrated with the information from other perceptual systems. Moreover, the multimodal system of orientation is adaptable. For example, if the vestibular system is damaged or removed, the orientation system can learn to function without it. To appreciate that SD can result from the normal reactions of the vestibular system to motion stimulation in three-dimensional flight, an understanding of vestibular anatomy and physiology is required.

C. Morphological and Physiological Considerations of the Semicircular Canals

The semicircular canals are the primary receptors for angular accelerations, independent of the distance from the center of rotation. The term semicircular canal is not an accurate description because each canal functions as a complete and independent fluid-filled torus. Each of the canals forms nearly $\frac{2}{3}$ of a torus, with the remaining third sharing a common cavity with the utricle. The lumen (space in the interior) of the canals is elliptical, with a mean diameter of 0.3 mm. In humans the lateral (also referred as horizontal) and posterior (also referred as posterior vertical or inferior) canals have a radius of curvature of 1.6 to 1.9 mm, whereas the superior (also referred as anterior vertical) canal has a radius of curvature of about 2.2 mm (Ref. 6.) The planes of the three semicircular canals (the lateral, posterior, and superior canals) are approximately orthogonal. When the head is held naturally erect, the fore-aft diameter of the lateral canals is pitched up by an angle of 25–30 deg with respect to the Horsley–Clark stereotaxic plane, the plane through the lower margins of the orbit of the eye and the auditory meatus (external ear canal). The posterior canals lie in an almost vertical plane, whereas the superior canals lie in a plane inclined at an angle of approximately 15 deg to the vertical. Both the posterior and superior canals lie roughly at 45 deg from the frontal plane. Whereas the planes of the lateral canals of the two ears are parallel, the plane of the posterior canal of one ear is nearly parallel to the plane of the superior canal of the contralateral ear but orthogonal to the plane of the posterior canal of the contralateral ear.[7]

Neurophysiological findings have suggested that any head movement exciting a canal on one side of the head inhibits the corresponding canal on the other side. It is the difference in the responses of synergic canals that is interpreted by the brain as an angular head motion. Hence, the vestibular system is said to function as a "push–pull" balance system.[8] The disposition of the canals into three approximately orthogonal planes, with the canals in the two ears acting synergistically, permits generation of afferent signals indicating angular acceleration about any axis. However, the canals on one side are not exactly orthogonal, and synergistic pairs are not precisely parallel; therefore, there is no plane of rotation that stimulates only one pair of canals. In addition, the semicircular canals are not aligned with the respective interaural (pitch or y), dorsoventral (yaw or z), and naso-occipital (roll or x) axes of the head. However, they work in harmony to signals in rotational motion about any or all three of the Cartesian coordinate axes.

Each canal is filled with endolymph, which by virtue of its inertia flows through the canal whenever a component of the angular acceleration of the head is in the plane of the canal. Flow of the endolymph deflects the cupula, a gelatinous mass of mucopolysaccharides that forms a moveable diaphragm across the canal at a swelling near the junction of the utricle called the ampulla, as seen in Fig. 3. The ampulla contains the sensory epithelium called the crista ampullaris. It is believed that the cupula normally functions as a fixed, weakly elastic diaphragm rather than a hinged door as suggested by Steinhaussen[9,10] and Dohlman.[11] In frogs, this has been convincingly supported by a movie of cupula movements during sinusoidal rotation of the semicircular canal.[12] Instead of acting like a hinged membrane, the cupula remains attached at both extremities, bulging like a fixed, elastic diaphragm in the direction of fluid movement. Based on physical principles, exceedingly small displacements are to be expected. Therefore, the cupula could well be attached all around its margins without significant modification of the canal's hydrodynamic response.[13]

The neural transduction function is carried out by the cupula and the crista ampullaris. Figure 3a is a schematic of an idealized semicircular canal. The crista ampullaris contains many multiciliated hair cells, each with a single kinocilium and some 60 to 100 stiff stereocilia arranged in a regular pattern that protrude into the cupula as shown in Fig. 4 (Ref. 14.) Endings of the vestibular afferent fibers are in close contact with the hair cells. The cell bodies of the 19,000 neurons supplying the crista ampullaris and the maculae (to be discussed in Sec. III.G) on each side of the head are located in the vestibular ganglion. The vestibular nerve joins afferent fibers from the cochlea to form the eighth cranial nerve or statoacoustic nerve.

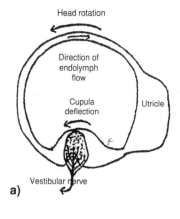

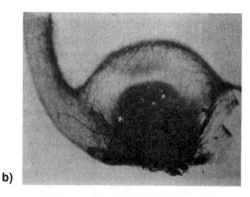

Fig. 3a   Idealized semicircular canal showing the direction of head rotation and the direction of endolymph flow.
Fig. 3b   Photograph of a dissected ampulla showing the membranous canal and the crista ampullaris.

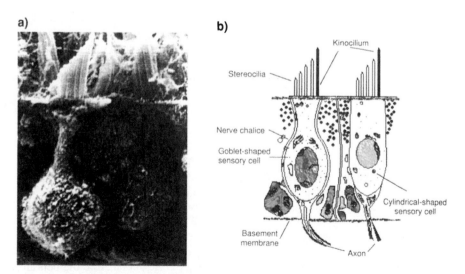

Fig. 4   Vestibular epithelium showing the two types of hair cells (goblet-shaped and cylindrical-shaped) and their innervations: a) electronmicrograph and b) schematics.

Each vestibular nerve terminates in one of four portions (lateral, medial, superior, and inferior) of the ipsilateral vestibular nucleus in the brain stem and in the flocculonodular lobe of the cerebellum. Second-order neurons descend down the spinal cord from the vestibular nuclei in the vestibulospinal tracts and ascend through the medial longitudinal fasciculi to the thalamus and on to the motor nuclei of the extraocular nerves that control eye movements and eventually terminate in the primary vestibular projection area of the cerebral cortex.

Lowenstein and Wersäll[15] first pointed out the relationship between the morphological and functional polarization of the hair cells. According to the Lowenstein–Wersäll theory, bending of the stereocilia towards the kinocilium during deflection of the cupula causes excitation (depolarization) and an increase in the discharge of vestibular afferents. Bending of the stereocilia away from the kinocilium causes inhibition (hyperpolarization), decreasing the resting discharge of the vestibular nerve.[16,17] During a leftward head rotation, deflection of the cupula toward the utricle (utriculopetal) in the left lateral canal increases the firing rate in the left ampullary nerve, while deflection away from the utricle (utriculofugal) in the right lateral canal decreases the firing rate in the right ampullory nerve. In the superior and posterior canals, utriculofugal cupula deflection increases firing rate, while utriculopetal cupula deflection decreases it. Therefore, nerve fibers running from each ampulla, projecting in turn to the vestibular nuclei at the brain stem via the eighth nerve, are the means by which information about angular motion of the head is relayed to the central nervous system. A schematic of the vestibular sensory cells and neural elements, including the kinocilium and stereocilia, is illustrated in Fig. 4b.

The neural pathways that connect the vestibular apparatus with the brain and spinal cord are complex. Readers are encouraged to refer to the *Mammalian Vestibular Physiology* by Wilson and Melvill Jones[18] for details. The vestibular nuclei consist of the superior, lateral (Dieters'), medial, and descending (inferior) nuclei. These nuclei also receive and serve to coordinate visual and somatic information. The vestibular nuclei, in turn, project neural signals to the cerebellum, oculomotor nerves, and spinal cord, where such signals excite the vestibulo-ocular reflex and the reflex contraction of limb and body muscles. Both vestibular afferent fibers and axons of neurons in the vestibular nuclei reach the vestibulocerebellum where inhibitory Purkinje cells and excitatory fastigial neurons exert their influence on the vestibular nucleus neurons. The activity of the vestibular nuclei is continually under cerebellar control.

Cumulative evidence[19,20] suggests that the vestibulo-cortical pathway coursing through the thalamus is concerned with the control of body position and orientation in space. Evidence for a vestibulo-thalamic projection is supported by electrophysiological studies in alert monkeys, where units in the thalamus exhibit consistent activity changes during sinusoidal rotation.[21] These thalamic units can also be activated by proprioceptive stimuli. Various regions of the cerebral cortex that receive vestibular inputs[22,23] have also been identified in the monkey. These regions include portions of the intraparietal cortex (area 2v), the central sulcus (area 3av), the posterior end of the insula (the parieto-insular vestibular cortex, or area PIVC), and the medial superior temporal visual area (MST). Recently, using functional magnetic resonance imaging during caloric,[24] galvanic,[25] and optokinetic[26,27] stimulation, human analogues of the areas as just described were identified. It is suggested that at least some of these areas, such as MST, PIVC, and 2v, contain multimodal neurons that respond to vestibular and visual or somatosensory stimulation.

D.   Semicircular Canal Dynamics

Angular acceleration of the head in the plane of a particular semicircular canal results in net flow of endolymph relative to the canal walls in the direction opposite to that in which the head is turning. This is because of the inertia of the endolymph, which initially tends to stand still as the canal rotates. The movement of the endolymph causes the cupula to deflect, with a latency defined as the time taken for the deflection to reach $1/e$ (e is the exponential constant $= 2.718$) of its maximum value after an acceleration of the head. This inertial (short) time constant of the cupula is in the order of 3–5 ms, based on physical measurements in humans[28] and in recordings of the latency of responses in the primary afferents of monkeys.[29] However, if the rotation continues at a constant velocity the endolymph quickly begins to rotate at the same speed as the canal, because of the elasticity of the cupula and the friction between the endolymph and the canal walls. As a result, the cupula returns to its resting position during constant velocity rotation. The time taken for the cupula to regain its nominal resting position after cessation of the stimulus is the elastic (long) time constant. A direct measurement is unavailable, but from the persistence of nystagmic (involuntary) eye movements to vestibular stimulation and the subjective response decline using magnitude estimation it has been estimated at 10–20 s for the lateral canal.[30–32] These values are greater than would be predicted from the mechanical properties of the semicircular canals. In other words, the estimated elastic time constant does not reflect the restoration time of the cupula but the time taken for the neural events to subside. The difference represents a preservation of the raw vestibular signal in the brain, which has been proposed as the velocity-storage integrator mechanism.[33,34] One of the fundamental functions of the velocity-storage integrator is hypothesized to be related to the central estimation of head-angular velocity with respect to a gravity-centered reference system.[35,36] Presumably, the elastic time constant also plays an important role in the latency of vection (the visually induced sensation of self-motion), which is also in the order of 10 s (see Chapter 3, Sec. IV.A).

Deflection of the cupula is produced by changes in head velocity within the physiological range of 0.1–5.0 Hz in humans.[18] The canal-cupula-endolymph system behaves in many ways like a heavily damped torsion pendulum, and some psychophysiological effects are predictable from the differential equation describing its behavior.[28] This mathematical model of semicircular canal function was presented first by Steinhaussen[10] and reviewed by Mayne,[37] Goldberg and Fernandez,[8] and Howard.[38] In summary, when a person rotates the head with an angular acceleration of α in the plane of a particular semicircular canal the approximate force acting on the cupula is related to the displacement by

$$H\alpha(t) = K\theta + \Upsilon(\mathrm{d}\theta/\mathrm{d}t) + H(\mathrm{d}^2\theta/\mathrm{d}t^2) \tag{1}$$

where H is a mass-dependent, effective moment of inertia of endolymph and cupula; α is the angular acceleration of head rotation; K is a position-dependent, elastic-restoring factor on the cupula after it is displaced from its neutral position; θ is the angular displacement of endolymph and cupula; Υ is a velocity-dependent, damping constant reflecting the viscous drag exerted by the canal wall as the endolymph flows past it; and t is the elapsed time taken.

Because the lumen of a human vestibular canal is about 0.3 mm in mean diameter, its viscous resistance is high for moderate velocities, and the mass of the endolymph is small. The elasticity of the cupula is small compared its viscous resistance. Therefore, the torsion pendulum equation can be simplified as

$$H\alpha(t) = \Upsilon(d\theta/dt) \tag{2}$$

Because H and Υ are constants, at moderate velocities head acceleration is proportional to the angular velocity of the cupula. Equation (2) can be rewritten as

$$\alpha(t) \propto d\theta/dt. \tag{3}$$

Integrating Eq. (3) with respect to time (i.e., $\int \alpha(t) = \int d\theta/dt$) results in

$$\omega \propto \theta \tag{4}$$

where ω is the angular velocity of the head. Therefore, it is the angular velocity of the head rather than acceleration that is proportional to the angular displacement of the cupula. *Therefore, at the velocities and durations of normal head rotations the canals act as integrating accelerometers.* When the head rotates very slowly, the viscous resistance becomes smaller than the inertial resistance, so that $H(d^2\theta/dt^2)$ becomes the dominant factor and the response of the system is proportional to the acceleration of the head; this is also the case at higher frequencies too.

Therefore, consistent with the dynamic model of the semicircular canals just described, angular acceleration of the head in one direction is regularly followed by deceleration as the head is moved sinusoidally through relatively small angles. In this case the semicircular canals evoke appropriate sensations of motion and compensatory eye movements to the motion undergone by the head. The two opposed deflections of the endolymph and cupulae (as well as the two opposed neural events associated with acceleration and deceleration) tend to nullify each other by the end of the motion, leaving little residual deflection or aftereffects. However, the situation is quite different when we are exposed to angular accelerations of longer duration and when vision is not available. Following an initial acceleration to a constant rotational speed, the subjective sensation of rotation gradually subsides after 20–30 s. After a short delay most subjects will perceive a slow rotation in the opposite direction, which soon disappears. A sudden cessation of rotation will give rise to a sensation of rotation in the opposite direction, which persists for about 30 s and is followed by a sensation of slow rotation in the original direction of motion that eventually disappears.

E.   Thresholds for Angular Motion Perception

For an angular acceleration less than 10 s in duration to be perceived, the product of the intensity of acceleration in deg/s^2 and the time (in seconds) of application must be equal to 2.5. This is known as Mulder's law and is expressed as

$$\alpha\tau = 2.5\,\text{deg/s} \qquad (5)$$

where α is magnitude of acceleration and τ is time of application.

In other words, the weaker an angular acceleration (up to a certain threshold limit), the longer it must affect the perceiving subject. The limits of perception of an angular acceleration are determined not only by the value of the acceleration but also by its duration.

Guedry[39] provides an excellent review on the thresholds of perception of angular and linear acceleration. Most of the sensitivity studies, using subjective indications to determine threshold, describe the rotation of a subject about the yaw axis. As a result, there is a limited amount of information describing the sensitivity to angular accelerations about the pitch and roll axes. In general, available data suggested that z-axis thresholds are higher than x- or y-axis thresholds.[40] The values obtained also depend on individual differences among subjects; different psychophysical procedures and various rotation devices were employed in determining the thresholds.

The stimulation of the canal is dependent on the magnitude of the angular acceleration and the time for which it is applied; these parameters must be taken into account when determining threshold. Because the somatosensory system also responds to fast transients and vibrations, its contribution cannot be neglected. For sustained angular acceleration longer than 10 s about the yaw axis, the mean threshold values were reported as 0.035–4.0 deg/s^2 (Ref. 41). Another study indicated that the thresholds of vestibular perception for yaw, roll, and pitch rotation under sustained acceleration are 0.14, 0.5, and 0.5 deg/s^2 respectively.[42] The threshold for direction detection of a transient angular movement with durations of 1–5 s about the z axis (sitting upright) is 1.5 deg/s and is significantly lower than for angular stimuli about the y axis (lying on the side) and x axis (lying supine) at 2.07 and 2.04 deg/s, respectively.[43] In everyday life prolonged rotation seldom occurs. The duration of the stimulus is usually shorter than the time constant of the cupula-canal-endolymph system, and hence the threshold of the sensation of rotation is related to the magnitude of the velocity change rather than the acceleration. In flight, the acceleration thresholds are likely to be much higher than measured in laboratory settings because of the more stressful environment. The pilot is preoccupied with the control and navigation of the aircraft, communications, and mission execution. These activities can distract him or her from the task of orientation and motion detection and serve to increase the thresholds of motion perception. By contrast, the presence of a subject-fixed target light substantially lowers angular-motion thresholds because of the oculogyral illusion (see Chapter 7, Sec. II.B.4). In addition, thresholds are lower with increasing frequency of angular movement, a dynamic that mirrors the increasing sensitivity shown by primary vestibular afferents with increasing frequency.

F. Limitations of the Semicircular Canals in Flight

Based on the canal dynamics already described, when flying straight and level, the cupulae are in their neutral positions (not being deflected in any direction).

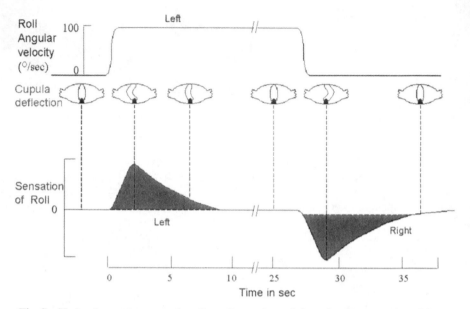

Fig. 5 **Hydrodynamic properties of canal-cupula-endolymph system, as viewed from behind the pilot (modified from Ref. 44).**

When the pilot rolls to the left, the cupulae in the vertical canals will, after the inertial time constant of 3–5 ms, be deflected by the angular acceleration in the roll axis and will generate a signal reflecting angular velocity in that axis. A corresponding sensation of rotation to the left peaks for approximately 4 s. During a prolonged constant-velocity rotation, the cupulae of the stimulated canals return to their neutral position, and the subjective velocity and the corresponding sensation of rotation disappear within 10 s. On stopping the roll suddenly, the cupulae are initially deflected through angles equal but opposite to the original angular velocity, and the corresponding sensation is of rotation to the right. Subsequently, the cupulae return along an approximately exponential time course back to their neutral position. The hydrodynamic properties of the canal-cupula-endolymph system during a sustained roll and upon cessation of the roll maneuver are depicted in Fig. 5.

Because of the different physical dimensions of the lateral and vertical canals, one would expect characteristic differences in the cupular response between these canals during and after acceleration. Canals in the vertical plane have lower sensitivities and shorter time constants than do the lateral canals. The time course of cupular return has been estimated by postrotational decay of the resulting illusory sensation of rotation and by following the slow-phase angular velocity of compensatory nystagmus. The postrotational decay of nystagmus was found to be shorter in roll (4 s) than in pitch (7 s) and yaw (16 s) (Ref. 45). Shorter time constants suggest that the response-decay rate following angular acceleration is greater. The subjective response to yaw rotation was also confirmed to be 16 s as compared to

7 s for pitch rotation.[46] The sooner the cupula returns, the sooner the sensation of rotation stops, even if actual rotation is physically occurring. Therefore, in the case of pitch and roll, there is a greater underestimation of velocity. Using the above time-constant values, for a 360-deg roll (point roll or barrel) taking 6 s and having a constant angular velocity of 60 deg/s throughout, the apparent rate of roll will have fallen to 18 deg/s at the end of the maneuver, and the total perceived roll displacement will only amount to approximately 230 deg. Therefore, if the pilot starts the roll from an erect position he or she will feel still upside down after one complete turn, assuming that visual and otolith inputs are not available. Teleologically, we are better "programmed" for lengthy yaw rotation than for pitch and roll rotation. Moreover, SD caused by rapid roll rotation in flight can be attributed to the failure of the neuromuscular mechanism to follow the sequence of events, resulting in impaired cardiac function and involuntary oculomotor response about the nasooccipital x axis.[47]

In short, the limitations of the semicircular canals in the perception of angular acceleration can be summarized as follows: 1) a limited threshold of vestibular perception: 0.14, 0.5, and 0.5 deg/s^2 for sustained yaw, roll, and pitch motion and 1.5, 2.1, and 2.0 deg/s for transient (<5-s duration) movements in yaw, roll, and pitch; 2) a perceived angular velocity that is progressively less than the actual angular velocity during prolonged rotation; 3) an absence of sensation of rotation during constant velocity rotation; 4) an apparent sensation of rotation in the opposite direction during deceleration; 5) a persistent apparent sensation of rotation in the opposite direction, after physical rotation has actually stopped; 6) a greater chance in developing error in roll than in pitch, which in turn is greater than in yaw; and 7) a rotation-induced involuntary oculomotor response that destabilizes the retinal image.

G. Morphological and Physiological Considerations of the Utricles and Saccules

The utricle and saccule, connected by small ducts at an acute angle, are identical histologically and are often referred to as the otolith organs or otoliths. The otolith organs respond to the magnitude and direction of linear acceleration and to head tilts relative to gravity. The sensory epithelium of the otolith organ is known as the macula. The macula contains supporting cells and hair cells with bundles of cilia that project into the otolithic membranes or otoconial membranes (Fig. 6). These membranes consist of a gelatinous substrate in which are embedded otoconia (calcium carbonate crystals). The octoconia are denser, with a specific gravity of 2.94 (Ref. 48) than the endolymph and surrounding gelatinous substrate. The deflection of the cilia of the hair cells in the otoliths depends upon the relative motion or position of the otoconia with respect to the supporting substrate. The effective stimulus for the otoliths is the tangential shearing force acting in the plane of the macula.[49] Therefore, the action of gravity or linear acceleration on the otoconia results in displacement of the otolithic membrane and consequent bending of the cilia of the hair cells. Bending of the cilia generates changes in the activity of the vestibular branch of the eighth nerve, innervating the macula. When the head is upright, there is a resting frequency of impulses generated by

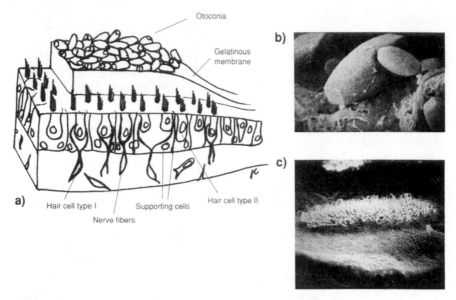

Fig. 6a Schematics of the sensory epithelium of the utricular macula.
Fig. 6b Electronmicrograph of the otoconia or calcium carbonate crystals.
Fig. 6c Freeze-dired preparation of the utricular macula showing the cilia of the hair cells.

the hair cells and a spontaneous resting discharge in the utricular and saccular nerves, just as in the ampullary nerves. However, static otolith information has no utility in weightlessness. During the weightless phase of parabolic flight maneuvers, it is relatively common to feel upside down (inversion illusion) in relation to the aircraft or to feel that both one's body and the aircraft are inverted (see Chapter 6, Sec. III.A.3). Visual, tactile, and cognitive factors also play important roles in the inversion illusion.[50] When the head is tilted on Earth, the resting frequency of the otoliths is altered to signal the new position of the head relative to the gravitational vertical. The behavior of the otolith afferents has also been described,[51] and some studies have addressed the response of central neurons to otolith stimulation.[52,23] However, the proposed utricular shear mechanism may not explain all of the increased perceived tilt under high-G load. One appealing explanation proposed by Correia et al.[54] is that once the hair cells are bent by a shear component of specific force any subsequent compressive component would result in further bending of the hair cells. This action could increase the afferent signal and presumably increase the perceived tilt under high-G loading.

1. Utricular Macula

The utricular macula lies on the floor of the utricular sac in the approximate plane of the lateral semicircular canals, although its anterior end turns even more upwards. The directional sensitivities of sensory cells on either side of a dividing crest known as the striola are of opposite polarity, with the kinocilia on hair cells on either side oriented towards each other.[55] Common to both utricular and saccular macula, a functional-polarization vector presumably reflecting the morphological polarization of the hair cells that it innervates characterizes each otolith neuron. As in the hair cells in the crista ampullaris, accelerations that cause the displacements of the hair bundles toward the kinocilium result in a depolarization of the cell membrane and an increase in the frequency of afferent neural discharge. Oppositely directed accelerations result in a corresponding decrease of neural discharge. Implicit in the Lowenstein–Wersäll theory (Sec. III.C) is the notion that displacements of the hair bundles at right angles to the polarization axis should be ineffective.

During yaw rotation, which places the utricular plane in the plane of rotation, the rotational component of the motion presumably stimulates an equal number of cells with opposite polarization axes in each utricle on the two sides of the head, therefore resulting in a zero output. Because the centrifugal component of the rotation produces equal but opposite stimulation of the utricles, it is suggested that these opposed inputs from the two sides are cancelled in the vestibular nuclei. Therefore, the otolith organ has been found to be unaffected by intense angular acceleration.[56] Tilting of the head from a vertical position in any direction results in the bending of cilia of at least some of the hair cells. Therefore, the utricular macula is most effective in detecting the gravitational vertical when the head is laterally upright and inclined approximately 25–30 deg forward in a normal gravity environment (as the plane of the utricular macula is approximately parallel to the plane of the lateral canal; Sec. III.C). It is least effective when the head is tilted close to and beyond 90 deg to the vertical. A review of the linear and nonlinear force-response properties of otolith neurons to static head tilt is provided by Goldberg and Fernandez.[8]

In addition to responding to the direction and magnitude of the Earth's gravitational field, the otoconia are displaced whenever the head is subjected to linear acceleration. Therefore, there is a fundamental ambiguity in the signals from the otolith organs. Following Einstein's Equivalence Principle, the otoliths cannot distinguish between gravitational forces and sustained inertial reaction forces resulting from linear acceleration. For instance, the effect of a sustained horizontal linear acceleration of value a, acting in the plane of the inertial utricles, is theoretically indistinguishable in magnitude from the effect of holding the head at an angle ϕ to the vertical, whose sine function is equal to a. In other words, the otoliths indicate the orientation of the head relative to the gravitoinertial force (GIF). The output of the otolith organs is interpreted as a body tilt rather than a linear acceleration if the latter is prolonged, and no vision is available (see Fig. 7). However, other sensory inputs as well as past history of motion exposure can be useful in clarifying the otolith signals.

The Torsion Pendulum Model can also be applied to the dynamic characteristics of the otolith organ. Howard[38] noted that the shearing force acting on the otolith organ is the product of the excess mass of the statoconial membrane (mass of the membrane minus the mass of an identical volume of endolymph) and the linear acceleration acting in the plane of the macula. The resistance stemming from the

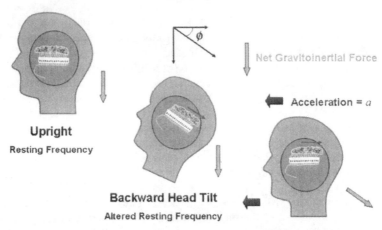

Fig. 7   Otolith ambiguity during sustained acceleration. The inertial G effect of a horizontal acceleration a**, acting in the plane of the utricles, is indistinguishable from the effect of tilting the head through the angle whose sine is** a**.**

elasticity, viscosity and mass of the otolith system opposes this shearing force [Eq. (6)].

$$\beta a\,(t) = \kappa\chi + \gamma(\mathrm{d}\chi/\mathrm{d}t) + m(\mathrm{d}^2\chi/\mathrm{d}t^2) \qquad (6)$$

where β is the excess mass of the statoconial membrane, a the linear acceleration acting on the plane of the macula, κ the elastic (position-dependent) resistance, γ the viscous (velocity-dependent) resistance, m the mass (acceleration-dependent) resistance, χ the linear
displacement of the otoliths, and t the time.

2.   Saccular Macula

The cavity of the utricle is linked with that of the saccule by way of the utriculo-saccular duct. The plane of the saccular macula, on the medial wall of the saccule, is perpendicular to that of the utricle, suggesting that the saccule should be more sensitive to vertical (dorsoventral) acceleration than to horizontal (naso-occipital or interaural) acceleration. It is assumed that the human utricular macula is mainly stimulated by shearing forces acting parallel to the horizontal plane and the saccular macula predominantly by shearing force acting parallel to the vertical plane. However, exact information on the orientation and position of the human macular surfaces is sparse.

Unlike in the utricluar macula, the hair cells on either side of the striola in the saccule have kinocilia oriented away from each other rather than toward each other. There are other important differences between utricular and saccular units, aside from their polarization directions. The human saccule has only 19,000 receptors as compared to the 33,000 of the utricle.[57] Saccular neurons have, on average, half the sensitivity to specific force changes, as well as half the resting discharge.[49] They also show a marked nonlinearity, with decreased sensitivity in the inhibitory direction for specific force magnitudes exceeding 0.6 G. The precise location of this nonlinearity remains speculative, but Fernandez and associates suggest that it is at the hair-cell level.

The precise function of the mammalian saccule remains a matter of discussion. As mentioned earlier, it is generally accepted that the saccule plays a role in detecting linear acceleration along the dorsoventral axis, thereby contributing to spatial orientation. Supporting evidence is provided by neurophysiological studies. Fernandez and Goldberg[51] identified two classes of peripheral neurons innervating the otolith organs of the squirrel monkey: one (142 units) whose vectors lay near the plane of the utricular macula and the other (115 units) with vectors near the plane of the saccular macula. The large number of saccular vectors obtained from combinations of static gravitational stimuli provided convincing evidence that saccular afferents serve the same general equilibrium function as the utricular ones, at least in the squirrel monkey.

The influence of the saccular macula in conscious spatial orientation in humans is less clear. Malcolm and Melvill Jones[58] and Melvill Jones and Young[59] showed that oscillatory gravitational acceleration along the dorsoventral z axis of the body, which primarily stimulates the hair cells of the saccule, leads to uncertain and usually erroneous perception of the direction of motion. The authors suggested that the paucity of vertical representation in the saccular otoliths could be largely responsible for the particular difficulty attached to sensing body motion in a vertical direction, although central processing could also be involved.

Another uncertainty regarding the saccule stems from the fact that ablation of the mammalian (squirrel monkey) saccule does not lead to any marked postural or locomotor deficits.[60] Furthermore, it is not known how saccular inputs are used in tilt estimates. As mentioned before, the receptors are stimulated when the relatively dense otolithic membrane glides over the sensory epithelia in a tangential direction. Each receptor cell has a direction of maximum excitability, this being the direction of shear of the otolith membrane that causes the greatest increase in the frequency of action potentials in the first-order afferent neuron.[15] Based on this interpretation, and the histological data of the guinea pig, vertical acceleration will generate little response from the utricular organs because they lie close to the horizontal plane and a maximal response from the saccular organs because their planes are close to the vertical plane. However, recent work by Curthoys et al.[61] suggests that both the utricular and saccular maculae in the guinea pig have pronounced curvature so that vertical shear forces might well stimulate regions of both the utricular and saccular maculae. Other experimental results suggest that utricular ablation would destroy the integrity of both the semicircular canal and utricle, but this is less true of saccular ablation, thereby resulting in less equilibrium disturbance.

Historically, the saccule has also been linked to sound and vibration detection. In fishes and amphibians parts of the vestibular apparatus are involved in audition. Recently, it has been shown that in cats a sizeable fraction of vestibular afferents with irregular activity was acoustically responsive. Labeling experiments demonstrated that these acoustically responsive afferents innervate the saccule, have cell bodies in Scarpa's ganglion, and project to central regions both inside and outside the traditional boundaries of the vestibular nuclei.[62] Further evidence also suggests that acoustically responsive afferents trigger acoustic reflexes of the sternocleidomastoid muscle in humans,[63,64] and measurement of such reflexes can provide a relatively simple test for saccular dysfunction.

H. Thresholds for Linear Motion Perception

In a static environment the otoliths accurately detect head orientation with respect to the apparent vertical. However, this ability is modified by habituation, for example, during a prolonged stay in the tilted position, that presumably occurs in the central interpretation of the otolith signal. The perception of linear motion has been less extensively studied than the perception of angular movements, because of the greater difficulty with which controlled whole-body linear motion stimuli can be generated without mechanical and acoustic cues. In general, the threshold for the detection of linear movement of the body is higher than for detection of head movement. The thresholds for the detection of discrete translational movements are higher than the threshold for the detection of sustained oscillatory motion, and the threshold decreases with increasing frequency.[40] Between 0.016–0.25 Hz, the otolith organs function as linear velocity indicators. The importance of cues other than those from the otoliths in the perception of linear acceleration cannot be absolutely excluded. For example, tactile receptors associated with kinesthetic information from the limb act in a fashion similar to that of otolith organs. For frequencies above 1 Hz, orientation perception reflects a combination of visual, otolith, and somatosensory influences. However, for frequencies below 1 Hz somatosensory mechanoreceptors do not appear to contribute to the perception of movement.[65]

According to the comprehensive review by Guedry,[39] there is a wide scatter of experimental data concerning threshold values below 1 Hz. This could be explained by differences in the orientation of the subjects to the gravitational vertical and to the stimulus vector or by the differences in the apparatus and psychophysical method employed. During sustained horizontal linear (step) acceleration, detection thresholds for the direction of discrete movement were 0.01 m/s^2 (0.001 G) when the subject was supine and 0.06 m/s^2 (0.006 G) when the subject was upright. The difference in threshold has been attributed to the angle of the imposed acceleration relative to the average utricular shear plane.[42] The mean threshold for the detection of discrete transient movements in the horizontal plane was found to be significantly higher in the Z-body axis (0.15 m/s^2) than X-body axis (0.06 m/s^2) and Y-body axis (0.06 m/s^2), increasing sensitivity with decrease in duration of transient linear movement of primary afferents. The greater sensitivity of the subjects in the x and y axes than z axis was attributed to the differences in the geometrical position of the utricules and saccules.[66] As mentioned earlier, linear acceleration in the x and y axes predominantly acts as a shear stimulus on the utricular maculae, whereas z-axis accelerations predominantly stimulate the saccular maculae. The threshold for the detection of linear motion was corroborated by Borel et al.[67] in head-free subjects, the threshold for linear acceleration along the y axis in darkness is reported to 0.004 m/s,^{2} and the threshold for the perception of the direction of motion is about 0.007 m/s^2. It appears that weaker linear stimuli led to motion detection but resulted in erroneous estimation of the direction of motion. Such an ambiguity in the perception of motion has already been described during vertical motion with subjects sitting upright (Sec. III.G.2).

There is limited information on the effect of Earth orientation on the threshold of linear motion. Walsh[68,69] reported that the threshold for perceiving vertical oscillation along the x axis (lying supine or prone) and y axis (lying on the right or left side) is higher than for horizontal oscillation along the same axes (i.e., sitting upright facing direction of motion for x and sitting sideways for y).

I. Limitations of the Otoliths in Flight

When the linear acceleration and gravity vectors are summated during flight, the new direction can be interpreted by the pilot as the true vertical, depending upon his or her perceptual and intellectual assessment of how this position was attained. In time, pilots realize that the resultant gravitoinertial vector can be mistaken for vertical when the resultant vector is actually tilted relative to the Earth. For example, during takeoff in an aircraft a strong forward acceleration of the aircraft can be interpreted as pitching upward, resulting in an overestimation of the actual pitch angle during ascent. This is the somatogravic illusion, which is discussed in detail in Chapter 6, Sec. III.A. If the visual horizon is obstructed, as when the aircraft is in the clouds or during night takeoff from aircraft carriers, the pilot may correct for the apparent upward pitch by pitching the aircraft down and then flying it into the ground or water. These observations highlight the fundamental importance of vision during sustained motion.

Despite the ambiguous response to inertial accelerations by the primary otolith afferents during translational motion and tilting movements, the oculomotor responses are appropriately compensated for the correct translational component of head movement (to be discussed in Sec. IV.B). Two neural computational strategies have been proposed to distinguish between head orientation (gravitational acceleration) and linear head translation (inertial acceleration). The multisensory integration hypothesis suggests that information from the semicircular canals, otolith organs, and other sensory inputs are all required to distinguish between head tilt and translation.[39,70] Alternatively, the frequency-segregation hypothesis suggests that high-frequency accelerations are interpreted as translations, whereas low-frequency accelerations are interpreted as tilts.[71] Recent evidence in the rhesus monkey[72] indicates that semicircular input is essential in resolving the tilt-translation ambiguity centrally. When the semicircular canal is inactivated, horizontal eye movements (appropriate for translational motion) could no longer be correlated with head translation. For frequencies greater than 0.1 Hz—in which range the vestibulo-ocular reflex (to be discussed in Sec. IV.A) is important for gaze stabilization—it appears from Angelaki et al.'s study that the oculomotor system discriminates between head translation and tilt primarily using the multisensory integration strategy rather than frequency segregation of otolith afferents. In other words, neural computation requires linear acceleration information from the otolith receptors as well as angular velocity signals from the semicircular canals to correctly estimate the source of linear acceleration and to elicit appropriate eye movement responses.

The limitations of the otoliths can be summarized as follows: 1) no transduction of linear velocity, but only linear acceleration; 2) an inherent inability to distinguish between gravity and sustained linear acceleration of the body; 3) accuracy for determining the direction of the vertical only with the head upright pitched forward

25–30 deg, because the utricular macula and lateral semicircular canals are pitched up by 25–30 deg with respect to the Horsley–Clark plane; 4) a limited threshold (Y and $X = 0.005–0.01$ G; $Z = 0.01–0.1$ G); and 5) a higher threshold and greater error in detecting vertical motion.

IV. Vestibular Contribution to Gaze Stability

A. Angular Vestibulo-Ocular Reflex

Our eyes are the most important sense organs that provide information about the orientation of the body with respect to the immediate environment and the position and attitude of the aircraft relative to the surface of the Earth. When flying in conditions of good visibility, the task of determining the orientation of the aircraft is relatively straightforward. It is primarily an extension of the perceptual skills first acquired in childhood (natural orientation). In conditions of poor visibility (when flying in clouds or at night), pilots must determine aircraft orientation from cockpit instruments. In the latter case the visual information lacks the naturalness and the strength of external visual cues, and symbolic information also requires correct interpretation (synthetic orientation).

In general, the maintenance of visual orientation in a dynamic environment is greatly enhanced by the fact that the retinal image is stabilized. Decreases in visual acuity begin to occur once the velocity of inappropriate eye movements exceeds 3–5 deg/s. One of the most serious threats to the stability of the retinal image comes from the observer's own head movement. Because natural head movements are of high frequency, the visual system—encumbered by relatively slow retinal processing (about 70 ms)—cannot produce compensatory eye movements that stabilize the retinal image. On the contrary, the vestibulo-ocular reflex has a latency of less than 16 ms and promptly produces slow-phase eye movements that compensate for head rotations. Therefore, during angular acceleration about the yaw axis (e.g., to the right) the slow-phase compensatory eye movements will be to the left so that the angle of gaze does not change and the image of the world remains relatively stationary upon the retina. If the slow component is to the left, it follows that the return eye movement (fast phase) is to the right. This compensatory action is termed the angular VOR, and it almost perfectly compensates for head oscillations that occur during walking, running, or simply shaking one's head. Eye stabilization is normally brought about by the combined action of optokinetic and vestibular influences. Normal head and body movements produce alternating accelerations of opposite signs with short intervals between. As a result, the slow-phase VOR eye movements are temporary and lead to a stabilized image. Compensation for yaw and pitch rotation is quite efficient with a gain of 0.7–1.0, but it is less efficient for roll rotation, where the gain is about 0.5 or less. The horizontal angular VOR is mediated most directly by a three-neuron arc consisting of the primary afferent, a secondary neuron usually found in the ipsilateral rostral medial vestibular nucleus, and the oculomotor neuron (see Fig. 8). The involvement of these neurons in the angular VOR has been well characterized (see Ref. 73 for a review).

The vestibulo-ocular reflex is now quantifiable in three dimensions, and it has been employed to study the interaction between the horizontal VOR and head

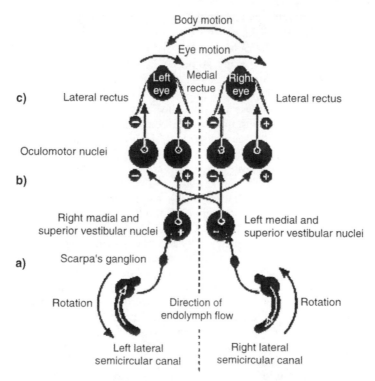

Fig. 8   Schematic drawing of how the angular vestibulo-ocular reflex is mediated by a three-neuron arc: a) primary vestibular afferent, b) ipsilateral rostral medial and superior vestibular nucleus, and c) the oculomotor neuron stage.

orientation. Tilting the head out of the horizontal plane of rotation immediately after cessation of motion results in postrotatory horizontal nystagmus, vertical nystagmus following roll tilt to the left or right, and torsional nystagmus following pitch-tilt downwards or upwards. The axis of eye rotation always shifts toward alignment with gravity following postrotatory tilt, which suggests neural processing is required to resolve the sensory conflict.[74] Similarly, postrotatory eye movements after passive head tilt indicate that while the initial VOR response is expressed in a head-fixed frame determined by the orientation of the semicircular canals the late component appears to undergo a central transformation from head-fixed to gravity-centered coordinates.[35] In other words, stabilization of the VOR is meant for Earth-fixed but not head-fixed targets. Central representation of the angular motion signals in gravity-centered coordinates contributes to the ease of multisensory integration and motor control.

Early studies suggested that the angular VOR is cancelled by using the smooth pursuit system. It is believed that when subjects cancel their VOR by observing a target that moves with the head vestibular eye movements result in a slip of the retinal image, which will, in turn, activate smooth pursuit. This is based on the observation that smooth pursuit and VOR cancellation have similar frequency responses and the fact that patients with smooth pursuit deficits generally exhibit cancellation deficits as well. In general, ocular following, or smooth pursuit, contributes little to the cancellation above 1 Hz and nothing above 2 Hz.

In flight, however, where the aircraft movements are frequently of much larger amplitude and longer duration, the concerted action of optokinetic and vestibular influences can break down, owing largely to the limitations of the vestibular sensors. During motion, the instrument displays in aircraft and other moving platforms can move in unison with the head. If there is a tight coupling between the head and the display during such movement, the VOR will interfere with reading the display at certain peak angular velocities and frequencies. In this case involuntary nystagmus as a result of vestibular stimulation can occur. Consider the case of leftward rotation about the yaw axis. During initial acceleration to the left, the eyes drift to the right (slow phase). As the head continues to turn, the eyes recenter by a saccadic eye movement to the left (fast phase) with a velocity of 300 to 800 deg/s and then recommence the drift to the right. The slow and fast phases create a sawtooth pattern. Nystagmus is named by the direction of the fast component and by the plane of movement. In the preceding example it is called left horizontal nystagmus. During the period of constant velocity, the slow-phase eye velocity abates and becomes less effective in assisting the eye in fixating Earth-fixed targets. During deceleration, the reversed direction of nystagmus and its persistence after stopping continue to impair vision for both Earth-fixed and head-fixed targets. Figure 9 illustrates a typical vestibular nystagmus tracing using electronystagmography with slow phase to the right (upward tracing) and the fast phase to the left (downward tracing).

The nystagmus of a pilot with vision restricted to the interior of the cockpit is partly suppressed by a visible head-fixed display. Even with visual suppression,

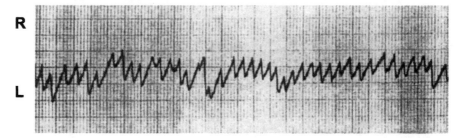

Fig. 9 Example of vestibular nystagmus. It always has two components: 1) the slow phase, which is the compensatory eye movement generated by signals arising from the vestibular apparatus; and 2) the fast phase, which is a saccade in the direction opposite to that of the slow phase. The direction of nystagmus is designated according to the direction of the fast phase. In this example the head is accelerated about the spinal axis to the left, and the head movement is said to be "in" the horizontal plane; endolymph movement is in the lateral (horizontal) semicircular canals, and the eye movement is horizontal. The compensatory (slow phase) of nystagmus is to the right, because that is the eye movement that will compensate for a head movement to the left. It then follows that the fast component is to the left.

however, the maximum slow-phase velocity could still be greater than 3–5 deg/s, which is sufficient to degrade visibility of fine details on instruments briefly until the partly suppressed nystagmus abates. Disruption of ocular stabilizing reflexes can result in the instability of the retinal image, resulting in oscillopsia or loss of situation awareness. Oscillopsia can be likened to a television image with a vertical or horizontal hold, resulting in a jostling, to-and-fro, or up-and-down visual motion. Reduction in visual acuity is related to the magnitude of the angular acceleration, the amount of resulting nystagmus, and the subject's ability to control the nystagmus. It is often reported that, aircraft at higher rates of rotation, pilots can neither fixate upon the instruments nor upon the external visual field.

Blurring of vision as a result of torsional nystagmus during x-axis rotation has been reported to be weak in comparison to that resulting from rotation in the y and z axes. However, experimental evidence[75] suggests that the inappropriate torsional nystagmus produces an apparent deflection of the horizon indicator (an apparent flicking back and forth) during and after roll maneuvers involving high peak angular velocities. This perceptual aberration could be disturbing to a pilot attempting to use the horizon indicator and could lead to a suspicion of instrument malfunction. Melvill Jones[76] obtained video recordings of pitch, roll, and yaw eye movements of pilots during eight-turn spins in flight. The results suggested that compensatory eye movements during the maneuver failed to stabilize the retinal image, with the greatest discrepancies in the roll plane. During a roll, the pilot is looking forward, and the associated nystagmic eye movements caused by vestibular and optokinetic stimuli will be rotational ones about the nasooccipital x axis. Such eye movements will initially be useful to maintain a stable retinal image. However, their usefulness progressively decreases as rotation continues, until a stabilized retinal image is no longer possible. On stopping the roll, torsional nystagmus will be induced by stimulation of the semicircular canals, and the pilot will see an apparent rotation of the horizon, even when physical rotation has ceased.

B. Translational Vestibulo-Ocular Reflex

The VOR has traditionally referred to the eye movements in response to head rotation, a canal-mediated effect. Although considerable attention has been given to vestibulo-ocular interaction during angular motion of the head as might occur during an aircraft spin, less attention has been given to vestibulo-ocular interaction during linear motion (translation) of the head. The usefulness of the translational VOR as a compensatory reflex for linear head movement has been much debated in the last 30 years. Such interaction might occur while viewing a stationary or moving display during vertical takeoff and landing operations.[77]

The compensatory eye movements induced by translational acceleration along the naso-occipital x, interaural y, and dorsoventral z axes are termed the translational (or linear) vestibulo-ocular reflex. The translational VOR was believed to be negligible in humans until Buizza et al.[78] showed that for geometric reasons the gain of this reflex should be a function of target distance. Paige[79] and Schwarz et al.[80] showed that the translational VOR could be substantial in humans if the target distance is not large. Because most natural head movements are a combination of linear and angular motion, it is important to understand how these two distinct components of the vestibular system interact centrally in order to produce appropriate eye movements. Such considerations are particularly important for pilots because of the translational accelerations experienced during flight. This is especially obvious when one recalls that the centripetal and tangential accelerations occurring when flying high-performance aircraft are actually translational, not pure angular, accelerations. Given the large translational accelerations experienced by pilots, proper functioning of the translational VOR is clearly essential for these individuals. Because otolith functioning is essential for proper determination of the direction of the gravity vector, failures within the otolith system have the potential to cause serious SD. However, little is presently known about the central pathways that mediate the translational VOR and about the convergence of canal and otolith inputs in the generation of a net translational VOR response.

When flying high-performance jets, a translational VOR along the naso-occipital axis can be invoked. Recently Tomlinson et al.[81] reported that translational VOR along the naso-occipital axis, in the horizontal plane, is a highly robust reflex, particularly at high frequencies (>1 Hz). The magnitude of the latency of the reflex is less than 20 ms (Fig. 10), far less than previously believed. Because of a much longer latency of visual following mechanisms, suppression of these reflexive eye movements by smooth pursuit is not possible until at least 130–150 ms after movement onset. Because peak eye velocities of more than 80 deg/s were attained within less than 100 ms following movement onset, visual degradation should be severe. This short latency can have important consequences in flight situations, as sudden accelerations at frequencies greater than 2 Hz will induce reflexive eye movements that will function to destabilize vision.

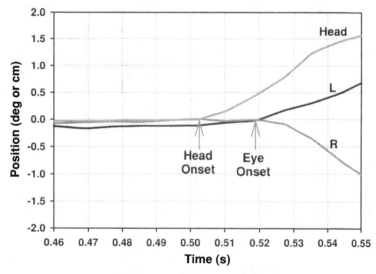

Fig. 10 Latency of the translational VOR. The eyes begin to converge less than 20 ms after the onset of head movement.

There are two proposed gaze strategies during linear motion. Tomko and Paige[82] measured translational VOR during horizontal motions along the interaural, naso-occipital, and the intermediate axes at a frequency of 0.5 Hz. This paradigm allows for the reorientation of the head and otoliths relative to linear motion. It was observed that regardless of eye position in the head or head orientation relative to motion, the translational VOR behaves according to the kinematic requirements of compensatory eye movements when subjects were exposed to linear motion along the x, y, and z axes. For example, when horizontal gaze shifts from right to left, but vertical gaze remains down, the horizontal eye movement component shifts from 0 to 180 deg in phase while the vertical responses remains fixed. Based on this evidence, it was proposed that eye-position information must integrate with otolith inputs rapidly, accurately, and continuously to determine gaze relative to the axis of motion, in order to account for the rapidity with which the reflex must adjust its response characteristics. By comparing the measurement of gaze displacement at the end of linear motion (along the naso-occipital and interaural axes) and the relative displacement of the target, Israel and Berthoz[83] demonstrated that healthy human subjects could correctly estimate the distance that they have been transported along in complete darkness. Anticipation of the target on the outward path, and not on the return, is in accord with the model of double integration of the otolith signal, suggesting that linear path integration is the basic sensory mechanism.[84] [Central filtering is required to distinguish between translational and gravitational acceleration: low frequency is used as an estimate of gravity, whereas high frequency is interpreted as translation (see Sec. III.I). A double integration of the high-frequency component could then provide an approximation of position in space.]

The interaural translational VOR has also been investigated in humans. It has been shown that transient linear accelerations of 0.08 and 0.17 G evoked compensatory slow phases whose velocities were enhanced in proportion to acceleration magnitude and target proximity.[85] More recently, it was demonstrated that during interaural translations subjects are able to cancel their translational VOR very effectively at 2 Hz (by visual fixation) and can reduce their reflex sensitivity by about 25% at 3 Hz.[86] The robust and short-latency nature of the translational VOR along the interaural axis should be considered in any environment involving high translational accelerations. When viewing targets located at optical infinity, the eye movements evoked by such accelerations are inappropriate. As just mentioned, the translational VOR along the naso-occipital axis is also very robust, although the evoked eye movements were generally much smaller. Given this, as well as the recent observations that the translational VOR along the interaural axis can be cancelled up to 3 Hz (see Fig. 11), naso-occipital accelerations are unlikely to pose many instrument readability problems for pilots. The cancellation of this reflex is far better than might have been expected. Thus, when viewing near targets that move with the head, such as the heads-up display (HUD) in high-performance aircraft, the displays should remain readable so long as the acceleration remains below 3 Hz, especially if the symbols are kept large. However, if translational accelerations exceed 3 Hz, particularly in the interaural direction where the evoked eye movements are large, the ability to read instruments might be seriously compromised. A special consideration of the impact of interaural translation on SD is included in Chapter 11, Sec. III.

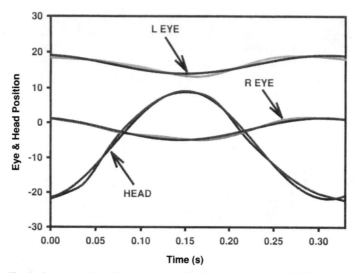

Fig. 11　Typical eye and head movements during (interaural) tVOR cancellation at 3 Hz with a 20-cm target. Note that the subject was able to maintain vergence. The eye position is in degrees and the head position is in centimeters. The dark lines are the best-fit sinusoids.

V.　Interactions Between the Semicircular Canals and Otoliths

The semicircular canals detect angular accelerations relative to the head during head movement and contribute sensory input for appropriate reflex action relative to the axis of motion. Perception of how this axis is oriented relative to gravity depends upon sensory inputs from the otoliths and the somatosensory systems (to be discussed in Sec. X), and appropriate reflex action relative to the Earth depends upon the synergistic integration of these other systems with the semicircular canals. The otoliths provide both static and dynamic orientation information relative to gravity and contribute to the perception of tilt and linear acceleration. The perception of linear acceleration is derived from a combination of change in position information from the otoliths and the absence of angular velocity information from the canals.

There are major differences in the vestibulo-ocular and psychophysical reactions to rotations about axes that are vertical or horizontal with respect to the Earth.[87] A constant velocity rotation about an Earth-vertical axis does not lead to a maintained response. In contrast, when the subject is rotated about an Earth-horizontal axis, as on a barbecue spit, there is a persistent unidirectional nystagmus superimposed on a sinusoidal (direction-changing) component and a corresponding sensation of turning. The effects depend on the continual reorientation of the head relative to gravity, and the sinusoidal component most likely has an otolithic origin. Following the cessation of a prolonged rotation about a horizontal axis, nystagmus and the subjective sensation of rotation disappear rapidly, in contrast to the extended postrotational decay following rotation about a vertical axis.[88] These studies have also shown that following sustained vertical-axis rotation postrotational tilts away from the Earth vertical induce an attenuation of the nystagmus, previously known as "dumping" when the graviceptor cues are inconsistent with rotation cues. Based on studies described next, the idea of dumping might not be appropriate as the nystagmus is shown to transfer to other axes as the nystagmus is increased rather than attenuated in some axes.

Earlier studies in humans[89] and more recent studies in squirrel monkeys[72,90] demonstrated that information from the semicircular canals influences the interpretation of graviceptor cues. For example, in monkeys, a 45-deg postrotational tilt induced a percept of linear acceleration and evoked an induced VOR that contributed to the total VOR. Similarly, when human subjects are tilted after being rotated at a constant velocity about an Earth-vertical axis the eye movement response evoked by such postrotational tilt also includes a component that compensates for the estimated linear acceleration even when no linear acceleration occurs.[91] Merfeld et al.[91] suggest that illusory tilt can be elicited by information from the semicircular canals and that these measured responses are consistent with an internal neural model that serves to resolve sensory ambiguity (see Sec. III.I).

Furthermore, in response to combined lateral translations and head tilt about the roll axis it was found that the VOR in rhesus monkeys generates robust compensatory horizontal eye movements. The response is independent of whether or not the interaural translation component is canceled out by a gravitational component caused by the roll-tilt, but it depends on functional semicircular canals.[92] The evidence suggests that the vestibular system controls both head tilt and velocity with respect to a gravity-centered reference system and that the brain uses both otolith and semicircular canal signals to estimate head motion relative to gravitational space. These findings are consistent with the postulate that when tilted away from the Earth vertical the transient angular motion is detected primarily by the semicircular canals and the persistent changed body position is sensed by the otolith sensor. Similarly, the absence of an expected canal input during linear acceleration allows us to infer acceleration rather than head tilt initially; at longer intervals when the canal signal would normally dissipate, the sense of acceleration gradually turns into a sensation of head tilt. Because sensory systems often provide ambiguous information, it is likely that neural processes are used by the different sensory systems to resolve such ambiguities.

VI. Visual-Vestibular Interaction

Visual-vestibular interaction is a process by which the visual and vestibular signals inform us of our position and motion in space and serves as a model for the study of intersensory conflict and integration. In studying visual-vestibular interactions, psychophysical results on motion perception, postural reactions, and eye movements are correlated with single-unit activity in the peripheral nerves, brain stem, and cortex. During head rotation, visual-vestibular interaction reflects synergistic influences of vestibular and visually guided eye movements, in which a high-pass filtered angular VOR combines with low-pass filtered visual-following mechanisms (see also Chapter 3). It is proposed that a similar mechanism applies during linear head motion. Otolith responses to translation are high-pass filtered and extend beyond the capacity of visual-following mechanisms.[71] Interest in the practical applications of visual-vestibular interactions grew out of the problems of blind flying and pilot disorientation in the early days of aviation and increased with the introduction of manned space flights in the 1960s, with the development of space shuttle flights and in anticipation of projected long-duration flights to Mars and elsewhere.

A mismatch between simultaneous inputs from the sensory systems can elicit a displeasing distortion of static orientation and an erroneous perception of self-motion or object motion. Normally, the surrounding visual scene moves in the opposite direction to head movements. When we rotate our head to the right about the yaw axis, the visual scene moves to the left and vice versa, but when the aircraft banks to the right and the pilot is devoid of external vision (as when flying in clouds) the visual scene of the cockpit does not bank to the left but rather is fixed with respect to the aircraft and will appear to move in the same direction (e.g., the oculogyral illusion, Chapter 7, Sec. II.B.4). Therefore, the visual information signals no motion, but the vestibular and somatosensory cues signal banking to the right. This is an example of visual-vestibular mismatch, and the solution to the pilot is to rely on the interpretation of the flight instruments.

A well-established phenomenon arising from visual-vestibular interaction is circularvection, a sensation of self-rotation in a stationary subject exposed to a rotating visual field. As discussed in Sec. III, the vestibular system cannot detect self-motion at constant velocity and thus requires supplementary visual information. The perception of self-motion during constant velocity movement in an inertial frame is generally dependent on the visually induced sensation of motion. This phenomenon has practical applications in the design of flight simulators and in the understanding of some SD illusions. The visual requirements for circularvection and the effects of visual motion on the oculomotor system are discussed in Chapter 3, Sec. IV.A.

Findings that pseudo-Coriolis effects can be induced by head tilts during visually induced motion provide further evidence for a functional visual-vestibular convergence.[93] Pseudo-Coriolis occurs when a sense of rotation is visually induced without actual motion; when this apparent sensation of self-motion is combined with head movements, it results in a similar effect as one would have felt during Coriolis stimulation (Chapter 6, Sec. II.B). Moreover, electrophysiological evidence[94] demonstrates that the thresholds for object motion detection are significantly increased during circularvection. The similarity of sensations engendered by visual and vestibular stimuli suggests that visual and vestibular neural signals converge at some site in the central nervous system. Visual-vestibular convergence has been shown to occur in the vestibular nuclei, thalamic, cerebellum, subnuclei, and vestibular cortex. For example, optokinetic stimulation has been found to induce a direction-specific modulation of the resting discharge of single cells in the vestibular nuclei of goldfish, rabbits, and rhesus monkeys.[93,95–98] The directional specificity of these neurons is generally opposite for visual and vestibular stimuli. For low-frequency angular oscillation (0.1 Hz) about the Earth-vertical axis, visual cues largely determine the activity of the vestibular nuclei units. The vestibular nuclei activity is driven almost entirely by the vestibular system at frequencies beyond 1.0 Hz, whereas both visual and vestibular inputs play a role at frequencies from 0.1–1.0 Hz (Ref. 99). A recent study[100] using positron emission tomography demonstrated that visual motion stimulation resulting in circularvection not only activates the medial parietal-occipital visual area bilaterally, but it also simultaneously deactivates the parieto-insular vestibular cortex (see also Chapter 3). This finding suggests a reciprocal inhibitory visual-vestibular interaction as a multisensory mechanism for self-motion perception (see Chapter 3, Sec. V).

A similar interaction between visual and otolith inputs is known as linearvection. Detection of suprathreshold vestibular stimulation was impaired by a simultaneously moving visual pattern inducing linearvection,[101] which demonstrated the dominant influence of visual input on vestibular thresholds. As described earlier, the otolith organs respond to higher-frequency stimuli than visual inputs in detecting self-motion, as sustained tilt is detected at low frequencies by the otolith organs. The idea that visual inputs might complement otolith inputs is also supported by the finding that neurons in the cat's vestibular nucleus receiving afferents from the otoliths respond to translational self-motion and also to translational movement of a large visual field relative to the stationary animal.[102]

VII.   Vestibular Influence on Cardiovascular Control

G-transition effects often accompany changing orientation during some flight maneuvers. These are defined as the spectrum of physiological and psychophysical effects induced by rapid changes in gravitoinertial forces, alternating between hypogravity (<1 Gz) and hypergravity (>1 Gz) and vice versa.[103] The effects of changing from hypogravity to hypergravity include reduced cardiovascular G-tolerance and reduced efficiency in physiologic recovery mechanisms. The effects of the reverse, that is, hypergravity to hypogravity transitions, include pronounced disorientation, delayed recovery from G-induced loss of consciousness or blackout (if the pilot succumbed to these conditions already), and increased discomfort.[104,105] Von Beckh[105] referred to the reduced G-tolerance and greater strain as "a logical consequence of the transition from hypogravity to hypergravity." Regarding SD during G-transitions, he speculated that it was caused by incorrect vestibular cues. More recently, it has also been reported that, following exposure to $-Gz$ and off-axis $+Gz$ in flight, some pilots experience sudden onset of vertigo and SD.[106] The condition is commonly referred to as "wobblies" by pilots or as vector-related vertigo (see Chapter 6, VII.C). Furthermore, there is some evidence on interaction between G tolerance and vestibular stimulation. Upon recovery from a prolonged and rapid roll (greater than $200°/s$), it was documented that susceptible pilots experienced both SD and reduced G tolerance, leading to blackout at an unusually lower G level.[47,107] As early as 1943, vestibular stimulation was shown to induce a significant fall in blood pressure and reduction in pulse rate.[108] It is reasonable to assume that a similar mechanism might be responsible for the reduced G threshold.

Recent animal studies provide convincing evidence that the vestibular system is involved in compensating for posture-related changes in blood pressure. Decerebrate cats with intact vestibular pathways[109,110] demonstrated an increase in sympathetic nervous system output during pitch rotation, but not during roll rotation. These cats also underwent removal of other key structures of the CNS (e.g., upper cervical root transection, cerebellectomy, baroreceptor denervation, and vagotomy). Bilateral transection of the vestibular nerves in paralyzed, anesthetized cats impairs hypotension compensation.[111] The gain of the vestibulo-sympathetic reflexes during pitch rotation is constant across stimulus frequencies and is in phase with the change in head position, implying that the vestibular influence is primarily of otolith origin. Anatomically, direct connections between pertinent areas of the brain (e.g., vestibular nuclei, locus coeruleus, and brainstem pathways) controlling the sympathetic nervous system have been mapped.[112] Neurons have been identified in the medial vestibular nucleus where pitch responses predominate, suggesting that the medial vestibular nucleus might also be an important relay for information about orientation within the pitch plane.[113]

In humans, the observation that galvanic and caloric stimulation can bring about significant changes in blood pressure and pulse rate[108,114,115] has been extended to Coriolis and pseudo-Coriolis stimulation.[116–118] However, these stimuli also provoked nausea and discomfort that have led to cardiovascular effects (psychologically or otherwise). Clinical observations indicate that a significant number of patients with peripheral vestibular disease are susceptible to orthostatic hypotension after standing up, following a sustained supine posture.[119] Fore, aft, or lateral linear acceleration produced an increase in systolic blood pressure (7–9 mm Hg) in normal subjects sitting upright but to a lesser extent in "idiopathic" vestibular patients whose eye movement response to either caloric or rotational stimuli was <10% of the normal population.[120] An immediate increase in muscle sympathetic nerve activity with head-down neck flexion suggests a vestibulo-sympathetic reflex effect[121,122] because the change in muscle sympathetic nerve activity is one of the important compensatory mechanisms in maintaining arterial pressure. There is some evidence that orthostatic hypotension induced by head-down to head-up tilt in pitch orientation is more effectively compensated than head tilt in roll.[123] This is not surprising from an evolutionary standpoint because we often pitch forward but seldom have to roll more than 5–10 deg. Further, this movement is limited to the upper torso; in other words, teleologically we are not "hard wired" to roll. On the other hand, the greater sensitivity to pitch might be a residue of the transformation of our hominid ancestors from a quadrupedal posture to a tree-climbing one.

Other forms of vestibular stimulation also affect cardiovascular responses in humans. For example, high-speed yaw rotation (120 rotations per minute) caused progressive tachycardia, narrowing of pulse pressure, a drop in mean arterial pressure, and, inferentially, a drop in cardiac output.[124] It was shown that high angular acceleration (with peak acceleration at 125 deg/s^2) of the head about the yaw axis reduces the baseline baroreflex responsiveness by 30%, inhibits vagally mediated baroreflex control of heart rate, and impairs orthostatically induced tachycardia.[125] The attenuating effect of vestibular stimulation on baroreflex function could potentially compromise blood pressure regulation and cerebral perfusion during rapid G transition exposures. In flight, the extent to which vestibular stimulation can impair G-tolerance has yet to be determined.

Excessive blood pooling in the lower body during $+G_z$ positive acceleration or other vertical movement is associated with reduced or uneven blood flow within the intracranial circulation. A steep gradient in blood pressure is normally present between the aorta and the terminal arterioles of the brain stem. If systemic pressure drops, the arterioles are deprived of blood flow. The vestibular nuclei might be vulnerable to this form of ischemia. The interaction between SD and acceleration is an important issue because next-generation thrust-vectored superagile aircraft provide greater multiaxis maneuver capability (see Chapter 11, Sec. III).

VIII. Vestibular Habituation

A significant concern regarding the vestibular system and SD has been centered on the possibility of abolishing or reducing undesirable vestibular responses by repeated exposure to appropriate stimulus conditions. The term habituation is used here referring to the reduced response upon repeated exposure to angular or linear acceleration. On the other hand, adaptation can generally be referred to as the process by which we become adjusted to a new environment. It is well-known that experienced pilots, like figure skaters and ballet dancers, learn to suppress inappropriate vestibular responses. Aschan[126] reported that during flight training fighter pilots progressively build up a resistance to vestibular stimuli, as measured by clinical rotary tests, and that conversely this resistance is lost after a period away from flying. In general, experienced fighter pilots have shorter postrotatory sensations and shortened postrotatory nystagmus following specific angular decelerations[126] and Coriolis stimulation[127] than do nonpilots and pilots with infrequent flying duties. Significant differences in postural control ability among fighter pilots, helicopter pilots, and candidates for flight training have also been observed.[128] However, the implication that fighter pilots make less movements in maintaining balance could be attributed to other confounding variables, for example, training might have affected the postural-control mechanism independently of any vestibular effects. Although differences between pilots and nonpilots have been reported for subjective responses to repeated angular acceleration, habituation to linear motion sensitivity has not been demonstrated.[129]

In the laboratory there is abundant evidence that repetitive vestibular stimulation (yaw rotation) can lead to a reduction of postrotatory nystagmus, subjective reactions, and the oculogyral illusion. A comprehensive review is provided by Collins.[130] For example, in humans there is a 30% decline in the slow phase of nystagmus resulting from unidirectional rotation. Several lines of evidence suggest that habituation is a form of learning because vestibular habituation can only result from unusual stimulation (caloric and unidirectional stimulation) outside the normal frequency range of velocity transduction in humans (0.1–5.0 Hz). Sinusoidal rotation provides no conflict between vestibular and visual input, and there are no postrotatory effects by which such conflicts could arise. The habituation phenomenon also fails to describe adequately the dynamic processes that occur under certain conditions as a result of repeated vestibular stimulation. For example, the horizontal VOR is also capable of a remarkable degree of adaptation[131]; human subjects wearing reversing prisms for several days show a substantial reduction in the gain of the VOR and a phase reversal of the reflex. When the prisms are removed, the phase returns to near normal within a few hours, whereas the restoration of the gain required a few weeks. Subjective orientation and motor control were also shown to be appropriate in both the normal and reversed visual conditions.

An issue of both theoretical and practical interest, especially regarding motion sickness and SD, is the extent to which habituation to one kind of vestibular stimulation can transfer to other kinds of stimulation. In this case habituation is used to describe the situation where a change in susceptibility to airsickness or SD in-volves conscious mental activity, such as learning the characteristics of the motion environment to predict future movements. It has been shown that individuals who are subjected to a motion stimulus that provokes nausea and vomiting tend, with repeated exposure, to become increasingly resistant to its nauseogenic effect. This habituating response has been seen in a variety of situations, such as onboard ships, in spaceflight, and in the laboratory. For example, habituation to Coriolis stimula-tion in the laboratory has been shown to demonstrate a gradual decline in Coriolis effects, for example, a reduction in the perceived orientation change, a reduction in the unpleasant sensations, and an increase in tolerance to the nauseogenic effects of the cross-coupled stimuli (Chapter 6, Sec. II.B). During yaw rotation, when head tilting was practiced in a given direction, the symptoms gradually subsided but only for the practiced direction.[132] The preceding evidence suggested that there are central modifications (or recalibration) of reflexes and sensations originating from semicircular canal stimulation. The gradual decay of otolith neurons during sustained tilt, that is, short-term adaptation,[49] also suggests central modification of otolith activity. Certainly, prolonged exposure to hypergravity adapts the otolith organ at least temporarily.

The suggestion of vestibular exercises (achieved through gymnastics) to reduce susceptibility to airsickness has been proposed by Popov.[133] However, the phe-nomenon of vestibular habituation or possible adaptation raises many questions that have not been resolved. This is partially because acquisition of habituation shows individual variation. The factors that determine the rate of habituation are unknown. As just discussed, habituation can occur to a specific combination of motion cues and not to all provocative stimuli. In addition, the neurophysiological mechanisms that underlie habituating responses are unknown. The potential for long-term adaptation is also unclear. Certainly, the adaptation hypothesis cannot explain adequately the manner in which motion sickness susceptibility varies with exposure to provocative motions. Whether habituation to certain SD illusions could improve the ability to overcome them remains to be investigated.

IX.   Alignment with the Gravitational Vertical

It is generally agreed that control of self-motion and orientation in space depends on vestibular information that is supplemented by visual and somatosensory mo-tion cues. For example, in the perception of vertical orientation, incoming otolith signals convey the orientation of the head with respect to the GIF. When verticality is assessed by means of a visual task, the orientation of the retina with respect to the head is predominant, at least for large tilt angles. A luminous vertical or hori-zontal line in a totally dark setting appears to tilt when the head is tilted about the naso-occipital axis. When the head tilt is greater than about 70 deg, the luminous line appears to be tilted in the opposite direction up to a maximum of about 10 deg. The effect is known as the Aubert (or A) effect, named after its discoverer,[134] and it is consistent with the perceptual underestimation of a large head tilt. For smaller angles of head tilt (less than 30–40 deg), the luminous line appears to be tilted in the same direction, and the effect is known as the Müller (or E) effect. The Müller effect is what one would expect from an overestimation of the head tilt. There are wide individual differences in the Aubert and Müller effects, with many subjects experiencing only the Aubert effect. These two effects might be of some significance regarding spatial orientation during night flying, although it is uncommon that pilots would tilt their head up to 70 deg.

There have been a number of attempts to explain the Aubert and Müller effects, but there is no satisfactory agreement on the overall mechanism. A comprehensive review of the subject can be found in Howard[135] and more recently in Bronstein.[136] The interaction between the magnitude of the Aubert and Müller effects and the degree of body tilt resembles a sine function. It was suggested that the effects are related to the shearing force acting on the utricular macula, which is also a sine function of body tilt.[137] It has frequently been overlooked that during the initial portion of the head tilt there are stimuli from the neck receptors, semicircular canals, and utricles as well as haptic receptors. When the canal stimulation subsides, the tilt percept is maintained by the neck receptors and the utricle. More recently, Mittelstaedt[138,139] has indicated that under certain circumstances, when other receptors are absent or when their inputs are ambiguous, the visceral receptors can influence the perception of verticality. Clear dissociation of the subjective postural vertical and subjective visual vertical was found in patients with acute unilateral vestibular disorders, and it could also be induced in normal subjects by visual motion stimuli in the roll plane.[136] Prolonged lateral body tilt was shown to bias the A effect and the subjective postural vertical in both normal subjects and vestibular patients, suggesting that these effects are likely mediated by somatosensory as well as otolith inputs. The subjective visual vertical was found to be tilted in the direction of the motion, but the subjective postural vertical was not. These findings suggest that different sensory modalities convey different and sometimes conflicting information concerning verticality. It is likely that the internal representation of verticality involves multisensory inputs.

It has been proposed that ocular counterrolling could account for part of the Aubert effect. Ocular counterrolling is the reflex rotation of the eyes about their visual axes in a direction opposite to head movement when the head is rolled about the naso-occipital axis. The eyes can counterroll up to 10% of the head tilt angle. The static component of ocular counterrolling is the displacement of the eyes from their normally vertical orientation when the head is held tilted relative to gravity. It is now considered to be mediated by the utricles[140,141] and has been used as a relatively pure indicator of utricular function. The proposed relationship of ocular counterrolling to the Aubert effect is unclear since both subjects with normal vestibular function and subjects with bilateral loss of vestibular function demonstrated both the Aubert and Müller effects. On the other hand, subjects with bilateral vestibular loss do not demonstrate ocular counterrolling.[142]

Despite the A and E effects, the perceived horizon appears relatively stable because stability of body orientation and dynamic postural control are maintained through the integration of afferent and efferent inputs involving the sensorimotor systems. The hierarchical organization permits modification with respect to the relative importance of each sensory modality in maintaining posture under specific environments. For example, it has now been demonstrated that when pilots bank the aircraft during visual meteorological conditions (VMC) they consistently tilt their head in the opposite direction of the bank in an attempt to stabilize the horizon on the retina.[143,144] The head tilt is presumably caused by the optokinetic cervical reflex

(OKCR), driven by rotation of the peripheral visual field. Similarly, optokinetic torsion during head tilt also contributes to the stabilization of the horizon (see Chapter 3, Sec. IV.A.3.). Finally, as discussed earlier in Sec. V, central resolution of gravitoinertial signals has now been established based on the evidence that the VOR is aligned with the horizon during posttranslation head tilt.

X.   Vestibulospinal vs Corticospinal Motor Mechanisms

The vestibular system plays an important role in the regulation of body posture. Activation of the labyrinth leads to a variety of reflexes of the body and limb musculature that result in stabilization of the head and body. In humans, for example, the Fukuda test of vertical writing[145] and its modifications[146,147] demonstrated that the vestibulospinal tract can be evoked by relatively weak rotatory or caloric stimulation that cannot induce nystagmus. The deviation in writing induced by mild labyrinthine stimulation can be explained as a result of changes in the tonus of the upper extremity musculature caused by impulses originating from the vestibular apparatus and passing through the vestibulospinal tract.

The principal motor pathway from the brain stem to the spinal cord includes two vestibulospinal tracts that originate in the vestibular nuclei: a lateral vestibulospinal tract (LVST) and a medial vestibulospinal tract (MVST). They are located in the anteromedial column of the spinal cord, and they excite motor neurons located primarily in the medial portion of the anterior horn. Two reticulospinal tracts—an excitatory pontine reticulospinal tract and an inhibitory medullary reticulospinal tract—terminate on the medial motor neurons of the anterior horn. Embedded within the lateral vestibulospinal tract and the pontine reticulospinal tract are the tectospinal tract originating in the mesencephalon and the interstitiospinal tract originating within the reticular formation. Motor neurons in the anterior horn control the axial musculature of the body and the girdle musculature of the shoulders and hips and the proximal portion of the limbs.

Vestibular signals are sent to the vestibular nuclei and on to the spinal motor centers of the LVST and MVST and to the reticulospinal tract. Together, these descending tracts constitute the medial brainstem pathways, whose important role in the regulation of posture, by action of the proximal and axial muscles, was described by Lawerence and Kuypers.[148,149] This complex of pathways and motor neurons provides contraction of the antigravity muscles while inhibiting the flexor muscles to prevent their opposition to the antigravity muscles. The medullary reticulospinal tract tends to inhibit the antigravity muscles while providing some degree of excitation to the flexors. The vestibular nuclei have reciprocal connections with the spinal cord. Ascending spinal inputs include direct spinovestibular fibers, some of which are collaterals of spinocerebellar pathways. Other spinal inputs are provided by indirect pathways that might be responsible for the influence of natural stimulation, such as joint receptors.[150]

The organization of the central nervous system and the subcortical mechanisms controlling posture and locomotion suggests that the CNS is not limited to information processing about the position of the body and its relation to its environment. It is also informing other parts of the nervous system about what it is doing before any motor response has been effected. The corticospinal pyramidal tract not only generates motorneuron activity to voluntarily control skeletal muscles, but it also sends collateral branches to influence sensory activity in dorsal column nuclei.[151] Sensory stimuli are conveyed to the CNS over specific pathways, with variable latency depending upon the length and complexity of the sensory route. For example, visual information affects premotor pyramidal tract neurons after a relatively long interval (more than 100 ms), whereas impulses from tendons and joint receptors reach the premotor region more promptly (in less than 25 ms). By the time the pyramidal tract neurons become active, the incoming information has been processed and modulated in the spinal cord, brainstem, thalamus, sensory cortex, association cortex, and in the column of neurons where the pyramidal tract neuron is situated. The pyramidal tract output can also enhance its own afferent input. When the cortical motor neurons discharge, they act directly upon motor neurons of the spinal cord as well as nerve cells in their own cortical column, the basal ganglia, and the cerebellum. Presumably, the circuits through the basal ganglia are for the modification of posture in preparation for the execution of an intended motor command. The cerebellum serves to modulate and stabilize the movement, and the reticular formation provides an overall gain control. During the movement, information is returned to the brain from receptors in muscle, tendon, joint, and skin receptors. Neural integration occurs in the spinal cord and brain stem, and signals are projected to the cerebellum (through the spinocerebellar and vestibulo-cerebellar tract) and transmitted to the thalamus, sensory, and motor cortex.

The vestibulospinal reflex was proposed as one of the potential contributing factors to the giant-hand phenomenon, a false sensation that the aircraft control system is malfunctioning because a giant hand is perceived to be guiding the aircraft.[152,153] This phenomenon is discussed in more detail in Chapter 6, Sec. VII. Under some circumstances, vestibulospinal feedback can even affect the perceptual experience, as exemplified by the difference between the aftereffects of active and passive whole-body rotation. After prolonged active rotation the aftersensation is not one of turning in the opposite direction as would be predicted from the semicircular canal response, but rather of turning in the same direction as the preceding turning motion.[154] If the body is relaxed in the laboratory, the head, torso, and legs tend to twist in the same direction as previous turns. The phenomenon has been termed the antisomatogyral illusion.[155] It demonstrates that unusual vestibular stimuli can induce reflexive motion of the head, torso and limbs that may not be appreciated by the subject, yet they can influence performance. Presumably, during prolonged active rotation, cupula deflection decays toward the neutral position with superimposed cyclic variation related to perturbation in head velocity. Upon deceleration, because of the time-dependent decay, it produces a cupular overshoot and an opposite vestibulospinal effect. The prolonged active turning could also lead to vestibular preprogramming of insufficient torque to stop the body. A derangement of normal neuromuscular mechanisms as a result of vestibular stimulation is also possible. The difference in after-sensation can have potential implications for the perceptual experiences of pilots who actively generate unusual vestibular stimuli in flight maneuvers and continue to control the aircraft after maneuvers are completed.

There is also a difference in the dynamics of eye movements induced by active vs passive rotation. Nystagmus induced by active rotation of the body has a higher gain; presumably, the vestibular responses are augmented by those induced by trunk and leg movements. Accordingly, postrotatory vestibular nystagmus was shown to be reduced after active rotation because the somatosensory after-nystagmus (as described in Sec. XI.C) is opposite in direction.[154] It suggests that proprioceptive feedback associated with active turning and stopping can augment perrotatory vestibular nystagmus and suppress postrotatory vestibular nystagmus. The alternative explanation for the difference is that our CNS monitors the effort of will (efference copy) and sends this information (as a corollary discharge) to the sensory systems.

Despite the antisomatogyral effect, observed in the laboratory, it should be noted that pilots do experience graveyard spins. The graveyard spin is a false sensation of rotation about the vertical (yaw or dorsoventral) axis (see Chapter 6, Sec. II.A). In one survey[156] even experienced instructor pilots reported this illusion. Moreover, having control of the aircraft does not prevent even more commonly experienced postrotatory sensations and nystagmus. Nevertheless, experienced pilots "fly subconsciously," maintaining and correcting the equilibrium of their aircraft automatically. They do not resist gyration, but rather spontaneously adjust their bodies to follow the changes of position in order to maintain orientation. It is proposed that experienced pilots develop what is referred to as fusion, in which the aircraft is said to become a mere extension of their voluntary control of motion.[44] Therefore, the sensations of experienced pilots are probably shaped by their active control functions and are different from those that are engendered by passive stimulation in laboratory devices. This could partially account for why experienced pilots are much more disturbed by fixed-base flight simulators with moving visual scenes than are novice pilots. Therefore, it is likely that the pilot's active control of his aircraft reflexively shapes his perceptual experience, which highlights the importance of maintaining flying practice.

Recent studies of the OKCR during VMC flights could serve as an example of the preceding postulate. As discussed in Sec. IX, both simulator[144] and in-flight studies[143] suggest that the OKCR affects pilots differently while actively flying (active group) or in a passive supervisory role (passive group). It was reported that pilots who were not actively flying, but were in a supervisory role, had a greater onset rate of head tilt than the actively flying pilots.[157] A number of explanations for the OKCR attenuation in the active group were proposed, including greater cognitive activity and motor output in maneuvering the control stick in the active pilot group.

XI.   Somatosensory Input to Orientation

A.   Proprioceptive and Tactile Sensors

Altered gravitoinertial force patterns that elicit vestibular illusions also stimulate the somatosensory receptors and impose changing sensorimotor control demands on body posture and movements. The somatosensory system consists of proprioceptors and cutaneous tactile sensors. Proprioception, or kinesthesis, includes the subcutaneous and kinesthetic muscle-activity sensors, which enable an individual to determine body position, movements in space, and the level of force that must be exerted to make a movement and to maintain the position of a joint against a resisting load. When combined with other senses such as vision, proprioception

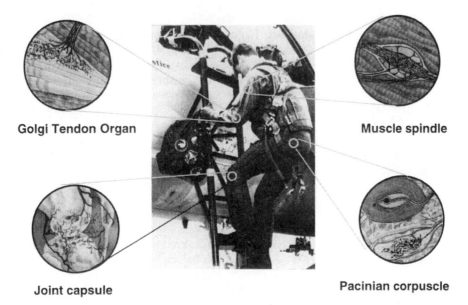

Golgi Tendon Organ

Muscle spindle

Joint capsule

Pacinian corpuscle

Fig. 12   Key proprioceptors and tactile sensors.

provides feedback for skilled movements. In most vertebrates the proprioceptive and tactile systems are the first sensory systems to develop because early in development the somatosensory system requires information concerning the direction of the gravity vector to properly control the antigravity muscles.[158] Muscle and joint senses contribute to the maintenance of equilibrium; in fact, the information received from the control stick is, next to vision, probably the most important factor in the maintenance of equilibrium in flight. The resultant GIF vector increases or decreases the stretching of muscles, particularly the extensor muscles of the neck, head, trunk, and limbs. This action produces changes in reflexes that maintain the body's normal spatial relationship to gravity. The force of gravity also produces sensations of pressure, and the resultant GIF also changes the information supplied by the cutaneous receptors by altering the normal distribution of these sensations. Finally, the somatosensory system is intimately related to the perception of acceleration (G-force). Therefore, the importance of the somatosensory system in the flight environment should not be overlooked. Figure 12 illustrates the key proprioceptive and cutaneous receptors that are involved in spatial orientation in flight.

Major proprioceptors are located in the muscle, tendons, and joint capsules. In the muscle the stretch receptors are primarily located in the intrafusal fibers in the muscle spindles innervated by gamma motor neurons and arranged in parallel with the larger extrafusal muscle-fiber group, which is innervated by alpha motor neurons. The annulospiral and flower-spray endings in the intrafusal fiber signal changes in the state of voluntary muscle stretch. If the muscle and the muscle spindles it contains are stretched, then action potentials are transmitted to the CNS from the annulospiral and flower-spray endings. The frequency of the action potentials is proportional to the degree of stretching. As the muscle spindle is stretched and becomes longer, the impulse frequency in its fiber increases. If the muscle shortens by contraction of the extrafusal fibers, the tension on the muscle spindle is relaxed, and the discharge rate will decrease. Hence the muscle spindle signals the length of the muscle. A series of experiments by Goodwin et al.[160] demonstrated clearly the role of the muscle spindle in the perception of limb position and movement. The otolith-spinal modulation of the antigravity musculature of the body affects both alpha and gamma motor neuronal activity that determine the gain of the muscle spindle. It has been demonstrated that high levels of spindle activity in a vibrated muscle, with respect to the alpha and gamma motorneuron innervation, are interpreted as stretch. This "stretch" is referred to the joint or joints about which the vibrated muscle acts. By vibrating the appropriate muscles, it is possible to illicit illusory motion of the body in any desired direction.[161] More recently, it has also been shown that during a limb movement controlled by contraction of the lengthening muscle, muscle spindle information from the lengthening muscle continues to play an important role in the accurate perception of limb movement and position sense.[162]

Lackner[163] suggests that the skeletal muscular control is actively tuned to the 1-G terrestrial force background and that the muscle spindle is crucial for the adaptive tuning. In altered gravitoinertial environments, as in weightlessness or during a high-G turn when total limb weight is increased, the normal relationship among patterns of alpha and gamma motorneuron activity, muscle spindle discharge level, and the resulting movement of the body is altered, leading to erroneous information about limb position and control. In weightlessness, the otolith influence is diminished, possibly leading to a decrease in the gain of the spindle and a degradation of position sense.

A second type of stretch receptor, located in the tendons, is called the Golgi tendon organ. The receptors are arranged in series with the extrafusal musculature and respond to changes in tension. Both muscle spindles and Golgi tendon organs provide a sensory basis for myotatic (spinal) reflexes to stabilize a joint, and they help to maintain the foundation of posture and locomotion. However, proprioceptive stimulation does not necessarily result in a corresponding conscious perception. Because of the different arrangement of the muscle spindles and tendon organs, they produce different patterns of nerve impulse discharge when the muscle contracts. For example, if a muscle is stretched near its resting length, most spindle afferents responded readily to stretch, whereas the Golgi tendon organ afferents produce very poor stretch responses.[164] This situation results from the fact that the thresholds of tendon organs are higher than those of the muscle spindles. Moreover, for a given length, the discharge frequency of the tendon organ is always lower than that of the muscle spindle.

The joint capsules contain Ruffini-like (spray-type) receptors and Golgi tendon organs in ligaments that are slow adapting, as well as a small number of Paciniform corpuscles. Few slowly adapting Pacinian corpuscles and free-nerve endings are found in the connective tissue enclosing the joint. The joint capsules are compressed and stretched as the joint moves. It has been suggested that mechanoreceptors in the joint capsule signal the position of a joint as well as the direction and velocity of its movement, but not the force acting on it.[165] Specifically, the receptor discharge rate for a certain joint position reflects both the position of the joint at the end of the movement and the velocity of movement. However, recent research[166] suggests that joint-receptor afferents lack the spontaneous activity recorded in other receptors, such as in skin and muscle, and they do not contribute significantly to the conscious perception of limb position during active movement. The threshold for the knee joint is 0.5–0.7 deg, when movement is made at 1–2.5 deg/s. As just mentioned, convincing evidence suggest that muscle spindles are involved in proprioception although they might play a lesser role during passive movements. Therefore, a primary factor in the perception of joint angles relates to the interpretation of muscle–spindle afferent signals in relation to alpha and gamma patterns of muscle coactivation. In addition, cutaneous mechanoreceptors in the dorsal skin of the human hand and finger joint are shown to provide the CNS with detailed kinematic information for movements of the hand.[167] When a conflict is artificially created between the input pattern from skin mechanoreceptors and that of muscle–spindle afferents, humans seem to primarily judge finger joint movements and postures on the basis of sensory cues from the skin.[168] The neurophysiological evidence that afferent information from skin mechanoreceptors is important for proprioception has been extended to other body parts: e.g., the human thigh. Afferent information from the slowly adapting receptor (SA III) in the hairy skin of the human thigh was shown to effectively encode both static and dynamic aspects of passively imposed knee-joint movements.[169]

In summary, muscle-spindle and joint receptors provide the pilot with feedback about the motion of aircraft through force or displacement of the control stick or rudder pedals. However, it should be noted that proprioceptive receptors do not respond to a single physical stimulus because velocity, tension, and orientation to gravity all affect the receptor simultaneously. Furthermore, input from the body's pressure receptors and the otolith organs both help in detecting inertial forces resulting from linear acceleration. Sensory inputs from these two sources generally agree, even if the sensation is erroneous. For example, illusions related to stimulation of the otolith organs, such as the somatogravic and inversion illusions (see Chapter 6, Sec. III), are usually reinforced by "seat-of-the-pants" sensations. Consequently, it has been suggested that the CNS utilizes a combination of sensory inputs from various receptors as a basis for the kinesthetic sense, which supports the notion that proprioception is not a unitary sense such as vision and audition.[170]

B. Somatoreceptors (Touch and Pressure)

The subcutaneous pressure receptors are capable of informing individuals of their position in relation to the Earth, if they are in contact with Earth-bound objects. The pressure receptors are stimulated by the pressures created on the gluteal region when sitting, on the feet when standing, or on the back when lying down. They provide the seat-of-the-pants sensation often referred to in flying. Although early aviators believed they could determine their aircraft's position by the seat-of-the-pants, they were often fatally mistaken. Forces encountered in the flight environment can lead to completely erroneous percepts, if these pressure receptors are relied on for orientation (for example, pressure on the pilot's back and gluteal region during forward acceleration). Somatosensation is not designed to orient individuals in three-dimensional space but rather to inform them of the relative motion and position of their body parts.

The three main types of mechanoreceptors are the intensity, velocity, and acceleration detectors. Similar to the proprioceptors, several types of mechanoreceptors are simultaneously stimulated by the mechanical stimuli encountered in everyday life. For example, sensations of touch and pressure on the soles of the feet, the gluteal surface, and other parts of the skin are mediated by several mechanoreceptors in the skin and underlying tissues. These mechanoreceptors include 1) very rapidly adapting lamellated Pacinian corpuscles for vibration and transient touch, 2) moderately adapting Meissner corpuscles for the detection of the velocity of skin deformation, 3) slow-adapting, spray-type Ruffini endings for sustained touch and pressure, and 4) moderately slow-adapting Merkel's disks for static displacement and velocity. The tactile feedback from the controls of the aircraft is of great value to the pilot, although as stated earlier, flying by the seat of the pants can be deceiving. Touch has been proposed as a warning mechanism in future cockpit design, by enabling part of the control stick to stimulate touch receptors and attract the pilot's attention. This technology is used in warning systems such as "stick shakers," in which the control stick is shaken violently to warn against an impending stall. More recently, Rupert[171] has demonstrated that tactile cues, spatially distributed on the body surface, can signal aircraft orientation to pilots during dynamic flight conditions. This technology is discussed in Chapter 11, Sec. IV.B.2.

C.   Interactions Between the Somatosensory and Other Sensory Systems

As mentioned earlier, the important influence of somatosensory cues on human spatial orientation has not always been recognized, although experimental evidence on the active "stepping-around" phenomenon suggests a somatosensory-vestibular convergence at the vestibular nuclei and the thalamus. Apparent stepping around in the dark (without actual displacement and consequently no stimulation of the peripheral vestibular system) can induce sensation of self-motion, with concomitant nystagmus,[172] and it evokes Coriolis-like effects[173] (see Section XI.D). Limb movements that are directionally concordant with muscle torque in generating body motion also yield arthrokinetic effects, which augment perrotational nystagmus and sustain the sensation of turning.[174] Similarly, arthrokinetic motion information from the upper limb in blindfolded stationary subjects generates convincing linear vection and overrides discordant suprathreshold vestibular input.[175] These studies suggest that afferent somatosensory information from muscle, joint receptor, and cutaneous mechanoreceptors of the human upper limb and thigh are sufficient to induce apparent sensation of motion and that arthrokinetic information has a predominant effect on the perceived direction of self-motion under certain circumstances. Anatomically, convergence of vestibular and somatosensory signals at the cortical level has been established[176] and is of functional importance because both systems provide information about position and movements of the body.

A wide range of situations has been identified in which touch and pressure cues have a profound influence on human spatial orientation. Recent studies[177,178] have shown that spatial information about body posture derived from fingertip contact with a stationary surface, coupled with other proprioceptive information, serves as an indicator for body sway. In bilateral labyrinthine-defective subjects, light touch of the index finger with a stationary surface during quiet stance can serve as an effective substitute for vestibular function in minimizing postural sway.[179] Tactile and pressure receptors also inform the individual of contact with other objects, such as the aircraft seat and control stick, and by inference, the Earth. When good visual information is unavailable, intense periodic touch and pressure stimulation to the body surface can determine the apparent orientation of the body, overriding the contribution from the otolith receptors. On the other hand, the unusual force patterns that elicit vestibular illusions also stimulate the tactile and proprioceptive receptors of the body and impose altered sensorimotor demands on the coordination of body posture and movements. It has been documented that non-1-G background force levels, that lead to alterations in the effective weight of the head, limbs, and body, can, in turn, alter the apparent feel of controls.[180,181]

Two of the sensory organs that are involved with spatial orientation, namely, the vestibular apparatus and the eyes, are situated in the head. The head is free to move (to a certain extent) relative to the body, which suggests the necessity for an adequate integration with the somatosensory system to maintain space constancy. Experimental evidence indicates that vestibular and neck-input exert opposite influences on posture.[182] In particular, roll tilt (head displacement) increases the contraction of ipsilateral limb extensors, whereas rotation of the body over a stationary head (neck displacement) produces relaxation of the same muscles. Similarly, unilateral labyrinth deafferentation produces a postural asymmetry characterized by head and body tilt towards the side of the lesion, hypotonia in the extensor muscles of the ipsilateral limbs, and hypertonia in the extensor muscle of the contralateral limbs. These findings suggest that the interaction between the somatosensory and vestibular system also serves to determine head position.

As discussed in Sec. III.I, in order to perceptually discriminate between inertial and gravitational acceleration, multisensory integration at the CNS level is required. Mayne[70] proposed that this is achieved by central filtering: a simple first-order low-pass filter is used as an estimate of gravity to determine spatial orientation with respect to the vertical, whereas the high-frequency component is interpreted as translational acceleration. [A low-pass filter greatly attenuates high-frequency input but passes low-frequency inputs (e.g., the constant force of gravity) with little loss of amplitude.] The somatogravic effect as measured by the subjective vertical was reexamined using counter-rotation (so as to eliminate angular motion) in a short-arm centrifuge to overcome the problem of interacting angular motion.[183] Specifically, the phase relationship between the gravitoinertial force vector and the subjective vertical was reexamined.[184] To derive the linear motion, gravity should be subtracted from the gravitoinertial force vector as sensed by the somatosensory system by employing a simple first-order low-pass filter. Accordingly, the estimate of the subjective vertical should lag behind the shift of the GIF. However, there is no evidence that the simple first-order low-pass filter is sufficient to explain the tilt sensation during linear acceleration, as reflected by the inconsistent phase response between the subjective vertical indication and the gravitoinertial force vector exhibited by the subjects.[184] The results suggested that the somatosensory system, neglected in previous somatogravic studies, might play an important role. The relatively fast adaptation to pressure exerted on the body surface[185] suggests that the somatosensory afferents behave like a high-pass filtered specific force. Graybiel and Clark[186] reported that labyrinth-defective subjects used somatosensory cues in perception of bodily position and that performance improved with the practice. Therefore, these studies provide further evidence that the perception of subjective vertical is determined by a combination of individually weighted vestibular and somatosensory afferents.

D. Somatosensory (Arthrokinetic) Nystagmus

Based on available evidence described in the preceding section, it is not surprising that purely somatosensory nystagmus, in the absence of concurrent vestibular and optokinetic stimulation, can be generated. Bles and Kapteyn[172] recorded nystagmic eye movements in subjects who stepped on a small rotating platform in darkness at such a rate that they did not actually move. Arthrokinetic nystagmus can also be evoked in stationary subjects seated in darkness inside a rotating drum, tracking the rotating cylinder by placing their hands on its inner wall.[187] Both types of nystagmus have a latency of several seconds after stimulus onset and a gradual buildup of slow-phase velocity. The direction of the nystagmus is in the compensatory direction (stabilizing the visual surround), as if subjects had been actually moving. Upon stopping, the nystagmus persists in the same direction for a minute or so. Patients with bilateral labyrinthine deficits exhibit characteristic abnormalities of somatosensory nystagmus, with rapid onset and rapid buildup to slow-phase velocity and an absence of after-nystagmus.[188] This is presumably caused by the lack of conflicting signals from an intact vestibular system. Arthrokinetic enhancement of smooth ocular tracking during linear motion has also been described.[189]

XII. Auditory Input to Orientation

Details concerning the anatomy and physiology of the organ of hearing (the cochlea) will not be discussed here. However, the functions of the auditory sensory system regarding spatial orientation, and current research into using acoustic orientation indicators as a potential SD countermeasure, are briefly described next.

A. Auditory Orientation Information

One of the functions of the organ of hearing is sound localization. The determination of the direction from which sound emanates depends upon detecting the difference in time of arrival of the stimuli in the two ears. It also depends on the consequent difference in the phase of the sound waves at the two ears, as well as the loudness on the side closest to the source. It has been shown that stationary auditory information presented adjacent to each ear can affect body and head sway in sighted and congenitally blind human subjects.[190]

Illusions of self-rotation, accompanied by nystagmus with slow phase in the direction opposite that of the apparent self-rotation can be induced in a stationary subject in the dark with a rotating sound field.[191] "Internal" sound fields, created by dichotic stimulation, are effective as well as external sound sources. However, when the contours of the laboratory were visible to the subject, auditory stimulation elicited neither illusory self-rotation nor nystagmus. These findings are partially confirmed by Marme-Karelse and Bles[192] in that apparent self-rotation can be induced by a single sound source attached to a rotating drum, but the effect is much less than those induced by visual stimuli.

Binaural sound localization is of limited use in determining orientation in flight because of high ambient noise levels and internal sound reflection, especially within the small confines of some cockpits. Noise also emanates from the interaction of the aircraft and the air through which it is moving (boundary-layer noise and noise from the aircraft). Aircraft noise is derived from power sources including transmission systems, propellers (e.g., on helicopter rotors), and jet efflux. The contribution of these various sources to total noise will largely depend on the type of aircraft, phase of flight, and location of the listener. As a comparison, normal speech has a level of about 70 dB, whereas high-performance military aircraft and helicopters can produce internal noise levels of up to 120 dB. Levels above 125 dB are painful, and rupture of the tympanic membrane is estimated to occur at about 160 dB.

There is some evidence that suggests that real or apparent motion, similar to that encountered in vehicular travel, can affect an individual's ability to process binaural time differences.[193] In addition, the localization of a sound source in terms of a Cartesian reference frame is influenced by the change in direction of the resultant force.[194] This phenomenon has been termed the audiogravic illusion and will be discussed in Chapter 6, Sec. V.

Although significant information about aircraft position and flight trajectory can be obtained over the radio during flight operations, such information mainly provides geographic orientation. In some cases noise generated by the boundary layer and the engine can contribute to the perception of velocity by means of the frequencies and intensities of airspeed and can contribute to the perception of pitch attitude and angle of attack.

B. Acoustic Orientation Research

In theory, acoustic displays of primary flight parameters allow pilots to maintain spatial orientation of the aircraft while visually occupied with other tasks. The potential of a stereophonic acoustic orientation instrument (AOI) to help maintain aircraft control when pilots' vision is either occupied or temporarily incapacitated was examined in two studies. An AOI has been demonstrated to be effective, both in a simulator[195] and in a research aircraft,[196] in allowing blindfolded pilots to maintain control of aircraft bank angle and, to a lesser extent, maintain vertical velocity. However, under conditions of heavy workload, when the pilot must complete certain secondary tasks requiring visual and cognitive activity, the presence of the additional auditory signals can compromise secondary task performance.[195]

With the development of powerful digital-signal-processing techniques and using head-related transfer functions (see Chapter 11, Sec. IV.B.1.), virtual three-dimensional auditory displays can be generated in real time with minimal mental transformation or interpretation.[197] The primary advantage of three-dimensional auditory cues is that there is a direct correspondence with the spatial information desired during spatial localization. The pilot can use the information directly without visual processing, so that it is fairly easily processed in parallel with other visually demanding tasks.

Basic research in the design and the effectiveness of three-dimensional auditory displays has been performed. Broadband signals encompassing frequencies from 1 to 13 kHz have been identified to accurately localize signals actually presented from a range of spatial locations.[198] The ability to localize a virtual auditory source was evaluated under varying levels of sustained ($+G_z$) acceleration.[199] No significant increases in localization error were found between $+1.0$ and $+5.6$ G_z, but significant errors occurred at the $+7.0$-G_z level. Flight-test results of three-dimensional audio technology demonstrated successful audio-cued target acquisition. Relative to a no-visual and no-sound condition, pilots subjectively reported a decrease in target acquisition times, an improvement in speech intelligibility, an increase in situational awareness, and a decrease in pilot workload.[200]

In the presence of visual displays, however, the three-dimensional auditory display did not demonstrate a significant effect in enhancing spatial awareness.[201] The preference for the visual display might be caused by limitations in the level of integration with three-dimensional audio. In simulated flight, when paired with a two-dimensional visual display, the three-dimensional auditory display was demonstrated to be effective as a radar display.[202] Although the ability to distinguish left from right can be quite accurate in adverse situations, the accuracy of elevation judgments decreases and front/back confusion increases with relatively small deviation from ideal conditions.[203] These studies suggest that further development of three-dimensional auditory technology is required to reach the performance level of advanced three-dimensional visual displays.

A number of outstanding issues that need to be explored include the degree to which spatial auditory cues provide predominant sensory information when conflicting vestibular or visual cues are present during spatial disorientation. Similarly, the selection of an auditory display that is distinguishable from other auditory cues and background noise in the cockpit needs to be investigated. Most of the studies supporting three-dimensional audio displays have been conducted in controlled laboratory or in-flight settings. It is not clear if the reported performance enhancement can be transferred into the dynamic real-world flight environment. It is also necessary to establish that spatial auditory cues for orientation can be effectively utilized by pilots in conjunction with other flight tasks. Thus, the usefulness of the three-dimensional auditory display as an acoustic attitude indicator and the optimization of its use in aircraft require further research (see Chapter 11, Sec. IV.B.1).

XIII.   Cortical Input to Spatial Orientation

Many of the sensory cues that we receive are subconscious, especially the vestibular, kinesthetic, and ambient visual cues; conversely, focal visual cues and audition are processed mainly in the conscious domain. Our intellectual response might be in the subconscious or conscious domain. Although our conscious thoughts often overrule our subconscious ones, irrational fear or anxiety can still occur. Fatigue, fear, anxiety, mental stress, and inexperience in instrument flying are predisposing factors in the perception of SD illusions and their effects on aircraft control (see Chapter 4, Sec. II). Because fatigue and altered circadian rhythms modify physiological responses, it is not surprising that performance measures during simulated disorientation in the flight simulator were found to be significantly degraded after sleep deprivation.[204] The performance tests include mood, alertness, cognition, spatial orientation, postural stability, flight accuracy, and recovery. All of the cognitive assessments used in this study were visually based tasks, and it is possible that visibility problems could partially account for the degradation in both flight and cognitive performance. Sleep deprivation also resultes in increased sensitivity to Coriolis stimulation and interference with the vestibular habituation process.[205,206] In addition, a pronounced increase in the latency of signaling the onset of turning during Coriolis stimulation suggests that performance capabilities were affected.

Sensory localization relative to the body vs orientation in space were thought to be independent processes. However, recent research[207,208] suggests that localization relative to the body and orientation in space are interdependent processes in the CNS. For example, exposure to weightlessness affects the control and appreciation of body position and orientation. During weightlessness, perception of one's own orientation is dependent on the presence and absence of contact cues and whether part of the body is visible with respect to the architecturally defined horizontal and vertical reference of the vehicle. Limb position sense is degraded as a result of a decreased otolith-spinal modulation of the antigravity musculature. Finally, cognitive factors and previous exposure (experience) to the weightless environments also play an important role. Adaptive changes to weightlessness are initiated when sensorimotor error exceeds a certain limit and results in postural remapping of the changing position of eye in the head or head on the trunk. These postural remappings produce changes in sensory localization that are compensatory for the weightless state that initiated the process of adaptation. Based on this evidence, Lackner and associates hypothesized that CNS processing of sensory information about the gravitoinertial environment conjointly determines sensory localization and spatial orientation. The multisensory, motor, and cognitive strategies used in adaptation to weightlessness are not unique as similarities to the adaptation to an increased force environment can be drawn. Typical SD mishaps in flight occur when the visual orientation system is compromised not only because of reduced visibility, prolonged rotation, or a changing gravitoinertial vector but also during periods of temporary distraction, increased workload, and visual flight rule–instrument flight rule (VFR–IFR) transition. The CNS must recompute orientation with the only information at its disposal, which are the continuous but erroneous vestibular and somatosensory inputs.

Behavioral, neuroanatomical, and neurochemical evidence of the role of cerebral cortical processing in human spatial orientation was reviewed by Previc.[209] A brief summary on the cortical processing of the vestibular and somatosensory system is described next. The brain mechanisms that mediate our perceptual-motor interaction are said to operate within the domains of four major cortico-behavioral systems: a dorsolateral peripersonal, a ventrolateral focal-extrapersonal, a ventromedial action extrapersonal, and a dorsomedial ambient-extrapersonal space (see Chapter 3, Sec. V.B). Although vision remains the primary sensory system, the degree of visual dominance varies across the four systems. Vestibular and somatosensory systems contribute significantly in the peripersonal and ambient-extrapersonal realms. Within the dorsolateral peripersonal system vestibular information provides the position of the head in space and is integrated with the optokinetic, vestibulo-ocular, pursuit, and vergence eye movements. The somatosensory system provides information concerning the positions of the eyes, head, upper limb, and torso movement. Available evidence suggests that integration of the visual, vestibular, and somatosensory information takes place mainly in the posterior parietal lobe.[209]

The cortical component of the ambient extrapersonal system is least understood and least differentiated. Within the dorsomedial ambient-extrapersonal space the vestibular system provides inertial information concerning the direction of the head relative to gravity in order to stabilize oculomotor function in space by means of the OKCR and VOR. Somatosensory inputs provide information concerning the proper orientation of specific body parts relative to gravity and the control of the lower limb movements. Somatosensory information is processed in the anterior parietal lobe. The cortical projection of vestibular inputs was discussed in Sec. III.C; it includes the dorsomedial portion of the superior parietal lobe and the retroinsular cortex in the parietal-temporal junction, and the main integration centers for vestibular, optokinetic, and somatosensory inputs. Finally, dopaminergic cortical systems are implicated in locomotion and motivation in extrapersonal space, whereas noradrenergic (arousal, attention) and serotonergic (arousal, autonomic control) systems are hypothesized to facilitate peripersonal function. The reader is encouraged to refer to Previc[209] for details.

XIV. Summary

In terrestrial environments our perception of position, motion, and attitude with respect to the fixed frame of reference provided by the gravitational vertical and the surface of the Earth is based on the neural integration of concordant, complementary, and redundant information from the visual, vestibular, somatosensory, and, to a lesser extent, auditory systems. The successful maintenance of orientation depends on the availability of reliable sensory information, the proper integration of these sensory inputs in the CNS, the formulation of appropriate patterns of response, and finally, the effective execution of such responses by the body musculature. Unfortunately, the relative contributions and reliability of the various sensory systems involved in the perception of one's orientation are significantly altered when exposed to unusual gravitoinertial environments such as in flight, space, and underwater. Vestibular and somatosensory information can no longer be relied upon, owing to continuous variations in both magnitude and direction of the gravitoinertial vector and to the prolonged rotational movements to which a pilot is normally exposed. Consequently, all responsibility for acquiring reliable information depends on vision, although this sensory modality is not immune to illusory and erroneous perceptions (see Chapter 7). The integration of information in the CNS is complicated by the necessity of sifting reliable from unreliable signals and by the fact that the motion of the aircraft has six degrees of freedom. The effective muscular response must be directed through new channels to maintain aircraft control, rather than maintaining balance and posture. As a result, pilots are forced to deal with flight-control challenges that are not always matched with their natural and learned aptitude. Other factors that predispose pilots to SD include their level and currency of instrument training (see Chapter 8) and their physical and mental state (see Chapter 4). In the absence of underlying pathology, SD should be regarded as an extension of a normal physiological response to an altered gravitoinertial environment. The implication is that SD cannot be avoided or entirely prevented. However, training, flight displays, and other technologies can mitigate the effects of SD on flight performance and improve flight safety.

References

[1]Benson, A. J., and Barnes, G. R., "Vision During Angular Oscillation: The Dynamic Interaction of Visual and Vestibular Mechanisms," *Aviation, Space, and Environmental Medicine*, Vol. 49, 1978, pp. 340–345.

[2]Reschke, M. F., Bloomberg, J. J., Harm, D. L., Paloski, W. H., Layne, C., and McDonald, V., "Posture, Locomotion, Spatial Orientation, and Motion Sickness as Function of Space Flight," *Brain Research Reviews*, Vol. 28, 1998, pp. 102–117.

[3]Parker, D. E., Reschke, M. F., Arrott, A. P., Homick, J. L., and Lichtenberg, B. K., "Otolith Tilt-Translation Reinterpretation Following Prolonged Weightlessness: Implications for Preflight Training," *Aviation Space and Environmental Medicine*, Vol. 56, 1983, pp. 601–606.

[4]Melvill Jones, G. M., and Milsum, J. H., "Spatial and Dynamic Aspects of Visual Fixation," *IEEE Transactions on Biomedical Engineering*, Vol. 12, 1965, pp. 54–62.

[5]Fernandez, C., and Goldberg, J. M., "Physiology of Peripheral Neurons Innervating Otolith Organs of the Squirrel Monkey. III. Response Dynamics," *Journal of Neurophysiology*, Vol. 39, 1976, pp. 996–1008.

[6]Curthoys, I. S., Blanks, R. H. I., and Markham, C. H., "Semicircular Canal Functional Anatomy in Cats, Guinea Pigs, and Man," *Acta Otolaryngologica*, Vol. 83, 1977, pp. 258–265.

[7]Blanks, R. H., Curthoys, I. S., and Markham, C. H., "Planar Relationships of the Semicircular Canals in Man," *Acta Otolaryngology*, Vol. 80, 1975, pp. 185–196.

[8]Goldberg, J. M., and Fernandez, C., "The Vestibular System," *Handbook of Physiology: Volume III*, edited by I. Darian-Smith, Oxford Univ. Press, Oxford, England, U.K., 1983, pp. 7–1022.

[9]Steinhaussen, W., "Uber den Nachweis der Bewegung der Cupula in der Intakten Bogengangsampulle des Labyrinthes bei der Naturlichen Rotatorischen und Calorischen Reizung," *Pfugers Arch. Ges. Physiol.*, Vol. 228, 1931, pp. 322–328.

[10]Steinhaussen, W., "Uber die Beobachtung der Cupula in den Bogengangsampullea des Labyrinths des Lebenden Hechts," *Pfugers Arch. Ges. Physiol.*, Vol. 232, 1933, pp. 500–512.

[11]Dohlman, G. F., "The Shape and Function of the Cupula," *Journal of Laryngology and Otology*, Vol. 83, 1969, pp. 43–53.

[12]McLaren, J. W., and Hillman, D. E., "Displacement of the Semicircular Canal Cupula During Sinusoidal Rotation," *Society for Neuroscience Abstracts*, Vol. 3, 1977, p. 544.

[13]Oman, C. M., and Young, L. R., "The Physiological Range of Pressure Difference and Cupula Deflection in the Human Semicircular Canal," *Acta Otolaryngology*, Vol. 74, 1972, pp. 324–331.

[14]Engstrom, H., Ades, H. W., and Hawkins, J. E., Jr., "Structure and Functions of the Sensory Hairs of the Inner Ear," *Journal of Acoustic Society*, Vol. 34, 1962, pp. 1356–1362.

[15]Lowenstein, O., and Wersäll, J., "A Functional Interpretation of the Electron Microscopic Structure of the Sensory Hair Cells in the Cristae of the Elasmobranch Raja Clavate in Terms of Directional Sensitivity," *Nature*, Vol. 184, 1959, pp. 1807–1810.

[16]Lowenstein, O., "The Functional Significance of the Ultrastructure of the Vestibular End Organs," *Second Symposium on the Role of the Vestibular Organs in Space Exploration*, NASA SP-115, Washington, D.C., 1966, pp. 73–90.

[17]Wersäll, J., and Lundquist, P. G., "Morphological Polarization of the Mechanoreceptors of the Vestibular and Acoustic Systems," *Second Symposium on the Role of the Vestibular Organs in Space Exploration*, Vol. 15, NASA, Washington, D.C., 1966, pp. 57–72.

[18]Wilson, V., and Melvill Jones, G., *Mammalian Vestibular Physiology*, Plenum, New York, 1979.

[19]Deecke, L. D., Schwarz, D. W. F., and Fredrickson, J. M., "Nucleus Ventroposterior Inferior (VPI) as the Vestibular Thalamic Relay in the Rhesus Monkey. I. Field Potential Investigation," *Experimental Brain Research*, Vol. 20, 1974, pp. 88–100.

[20]Schwarz, D. W. F., and Fredrickson, J. M., "Rhesus Monkey Vestibular Cortex. A Bimodal Primary Projection Field," *Science*, Vol. 172, 1971, pp. 280–281.

[21]Büttner, U., and Henn, V., "Thalamic Unit Activity in the Alert Monkey During Natural Vestibular Stimulation," *Brain Research*, Vol. 103, 1976, pp. 127–132.

[22]Fredrickson, J. M., Figge, U., Scheid, P., and Kornhuber, H. H., "Vestibular Nerve Projection to the Cerebral Cortex of the Rhesus Monkey," *Experimental Brain Research*, Vol. 2, 1966, pp. 318–327.

[23]Guldin, W. O., and Grusser, O. J., "Is There a Vestibular Cortex?" *Trends Neuroscience*, Vol. 21, 1998, pp. 254–259.

[24]Bottini, G., Sterzi, R., Paulesu, E., Vallar, G., Cappa, S. F., Erminio, F., Passingham, R. E., Frith, C. D., and Frackowiak, R. S. J., "Identification of the Central Vestibular Projections in Man: a Positron Emission Tomography Activation Study," *Experimental Brain Research*, Vol. 99, 1994, pp. 164–169.

[25]Lobel, E., Kleine, J. F., Le Bihan, D., Leroy-Willig, A., and Berthoz, A., "Functional MRI of Galvanic Vestibular Stimulation," *The Journal of Neurophysiology*, Vol. 80, 1998, pp. 2699–2709.

[26]Fasold, O., Wenzel, R., von Brevern, M., Kuhberg, M., Lempert, T., and Villringer, A., "Overlaps Between Visual and Vestibular Cortical Areas in Humans as Identified by fMRI," NeuroImage Human Brain Mapping 2000 Meeting, Poster # 689, 2000.

[27]Previc, F. H., Liotti, M., Blakemore, C., Beer, J., and Fox, P., "Functional Imaging of Brain Areas Involved in the Processing of Coherent and Incoherent Wide Field-of-View Visual Motion," *Experimental Brain Research*, Vol. 131, 2000, pp. 393–405.

[28]Van Egmond, A. A., Groen, A. J., and Jongkees, L. B. W., "The Mechanics of the Semi-Circular Canal," *Journal of Physiology*, Vol. 110, 1949, pp. 1–17.

[29]Fernandez, C., and Goldberg, J. M., "Physiology of Peripheral Neurons Innervating Semicircular Canals of the Squirrel Monkey II. Response to Sinusoidal Stimulation and Dynamics of Peripheral Vestibular System," *Journal of Neurophysiology*, Vol. 34, 1971, pp. 661–675.

[30]Baloh, R.W., Honrubia, V., Yee, R., and Hess, K., "Changes in the Human Vestibulo-Ocular Reflex After Loss of Peripheral Sensitivity," *Annals of Neurology*, Vol. 16, 1984, pp. 222–228.

[31]Cohen, B., Henn, V., Raphan, T., and Denett, D., "Velocity Storage, Nystagmus, and Visual-Vestibular Interactions in Humans," *Annals of New York Academy of Science*, Vol. 374, 1981, pp. 421–433.

[32]Weissman, B. M., Discernna, A. O., Ekelman, B. L., and Leigh R. J., "The Effect of Eyelid Closure and Vocaliztion upon the Vestibulo-Ocular Reflex During Rotational Testing," *Annals of Otology, Rhinology, and Laryngology*, Vol. 98, 1989, pp. 548– 550.

[33]Raphan, T., Matsuo, V., and Cohen, B., "A Velocity Storage Mechanism Responsible for Optokinetic Nystagmus (OKN), Optokinetic Afternystagmus (OKAN) and Vestibular Nystagmus," *Control of Gaze by Brain Stem Neurons*, edited by R. Baker and A. Berthoz, Elsevier/North-Holland, Amsterdam, 1977.

[34]Raphan, T., Matsuo, V., and Cohen, B, "Velocity Storage in the Vestibulo-Ocular Reflex Arc (VOR)," *Experimental Brain Research*, Vol. 35, 1979, pp. 229–248.

[35]Angelaki, D. E., and Hess, B. J. M., "Inertial Representation of Angular Motion in the Vestibular System of Rhesus Monkeys. I. Vestibuloocular Reflex," *Journal of Neurophysiology*, Vol. 71, 1994, pp. 1222–1249.

[36]Raphan, T., and Cohen, B., "Organizational Principles of Velocity Storage in Three

Dimensions: The Effect of Gravity on Cross-Coupling of Optokinetic After Nystagmus," *Annals of the New York Academy of Science*, Vol. 545, 1988, pp. 74–92.

[37]Mayne, R., "The Dynamic Characteristics of the Semicircular Canals," *The Journal of Comparative and Physiological Psychology*, Vol. 43, 1950, pp. 309–319.

[38]Howard, I. P., "Sensory Processes and Perception The Vestibular System," Boff K. R. Boff, L., Kaufman, and J. P. Thomas, *Handbook of Perception and Human Performance*, Vol. I, edited by Wiley, New York, 1996.

[39]Guedry, F. E., "Psychophysics of Vestibular Sensation Chapter 1," *Handbook of Sensory Physiology*, Vol. 6, edited by H. H. Kornhuber, Springer-Verlag, Berlin, 1974, pp. 3–154.

[40]Gundry, A. J., "Thresholds of Perception for Periodic Linear Motion," *Aviation, Space, and Environmental Medicine*, Vol. 49, 1978, pp. 679–686.

[41]Clark, B., "Threshold for the Perception of Angular Acceleration in Man," *Aerospace Medicine*, Vol. 38, 1967, pp. 443–450.

[42]Meiry, J. L., "*The Vestibular System and Human Dynamic Space Orientation*," Master's Thesis, Massachusetts Inst. of Technology, Cambridge, MA, 1965.

[43]Benson, A. J., Hutt, E. C. B., and Brown, S. F., "Threshold for the Perception of Whole-Body Angular Movement About a Vertical Axis," *Aviation Space and Environmental Medicine*, Vol. 60, 1989, pp. 205–213.

[44]Benson, A. J., "Spatial Disorientation—general Aspects, Spatial Disorientation—Common Illusions, & Motion Sickness," *Aviation Medicine*, 3rd ed., edited by, J. Ernsting, A. Nicholson, and D. Rainford, Butterworth Heinemann, Oxford, England, U.K., 1999, pp. 419–471.

[45]Melvill Jones, G., Barry, W., and Kowalsky, N., "Dynamics of the Semicircular Canals Compared in Yaw, Pitch and Roll," *Aerospace Medicine*, Vol. 35, 1964, pp. 984–989.

[46]Guedry, F. E., Jr., Stockwell, C. W., and Gilson, R. D., "Comparison of Subjective Responses to Semicircular Canal Stimulation Produced by Otation About Different Axes," *Acta Otolaryngology*, Vol. 72, 1971, pp. 101–106.

[47]Melvill Jones, G., "Disorientation due to Rapid Rotation in Flight," *Medical Aspects of Flight Safety*, edited by E. Evard, P. Bergeret and P. M. van Wulfften Palthe, Pergamon, London, 1959, pp. 92–101.

[48]Engstrom, H., "The First Order Vestibular Neurons," *Fourth Symposium on the Role of the Vestibular Organs in Space Exploration*, NASA, Washington D.C., 1998, pp. 123–135.

[49]Fernandez, C., Goldberg, J. M., and Abend, W. K., "Responses to Static Tilts of Peripheral Neurons Innervating Otolith Organs of the Squirrel Monkey," *Journal of Neurophysiology*, Vol. 35, 1972, pp. 978–997.

[50]Lackner, J. R., "Sense of Body Position in Parabolic Flight," *Sensing and Controlling Motion: Vestibular and Sensorimotor Function*, edited by B. Cohen, F. Guedry, and D. Tomko, Annals of the New York Academy of Sciences, Vol. 656, 1992, pp. 329–339.

[51]Fernandez, C., and Goldberg, J. M., "Physiology of Peripheral Neurons Innervating Otolith Organs of the Squirrel Monkey. II. Directional Selectivity and Force Response Relations, *Journal of Neurophysiology*, Vol. 39, 1976, pp. 985–995.

[52]Sasaki, M., Hiranuma, K., Isu, N., and Uchino, Y., "Is There a Three Neuron Arc in the Cat Utriculo-Trochlear Pathway?" *Experimental Brain Research*, Vol. 86, 1991, pp. 421–425.

[53]Xerri, C., Bartholomy, J., Harlay, F., Borel, L., and Lacour, M., "Neuronal Coding of Linear Motion in the Vestibular Nuclei of the Alert Cat. I. Response Characteristics to Vertical Otolith Stimulation," *Experimental Brain Research*, Vol. 65, 1987, pp. 569–581.

[54]Correia, M. J., Hixson, W. C., and Niven, J. I., "On Predictive Equations for Subjective Judgements of Vertical and Horizontal in a Force Field," *Acta Oto-Laryngology*, Supplement 230, 1968, pp. 1–20.

[55]Spoendlin, H. H., "Ultrastructural Studies of the Labyrinth in Squirrel Monkeys," *The Role of the Vestibular Organs in the Exploration of Space*, NASA SP-77, Washington, D.C., 1965, pp. 7–22.

[56]Goldberg, J. M., and Fernandez, C., "Responses of Peripheral Vestibular Neurons to Angular and Linear Accelerations in the squirrel Monkey," *Acta Otolaryngology*, Vol. 80, 1975, pp. 101–110.

[57]Rosenhall, V., "Vestibular Macular Mapping in Man," *Annals of Otology*, Vol. 81, 1972, pp. 339–351.

[58]Malcolm, R., and Melvill Jones, G., "Erroneous Perception of Vertical Motion by Humans Seated in the Upright Position," *Acta Otolaryngology*, Vol. 77, 1974, pp. 274–283.

[59]Melvill Jones, G., and Young, L. R., "Subjective Detection of Vertical Acceleration: a Velocity-Dependent Response," *Acta Otolaryngology*, Vol. 85, 1978, pp. 45–53.

[60]Igarashi, M., and Kata, Y., "Effect of Different Vestibular Lesions upon Body Equilibrium Function in Squirrel Monkeys," *Acta Otolaryngology*, Suppl. 330, 1975, p. 91.

[61]Curthoys, I. S., Betts, G. A., Burgess, H. G., MacDougall, H. G., Cartwright, A. D., and Halmagyi, G. M., "The Planes of the Utricular and Saccular Maculae of the Guinea Pig," *Otolith Function in Spatial Orientation and Movement*, Annals of the New York Academy of Sciences, Vol. 871, edited by B. Cohen & B. J. Hess, New York Academy of Sciences, New York, 1999, pp. 27–34.

[62]McCue, M. P., and Guinan, J. J., "Sound-Evoked Activity in Primary Afferent Neurons of a Mammalian Vestibular System," *The American Journal of Otology*, Vol. 18, 1997, pp. 355–60.

[63]Colebatch, J. G., and Halmagyi, G. M., "Vestibular Evoked Potentials in Human Neck Muscles Before and After Unilateral Vestibulat Deafferentation," *Neurology*, Vol. 42, 1992, pp. 1635–1636.

[64]Colebatch, J. G., Halmagyi, G. M., and Skuse, N. F., "Myogenic Potentials Generated by a Click-Evoked Vestibulocollic Reflex," *Journal of Neurology, Neurosurgery, Psychiatry*, Vol. 57, 1994, pp. 190–197.

[65]Walsh, E. G., "Role of the Vestibular Apparatus in the Perception of Motion on a Parallel Swing," *Journal of Physiology*, Vol. 155, 1961, pp. 506–513.

[66]Benson, A. J., Spencer, M. B., and Stott, J. R. R., "Thresholds for the Detection of the Direction of Whole-Body, Linear Movement in the Horizontal Plane," *Aviation Space and Environmental Medicine*, Vol. 57, 1986, pp. 1088–1096.

[67]Borel, L., Le Goff, B., Charade, O., and Berthoz, A., "Gaze Strategies During Linear Motion in Head-Free Humans," *Journal of Neurophysiology*, Vol. 72, 1994, pp. 2451–2466.

[68]Walsh, E. G., "The Perception of Rhythmically Repeated Linear Motion in the Horizontal Plane," *British Journal of Physiology*, Vol. 53, 1962, pp. 439–445.

[69]Walsh, E. G., "The Perception of Rhythmically Repeated Linear Motion in the Vertical Plane," *Quarterly Journal of Experimental Physiology*, Vol. 49, 1964, pp. 58–65.

[70]Mayne, R., "A Systems Concept of the Vestibular Organs," *Handbook of sensory physiology IV/2: Vestibular System*, edited by H. H. Kornhuber, Springer-Verlag, Berlin, 1974, pp. 493–580.

[71]Paige, G. D., and Tomko, D. L., "Eye Movement Responses to Linear Head Motion in the Squirrel Monkey. II. Visual-Vestibular Interactions and Kinematic Considerations," *Journal of Neurophysiology*, Vol. 65, 1991, pp. 1183–1196.

[72]Angelaki, D. E., McHenry, M., Dickman, J. D., Newlands, S., and Hess, B., "Computation of Inertial Motion: Neural Strategies to Resolve Ambiguous Otolith Information," *Journal of Neurosciences*, Vol. 19, 1999, pp. 316–327.

[73]Robinson, D. A., "The Use of Control Systems Analysis in the Neurophysiology of Eye Movements," *Annual Review of Neuroscience*, Vol. 4, 1981, pp. 463–503.

[74]Merfeld, D. M., Young, L. R., Paige, G. D., and Tomko, D. L., "Three Dimensional Eye Movements of Squirrel Monkeys Following Postrotatory Tilt," *Journal of Vestibular Research*, Vol. 3, 1993, pp. 123–139.

[75]Lentz, J. M., and Guedry, F. E., Jr., "Apparent Instrument Horizon Deflection During and Immediately Following Rolling Manoeuvres," *Naval Medical Research and Development Command, Rept. MF585.24.004-9022*, 1981, pp. 1–10.

[76]Melvill Jones, G., "Predominance of Anti-Compensatory Oculomotor Response During Rapid Head Rotation," *Aerospace Medicine*, Vol. 35, 1964, pp. 984–989.

[77]Correia, M. J., Luke, B. L., McGrath, B. J., Clark, J. B., and Rupert, A., "The Role of Linear Acceleration in Visual-Vestibular Interactions and Implications in Aircraft Operations," *AGARD CP-579: Neurological Limitations of Aircraft Operations: Human Performance Implications*, 1995, pp. K2-1–K2-5.

[78]Buizza, A., Avanzini, P., and Schmid, R., "Visual-Vestibular Interaction During Angular and Linear Body Acceleration: Modeling and Simulation," *Mathematical and Computational Methods in Physiology*, edited by L. Fedina, B. Kanyr, B. Kocsis, and M. Kollai, Pergamon, Oxford, England, U.K. 1981, pp. 13–19.

[79]Paige, G. D., "The Influence of Target Distance on Eye Movement Responses During Vertical Linear Motion," *Experimental Brain Research*, Vol. 77, 1989, pp. 585–593.

[80]Schwarz, U., Busettini, C., and Miles, F. A., "Ocular Responses to Linear Motion are Inversely Proportional to Viewing Distance," *Science*, Vol. 245, 1989, pp. 1394–1396.

[81]Tomlinson, R. D., Cheung, B., and Blakeman, A., "Responses of the Naso-Occipital Vestibulo-Ocular Reflex in Normal Human Subjects," *IEEE Engineering in Medicine and Biology*, Vol. 19, 2000, pp. 43–46.

[82]Tomko, D. L., and Paige, G. D., "Linear Vestibuloocular Reflex During Motion Along Axes Between Nasoocipital and Interaural," *Annals of the New York Academy of Science*, Vol. 656, 1992, pp. 233–241.

[83]Israel, I., and Berthoz, A., "Contribution of the Otoliths to the Calculation of Linear Displacement," *Journal of Neurophysiology*, Vol. 62, 1989, pp. 247–263.

[84]Israel, I., Chapuis, N., Glasauer, S., Charade, O., and Berthoz, A., "Estimation of Passive Horizontal Linear Whole-Body Displacement in Humans," *Journal of Neurophysiology*, Vol. 70, 1993, pp. 1270–1273.

[85]Gianna, C. C., Gresty, M. A., and Bronstein, A. M., "The Human Linear Vestibulo-Ocular Reflex to Transient Accelerations: Visual Modulation of Suppression and Enhancement," *Journal of Vestibular Research*, Vol. 10, 2000, pp. 227–238.

[86]Tomlinson, R. D., Cheung, B., and Blakeman, A., "Responses of the Translational Vestibulo-Ocular Reflex in Normal Human Subjects During Attempted Cancellation," *IEEE Engineering in Medicine and Biology, in press* (to be published).

[87]Guedry, F. E., "Orientation of the Rotation Axis Relative to Gravity: Its Influence on Nystagmus and the Sensation of Rotation," *Acta Otolaryngology*, Vol. 60, 1965, pp. 30–48.

[88]Benson, A. J., and Bodin, M. A., "Interaction of Linear and Angular Accelerations on Vestibular Receptors in Man," *Aerospace Medicine*, Vol. 37, 1966, pp. 144–154.

[89]Stockwell, C., and Guedry, F., "The Effect of Semicircular Canal Stimulation During Tilting on the Subsequent Perception of the Visual Vertical," *Acta Otolaryngology*, Vol. 70, 1970, pp. 170–175.

[90]Merfeld, D. M., and Young, L. R., "The Vestibulo-Ocular Reflex of the Squirrel Monkey During Eccentric Rotation and Roll Tilt," *Experimental Brain Research*, Vol. 106, 1995, pp. 111–122.

[91]Merfeld, D. M., Zupan, L., and Peterka, R. J., "Humans use Internal Models to Estimate Gravity and Linear Acceleration," *Nature*, Vol. 398, 1999, pp. 615–618.

[92]Hess, B. J. M., and Angelaki, D. E., "Inertial Processing of Vestibulo-Ocular Signals," *Otolith Function in Spatial Orientation and Movement*, edited by B. J. M. Hess and B. Cohen, Annals of the New York Academy of Sciences, Vol. 871 New York Academy of Sciences, New York, 1999, pp. 148–161.

[93]Dichgans, J., and Brandt, T. H., "Optokinetic Motion Sickness and Pseudo-Coriolis Effects Induced by Moving Visual Stimuli," *Acta Otolaryngologica*, Vol. 76, 1973, pp. 144–149.

[94]Probst, T., and Wist, E. R., "Electrophysiological Evidence for Visual-Vestibular Interaction in Man," *Neuroscience Letter*, Vol. 108, 1990, pp. 255–260.

[95]Allum, J. H. J., Graf, W., Dichgans, J., and Schmidt, C. L., "Visual-Vestibular Interactions in the Vestibular Nuclei of the Goldfish," *Experimental Brain Research*, Vol. 26, 1976, pp. 463–485.

[96]Dichgans, J., Held, R., Young, L. R., and Brandt T., "Moving Visual Scenes Influence the Apparent Direction of Gravity," *Science*, Vol. 178, 1972, pp. 1217–1219.

[97]Dichgans, J., and Brandt, T. H., "Visual-Vestibular Interaction and Motion Perception," *Cerebral Control of Eye Movement and Motion Perception*, edited by J. Dichgans and E. Bizzi, S. Karger, New York, 1972, pp. 327–338.

[98]Henn, V., Young, L. R., and Finley, C., "Vestibular Nucleus Units in Alert Monkeys Are Also Influenced by Moving Visual Fields," *Brain Research*, Vol. 71, 1974, pp. 144–149.

[99]Zacharias, G. L., and Young, L. R., "Influence of Combined Visual and Vestibular Cues on Human Perception and Control of Horizontal Rotation," *Experimental Brain Research*, Vol. 41, 1981, pp. 159–171.

[100]Brandt, T., Bartenstein, P., Janek, A., and Dieterich, M., "Reciprocal Inhibitory Visual-Vestibular Interaction. Visual Motion Stimulation Deactivates the Parieto-Insular Vestibular Cortex," *Brain*, Vol. 121, 1998, pp. 1749–1758.

[101]Berthoz, A., Ravard, B., and Young, L. R., "Perception of Linear Horizontal Self-Motion Induced by Peripheral Vision (Linearvection)," *Experimental Brain Research*, Vol. 23, 1975, pp. 471–489.

[102]Daunton, N., and Thomsen, D., "Visual Modulation of Otolith-Dependent Units in Cat Vestibular Nuclei," *Experimental Brain Research*, Vol. 37, 1979, pp. 173–176.

[103]Cheung, B. and Bateman, W., "G-Transition Effects and Their Implications," *Aviation Space and Environmental Medicine*, Vol. 72, 2001, pp. 758–762.

[104]von Beckh, H. J., "Experiments with Animal and Human Subjects Under Sub and Zero-Gravity Conditions During the Dive and Parabolic Flight," *Journal of Aviation Medicine*, Vol. 25, 1954, pp. 235–241.

[105]von Beckh, H. J., "Human Reactions During Flight to Acceleration Proceeded by or Followed by Weightlessness," *Aerospace Medicine*, Vol. 30, No. 9, 1959, pp. 391–409.

[106]Williams, R. S., Werchan, P. M., Fischer, J. R., and Bauer, D. H., "Adverse Effects of Gz in Civilian Aerobatic Pilots." *69th Annual Aerospace Medicine Association Meeting, Proceedings*, 1998.

[107] Melvill Jones, G., "Review of Current Problems Associated with Disorientation in Man-Controlled Flight," Air Ministry Flying Personnel Research Committee, Rept. FPRC 1021, 1957.

[108] Spiegel, E. A., "Studies and Experimental Investigations in Connection with the Prevention and Treatment of Motion Sickness," *Bulletin of Subcommittee on Motion Sickness*, National Research Council, Dec. 1943.

[109] Woodring, S. F., Rossiter, C. D., and Yates, B. J., "Pressor Response Elicited by Nose-Up Vestibular Stimulation in Cats," *Experimental Brain Research*, Vol. 113, 1997, pp. 165–168.

[110] Yates, B. J., and Miller, A. D., "Properties of Sympathetic Reflexes Elicited by Natural Vestibular Stimulation: Implications for Cardiovascular Control," *Journal of Neurophysiology*, Vol. 71, 1994, pp. 2087–2092.

[111] Doba, N., and Reis, D. J., "Role of the Cerebellum and Vestibular Apparatus in Regulation of Orthostatic Reflexes in the Cat," *Circulation Research*, Vol. 34, 1974, pp. 9–18.

[112] Balaban, D., and Porter, J. D., "Neuroanatomic Substrates for Vestibulo-Autonomic Interactions," *Journal of Vestibular Research*, Vol. 8, 1998, pp. 7–16.

[113] Schor, R. H., Steinbacher, B. C., Jr., and Yates, B. J., "Horizontal Linear and Angular Responses of Neurons in the Medial Vestibular Nucleus of the Decerebrate Cat," *Journal of Vestibular Research*, Vol. 8, 1998, pp. 107–116.

[114] Powell, T. J., "Acute Motion Sickness Induced by Angular Accelerations," *Air Ministry Flying Personnel Research Committee, Rept.* FPRC 865, Royal Air Force, England, U.K., 1954.

[115] Spiegel, E. A., "Effects of Labyrinthine Reflexes on the Vegetative Nervous System," *Archives of Otolaryngology*, Vol. 44, 1946, pp. 61–72.

[116] Cheung, B., and Hofer, K., "Coriolis-Induced Cutaneous Blood Flow Increase in the Forearm and Calf," *Brain Research Bulletin*, Vol. 54, 2001, pp. 609–618.

[117] Johnson, W. H., Sunahara, F. A., and Landolt J. P., "Motion Sickness, Vascular Changes Accompanying Pseudo-Coriolis-Induced Nausea," *Aviation, Space, and Environmental Medicine*, Vol. 64, 1993, pp. 367–370.

[118] Sunahara, F. A., Johnson, W., and Taylor N. B. G., "Vestibular Stimulation and Forearm Blood Flow," *Canadian Journal of Physiology and Pharmacology*, Vol. 42, 1964, pp. 199–207.

[119] Ohashi, N., Imamura, J., Nakagawa, H., and Mizukoshi, K., "Blood Pressure Abnormalities as Background Roles for Vertigo, Dizziness and Disequilibrium," *Otorhinolaryngology*, Vol. 52, 1990, pp. 355–359.

[120] Yates, B. J., Aoki, M., Burchill, P., Bronstein, A. M., and Gresty, M. A. "Cardiovascular Responses Elicited by Linear Acceleration in Humans," *Experimental Brain Research*, Vol. 125, 1999, pp. 476–484.

[121] Hume, K. M., and Ray, C. A., "Sympathetic Responses to Head-Down Rotations in Humans," *Journal of Applied Physiology*, Vol. 85, 1999, pp. 1971–1976.

[122] Shortt, T. L., and Ray, C. A., "Sympathetic and Vascular Responses to Head-Down Neck Flexion in Humans," *American Journal of Physiology*, Vol. 41, 1997, pp. H1780–H1784.

[123] Cheung, B., Hofer, K., and Goodman, L., "The Effects of Roll Versus Pitch Rotation in Humans Under Orthostatic Stress," *Aviation Space and Environmental Medicine*, Vol. 70, 1999, pp. 966–974.

[124] Urschel, C. W., and Hood, W. B., "Cardiovascular Effects of Rotation in the Z Axis," *Aerospace Medicine*, Vol. 37, 1966, pp. 254–256.

[125] Convertino, V. A., Previc, F. H., Ludwig, D. A., and Engelken, E. J., "Effects of Vestibular and Oculomotor Stimulation on Responsiveness of the Carotid-Cardiac Baroreflex," *American Journal of Physiology*, Vol. 273, 1997, pp. R615–R622.

[126] Aschan, G., "Response to Rotary Stimuli in Fighter Pilots," *Acta-Otolaryngology*, Supplement 116, 1954, pp. 24–31.

[127] Dowd, P. J., Moore, E. W., and Cramer, R. L., "Effects of Flying Experience on the Vestibular System: a Comparison Between Pilots and Non-Pilots to Coriolis Stimulation," *Aerospace Medicine*, Vol. 37, 1964, pp. 45–47.

[128] Kohen-Raz, R., Kohen-Raz, A., Erel, J., Davidson, B., Caine, Y., and Froom, P., "Postural Control in Pilots and Candidates for Flight Training," *Aviation Space and Environmental Medicine*, Vol. 65, 1994, pp. 523–526.

[129] Brandt, U., Fluur, E., and Zylberstein, M. Z., "Relationship Between Flight Experience and Vestibular Function in Pilots and Non-Pilots," *Aviation, Space and Environmental Medicine*, Vol. 45, 1974, pp. 1232–1236.

[130] Collins, W. E., "Habituation of Vestibular Nystagmus with and Without Visual Stimulation," *Handbook of Sensory Physiology. Vestibular System. Psychophysics, Applied Aspects and General Interpretations*, edited by H. H. Kornhuber, Vol. 6, No. 2, Springer-Verlag, New York, 1974, pp. 369–388.

[131] Gonshor, A., and Melvill Jones, G., "Extreme Vestibulo-Ocular Adaptation Induced by Prolonged Optical Reversal of Vision," *Journal of Physiology (London)*, Vol. 256, 1976, pp. 381–414.

[132] Guedry, F. E., "Visual Control of Habituation to Complex Vestibular Stimulation in Man." *Acta Otolaryngologica*, Vol. 58, 1964, pp. 377–389.

[133] Popov, A. P., "Special Vestibular Training," *Fundamentals of Aviation Medicine*, edited by W. E. Voyachek, English translation by I. Steinman, Univ. of Toronto Press, Toronto, 1943, Chap. 19.

[134] Aubert, H., "Eine Scheinbare Bedeutende Drehung von Objekten bei Neigung des Kopfes Nach Rechts Oder Links," *Virchows Arch.*, Vol. 20, 1861, pp. 381–393.

[135] Howard, I. P., "*Human Visual Orientation*," Wiley, New York, 1982.

[136] Bronstein, A. M., "The Interaction of Otolith and Proprioceptive Information in the Perception of Verticality." *Otolith Function in Spatial Orientation and Movement*, edited by B. J. M. Hess and B. Cohen, Vol. 871, New York Academy of Sciences, New York, 1999, pp. 334–344.

[137] Schone, H., "On the Role of Gravity in Human Spatial Orientation," *Aerospace Medicine*, Vol. 35, 1964, pp. 764–772.

[138] Mittelstaedt, H., "Somatic Graviception," *Biological Psychology*, Vol. 42, 1996, pp. 53–57.

[139] Mittelstaedt, H., "The Role of the Otoliths in Perception of the Vertical and in Path Integration," *Otolith Function in Spatial Orientation and Movement*, Vol. 871, edited by B. J. M. Hess and B. Cohen, New York Academy of Sciences, New York, 1999, pp. 334–344.

[140] Diamond, S. G., and Markham, C. H., "Ocular Counterrolling as an Indicator of Vestibular Otolith Function," *Neurology*, Vol. 33, 1983, pp. 1460–1469.

[141] Takemori, S., Tanaka, M., and Moriyama, H., "An Analysis of Ocular Counter-Rolling Measured with Search Coils," *Acta Otolaryngology (Stockh)*, Suppl. 468, 1989, pp. 271–276.

[142] Kellogg, R. S., "Dynamic Counterrolling of the Eye in Normal Subjects and in Persons with Bilateral Labyrinthine Defects." *Symposium on the Role of the Vestibular Organs in Space Exploration*, NASA, SP-77, 1965, pp. 195–202.

[143]Merryman, R. F. K., and Cacioppo, A. J., "The Optokinetic Cervical Reflex in Pilots of High Performance Aircraft," *Aviation Space and Environmental Medicine*, Vol. 68, 1997, pp. 479–487.

[144]Patterson, F. R., Cacioppo, A. J., Gallimore, J. J., Hinman, G. E., and Nalepka, J. P., "Aviation Spatial Orientation in Relationship to Head Position and Attitude Interpretation," *Aviation Space and Environmental Medicine*, Vol. 68, 1997, pp. 463–471.

[145]Fukuda, T., "Vertical Writing with Eyes Closed. A New Test of Vestibulospinal Reaction," *Acta Otolaryngology*, Vol. 50, 1959, pp. 26–36.

[146]Miura, M., and Sekitani, T., "Follow-Up of Square Drawing Test in Vestibular Neuronitis," *Acta Otolaryngology Supplement*, Vol. 503, 1993, pp. 35–38.

[147]Stoll, W., "Vertical 'X' Sign Test," *Archives of Otorhinolaryngology*, Vol. 233, 1981, pp. 201–217.

[148]Lawerence, D. G., and Kuypers, H. G. J. M., "The Functional Organization of the Motor System in the Monkey. I. The Effects of Bilateral Pyramidal Lesions," *Brain*, Vol. 91, 1968, pp. 1–14.

[149]Lawerence, D. G., and Kuypers, H. G. J. M., "The Functional Organization of the Moor System in the Monkey. II The Effects of Lesions of the Descending Brain-Stem Pathways," *Brain*, Vol. 91, 1968, pp. 15–36.

[150]Fredrickson, J. M., Schwarz, D., and Kornhuber, H. H., "Convergence and Interaction of Vestibular and Deep Somatic Afferents upon Neurons in the Vestibular Nuclei of the Cat," *Acta Otolaryngology*, Vol. 61, 1965, 168–188.

[151]Evart, E. V., Bizzi, E., Burke, R. E., Delong, M., and Thach, W. T., Jr., "Central Control of Movement," *Neurosciences Research Program Bulletin*, Vol. 9, 1997, p. 1.

[152]Lyons, T. J., and Simpson, C. G., "The Giant Hand Phenomenon," *Aviation, Space and Environmental Medicine*, Vol. 60, 1989, pp. 64–66.

[153]Malcolm, R., and Money, K., "Two Specific Kinds of Disorientation Incidents: Jet Upset and Giant Hand," *The Disorientation Incident*, AGARD, Neuilly-Sur-Seine, France, Vol. 95, 1972, A10-1–A-10-4.

[154]Guedry, F. E., Mortensen, C. E., Nelson, J. B., and Correia, M. J., "A Comparison of Nystagmus and Turning Sensations Generated by Active and Passive Turning," *Vestibular Mechanisms in Health and Disease*, edited by J. D. Hood, Academic Press, New York 1978.

[155]Correia, M. J., Nelson, J. B., and Guedry, F. E., "Antisomatogyral Illusion," *Aviation, Space and Environmental Medicine*, Vol. 48, No. 9, 1977, pp. 859–862.

[156]Sipes, W. E., and Lessard, C. S., "A Spatial Disorientation Survey of Experienced Instructor Pilots," *IEEE Engineering in Medicine and Biology*, Vol. 19, 2000, pp. 35–42.

[157]Smith, D. A., Cacioppo, A. J., and Hinman, G. E., "Aviation Spatial Orientation in Relationship to Head Position, Altitude Interpretation, and Control," *Aviation Space and Environmental Medicine*, Vol. 68, 1997, pp. 472–478.

[158]Gottlieb, G., "Ontogenesis of Sensory Function in Birds and Mammals," *The Biopsychology of Development*, edited by E. Tobach, L. R. Avonsen, and R. Shaw, Academic Press, New York, 1971.

[159]Gillingham, K. K. and Previc, F. H., "Spatial Orientation in Flight," *Fundamentals of Aerospace Medicine*, 2nd ed., edited by R. L. DeHart, Williams and Wilkins, Baltimore, MD, 1996, pp. 309–397.

[160]Goodwin, G. M., McCloskey, D. I., and Matthews, P. B. C., "The Contributions of Muscle Afferents to Kinesthesia Shown by Vibration Induced Illusions of Movement and by the Effects of Paralyzing Joint Afferents," *Brain*, Vol. 95, 1972, pp. 705–708.

[161] Lackner, J. R., and Levine, M. S., "Changes in Apparent Body Orientation and Sensory Localization Induced by Vibration of Postural Muscles: Vibratory Myesthetic Illusions," *Aviation Space and Environmental Medicine*, Vol. 50, 1979, pp. 346–354.

[162] Inglis, J. T., Frank, J. S., and Inglis, B., "The Effect of Muscle Vibration on Human Position Sense During Movements Controlled by Lengthening Muscle Contraction," *Experimental Brain Research*, Vol. 84, 1991, pp. 631–634.

[163] Lackner, J. R., "Human Sensory-Motor Adaptation to the Terrestrial Force Environment," *Brain Mechanisms and Spatial Vision*, edited by D. J. Ingle, M. Jeannerod, and D. N. Lee, Martinus-Nijhoff, Dordrecht, The Netherlands, 1985, pp. 175–209.

[164] Edin, B. B., and Vallbo, A. B., "Dynamic Response of Human Muscle Spindle Afferents to Stretch," *Journal of Neurophysiology*, Vol. 63, 1990, pp. 1297–1306.

[165] Skoglund, S., "Joint Receptors and Kinasthesis," *Handbook of Sensory Physiology, III*, A. Iggo and O. B. Ilyinsky, edited by Springer-Verlag, New York, pp: 1002–1025.

[166] Sabbahi, M. A., Fox, A. M., and Druffle, C., "Do Joint Receptors Modulate the Motoneuron Excitability?" *Electromyography Clinical Neurophysiology*, Vol. 30, 1990, pp. 387–396.

[167] Edin, B. B., and Abbs, J. H., "Finger Movement Responses of Cutaneous Mechanoreceptors in the Dorsal Skin of the Human Hand," *Journal of Neurophysiology*, Vol. 65, 1991, pp. 657–670.

[168] Edin, B. B., and Johansson, N., "Skin Strain Patterns Provide Kinaesthetic Information to the Human Central Nervous System," *Journal of Physiology*, Vol. 487, 1995, pp. 243–251.

[169] Edin, B., "Cutaneous Afferents Provide Information About Knee Joint Movements in Humans," *Journal of Physiology*, Vol. 531, 2001, pp. 289–297.

[170] Schmidt, R. A., *Motor Learning and Performance: From Principles to Practice*, Human Kinetics Publishers, Inco, Champaign, Il, 1991.

[171] Rupert, A., "An Instrumentation Solution for Reducing Spatial Disorientation Mishaps," *IEEE Engineering in Medicine and Biology*, Vol. 19, No. 2, 2000, pp. 71–80.

[172] Bles, W., and Kapteyn, T. S., "Circular Vection and Human Posture. I. Does the Proprioceptive System Play a Role?" *Aggressologie*, Vol. 18, 1977, pp. 325–328.

[173] Bles, W., and de Wit, G., "La Sensation De Rotation et la Marche Circulaire," *Aggressologie*, Vol. 19, 1978, pp. 29–30.

[174] Guedry, F. E., and Benson, A. J., "Modification of Per- and Postrotational Responses by Voluntary Motor Activity of the Limbs," *Experimental Brain Research*, Vol. 52, 1983, pp. 190–198.

[175] Bles, W., Jelmorini, M., Bekkering, H., and de Graaf, B., "Arthrokinetic Information Affects Linear Self-Motion Perception," *Journal of Vestibular Research*, Vol. 5, 1995, pp. 109–116.

[176] Fredrickson, J. M. and Schwarz, D. W. F., "Cortical Projections of the Vestibular Nerve," *Handbook of Sensory Physiology*, edited by H. H. Kornhuber, Vol. 6 Springer-Verlag, Berlin, 1974, pp. 565–582.

[177] Holden, M., Ventura, J., and Lackner, J. R., "Stabilization of Posture by Precision Contact of the Index Finger," *Journal of Vestibular Research*, Vol. 4, 1994, pp. 285–301.

[178] Rabin, E., Dizio, P. A., Bortolami, S. B., and Lackner, J. R., "Haptic Stanilization of Posture: Influence of Fingertip Contact Localization in Relation to Axis of Instability," *Society of Neuroscience Abstract*, Vol. 23, 1997, pp. 610.6.

[179] Lackner, J. R., Dizio, P., Jeka, J., Horak, F., Krebs, D., and Rabin, E., "Precision Contact of the Fingertip Reduces Postural Sway of Individuals with Bilateral Vestibular Loss," *Experimental Brain Research*, Vol. 126, 1999, pp. 459–466.

[180]Lackner, J. R., and Dizio, P., "Altered Sensorimotor Control of the Head as an Etiological Factor in Space Motion Sickness," *Perceptual and Motor Skills*, Vol. 68, 1989, pp. 784–786.

[181]Lackner, J. R., and Dizio, P., "Gravitational Effects on Nystagmus and Perception of Orientation," *Representation of Three Dimensional Space in the Vestibular, Oculomotor and Visual Systems*, edited by B. Cohen and V. Henn, Annals of the New York Academy of Science, Vol. 545, 1989, pp. 93–104.

[182]Pompeiano, O., "Experimental Central Nervous System Lesions and Posture," *Vestibular and Visual Control on Posture and Locomotor Equilibrium: 7th International Symposium of the International Society of Posturography*, edited by M. Igrashi, and F. O. Black, 1985.

[183]Benson, A. J., and Barnes, G. R., "Responses to Rotating Linear Acceleration Vectors Considered in Relation to a Model of the Otolith Organs," *Fifth Symposium on the Role of the Vestibular Organs in Space Exploration*, NASA SP-314, 1970, pp. 221–236.

[184]Bos, J., Cheung, B., and Groen, E., "The Somatogravic Effect Without Concomitant Angular Motion," TNO Rept. TM-01-B002, 2001.

[185]Lechner-Steinleitner, S., "Interaction of Labyrinthine and Somatoreceptor Inputs as Determinants of the Subjective Vertical," *Psychological Research*, Vol. 40, 1978, pp. 65–76.

[186]Graybiel, A., and Clark, B., "Validity of the Oculogravic Illusion as a Specific Indicator of Otolith Function," *Aerospace Medicine*, Vol. 36, 1965, pp. 1173–1181.

[187]Brandt, T., Buchele, W., and Arnold, F., "Arthokinetic Nystagmus and Ego-Motion Sensation," *Experimental Brain Research*, Vol. 30, 1977, pp. 331–338.

[188]Bles, W., Kloren, T, Buchele, W., and Brandt, T., "Somatosensory Nystagmus: Physiological and Clinical Aspects," *Advance Oto-Rhino-Laryngology*, Vol. 30, 1983, pp. 30–33.

[189]de, Graaf, B., Bos, J. E., Wich, S., and Bles, W., "Arthokinetic and Vestibular Information Enhance Smooth Ocular Tracking During (Self-) Motion," *Experimental Brain Research*, Vol. 101, 1994, pp. 147–152.

[190]Easton, R. D., Green, A. J., Dizio, P., and Lackner, J. R., "Auditory Cues for Orientation and Postural Control in Sighted and Congenitally Blind People, *Experimental Brain Research*, Vol. 118, 1998, pp. 541–550.

[191]Lackner, J. R., "Induction of Illusory Self-Rotation and Nystagmus by a Rotating Sound Field," *Aviation, Space, and Environmental Medicine*, Vol. 48, 1977, pp. 129–131.

[192]Marme-Karelse, A. M., and Bles, W., "Circular Vection and Human Posture II. Does the Auditory System Play a Role?" *Agressologie*, Vol. 18, 1977, pp. 329–333.

[193]Cullen, J. K., Collins, M., Dobie, T. H., and Rappold, P. W., "The Effects of Perceived Motion on Sound-Source Lateralization," *Aviation, Space and Environmental Medicine*, Vol. 63, 1992, pp. 498–504.

[194]Graybiel, A., and Niven, J. I., "The Effect of a Change in Direction of Resultant Force on Sound Localization: the Audiogravic Illusion," *Psychophysiological Factors in Spatial Orientation*, edited by A. Graybiel, 1950.

[195]Lyons, T. J., Gillingham, K. K., Teas, D. C., Ercoline, W. R., and Oakley, C., "The Effects of Acoustic Orientation Cues on Instrument Flight Performance in a Flight Simulator," *Aviation, Space and Environmental Medicine*, Vol. 61, 1990, pp. 699–706.

[196]Gillingham, K. K., and Teas, D. C., "Flight Evaluation of an Acoustic Orientation Instrument (AOI). (Abstract)," *Aviation, Space and Environmental Medicine*, Vol. 63, 1992, pp. 441.

[197]Endsley, M. R., and Rosiles, S. A., "Auditory Localization for Spatial Orientation," *Journal of Vestibular Research*, Vol. 5, 1995, pp. 473–485.

[198]King, R. B., and Oldfield, S. R., "The Impact of Signal Bandwidth on Auditory Localization: Implications for the Design of Three-Dimensional Audio Displays," *Human Factors*, Vol. 39, 1997, pp. 287–295.

[199]Nelson, W. T., Bolia, R. S., McKinley, R. L., Chelette, T. L., Tripp, L. D., and Esken, R. L., "Localization of Virtual Auditory Cues in a High +Gz Environment," *Proceedings of the Human Factors and Ergonomics Society's 42nd Annual Meeting,* Human Factors Society, 1998, pp. 97–101.

[200]McKinley, R. L., Erickson, M. A., and D'Angelo, W. R., "3-Dimensional Auditory Displays: Development, Applications, and Peformance," *Aviation, Space and Environmental Medicine*, Vol. 65, Suppl. 5, 1994, pp. A31–38.

[201]Oving, A., van Breda, B., and Wrtkhoven, P. J., "Effects of Three-Dimensional Auditory Information on Spatial Situation Awareness of Pilots," NASA Technical Repts. TD98-0284, 1998.

[202]Bronkhorst, A. W., and Veltman, J. A., "Evaluation of a Three Dimensional Auditory Display in Simulated Flight," In *AGARD Conference Proceedings 596*, (AGARD, CP-596;) Audio Effectiveness in Aviation, AGARD, 1997, pp. 5-1–5-6.

[203]Gilkey, R. H., Simpson, B. D., Isabelle, S. K., Anderson, T. A., and Good, M. D. "Design Considerations for 3-D Auditory Displays in Cockpits," AGARD, CP-596, 1997, pp. 2-1–2-10.

[204]Leduc, P. A., Riley, D., Hoffman, S. M., Brock, M. E., Norman, D., Johnson, P. A., Williamson, R., and Estrada, A. (1999). 'The Effects of Sleep Deprivation on Spatial Disorientation," U.S. Army Aeromedical Research Lab., USAARL Rep. 2000–09, Fort Rucker, AL, 1999.

[205]Collins, W. E., "Some Effects of Sleep Loss on Vestibular Responses," *Aviation, Space and Environmental Medicine*, Vol. 59, 1988, pp. 523–529.

[206]Dowd, P. J., "Sleep Deprivation Effects on the Vestibular Habituation Process," *Journal of Applies Psychology*, Vol. 59, 1974, pp. 748–752.

[207]Lackner, J. R. and Dizio, P., "Multisensory, Cognitive, and Motor Influences on Human Spatial Orientation in Weightlessness," *Journal of Vestibular Research*, Vol. 3, 1993, pp. 361–372.

[208]Lackner, J. R., and Dizio, P., "Human Orientation and Movement Control in Weightlessness and Artificial Gravity Environments," *Experimental Brain Research*, Vol. 130, 2000, pp. 2–26.

[209]Previc, F. H., "The Neuropsychology of 3-D Space," *Psychological Bulletin*, Vol. 124, 1998, pp. 123–164.

Chapter 3

Visual Orientation Mechanisms

Fred H. Previc*

Northrop Grumman Information Technology, San Antonio, Texas

I. Introduction

S PATIAL orientation is carried out by many different sensory and motor systems in the brain, principally the visual, vestibular, somatosensory/proprioceptive, and ventromedial motor systems. Of the different sensory systems the visual system is arguably the most important for maintaining orientation, and in highly structured environments it predominates over the other sensory systems in a manner known as visual dominance.[1]

The predominance of visual orientational inputs stems from at least three major factors. First, visual inputs emanate from practically the entire three-dimensional space lying in front of us and do not emanate from localized points in the environment, as do sounds. Second, visual inputs provide a precise spatial mapping that offers, at least in central vision, a spatial resolution of ∼1 min of arc, which exceeds that of the auditory system by over an order of magnitude.[2] Third, visual inputs, unlike those from the vestibular system and, to a lesser extent, the somatosensory one, do not habituate during constant-velocity motion. Hence, the visual system continues to provide precise information concerning the spatial layout of the environment over time and is crucial in detecting motion and altitude above ground in nonaccelerating vehicles. Unlike many other creatures, humans do not possess effective atmospheric-pressure detectors and magnetoreceptors that sense altitude or position on Earth directly (see Ref. 3). Without good visual information our perceptual systems begin to break down, and our orientation in Earth-fixed space suffers. Such breakdowns are exemplified in circling behavior while walking upright and blindfolded in a 1-G field on earth,[4,5] in velocity underestimations when we pursue a slowly moving target,[6] and in orientational misjudgments when we are tilted relative to gravity or are subjected to a tilt of the gravitoinertial force vector away from zero (see Chapter 7).

This material is declared a work of the U.S. Government and is not subject to copyright protection in the United States.

* Senior Member, Technical Staff.

Conversely, the visual system is limited by the fact that it is a very sluggish system relative to the nonvisual orientational systems. Whereas the auditory system has 1-ms resolution in determining spatial location of a sound source and the vestibular system relays signals to the eye movement control centers in as little as 12 ms, visual signals require approximately 100 ms to reach the visual cortex. For this reason we can pursue visual targets at much higher sinusoidal velocities while moving our head, which evokes vestibular signals, than with our heads stationary and only visual pursuit being used. Whereas head-free tracking can effectively follow target velocities as high as 10 Hz, visual pursuit begins to suffer at frequencies as low as 0.5 Hz (Ref. 7; see also Chapter 2, Sec. VI).

As will be detailed in Sec. II, there are now believed to be multiple systems in humans that participate in various visual perceptual-motor functions in different realms of three-dimensional space.[2] The system that is believed to play the major role in maintaining orientation in Earth-fixed space is known as the ambient visual system. The term ambient refers to the fact that we are typically not consciously aware of the visual inputs that we use to infer our orientational status. It was first coined by Trevarthen[8] and Held[9] in reference to visual localization capabilities and, in an extrapolation of Schneider's[10] two-visual-system concept, was contrasted with the focal visual system, which was more involved in pattern vision in central vision. The two-modes-of-processing concept was later applied by Leibowitz and colleagues to a number of phenomena related to vehicle control and spatial disorientation.[11,12] Leibowitz and colleagues distinguished between the following:

> A *focal mode* which is concerned with object recognition and identification and in general answers the question of "what." Focal vision involves relatively fine detail (high spatial frequencies) and is correspondingly best represented in the central visual fields. Information processed by focal vision is ordinarily well-represented in consciousness and is critically related to physical parameters such as stimulus energy and refractive error.

and

> An *ambient mode* which subserves spatial localization and orientation and is in general concerned with the question of "where." Ambient vision is mediated by relatively large stimulus patterns so that it typically involves stimulation of the peripheral visual field and relatively coarse detail (low spatial frequencies). Unlike focal vision, ambient vision is not systematically related to either stimulus energy or optical image quality .... Presumably because they involve subcortical structures, the conscious concomitant of ambient stimulation is low or frequently completely absent (Ref. 11, p. B4-1).

Previc[2] later distinguished between two peripherally dominated perceptual-motor systems in the primate brain: an *action-extrapersonal* system used in navigation and orientation to objects in topographical space (e.g., location in a room) vs an *ambient-extrapersonal* system used in maintaining orientation in Earth-fixed (gravitational) space. It is this latter system that is most closely aligned with the function of spatial orientation as defined in this textbook (see Chapter 1, Sec. I) and with the other major sensory systems involved in spatial orientation (e.g., the vestibular and somatosensory/proprioceptive). This system will hereafter be

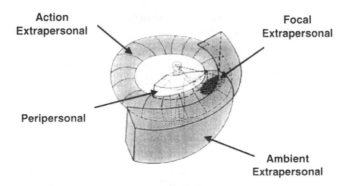

Fig. 1   Four behavioral realms in three-dimensional space. (Reproduced from Ref. 2.)

referred to as both the ambient extrapersonal system and the ambient system, with the visual portion of it known as the ambient visual system. By contrast, the *focal-extrapersonal* system in Previc's scheme will be considered synonymous with the focal visual or focal system. (It has also been argued[13] that two ambient visual systems exist—a primitive one dominated by inputs from the peripheral visual field and a "high-level" one that responds more to complex motion in the central visual field. Despite some quantitative differences in the way the central and peripheral portions of the retina process motion, as discussed later in Section IV.A, there is little evidence for a qualitative division of the ambient visual field.)

In the remainder of this chapter, the specific functions of the ambient visual system, the requirements for adequately stimulating it, and the neural networks subserving it, will all be discussed in detail.

II.   Nature of Three-Dimensional Space

According to a recent model,[2] the three-dimensional visual space around us can be compartmentalized into four major realms: a reaching space (*peripersonal*), an object-recognition space (*focal-extrapersonal*), a topographical space (*action-extrapersonal*), and an Earth-fixed space (*ambient-extrapersonal*) (see Fig. 1). These spaces are not rigid, in that focal-extrapersonal space—linked to the position of the eyes—can move in all three planes as the eyes move, whereas ambient-extrapersonal space represents the most distant portion of the visible world, whether that be the frame of a small room or the distant horizon outdoors.

Each of the systems dealing with a particular realm of three-dimensional space has its own preferred portion of space, its preferred sensory and motor pathways, and its unique coordinate system. For example, the peripersonal system and especially the focal extrapersonal system rely mostly on central vision, where reaching and object recognition take place. Indeed, the resolution of the retina decreases by an order of magnitude at 15 deg off axis[14] and cannot support detailed pattern recognition beyond this point. Whereas the peripersonal system primarily deals with visual inputs within binocular reaching space (2 m), the focal-extrapersonal system generally deals with objects ranging from slightly inside peripersonal space to distant space, depending on where the ocular fixation point lies in depth. Conversely, the action-extrapersonal and ambient-extrapersonal systems deal with our interactions within the entire visual field and require the inputs of peripheral vision. Action-extrapersonal space appears to be centered around 30 m in depth whereas the ambient-extrapersonal system relies on the most distant portion of the visible world. In terms of vertical biases, the peripersonal system controls reaching in lower-field, near-body space (where the arms reside), whereas the focal and action-extrapersonal systems are oriented toward more distant objects in the upper field (because more distant space is biased toward the upper field as a result of the slope of the ground plane up and away from us). The ambient visual system, on the other hand, relies on distant visual cues located below the horizon because we mainly use nearby ground objects to help gauge our motion in space[15,16] and ground texture to help to determine the slant of the world. The movement of a large portion of the distant field is also the most reliable indicator that self-motion has occurred in space, as local motion in distant space can represent movement of objects and motion in near space can be perceived as lying within the subject's inertial frame.

In terms of sensorimotor interactions, the focal-extrapersonal system is in many respects the simplest one, relying almost exclusively on visual inputs and oculomotor scanning.[2] The other systems all make use of bodily signals emanating from the vestibular and somatosensory/proprioceptive systems in addition to vision, as well as auditory ones in the case of the action extrapersonal system. The other systems also make use of movement circuits besides eye movements, for example, arm control by the peripersonal system, horizontal head control by the action-extrapersonal system, and control of the entire body (including the lower limbs) by the ambient-extrapersonal system.[2]

Finally, the four systems appear to use different spatial coordinate frames in interacting in three-dimensional space.[2] The peripersonal reaching system is tied mainly to a trunk- or shoulder-centered coordinate frame, the focal-extrapersonal system aligns the world in terms of retinotopic space linked to the position of the eyes in the orbit, the action-extrapersonal system is centered around the head, and the ambient-extrapersonal system revolves around the gravitational vertical and Earth horizontal. The four systems can operate somewhat independently of one another. For example, the reaching system is neither concerned with recognition of objects (because it mostly deals with objects that have already been recognized) nor with where the reached-for object is located within our larger topographical environment. Similarly, the focal-extrapersonal system is less concerned with where our arms are located in space or whether our posture is upright than in the bringing the searched-for object into our central vision (fovea) for inspection (e.g., foveation). Conversely, the action-extrapersonal system is less concerned with what a particular object looks like in detail than in orienting to it because of its general salience or using it as a spatial landmark to guide our locomotion. Finally, the ambient-extrapersonal system is less concerned with where we are located in a particular environment than in the orientation of our posture and movement relative to space in general.

Nevertheless, all systems are somewhat dependent on the ambient visual system. For example, reaching is affected by gravity, a perceptually stabilized visual world is necessary to process the details of objects, and the calculation of head position requires knowledge of how our body is positioned in space. In some respects, then, the ambient visual system serves as the bedrock for the other systems,[2] as evidenced by the fact that the ambient visual system interacts in a widely distributed manner with the rest of the brain (see Sec. V.B).

III. Function of Ambient Vision

The general function of ambient vision is to *stabilize the world perceptually in Earth-fixed coordinates*. Specifically, ambient vision provides us with a veridical three-dimensional spatial frame, including the distance and slant of the world, our tilt relative to it, and our motion within it. A number of cues are used by the ambient visual system to perform the preceding task, including motion flow, linear perspective, texture size and density gradients, motion parallax, brightness gradients, and aerial perspective. All of the important visual cues in ambient space are monocular, as the contribution of binocular vision is primarily within the first few meters surrounding us (i.e., peripersonal space). Indeed, a structured ambient visual world looks and behaves fundamentally the same whether one looks at it with one eye closed or with both eyes open, although binocular vision does improve spatial perception in impoverished environments.[17] The remarkable feature of ambient vision is that it essentially turns, in a preconscious manner, the various ambient visual cues into referents that then help to yield a stabilized and mostly veridical visual world. For instance, coherent visual motion over a wide field of view (FOV) allows us to perceive self-motion in a stable world; the convergence of lines in linear perspective helps us perceive depth in a Euclidean world in which the lines appear to remain parallel as they recede; and the rotation of the visual world on our retinas when we tilt our heads in the lateral plane leads us to perceive self-tilt in an upright world. In this sense ambient vision is very similar to what Gibson[18] termed the visual world, which he contrasted with the pictorial visual field:

> Pictorial seeing then differs astonishingly from ordinary objective seeing. The field is bounded whereas the world is not. The field can change in its direction-from-here but the world does not. The field is oriented with reference to its margins, the world with reference to gravity. The field is seen in perspective while the world is Euclidean..... In the field...shapes are deformed during locomotion, as is the whole field itself, whereas in the world everything remains constant and it is the observer who moves (Ref. 18, p. 42).

The way in which visual signals from the ambient system help stabilize the world remains somewhat mysterious, but a number of perceptual and motor responses have been implicated. For example, ambient visual scenes affect the position of the body via inputs to the vestibulospinal system[19] and influence head position by means of the optokinetic-cervical reflex, or OKCR.[20,21] Visual scenes further alter eye position by means of optokinetic nystagmus (OKN), whose slow phase compensates for motion of the head in the horizontal and vertical planes, and torsional eye movements that partly compensate for head tilts in the lateral plane.[22] Numerous models have postulated, therefore, that perceptual stability requires inputs from the ambient visual system.[23,24] However, no single optokinetic mechanism is in and of itself sufficient to stabilize the world, for example, the magnitude of optokinetic-cervical reflexes and torsional eye movements saturate at less than 20 deg in the roll plane,[20,22,25] the onset of visually mediated postural reactions is too slow (~1 s) to avoid substantial displacement of the visual world,[26] and even OKN requires time to build up.[1] It is generally held, therefore, that ambient visual inputs contribute mainly sustained, low-frequency signals to our spatial orientation system, whereas nonvisual systems provide a more transient signal to help stabilize our perceptual world in the immediate aftermath of self-motion (see Refs. 7 and 27).

The predominance of low-frequency signals in visual orientation is reflected in the visual frequencies and motions that are most likely to produce postural changes and the visually induced illusion of self-motion known as vection (see Sec. IV.A). The predominance of sluggish signals in visual orientation is further illustrated by the finding that the decomposition of visual motion caused by eye movements vs self-motion in space can only be accomplished visually when the oculomotor speed is below 2 deg/s. Above 2 deg/s, nonretinal information about the velocity and direction of the eye movements is needed to correctly infer one's heading in space.[28]

The effectiveness of ambient vision in stabilizing the perceptual frame is well documented when we are moving in a well-structured environment. For example, in experiments that manipulated the motion of the visual environment during head rotations, subjects could detect as little as a 2–3% offset of the visual world.[24] In a structured environment a good level of perceptual stability (~5%) during lateral head turns is achieved even for a relatively small FOV (40 deg). Similarly, the perceived vertical does not deviate from the actual one when our heads are tilted in a structured visual environment.[1] The tolerance for scene deviations during eye movements (8%) is slightly greater than for head movements, presumably because of weaker proprioceptive signals concerning eye movements[30] and a tendency during eye movements to attend to a small region surrounding the target.[31] The stability of the visual world is still less during fore-aft locomotion, with more stability occurring during the normal (forward) direction of locomotion.[29]

The stability of the visual world begins to disintegrate when briefly presented visual fields or those with small extents are used. This can easily be demonstrated by placing a tube in front of one's face and slowly moving one's head (and eyes) across the visual field. In contrast to a full-field viewing situation, the world will noticeably appear to move in the direction opposite to ones slow head movement. A breakdown in perceptual stability has also been shown to occur in the laboratory during slow pursuit movements, resulting in the occurrence of illusory movements of stationary small targets or briefly presented large visual backgrounds, known as the Filehne illusion.[6,24] During lateral (roll) head tilts, an illusory motion of a small line opposite to the head tilt, known as the Aubert or A effect, occurs for head tilts 60 deg or larger.[1] (A smaller and less consistent illusory target motion with the head, known as the E effect, occurs for head tilts between 30 and 60 deg; see Chapter 2, Section IX). The instability of the visual world in the absence of ambient vision is also dramatically evidenced after a long period of fixation on a small spot in an otherwise darkened environment, which leads one to erroneously perceive random gyrations of the spot (see Chapter 7, Sec. II.B.4 for a fuller discussion of the autokinetic illusion).

The stability of the structured world in full view is not absolute, however. Whenever we make a movement that is unplanned, such as pressing on and displacing our eyeball in its orbit when the other eye is closed, the world might appear to move because we have not provided an efferent signal to ignore the visual movement. Also, there can be noticeable "jumps" in the visual world during high-acceleration activities such as running and jumping, which produce what has been termed oscillopsia. Oscillopsia is not a problem for the average person moving about in our world, but it can be a more serious problem in persons with damage to their vestibular organs and in astronauts returning from space, whose otolith organs are less sensitive to (and hence, less able to compensate for) shifts in the head relative to gravity.[32] Yet another example of a "stability" failure is when we place our heads in an inverted position or wear inverting lenses or fly inverted; the world does not actually appear "upright" in this situation, although it might feel upright.[1,18] Indeed, a strong dominance of upright ambient visual inputs over discrepant gravitoinertial signals in the form of the somatogravic illusion only exists if the gravitoinertial tilt signals are 15 deg or less.[33] Beyond 15 deg of tilt, seated subjects begin to feel tilted even when a tilted visual room is level relative to them.[34] When standing upright and receiving powerful somatosensory input from the soles of their feet, most subjects feel a visual room to be tilted even at tilts of only 5 deg.[35]

A powerful ambient visual system is not always beneficial to us if it presents an image of the world that deviates from Earth-fixed space. This is shown in Fig. 2,

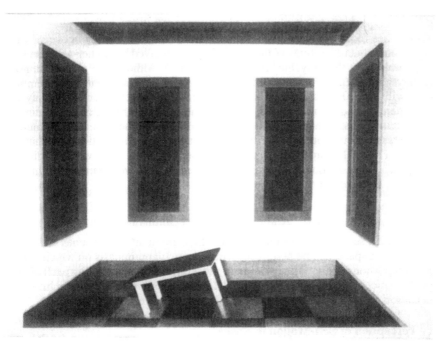

Fig. 2   Illustration of an Ames room that is actually slanted to the right but appears level (source unknown).

motion cues to judge his or her altitude above ground and fail to maintain proper clearance (see Chapter 7, Sec. II.A.4).

Whereas continuous visual motion is not required in topographical way-finding,[43] it is more important in perceiving and controlling our orientation in Earth-fixed space, as reflected in the breakdowns in postural control, manual control, and motion perception that occur in a flickering environment.[44–46] Optical-flow discrimination is reportedly one of the few basic visual measures that predicts flight performance.[47] The optical focus of expansion can be used by pilots in aim-point estimation during landing,[48] and dynamic changes in runway splay angle (the angle which the projected edges of the runway makes with a line perpendicular to the horizon) can be used during curved approaches.[49] However, other researchers have questioned the role of motion cues in landing performance.[50,51]

1. Vection

The flowfield is manifested as changes in the retinal image, which can then be used to infer self-motion through space. When visual motions recreate the optical flow patterns that normally accompany real-world motion in a particular axis, they often give rise to an illusion of motion in that same plane known as vection. In its classic form vection refers to the sensation of self-motion opposite to the movement of the visual scene, although vection can also occur to moving tactile and, to a lesser extent, moving sound sources (see Chapter 11, Sec. IV.B.1.c and IV.B.2.b). Vection was first investigated over 125 years ago by Mach,[52] who described the situation of a train passenger sensing illusory motion in response to the opposite movement of an adjacent railway car (Fig. 5). It can occur in response to yaw, pitch, and roll motion (in which cases it is referred as angular vection), as well as in response to linear motion in all three axes (in which case it is known as linearvection). Although similar in many respects, the three types of angular vection also exhibit some unique aspects. For example, yaw vection around the Earth-vertical axis (also traditionally termed circularvection) is arguably the strongest of the three types, mainly because there are no inputs from the otolith organs to contradict the vection. Pitch vection is more likely to be asymmetric than the other two types, with downward motion reputed to produce stronger vection than upward motion, possibly because of the ecological prevalence of downward terrain flow during forward motion. Roll vection is distinguished by its saturation at a much lower velocity (30 deg/s) than angular vection in the other two axes.[54]

The ability to accurately infer self-motion from visual scenes requires the ability to distinguish optical flow caused by the movement of one's body from movement of objects in the world or movements of the eyes. Indeed, when a moving scene slowly begins to produce vection after a latency of several seconds the external scene itself begins to slow down and might even appear to stop. Object motion is generally characterized by local discontinuities in the flow pattern (i.e., relative motion) and is therefore distinguishable from flow generated by self-motion, which is uniform across the entire visual field. Movement of the retinal image caused by saccadic eye movements is also distinguishable from optical flow

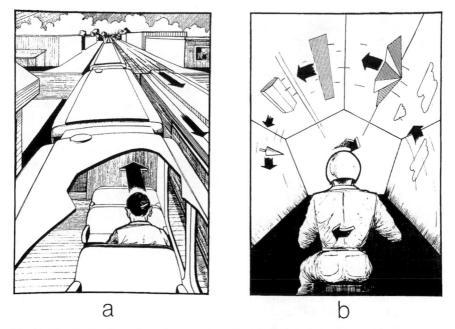

a   b

Fig. 5   Vection in the railroad car, as described by Mach. (from Ref. 53.)

during self-motion by its greater speed, but during slow pursuit movements the retinal image by itself is more difficult to discriminate from a heading change in space.[28]

Vection can lead to spatial disorientation (SD) in the aerial environment, especially during helicopter hovering (see Chapter 7, Sec. II.A.4). Among fixed-wing pilots, however, vection is rather infrequent because 1) most terrain optical flow is very slow, given the typically large distances between the aircraft and the ground and 2) most optical flow occurs in association with actual motion of the aircraft. Nevertheless, vection is still a very useful phenomenon to review because it sheds light on which properties of visual scenes are most important in influencing our orientation in space.

Despite our ability to characterize the optical flowfield mathematically and the fact that optical-flow rate provides an invariant measure of our self-motion in space, it is unlikely that the human brain actually performs such a formal, complex analysis. Rather, much evidence suggests that the human brain uses simpler metrics in determining the speed and direction of self-motion in the environment. For example, several studies suggest that the rate at which "edges" flow past us, which is controlled by a combination of texture density and speed of self-motion, is generally a more powerful cue to forward speed than is global optical-flow rate.[55,56] (Although edge rate per se is not sensitive to altitude but only to airspeed and changes thereof, a misperception of forward airspeed might nonetheless prevent a correct resolution of the already described flow-rate ambiguity resulting from the tradeoff between ground speed and eye heights above ground.) This is why we feel that we are going much slower than our actual speed on an expressway (few edges), whereas the reverse occurs on a small road through a forest (many edges). Texture-density effects have also been observed in the case of angular vection, where low-spatial-frequency gratings (containing fewer contours per degree of visual angle) are generally more effective than high-spatial-frequency gratings in generating vection, although this might not be as true for the central visual field.[57,58] Finally, our estimation of how fast we are approaching terrain appears to be mainly based on the expanding size of objects[59] or a combination of expanding size and edge rate[60] rather than a global analysis of the three-dimensional optical flow. Indeed, humans tend to misperceive a large object moving toward them at a slower speed as moving faster than a smaller object moving at a faster speed.[61]

2. Visual Requirements for Vection

This section will examine the visual requirements for generating vection and other motion-linked visual orientation phenomena. The following factors will be discussed: field-of-view effects, temporal frequency, spatial factors (including optical quality), and fixation and attentional issues.

Perhaps the most widely studied stimulus parameter related to vection is FOV. Most of these studies have examined the effects of the area or location of the stimulus and its eccentricity in two-dimensional space, but a substantial number have also studied how the radial distance of the stimulus affects the perception of vection. Most researchers who have studied FOV effects on vection have concluded that vection is dependent on the area of the stimulus,[62-64] although some researchers have claimed the peripheral field to be more important than the central field even when they are equated in area.[54,65,66] Because visual area increases by the square of distance from the center of the visual field, peripheral stimuli of the same lateral extent in terms of eccentricity clearly produce a greater amount of vection than do central stimuli, although this has not always been found.[67,68] Many commonly experienced vection episodes tend to occur when a large object in the peripheral visual field moves, although this might partly be because vection is strongest when we do not actually attend to the vection-inducing display as would be more likely in peripheral vision.

Although most laboratory studies have shown that little vection is produced by stimuli within the central 50 deg,[64,66] vection can be elicited even by a minimal real-world visual environment. For example, a pilot once relayed to me that he felt forward acceleration (i.e., getting closer) toward what he thought was an airplane with two tail lights during a night sortie; in fact, the "plane" turned out to be two aircraft, each with one tail light, that were separating. The roles of the central and peripheral visual fields can also differ depending on what type of motion is involved. For example, radially diverging flow is better seen by the central retina, which makes sense in that such flow typically occurs in the center of the visual field when we locomote forward and gaze in the direction of motion (see Fig. 4). Conversely, lamellar or parallel flow, which is typically seen at the observer's side during forward locomotion, is more powerful in the retinal periphery.[69] The lower thresholds for processing motion in the central retina[70] might help compensate for the fact that radial flow near the focus of expansion in central vision has a slower velocity than does lamellar flow in the periphery.[69] Lamellar flow might be more useful in judging acceleration and altitude, which might partly account for the importance of the visual periphery in producing vection and in controlling aircraft altitude and airspeed.[71]

In line with the reliance of ambient vision on the most distant portion of the visual world, it has been observed, in the case of scenes having competing radial distances, that scenes which are perceived as lying in the background dominate over ones perceived as foreground in terms of vection.[16,62,72–76] In particular, little or no vection can be elicited when observers view a moving foreground against a stationary background. Attesting to the higher-order perceptual nature of vection, the ability of visual backgrounds to suppress vection depends not on their actual distance but on their perceived distance.[77] In line with the ecological basis of vection, it has also been shown that the ability of stationary background scenes to suppress vection is greater for circularvection than for linear vection produced by expanding flow patterns.[77] This result is to be expected because the distant visual field does not move very much during locomotion (see earlier discussion), whereas the visual displacement during an angular motion is the same for both near and far objects.

In terms of temporal parameters, slowly moving or slowly changing visual scenes generally tend to produce the greatest amount of vection. According to Berthoz and colleagues,[78,79] linear vection in particular appears to resemble a temporally low-pass system, with a roll off around 0.1 Hz. In normal subjects the experience of exclusive self-motion in tilted rooms is eliminated when the room-motion frequency reaches 1 Hz (Ref. 35). This is not surprising in that vection in the laboratory typically requires 5–10 s to develop,[26,66] which would correspond to frequencies of 1 Hz or below. (Shorter latencies can occur with richly structured, real-world scenes, however.) Typically, both angular and linear vection also reach a saturation velocity before falling off with increasing visual speed (see Refs. 54, 68, 78, and 80), with roll vection peaking at a lower stimulus velocity ($\sim$30 deg/s) (Ref. 54) than yaw vection ($\sim$60 deg/s) (Ref. 80). The preceding findings confirm that the visual mechanisms mediating vection are not driven by transient motions. On the other hand, the fact that vection also tends to begin to "habituate" after 10–20 s indicates that its temporal response is not completely low pass.

Spatial and optical factors also exhibit an important influence on vection. As noted earlier, both global motion analysis and vection are influenced by the number of texture elements in a scene. When some texture elements in a scene are stationary, vection is a function of the number of elements that are moving, up to about 50% (Ref. 66). However, vection does not necessarily increase in magnitude with increasing texture density when all texture elements are in motion.[68] Higher spatial frequencies (associated with a greater number of edges) tend to produce greater faster vection[78] and a greater perceived speed in the vection-producing stimulus,[66] without necessarily increasing the magnitude of vection. As noted earlier, some evidence suggests that yaw vection is strongest at an intermediate spatial frequency,[57] with higher spatial frequencies playing a greater role in centrally mediated vection and lower spatial frequencies driving vection in the periphery.[58] This might be because the peripheral visual field, which is generally less sensitive to higher spatial frequencies, has more trouble organizing the high-frequency information into coherent stimulus motion. What is certain, however, is that the higher spatial frequencies (e.g., details) in a given stimulus are not needed to produce good vection. For example, degradation of a stimulus by reducing its overall luminance or contrast (by blurring) has little effect on the magnitude of vection,[79,81] although visually mediated postural stability might be somewhat reduced.

Finally, it must be recognized that vection is ultimately a higher-order perceptual (albeit largely preconscious) phenomenon that involves an inference concerning what is moving in the world. Hence, it is susceptible to where the observer is attending or fixating. Generally, vection is reduced when observers fixate upon the optokinetic scene. In this case observers are more likely to treat the scene as an object and perceive object-rather than self-motion.[23] On the other hand, if observers fixate upon a stationary object that is superimposed in front of the optokinetic scene, vection is markedly enhanced, with the scene appearing stationary and the object appearing to move with the observer. These different percepts are partly caused by the fact that there is more smooth retinal motion used for generating angular vection when the subject does not pursue the optokinetic stimulus, but they are also partly related to attentional factors. For example, if a subject merely attends but does not actively pursue the optokinetic background stimulus, the sensation of vection is reduced. This confirms our subjective experience in the real environment, in that vection illusions are most likely to occur when a large portion of the outside world begins to move when we are not attending to it.

3.   Other Effects of Ambient Visual Motion

In addition to vection, ambient visual motion influences a number of other phenomena, including shifts in the subjective vertical and straight-ahead, postural shifts mediated by vestibulospinal reflexes, manual biases, and at least two oculomotor reflexes. In general, postural reflexes appear to be more closely linked to the ambient visual mechanisms determining vection than some of the other phenomena.

When we view an optokinetic stimulus moving about an Earth-vertical vertical axis, we also tend to perceive the straight-ahead as deviated in the same direction as the stimulus motion.[82] This illusory shift of a static percept can be as much as 9 deg, for a wide-FOV stimulus rotating at 100 deg/s. A similar phenomenon occurs when we view a wide-FOV stimulus rotating around an Earth-horizontal axis in roll. In this case a deviation of the subjective vertical occurs, which reaches a maximum of about 15 deg. These deviations are in some cases linked to motor biases, such that path displacements in forward walking are comparable to the deviation of the straight-ahead during wide-FOV yaw stimulation[66] and manual biases to wide-FOV moving roll stimuli are also on the order of about 15 deg (Ref. 64).

Visually induced postural biases typically occur in the direction of scene motion, for example, a rightward body tilt occurs while the observer views rightward roll motion (Fig. 6). Postural biases have been shown to be very closely linked to mechanisms determining vection,[64] as would be expected given that both phenomena pertain to the movement of the overall body in space.[2] Like vection, visually induced postural changes are dominated by inputs from the peripheral retina and the more distant visual background.[64,73,83] Visually induced postural responses appear to dependent on the area of the moving stimulus,[64,84,85] although one study found a central advantage for equal-area stimuli.[86] Visual postural effects are also

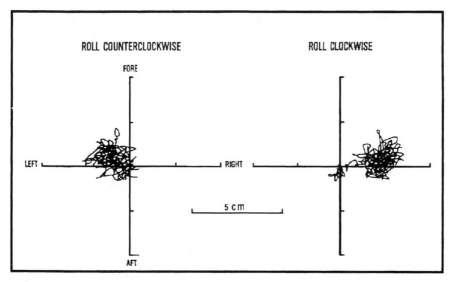

Fig. 6   Effects of counterclockwise and clockwise visual roll motion on postural sway. (Reproduced from Ref. 26.)

stronger for scenes with a high texture density (spatial frequency).[84] Like vection, visual postural responses are also influenced by the type of flow (e.g., radial vs lamellar) in the central and peripheral visual field.[69] Visually induced postural changes generally occur with a shorter latency than does vection,[26] but they exhibit a similar low-pass temporal response peaking about 0.1 Hz (Refs. 85–88). However, postural biases do not as closely match the shift of the subjective visual vertical in response to wide-FOV roll motion, in that the former only tend to be a few degrees (because the human body is inherently unstable and greater deviations would lead to frequent falls), whereas the visual vertical can deviate up to 15 deg (see preceding discussion).

The effects of visual scenes on manual control are different from those on postural control in several respects. First, manual control is relatively more influenced by central (<50 deg) visual motion,[64,89] and even a three-fold advantage in peripheral area leads to only a small manual bias favoring the peripheral visual stimulus.[64] However, both manual and postural effects are dominated by coherent visual motion beyond the plane of fixation. This makes sense in that manual reaching activity predominantly occurs in the central 60 deg of the visual field and to nearby targets, which one superimposes on the more distant ambient visual field (Ref. 2; Fig. 1). In terms of temporal frequency, visual effects on the manual system are dominated by higher frequencies than visually mediated postural effects and vection,[88] although they still are predominantly low frequency (peaking at <0.5 Hz).

The effects of visual motion on the oculomotor system can also be mediated by the ambient visual system, but only in some instances. One oculomotor response that might be related to ambient mechanisms is optokinetic torsion, the rotation of the eyes in the same direction as a moving roll stimulus (see Fig. 7). Like the optokinetic-cervical reflex, optokinetic torsion helps to stabilize the horizon during

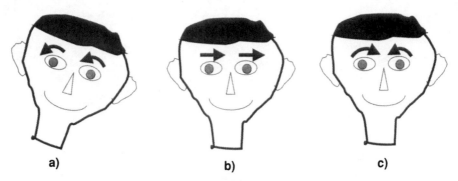

a)   b)   c)

Fig. 7   Three types of visually induced eye movements: a) torsion, b) horizontal nystagmus, and c) cyclovergence.

a postural tilt (in this case a head relative to gravity); also like the OKCR, optokinetic torsion saturates at ~15 deg. Optokinetic torsion is best when wide-FOV motion is presented to the observer,[90] and it exhibits a low-pass temporal response similar to vection.[22] Though closely related, vection and optokinetic torsion are not identical, however, as optokinetic torsion does not reverse its direction after a moving scene stops, whereas vection aftereffects do occur in response to a moving roll stimulus. Also, vection appears to be slightly more dominated by the visual periphery than is optokinetic torsion.

Another oculomotor system that is affected by wide-FOV visual motion is optokinetic nystagmus, which refers to the movement of the eyes in response to fronto-parallel linear motion and yaw and pitch angular motion (Fig. 7). The slow phase of OKN moves in the same direction of the visual stimulus and complements vestibularly generated slow-phase nystagmus (see Chapter 2, Sec. IV) in helping to stabilize the position of the eyes in space during head movements. Some researchers[57] have argued that OKN and vection are closely related, but most studies suggest that OKN is driven by a separate system. For example, OKN is severely diminished when the central 20 deg of the visual field is removed,[91] and it is dominated by motion in the plane of fixation.[92] Accordingly, OKN is driven by a coplanar and central (<50 deg) stimulus when the latter is placed in conflict with motion from a more distant and/or larger surround.[62,66] Another indication that OKN and vection are not closely related is that vertical OKN when created by visual pitching is usually asymmetric, with upward OKN slow phase faster than downward OKN,[93] whereas vection is not always asymmetric in the same direction as OKN.[93] [One explanation for the vertical OKN asymmetry relates to the already discussed slant of the ground plane away from us and the generally higher vestibular-ocular gains for near objects.[94] Optokinetic nystagmus to upward-moving scenes should have a higher gain because the slanted ground-plane comes "closer" to us (and thereby moves faster) when we tilt our heads downward than when we tilt our heads upward (resulting in downward movement of the visual world).]

B.   Perception of Self-Tilt in Space

A second important function of ambient vision is to convey how we are tilting in space. Whereas on Earth we use these inputs to maintain our upright posture

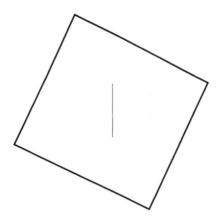

Fig. 8   Rod-and-frame illusion.

during standing and locomotion, pilots use this information to keep their aircraft upright while flying. As with ambient motion, tilted ambient scenes influence both perception (e.g., the sense of upright) as well as postural and oculomotor responses.

In terms of perception of the upright, tilted ambient scenes can influence both our perception of roll and pitch. In the case of roll, this percept is referred to as the *subjective vertical*. In the case of pitch, the percept has been referred to as the *visually perceived* (apparent) *eye level*.[95,96] It has already been noted that upright, structured visual scenes prevent misjudgments of the vertical when subjects are tilted; conversely, tilted visual scenes can lead to illusions of self-tilt. One of the classic demonstrations of how even modest scenes influence the subjective vertical is the rod-and-frame illusion.[97] In this illusion surrounding a vertical line with a visual frame (typically a luminous square) results in subjects setting the line (or perceiving vertical) in the direction of the frame tilt in order to make the line appear vertical (see Fig. 8). The rod-and-frame illusion, if carried out in an otherwise dark room, does not require a very large visual frame to achieve its effect; in fact, the rod-and-frame illusion typically reaches a maximum of about 5–10 deg for a frame diameter of about 20 deg. The rod-and-frame effect maximizes at 20–25 deg of tilt because increasing visual tilt makes the frame appear more like an upright diamond (which would be the case at 45 deg of tilt).

There is dispute among researchers whether the rod-and-frame effect truly represents an ambient visual effect. Some researchers have argued that this effect is an induction effect rather than a true ambient visual effect and is similar to other size, shape, and motion illusions in which a surrounding stimulus of one appearance or motion induces the opposite appearance or motion in an enclosed smaller stimulus that is neutral or stationary in appearance. Indeed, the induced-motion phenomenon in which a small spot appears to move opposite to a larger surround (e.g., a moon against moving clouds) has been shown to differ from other ambient visual phenomena in terms of both FOV (more influenced by central stimuli) and stimulus depth (more influenced by coplanar stimuli).[74,98] In support of the induction hypothesis, the rod-and-frame effect itself is clearly influenced by the size of the gap between the rod and the tilted frame, regardless of the size of the frame.[99]

Other researchers argue that the rod-and-frame effect is both an induced phenomenon at small frame sizes (<10 deg) and an ambient visual phenomenon when larger frame sizes are used. In support of this "dual" hypothesis, large frames have been shown to affect perceived head tilt in that seated subjects usually align their heads in the direction of the frame when instructed to align it with gravity.[100,101] However, the head and body tilts are typically much smaller (by about 50–75%) than the tilt of the rod, suggesting that ambient orientational influences cannot account for the entire rod-and-frame effect, even with larger frames. Moreover, Previc et al.[88] were unable to produce a postural bias in a standing subject even when a computer-generated scene with an extremely large (>100 deg) FOV was used, so that somatosensory input from the feet might be sufficient to break the visual effect. Ocular torsional effects have also been produced by large, static, tilted visual frames, but these are typically less than a degree,[103] which is considerably less than that produced by a scene moving in roll and far less than the magnitude of the rod-and-frame effect.

A stronger visual dominance has been achieved with tilted rooms, dating back to the "haunted swings" at fairgrounds in the late 1800s. Tilted rooms that are painted to seem furnished have proven capable of creating substantial self-tilts and shifts of the subjective vertical (see Sec. IV.D.1). Furnished rooms have been known to produce tilts of the visual vertical of as much as 15 deg (Ref. 104), whereas rooms that lack a clear polarity produce tilts of only a few degrees at most. Conversely, viewing a level room eliminates all sensations of tilt when subjects are exposed to gravitoinertial shifts of up to 15 deg (Ref. 33). The contribution of natural scenes to our upright sense is further confirmed by the fact that individuals who have been forced to live continuously in tilted buildings following earthquakes can tolerate room tilts of up to 4 deg relative to gravity,[105] despite the incongruence of their visual and graviceptor inputs. (Indeed, this author lived for many years in a hillside building that was slightly tilted, without ever noticing its tilt until it was subsequently discovered during a foundation survey.)

One postural reflex induced by visual roll tilt that has received a considerable amount of interest in recent years is the optokinetic-cervical reflex.[20,21] In a seated individual this reflex produces a tilt of the neck in the direction of the scene up to a maximum of about 15–20 deg (Refs. 20 and 25), which helps to keep the head aligned with the horizon during tilts of the body relative to gravity (see Fig. 9). Although the effects of FOV on the OKCR are not as clear cut as for whole-body postural effects and vection,[20] this reflex does not occur when pilots view a limited-FOV artificial horizon on the cockpit instrument panel. Hence, it is considered important for understanding the different orientational frames of reference used by pilots in controlling aircraft attitude during actual flight (see Chapter 9, Sec. III.A).

Ambient visual tilt effects have also been studied in the pitch plane, with similar results to the effects of tilted visual frames in roll. When subjects view a room tilted in pitch, a stationary light spot appears to be displaced opposite to the tilt of the room, for example, a downward-tilted back wall produces an upward perceived shift of the spot and vice versa.[106] Correspondingly, subjects perceive the level of their own eyes to move with the room; for example, a back wall that is tilted downward by about 20 deg will result in a lowering of perceived eye level by about a third of that amount.[106] Subjects shift their posture in the direction

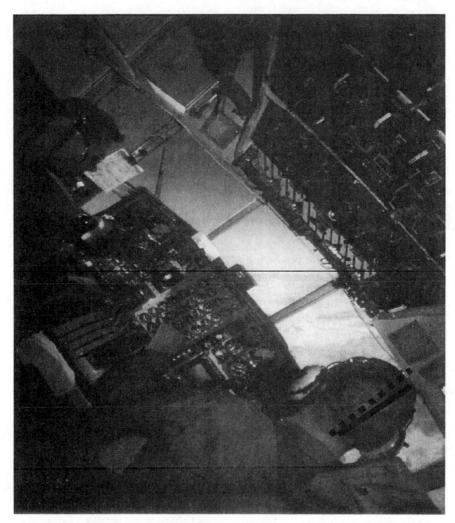

Fig. 9 Illustration of how the head is partially aligned with the background horizon (thin horizontal line across center of photo) during the optokinetic-cervical reflex (solid line on back of copilot's head represents orientation of aircraft; dashed line is orientation of head). (Photo reproduced with permission of Cmdr. Fred Patterson.)

of the pitched room by about the same amount when setting it to the perceived gravitational vertical.[107] Some of these visual-pitch effects evidently do not require a fully structured environment, as two upright parallel lines placed on an otherwise dark wall can, when pitched, prove as effective as a fully lit room in influencing perceived eye level. (This is not true of two horizontal lines when pitched, however.) The intersection of two vertically parallel but pitched lines on the central vertical meridia of the retinas is evidently a sufficient cue for perceived eye level.[106] However, two pitched lines do not approach the effectiveness of a

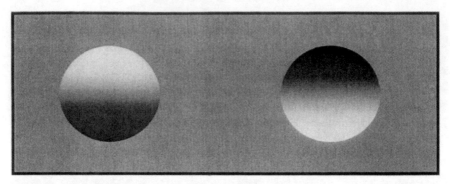

Fig. 10 Visual inversion illusion. An illustration of how we assume that light ordinarily emanates from above. The top-lit object appears as a convex sphere, whereas the bottom-lit object appears to be a concave depression.

structured pitched room in producing postural deviations.[107] (Even more dramatic is the effect of a wide-FOV, tilted outdoor scene. In Big Bend National Park in West Texas, one particular canyon—Santa Elena—rises over 450 m above the Rio Grande River. The formations on its massive walls are tilted, which from the entrance of the canyon gives rise to a powerful illusion that the narrow Rio Grande River in central vision is steeply tilted in the opposite direction!)

An extreme example of how visual scenes can affect our orientation in space is the visual inversion illusion. Although visual inversions are not readily achievable in a laboratory environment, reorientation illusions of close to 90 deg can occur in about half of adult subjects when they lie supine (on their back) and view a room whose floor lies directly above them.[34] In flight, visual inversion illusions are quite common and are usually caused by changes in the normal luminance gradient, often in conjunction with a reduction or reversal of the normal 1-G resultant gravitoinertial force. Ordinarily, the brightest portion of our world lies on top because of the elevated position of the sun; indeed, on a normal day the brightness of the sky is several times that of the ground just below the horizon. Our assumption that light shines from above is demonstrated in the two objects in Fig. 10. The object on the left appears as a sphere because it is lightest on top. Conversely, the object on the right appears concave because it is lightest on the bottom and is assumed to be open on top to let the light from above shine through. This normal luminance gradient outdoors can be reversed in certain weather conditions, however, which can lead to pilots experiencing dangerous inversion illusions during flight (see Chapter 7, Sec. II.A.3).

C. Perception of Distance and Slant

The final major function of ambient vision is to provide a veridical registration of the distance and slant of the ground plane in front of us. Slant refers to the angle of a surface relative to the fronto-parallel plane, that is, the plane orthogonal to the surface of the Earth and the viewer's straight-ahead line of sight, although some researchers prefer the term inclination when referring to tilt about an Earth-horizontal axis (i.e., toward or away from the observer). [One must distinguish between geographical slant (the slope of the terrain away from the normal plane

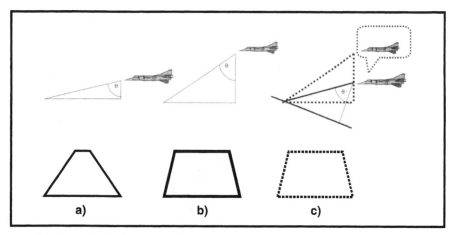

Fig. 11   Ambiguity of slant and distance approaching runways of equal length and width from the same range. The runway projection is shown below each figure: a) approaching a level runway at a low altitude, b) approaching a level runway at a high altitude, and c) approaching an up-sloping runway at an altitude lower than that of Fig. 11b. The altered slant angle in Fig. 11c produces a runway projection or splay angle (....) that is similar to what occurs when flying at a higher altitude above a normal surface plane (Fig. 11b) and can lead a pilot to overestimate altitude.

of the earth's surface) and optical slant (which also takes into account the visual angle between the eyes and the ground). Optical slant can occur in the absence of geographical slant.[108] Distance and slant information are especially important for judging altitude above ground while flying. The reason that they are considered together is because many of the same cues are used in judging both slant and depth (e.g., perspective). Unfortunately, there exists a fundamental ambiguity between the perception of surface slant and distance, which causes problems similar to the already noted optical-flow ambiguity in judging altitude above ground. As shown in Fig. 11, flying over upsloping terrain decreases the perspectival splay angle, as would normally be the case when flying at a higher altitude. Hence, flying over an upsloping surface tends to create the illusion of flying too high and a corresponding tendency to lower the altitude of the aircraft (see Chapter 7, Sec. II.B.3).

As with other ambient visual phenomena, distance and slant judgments can be quite poor in an impoverished visual environment. In such environments observers tend to overrely on the size and shape of familiar objects[108] because ordinarily changes in the retinal size and shape of objects reflect changes in their distance or slant relative to us (see Sec. IV.C.3 for a further discussion of size and shape constancy). Observers are also influenced by remembered spatial layout and specific distance tendencies derived in part from the resting state of accommodation and vergence (see Sec. IV.C.1). In a structured environment, on the other hand, observers' distance estimates tend to be close to veridical.[108]

1. Binocular Cues to Distance and Slant

The issue of how much and under what circumstances binocular cues contribute to ambient distance and slant perception has been debated for many decades. The major binocular cues involve 1) retinal disparity (the differently located images of a more or less distant object on the retinas of the left and right eyes, 2) convergence (the angle of offset between the visual axes of the two eyes, with increased convergence associated with fixation on nearer objects), and 3) accommodation (the focusing power of the lens, which is closely tied to convergence and increases with decreasing viewing distance). In general, binocular cues are believed to be most valuable for judging distances within peripersonal space (2 m),[2,37,109] which is why binocular cues are important in reaching and other manual behaviors.[110,111]

Retinal disparity is involved in perceiving both static depth and motion in depth, as well as surface slant. In principle, retinal disparity provides very precise estimates about the relative depths of objects, but it must be scaled by vergence information to provide absolute depth information[112] and is a somewhat sluggish system.[113] Indeed, retinal disparity (in the form of horizontal shear disparity) is a very poor cue for detecting sudden changes in surface slant, although it plays a more important role at longer inspection durations.[113] Horizontal retinal disparity is a cue primarily for detecting the depth and motion in depth of smaller targets,[114] although the vertical disparities resulting from different perspective views of a scene require much larger FOVs (see later discussion in this section). Retinal disparity is also of limited value at large distances; although under ideal conditions retinal disparity can extend out to 200 m, disparity information is believed to be of little value beyond ~50–75 m (Refs. 109 and 115). Indeed, it has repeatedly been shown that binocular vision is not required for normal landing performance in aircraft.[114]

Vergence is another binocular cue to the depth of objects, but absolute knowledge of vergence position has been shown to be of dubious utility in judging depth.[116,117] Indeed, individuals can make large tracking vergence movements without seeing any movement of a target in depth.[118] Like disparity cues, vergence information appears to be most useful when registering the depth of small, near targets.[119] Convergence can also influence depth judgments indirectly by means of changes in perceived size. This phenomenon, known as convergence micropsia,[120] relates to the perceptual minification of images as they come closer to us, which aids in maintaining size constancy of objects. However, convergence micropsia is only believed to affect perceptual judgments within a distance of ~1 m (Ref. 120).

It has also been claimed that accommodation, which is reflexively tied to convergence, can indirectly influence distance judgments by means of a similar phenomenon known as accommodative micropsia.[121] However, accommodative micropsia has been questioned on the basis of studies that have paralyzed accommodation during convergence,[122] and it has been argued that it affects size perception by 1–2% at most.[123] In any case there is little any evidence that accommodation affects perceived distance,[108,124] regardless of the specific mechanism. Accommodative micropsia and associated distance misjudgments are claimed to be a major problem associated with head-up displays because they are believed to direct the pilot's accommodation toward its resting state or "dark focus" (slightly <1 m) rather than at optical infinity.[125,126] It has even been claimed that the increased accommodation is a source of aircraft mishaps,[125,126] but other perceptual and attentional traps can account for the impaired ability to orient to the distant ground plane with these displays (see Chapters 7 and 9). [For example, it is difficult to focus on a distant object when a more proximal structured field (e.g., a splattered windscreen) is superimposed on it, in what is known as the Mandelbaum Effect.[127]]

One set of binocular cues that might be important for the registration of visual slant are the cyclodisparities resulting from the slant of the visual world as well as torsional misalignment and cyclovergence of the eyes (see Fig. 7c). It is generally agreed that the horizontal cyclodisparities (in which the shear gradient from the top to bottom of a slanted image is opposite in the two eyes) are useful in perceiving surface inclination. However, a more recent theory suggests that it is the difference between vertical and horizontal disparity shearing that contributes to our perception of slant.[128] The vertical disparities are best detected with wide-FOV stimuli,[119] which we use to torsionally align our eyes to the proper slant of the overall visual world.

Cyclodisparities are nullified by cyclovergence movements, which are disjunctive torsional movements of the eyes. In the example shown in Fig. 7c, known as incyclovergence, the left eye is rotated clockwise and the rightward one counterclockwise (from the standpoint of the observer). Cyclovergence is useful in a situation wherein the disparity of the two retinal images varies as a function of elevation and distance from the observer. In incyclovergence, for example, the image of the upper-most portion of a vertical plane is most likely to appear at a coplanar or uncrossed (far) disparity, whereas the image of the lower-most portion of the ground plane occurs at a crossed or "near" disparity. This results in the "top-away" slanted ground plane being in complete binocular registry. The fact that incyclovergence is stronger than the ecologically inconsistent excyclovergence[128] indicates that cyclovergence might be important in perceiving and adjusting for the top-away visual slant of the world. Several other pieces of evidence suggest that cyclovergence is related to ambient visual processing, including the fact that 1) it requires FOVs beyond 40 deg to be effective; 2) it exhibits a low-pass temporal response, being dominated by frequencies less than 0.1 Hz (Ref. 129); and 3) it is ordinarily not under voluntary, conscious control. Thus, it is possible that the capacity of the ambient visual system to perceive a parallel (Euclidean) ground plane despite its optical inclination might depend at least partly on the complex interplay of cyclodisparity information and cyclovergence state.

2. Monocular Cues to Distance and Slant

Beyond a few meters, the world looks essentially similar whether one is viewing it through one eye or both. This makes it clear that whatever are the contributions of binocular cues to our perception of three-dimensional space they are not critical to it. A good illustration of the predominance of monocular cues is the rotating Ames trapezoidal window (see Fig. 12). Rather than an object with transparent panes, this "window" is actually a trapezoidal figure whose monocular depth cues (perspective and shading) are incompatible with one of its edges appearing in front as it turns. Hence, if it is viewed from a few meters away, a three-dimensional Ames window does not appear to rotate 360 deg as it spins about its center vertical axis, but rather appears to alternately rotate back and forth 180 deg. Inside of this distance, the actual rotation of the figure can be discerned because of retinal disparity and other binocular cues.

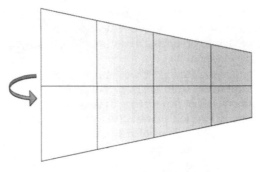

Fig. 12 Ames window, which when set in motion about its center vertical axis, appears to flap back and forth rather than rotate 360 deg because we cannot overcome the monocular cues that indicate the right portion of the window is in back.

The major static monocular cues to depth and surface slant are derived from the three-dimensional geometry of the visual world.[18] These cues include *linear perspective* (the convergence of parallel lines upon a radially distant vanishing point), *compression* or foreshortening (gradients that compress the more radially distant portions of distant space), and *texture density* (i.e., wider spacing of texture elements in the near ground plane). These three major monocular cues to depth are shown in Fig. 13. Element-size gradients are typically a combination of the effects of linear perspective and compression, as evidenced by the smaller grid elements in the top of the grid in Fig. 13. However, element size can also serve as a cue to depth when the observer changes his or her distance to a fronto-parallel surface lacking perspective and compression. Motion parallax is another cue based on the geometry of three-dimensional space and our motion through it, as already noted. Although motion parallax cues have a range slightly greater than that of

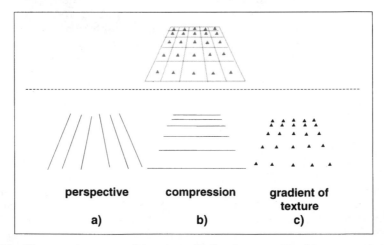

Fig. 13 Three major monocular cues to depth: a) perspective, b) compression, and c) gradient of texture. All are contained in the grid at top.

retinal disparity, their use is also mainly confined to peripersonal space.[108,109] Other monocular cues to depth such as luminance gradients, aerial perspective, height in field, and occlusion have also been implicated in distance perception.

One reason for regarding linear perspective, compression, and texture density as ambient visual cues is that we are not consciously aware of the slant of the world that is present on our retinas as we look out at the ground plane. Rather, we perceive the normal ground plane as a Euclidean (flat) surface extending outward to the horizon. A second reason for regarding perspective, compression, and texture density as ambient visual cues is that they tend to be less effective with very small FOVs,[130,131] although almost all monocular-depth cues have been studied with FOVs less than 50 deg. Finally, all three of these cues are available for distance judgments at the large distances at which the ambient visual system normally operates in the outdoor environment.[109]

Perspective is arguably the most powerful cue to distance, altitude, and slant, especially if there are clear lines present (as on a grid). Like optical flow, perspective is scaled for eye-height, with decreasing altitude resulting in larger splay angles.[132] The best-known example of how perspective affects perceived distance (as well as perceived size) is the corridor illusion, first described by Gibson[18] (see Fig. 14). Other examples are the illusory Ames room[36] and Ames windows, a terrain version affected judgments of aimpoint elevation during

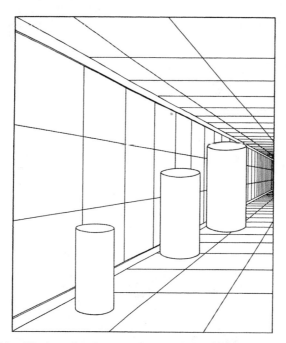

Fig. 14   Corridor illusion, showing the three major monocular cues to depth: perspective, compression, and gradient of texture. (Gibson, James J., *The Perception of the Visual World.* **Copyright © 1950 by Houghton Mifflin Company. Used with permission.)**

simulated landings.[133] Numerous studies have shown that perspective exerts a powerful effect on distance perception, although it cannot totally dominate over other distance cues.[108] One typical study showed that false perspective information simulating corridor lengths of 675 and 225 cm (when the actual corridor lengths were 450 cm) led to perceived lengths of 459 and 332 cm, respectively.[134] Grid textures that provide good perspective (as well as compression) information are much more effective than random textures in overcoming false retinal disparity gradients during slant perception,[113] at least for long, static exposures. Vertical textures containing meridian lines with good perspective cueing (Fig. 13c) have been shown to be best at influencing surface inclination judgments. However, perspective is not as effective when the texture is irregular.[113]

Compression has until recently been viewed as less effective than perspective in judging optical slant.[108] Generally, subjects tend to underestimate the amount of surface slant on the basis of compression alone, and their slant judgments are dominated by perspective cues when the latter is placed in conflict with them.[113,135] However, other findings indicate that compression can be effective in perceiving slant,[130] especially for curved surfaces.[136]

The least effective of the three most important static monocular depth cues appears to be texture-density. The use of texture-density cues alone leads to gross misperceptions of surface slant, with slant estimates attaining only about 20% of predicted value.[108] Relative to perspective and compression, texture density suffers the further disadvantage in that it requires the assumption that a surface texture is homogeneous; otherwise, changes in surface density can lead to reversals of the geometrically predicted texture gradient. When flying over a sparsely vegetated terrain, for example, local increases in elevation (e.g., ridges) would be expected to decrease texture spacing to a pilot flying at a constant altitude. However, the cooler temperatures and greater rainfall at higher elevations can actually produce the reverse—denser vegetation. Texture-density information can be most effective in surface slant and distance perception when it is able to complement perspective and compression cues.[136]

In simulated flying tasks perspective has clearly been shown to be the predominant cue. For example, a texture containing lines parallel to the direction of forward motion (such as in Fig. 13a) has been shown to be superior to a texture containing only lines perpendicular to the direction of forward motion (such as in Fig. 13b).[71,132,137] In actively controlling altitude, perspective lines by themselves can be even more effective than grid textures containing both types of cues. The advantage of perspective lines in controlling altitude might partly be caused by the fact that forward motion by itself creates substantial movement of a perpendicular (compressive) texture, thereby adding "noise" to the changes resulting from loss of altitude.[132] This is why in a hover task containing lateral as opposed to forward disturbances/motion perpendicular textures fare much better.[138] The advantage of perspectival splay is greater when compared to dot textures,[137,139] even if only two perspective lines are presented.[139]

The remaining monocular cues to depth vary in their range and degree of effectiveness.[109] Two cues—aerial perspective and luminance—are based on the decreased brightness and contrast of the more distant terrain. Aerial perspective[18] refers to the lowered contrast and bluish tint of terrain located in the distance, caused

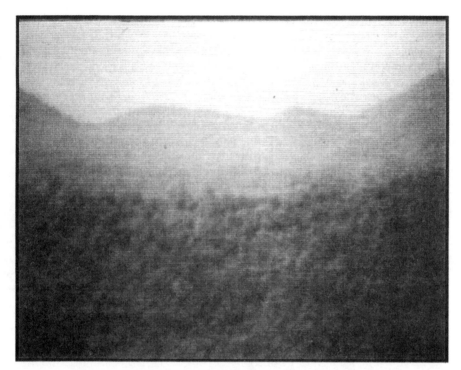

Fig. 15 Illustration of aerial perspective, which increases the brightness, reduces the contrast, and adds a bluish tint to the more distant terrain.

by greater atmospheric scattering of short-wavelength light. Aerial perspective is much reduced for thinner and less hazy atmospheres, for example, astronauts reported on the moon that distant mountains appeared much closer than they actually were. An example of aerial perspective is shown in Fig. 15. Luminance gradients also affect perceived perception,[140] although they play a less powerful role in depth judgments than they do in orienting to the upright, particularly in the daytime.[18] For example, because of aerial perspective and reduced shadowing in the distance distant hills might actually appear brighter than nearby ones (Fig. 15). However, a nighttime or otherwise impoverished scene with reduced brightness and contrast (e.g., a nighttime runway enveloped by mist or light fog) will appear farther away than is actually the case. This leads to serious problems in maintaining the proper approach and clearance during landing and while wearing night-vision devices (see Chapter 7).

Height in field and occlusion also contribute to our perception of distance. Height in field can be used as a depth cue because of the ecological tendency for the terrestrial ground plane to slope upward and away from us so that more distant objects are located higher in the visual field. Although height in field is a more powerful cue than once believed,[37] it has reportedly little value beyond 50–100 m (Ref. 109) in judging the distances of objects and might be less relevant in the aerial environment in which a pilot is oriented more perpendicularly to the ground plane. However, the perceived elevation of the horizon, in reference to the runway aimpoint, reputedly provides an important and essentially height-invariant cue to pilots in estimating their glide slope during landing.[50]

Occlusion is a powerful cue to depth at all distances, but it is only a cue to *relative* rather than absolute depth and it is useless when a surface plane as seen from above is flat and free of occluding surfaces. Occlusion is also limited when the occluding surface cannot be distinguished from the occluded surface because of sparse terrain, as an adequate terrain is required to perceive both the optical-flow and texture-gradient cues that distinguish surfaces from one another.

In summary, static monocular cues to slant and distance are very powerful and can easily override binocular cues to depth (especially beyond 2 m) and even optical flow cues. Of the static monocular cues, perspective splay (from parallel lines) and compression (from lines perpendicular to the direction of forward motion) exert the greatest influences over distance and slant judgments and appear to operate in a mostly ambient fashion. However, monocular cues such as known-size and perspective are based on assumptions about objects and terrain features that can, as discussed in the following section, lead to serious misjudgments concerning one's orientation relative to the ground.

3. Size and Shape Invariance in Judgments of Distance and Slant of Objects

One of the fundamental assumptions that we make about our perceptual world is that objects are inherently rigid, that is, they do not spontaneously change their size and shape, but rather exhibit constancy. This is particularly true of our focal visual system, which is responsible for recognizing objects rather than in determining their motion or orientation in space. If we from experience assume that an object is associated with a characteristic size and shape, then changes to its projective size and shape on the retina should be associated with changes in the angle or distance of our viewpoint. For example, a larger-than-normal projective shape would indicate that the object is closer to us. A highly trapezoidal shape would be construed as a rectangle that is tilted away from the frontal plane. These principles are known as the size–distance invariance and shape–slant invariance hypotheses.[108]

These invariances are far from perfect and are, at least in impoverished environments, consistently violated, for example, object slant tends to be grossly underestimated when only one or two monocular cues are available.[17,141,142] Nevertheless, there are clear instances when perceived size and shape do influence distance and surface–slant judgments in the aerial environment. The effect of abnormal size on distance judgments is greatest when the object is a familiar one and the judgment is made in a reduced-cue environment, for example, smaller-than-normal planes (e.g., drones) look more distant than larger-than-normal planes (e.g., C-5 cargo planes), contributing to a velocity overestimation in the former case and a velocity underestimation in the latter case.[143] This illusion has contributed to serious distance misjudgments in nighttime landings and other low-level flight situations (see Chapter 7, Sec. II). However, the distance misperception might be limited to the object itself and might not affect the overall scale of the surrounding room, if the latter is visible.[108] The shape–slant invariance has also been shown to be very weak, although it can also influence surface–slant judgments in reduced-cue environments[108] and affect glide-slope judgments during nighttime landings. For example, the projection of an upsloping runway, or the outline of a runway at night, might appear to have a greater perceived length-to-end-width ratio (i.e., will appear less trapezoidal) than a normal runway.[53,141] Because of shape-constancy, a pilot might presume not that the runway has changed in its projective shape but rather that he or she has changed his approach angle or distance to it (see Chapter 7, Sec. II.B.3 for a further discussion of illusory landing situations).

D. Simulating Ambient Vision

A major goal of research aimed at understanding the mechanisms of ambient vision is to be able to recreate it using artificial systems, such as spatial disorientation demonstrators (see Chapter 8, Sec. III). The fact that visual dominance occurs so readily in the real world under normal photopic (i.e., daylight) viewing conditions provides one important guidepost to synthetically creating a realistic ambient visual scene. The findings described throughout this chapter concerning self-motion perception, distance perception, and other ambient visual phenomena also provide insights as to what is needed to reproduce ambient vision. Despite all that is known concerning ambient vision and despite the supposed immersiveness of typical virtual reality displays, it has actually proven very difficult to recreate ambient vision except when using all but the most sophisticated computer-generated imagery or three-dimensional structured environments.

The difficulties in reproducing ambient vision are illustrated by the problems in overcoming one particular nonvisual disorientation illusion—the somatogravic illusion. This illusion is experienced in a forward-accelerating vehicle as a pitch-up sensation because of the backward tilt of the resultant gravitoinertial vector away from gravity (see Chapter 6, Sec. III.A). This illusion is easily broken when viewing a normal daylight scene through an aircraft window, but all attempts in novice subjects to break this illusion using SD demonstrators including the Advanced Spatial Disorientation Demonstrator (ASDD) at Brooks Air Force Base, Texas (see Chapter 8, Sec. III.D), have proven unsuccessful.[102,144,145] These failures have occurred despite the fact that ASDD possesses a very wide FOV (58 deg × 114 deg) and nearly collimated scene image.

1. Requirements for Synthetic Visual Systems

Based on knowledge of the cues required for generating ambient visual perceptions, there are at least five general requirements for a synthetic visual system to recreate the ambient visual world. First, such a system should possess a wide FOV, subtending at least 60 deg and preferably >100 deg in extent. Although real-world scenes do not have to subtend that much to dominate our orientational percepts and create a stable visual world, they, too, have a lower limit to their effectiveness (usually <10 deg) and are more influential as their area is increased. A major problem for artificial systems that "wrap around" is that they must be corrected for their spherical projection, that is, a scene that depicts roll motion around a horizontal axis while looking straight ahead must show vertical motion when looking 90 deg off axis. Second, artificial scenes should be generated at an optical or physical distance exceeding the effective range of most binocular mechanisms—optical infinity for a virtual scene and a distance of at least 5 m (and preferably larger) for projected scenes. As with real-world scenes, synthetically created scenes must be perceived as lying outside the observer's vehicle or frame of motion. For example, distant real-world images that are perceived as lying outside of one's frame of motion (such as the ground surrounding a runway, as seen through a small passenger window) can overcome a somatogravic illusion on takeoff much better than can a larger image that is perceived as lying within the observer's frame of motion (such as the bulkhead panel in the aircraft). However, a wide FOV and distant optical projection are not in and of themselves sufficient to duplicate ambient vision, as evidenced by the effects of different visual fields on the oculogyral illusion—the illusory motion of a head-fixed target during vestibular stimulation (see Chapter 7, Sec. II.B.4). In a recent study[146] an optically distant stripe pattern subtending >100 deg was no more successful than a near image subtending <40 deg in overcoming this illusion. Indeed, ramping up the planetary (angular) velocity of the ASDD to produce the desired centrifugal (inertial) force in recreating the somatogravic illusion leads to noticeable oculogyral illusions, despite the wide-FOV and optically distant projection of the ASDD's visual system.

The other three requirements pertain to the temporal and spatial resolution of the display and its overall scene content. Ideally, the temporal resolution should be as high as possible—a minimum of 30 Hz and preferably greater. Even though visual orientation systems are sluggish, artifacts (e.g., aliasing) introduced by insufficient temporal resolution can destroy the realism and believability of the computer-generated imagery. Likewise, temporal lags in head-slaved visual systems can destroy the realism of an out-the-window scene and must be kept within 100 ms or less.[147] Limited spatial resolution can also be detrimental if it leads to spatial aliasing and other artifacts; as with temporal resolution, the issue is not the resolution of the ambient visual system so much as a need to maintain image realism. Given that the human has a ~0.5 min of arc spatial resolution, the closer one can come to matching this limit is desirable. Approaching this resolution requires a very high pixel density—over 2000 per display for a typical small-window (40 deg or less) display—and proper blending of multiple displays to achieve a sufficient high-resolution yet wide-FOV image. Finally, an artificial scene must have sufficient content to both stimulate the ambient visual system and create the level of detail expected of a real-world, daylight scene. Structured visual scenes with many pictorial cues appear to work better than sparse visual displays.[148] In judging altitude in virtual or projected computer-generated imagery, the overall number of objects in a scene might be even more important than the amount of detail per object.[149]

Generally, moving rooms, tilt-translation devices, and other three-dimensional structures have been shown to achieve "visual dominance" to a greater extent than virtual devices. One such furnished room, used by Ian Howard and colleagues in their visual orientation studies, is shown in Fig. 16. Even tilt-translation devices that are composed of wooden boxes with painted grids can easily overcome a few degrees of tilt when the visual scene moves and subjects can reinterpret the tilt sensation as a result of linear acceleration. By contrast, no effects on tilt thresholds were found in a recent study using the ASDD's visual system and a scene depicting forward motion.[150] Of the computer-generated displays large dome and

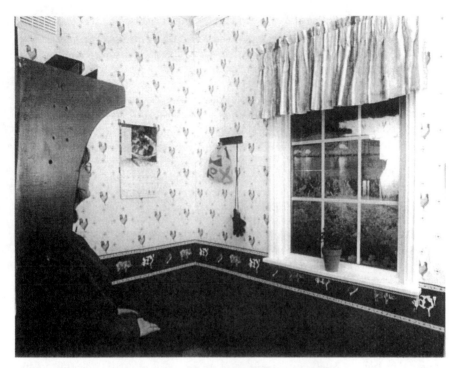

Fig. 16   Furnished room used by Ian Howard and colleagues in their visual orientation research. (Photo reproduced with permission of Dr. Ian Howard.)

other visual simulators appear to present a more compelling visual world than do helmet-mounted displays (HMD).[151] Indeed, high-fidelity simulated environments can generate ambient visual effects such as the optokinetic-cervical reflex, even if the subject is wearing night-vision goggles with their restricted FOVs and distorted optics.[25] Several problems continue to plague HMD from an orientational perspective, including inadequate spatial resolution, temporal lags during head movements, illusions and distortions caused by binocular misalignment, and sensorimotor aftereffects.[148,152]

Even helmet-mounted scenes can be effective if they are construed to represent the outside world, however. One study showed that angular sensations induced by a wide-FOV HMD scene that presented a camera view of the room in which the observer was seated were able to duplicate the Coriolis-induced pointing errors produced by actual motion.[153] What is most important for a synthetic scene is that it believably represents the movement of Earth-fixed space. Slight optical or other distortions do not appear to destroy the ambient capabilities of a scene as long as the observer *believes* the actual Earth-fixed space around him or her is being transmitted or rendered. On the other hand, a seemingly capable visual system that does not achieve this believability will not achieve adequate visual dominance and will fall prey to many motion-related visual illusions; hence, careful study must be undertaken with virtual visual systems before completely windowless cockpits become adopted in flight.[154]

2. Use of Focal Visual Displays to Simulate Ambient Vision

Given the difficulties in simulating ambient vision with large virtual scenes, small synthetic displays that engage the centrally dominated focal visual system (Sec. II) are even less likely to reproduce ambient visual functions. For example, attitude displays on the vast majority of current aircraft depict an artificial horizon that is conformal in roll to the actual horizon as viewed from the inside of the aircraft and are, therefore, termed inside-out displays. However, such generally small (<5 deg) displays evidently do not stimulate the optokinetic-cervical and other stabilization reflexes that real-world scenes do,[21] so that the artificial horizon is presumably not stabilized in the same manner as is the real horizon. This discrepancy leads many pilots to be confused about their roll attitude and is manifested in reversals of the control stick roll inputs in recovering from unusual attitudes[155,156] (see Chapter 9, Sec. II.A.1). Consequently, many researchers have proposed that attitude displays processed by the focal-extrapersonal system should reflect how the outside world is represented in our *mental model* of space, which contains a stable horizon, rather than attempt to simulate ambient vision directly. This belief has led to the development of attitude displays that show a moving aircraft symbol against a stable artificial horizon, as if viewed from behind the aircraft; hence, they are termed outside-into displays.[156]

Some display designers have attempted to use larger inside-out displays that span the entire cockpit, such as the peripheral vision horizon display.[157] However, such displays have not proven successful in eliminating attitude interpretation problems, including those associated with roll-reversal errors.[156] Inside-out attitude formats that present synthetic terrain information on collimated, "see-through" head-up displays.[158] can offer a more effective means of engaging natural ambient vision because their symbology contains prominent monocular depth cues (e.g., perspective, texture gradients) and is overlaid on the pilot's view of the outside world. However, no data currently exist to indicate that see-through synthetic terrain displays actually stimulate ambient visual reflexes in the absence of an outside view.

E. Individual Differences in Susceptibility to Ambient Vision

There is considerable variability among individuals as to the latency and strength of vection susceptibility to visual tilt (field-dependence), and other ambient visual phenomena. Much research has also been conducted to determine if particular groups of individuals differ in their ambient visual processing. However, the only common denominator that has thus far been found that can explain group differences in visual field-dependence appears to be the strength of nonvisual orientation signals, particularly those from the vestibular system.

One group difference that has been studied by many authors is the effect of gender on field dependence. Although male–female differences account for only a small percentage of the overall differences among individuals, the finding that females tend to be more field dependent than males has been replicated in 80% of the rod-and-frame studies reviewed by Allen and Cholet.[159] Males also exhibit a longer latency for circularvection[80,160] and reduced postural sway in response to visual motion.[161] Whether the greater field dependence of females stems from "weaker" vestibular inputs is not clear, but it is possible that males are exposed to greater vestibular stimulation both prenatally (because of greater testosterone-induced motor activity and turning) and postnatally (because of greater participation in sports).[162] Nonrighthanders are also reportedly less field dependent,[163] and this, too, might be related to the strength of their vestibular signals.[162] Finally, it has been shown that field dependence might be greater for both children under seven years of age[164] and in elderly individuals.[34,165,166] This might also be caused by vestibular factors, in that central vestibular processing has not yet fully matured in the children below the age of 10 and a decline of both peripheral and central vestibular function is known to occur in the elderly.[166]

The influence of vestibular inputs in determining the strength of vection is more clearly suggested by findings from two groups of individuals in whom vestibular function is impaired or altered: labyrinth-defective individuals and astronauts in the weightless environment. Individuals with bilateral vestibular loss experience heightened vection[35] and can, unlike normal subjects, readily perceive 360 deg of self-motion in pitch.[167] Patients with vestibular loss also show increased postural sway in response to wide-FOV scene motion.[35,168] In similar fashion, astronauts exposed to a weightless environment and decreased graviception show both increased vection,[169,170] self-tilt,[169] and visually induced postural sway.[32] The role of normal graviception cues in inhibiting vection and other ambient visual effects is further supported by the increased roll-and-pitch vection that occurs when subjects are positioned to the side or inverted rather than in their normal position relative to gravity.[93,171]

Because pilots must orient to the outside visual world rather than to their nonvisual orientation signals, which are typically not aligned with gravity because of the inertial forces during flight that shift the resultant gravitoinertial vector away from gravity (see Chapter 6, Section III), it might be presumed that they, too, are more visually field dependent. Two recent studies suggest that pilots rely more on visual inputs in overcoming the somatogravic and somatogyral illusions,[144,172] but a third study found no differences between pilots and nonpilots in the effects of visual scenes on their thresholds for perceiving roll-and-pitch tilt.[150] A greater field dependence among pilots is also suggested by the greater susceptibility of experienced pilots to simulator sickness,[147] a special type of motion sickness that is created by moving artificial scenes and that correlates positively with vection susceptibility.[173] Finally, there is preliminary evidence that pilots are posturally more susceptible to visual scene motion in conflict situations.[174] Obviously, further research is needed to determine conclusively if pilots rely more on visual orientation cues, but there is no evidence at this point to suggest that the reputedly greater field dependence of pilots is caused by abnormal vestibular processing in this population.[174-176]

V. Neurophysiology of Ambient Vision

Ambient visual functions are carried out in a large number of brain regions in humans and other mammalian species. Whereas nonprimate species use mostly primitive, subcortical pathways for maintaining ambient visual systems that closely parallel their nonvisual orientation systems, humans and other higher primates appear to have extensive cortical networks subserving ambient vision.

The visual system can be subdivided into different systems, depending on the functional specialization in question. One major division involves the cone system, which predominates in the fovea and is specialized for photopic (daytime) vision, color vision, and visual acuity. This system can be contrasted with the rod system, which is active only at low (scotopic) levels of illumination and is capable of greater spatial and temporal summation (and hence, lower thresholds for perceiving dim light). The cone–rod distinction is not all that relevant to the aerial environment in that pilots basically rely on their cone vision even at night, given that the color coding of cockpit instruments must be discernible at all times.

Of greater relevance to ambient visual orientation is the distinction between the parvo and magno systems of primates. These two systems, both of which are active at photopic levels of illumination, are named on the basis of where their retinal pathways terminate in the lateral geniculate nucleus—the upper four and lower two layers being referred to as parvocellular and magnocellular layers, respectively. Cells in the parvocellular layers exhibit a sustained response and show a greater spatial resolution and color specificity, whereas cells in the magnocellular layers respond more transiently and appear to be more involved in motion processing.[177] Thus, the parvo system in its cortical stages appears to be better suited to perform focal-extrapersonal processing in central vision, whereas the magno system appears more capable of performing the peripheral motion processing required for ambient vision.[2]

A. Subcortical Ambient Visual Centers

The primary subcortical centers for visual orientation are the vestibular nuclei, vestibulocerebellum, and the ventroposterior area of the thalamus. All of these structures are known to receive both wide-FOV visual and vestibular signals. Other subcortical regions such as the superior colliculus and putamen can also help to integrate visual and vestibular signals, but these are not as likely to be involved in ambient visual processing. For example, neurons in the superior colliculus do not possess the large, directionally selective receptive fields that are required for ambient vision.[2] On the other hand, the basal ganglia (and the putamen, in particular) can serve to integrate visual and nonvisual activity for predominantly focal and peripersonal functions rather than ambient extrapersonal ones; indeed, one study showed that visually mediated postural responses are actually heightened following lesions of the basal ganglia.[178]

The source of the signals to the ambient visual subcortical centers is not entirely clear; in nonprimates at least, it is likely that wide-FOV visual signals corresponding to the planes of the semicircular canals are transmitted by the accessory optic system (AOS) leading from the retina to the nucleus of the optic tract and into the midbrain tegmentum.[179] Although a recent brain imaging study[180] demonstrated that a region in the midbrain tegmentum that contains the posterior portion of the AOS in other species is intensely activated by wide-FOV coherent motion in humans, the AOS receives little, if any, direct retinal afferentation in primates.[179] Subcortical ambient visual centers, therefore, presumably receive the bulk of their visual inputs from cortical visual processing centers.[2]

Neurons in the vestibular nucleus and other brainstem areas have been shown to respond to vestibular, somatosensory, and wide-FOV visual signals.[19,181,182]

The visual responses of neurons in the medial vestibular nucleus tend to be more sluggish than their vestibular responses,[181] and the visual responses generally tend to complement the latter in terms of their directional sensitivity. For example, most neurons that respond to rightward acceleration prefer leftward visual motion, with the combination of the two stimuli increasing the firing of the neuron still further.[181,182] Because the more sluggish visual responses help overcome the typical phase lead of vestibular neurons at low temporal frequencies, the combined signal tracks the velocity of the motion stimulus much better.[182] No studies to date have implicated the vestibular nuclei in processing wide-FOV visual motion in humans, but this can relate to the limited spatial resolution of functional imaging techniques and the small size and variability in the location of the vestibular nuclei in humans.

The vestibular nuclei send a major projection to the vestibulocerebellum, which consists of the flocculus, paraflocculus, nodulus, uvula, and fastigial nucleus. The vestibulocerebellum is perhaps the major site of subcortical integration of the ambient visual and vestibular signals, as well as a major visual-vestibular integration center for the control of eye and head movements. In the pigeon neurons in the vestibulocerebellum respond to wide-FOV angular motion in axes that are located horizontally and at vertical angles of ~45 and ~135 deg relative to the midsagittal plane, that is, the planes of the semicircular canals.[183] A further visual-vestibular parallelism is found in the preferred directions of vestibulocerebellar neurons to visual translation, which correspond to those of the otolith organs.[183] Similar wide-FOV responses have been obtained from neurons in the AOS of the pigeon and rabbit, which is not surprising in that the AOS provides a major direct and indirect input into the ambient visual neurons of the vestibulocerebellum, at least in nonprimates. The role of the cerebellum in visual orientation has generally been confirmed by functional-imaging and postural-sway studies in humans. The vestibulocerebellum was strongly activated in a recent functional imaging study, which used wide-FOV visual roll stimuli.[184] Cerebellar lesions in humans are also known to increase overall postural sway, but the evidence is mixed as to whether they do so when visual stimuli are available.[178,185]

Ambient visual processing also occurs in the ventroposterior thalamus, which is believed to receive proprioceptive information and a direct projection from the vestibular nuclei. Buttner and Henn[186] showed that cells in this region respond to both sinusoidal rotation in darkness and, in about 50% of cases, to moving visual fields. No simple summation of the visual and vestibular responses occurred in this area, however.

B.   Cortical Ambient Visual Centers

Ambient visual functions in humans, particularly those that involve perceptual phenomena such as vection and judgments of the subjective visual vertical, are highly dependent on the integrity of the cerebral cortex. Even visually mediated postural reactions can, to a lesser extent, require visual cortical processing.[187] Until recently, little was known concerning the representation of ambient vision at the level of the cerebral cortex. Research conducted during the past decade, however, has considerably expanded our knowledge of where and how ambient vision is represented cortically.

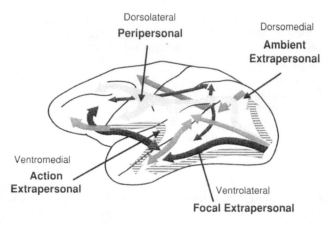

Fig. 17 Four cortical networks corresponding to the four behavioral realms shown in Fig. 1. Medially projecting pathways are shown in stripes. (Reproduced from Ref. 2.)

There appear to be many sites in the parietal and parietal-temporal areas of the cerebral cortex where visual-vestibular integration occurs.[188] However, not all of these sites are necessarily centers for ambient vision. Previc[2] put forth a model that posits four distinct cortical networks that correspond to the four behavioral realms described in Sec. II. These systems, projected onto the monkey cortex, are shown in Fig. 17. A dorsolateral cortical system is responsible for reaching and other peripersonal activities, and this system includes many sites of visual-vestibular interaction that are mainly involved in the control of smooth (pursuit and vergence) eye movements as the head moves during coordinated visual-manual activity. A ventrolateral system is involved in focal-extrapersonal activity, mainly in searching for and recognizing objects using parvo inputs. Neurons in this system have visual receptive fields confined to the central visual field and receive little vestibular inputs. A third system, coursing ventromedially into the parahippocampal gyrus and beyond, is concerned with topographical orientation. This system corresponds to the action-extrapersonal system and is involved in spatial navigation and spatial memory. It integrates vestibular inputs concerning the movement of the head in the horizontal plane (primarily emanating from the horizontal canals) with wide-FOV visual inputs to monitor where our location is in a specific spatial environment. Finally, a cortical system, termed the ambient-extrapersonal system, initially courses dorsomedially from the primary visual cortical areas and is especially responsive to wide-FOV visual motion; this system and its higher components in the temporal-parietal cortex appear to represent the major site of ambient visual processing in the cerebral cortex.

Evidence for the role of the medial-occipital and medial-occipital-parietal cortex in ambient visual functions comes from three major sources: primate studies, human brain-lesion studies, and functional brain imaging studies in humans. Many monkey studies have shown that the medially based visual pathways leading into the medial-parietal-occipital region represent the peripheral portions of the visual world and are sensitive to moving visual stimuli. These areas receive

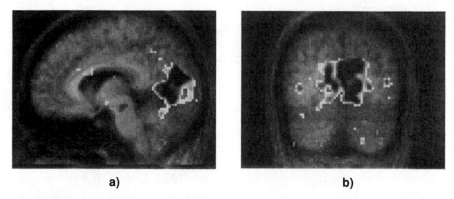

Fig. 18 Medial-occipital-parietal lobe activation (darkened area) to wide-FOV moving texture-fields: a) midsagittal view and b) coronal view from back of brain. (Reproduced from Ref. 184.)

their inputs mainly from the magno-visual pathways (see Ref. 2). Gattass et al.[189] were the first researchers to propose that these visual pathways subserved ambient vision. In a study of 26 patients with lesions to the occipital-parietal cortex,[190] about half reported a marked reduction in the magnitude of their vection sensations with horizontal stimulation, in addition to exhibiting impaired OKN and other optokinetic reflexes. The requirement of an intact occipital cortex in perceiving normal vection was further confirmed in a study of patients with hemianopias (half-field losses), who could experience normal vection with stimulation of their normal half-field but not with the half-field represented in their damaged cortex.[187] Finally, the role of the occipital-parietal cortex in ambient vision was confirmed by two recent functional brain imaging studies that used wide-FOV (>95 deg) visual motion. Both of these studies[184,191] used positron emission tomography (PET) and showed extensive activation of the occipital-parietal region to wide-FOV motion, regardless of whether it was random or coherent (see Fig. 18). These results confirm that the occipital-parietal region processes the elementary ambient motion signal but might not be responsible for processing the coherence of the visual stimulus itself, as would be required to perceive the direction of self-motion.[184] However, at least one study has shown that the medial-occipital-parietal cortex might specifically process vection-inducing visual motion.[192]

Activity in the dorsal portion of the occipital-parietal cortex correlates with activity in the posterior-temporal-parietal area,[184] which appears to be the single most important cortical region in the processing of the coherence (and direction) of the wide-FOV motion stimulus. This region lies behind the primary vestibular cortex, located in the posterior portion of the insular region lying at the junction of the parietal and temporal cortices in the lateral sulcus (Sylvian fissure).[193,194] This retroinsular region also receives input from somatosensory and even auditory spatial orientation sensory inputs.[195] The primary vestibular cortex receives from the aforementioned ventroposterior portion of the thalamus and is interconnected with at least four other processing sites located in parietal and frontal cortex.[194] Several pieces of evidence point to the importance of the retroinsular ventral temporal

Sylvian region, which lies anterior to the better known middle-superior-temporal region that receives both visual and vestibular signals in the monkey but which might be more involved in pursuit eye movements. First, at least two monkey studies have shown that the retroinsular region is replete with neurons that prefer large, moving textured fields.[194,195] Second, lesions to this area in humans have been shown to disrupt the perception of the subjective visual vertical[188] and vection.[187] Finally, functional brain imaging studies[180,184,191] have shown that the posterior temporal region is activated specifically by the coherence of the wide-FOV textured visual motion. In the Previc et al.[184] study the retroinsular activation consisted of an elongated area spanning 4 cm vertically from the base of posterior-parietal cortex to the middle of the posterior temporal lobe.

One interesting aspect of the cortical ambient visual system is that it seems to be reciprocally related to cortical vestibular activation. For instance, stimulation of the vestibular cortex has been shown to inhibit activity in visual cortical processing areas, whereas stimulation of visual cortical areas by wide-FOV moving textured fields can inhibit the primary vestibular cortex.[192] This finding might correlate with the hypothesis, expressed in Sec. IV.E, that the magnitude of vection is inversely proportional to the strength of the vestibular signal that would ordinarily inhibit it. Like the vestibular system's projection to the cerebral cortex,[194,196] that of the ambient visual system appears to be predominantly contralateral. Just as leftward turning excites primarily the left canal and right vestibular cortex,[194] so, too, does the complementary rightward visual yaw motion[197] stimulate mainly the right hemisphere.

All of the cortical systems shown are believed to have a frontal-lobe component to them, but this component remains poorly identified in the case of the ambient-extrapersonal system. Clearly, there are regions in the frontal lobes that respond to Earth-fixed orientation cues, as evidence by the illusions of inversion of the visual world that can occur following frontal as well as posterior (parietal-temporal) cortical lesions.[198]

The ambient visual network might eventually turn out to be much more widespread than the preceding account suggests. In two recent studies[184,197] that compared brain responses to opposite wide-FOV motions that activate one hemisphere more than another—including rightward and leftward yaw, which stimulate predominantly the right and left hemispheres, respectively—the lateralized activity that resulted was highly distributed across most of the cerebral cortex. This finding indicates that ambient visual processing, or at least the ambient visual output signal, can be found throughout the brain because of the need to first orient ourselves in relation to Earth-fixed space before we can properly ascertain the proper orientation of other elements within our perceptual world. This further confirms that ambient vision (and our spatial orientation system in general) might represent the "bedrock" of all perceptual-motor behavior.[2]

VI. Summary

This chapter has reviewed the basic mechanisms of visual orientation. The ambient visual system helps maintain our orientation in Earth-fixed space, and it generally dominates over other sensory orientation systems in full-field, structured visual environments. The three major perceptual influences of ambient vision are on our sense of self-motion in Earth-fixed space (vection), our perceived self-position in Earth-fixed space, and our perception of the slant and distance of the terrain around us. Although ambient visual cues are generally reliable on Earth, important cues such as optical flow and perspective are more ambiguous while flying at variable altitudes above ground. Besides contributing to spatial-orientational percepts, the ambient visual system also influences both postural control and the control of other motor systems (manual and oculomotor) that are less closely linked to orientation in space. Generally, ambient vision is dominated most by distant, wide-FOV scenes that appear highly realistic, but what is most important is that the observer believes the visual scene to be linked to Earth-fixed space. Certain individuals lacking strong input from their vestibular system appear to be especially susceptible to the influence of visual scenes, and it is also possible that other groups such as pilots might rely more on ambient vision despite apparently normal vestibular systems. Although ambient vision is largely a preconscious system that does not require a great deal of attentional resources, it nevertheless appears to be mostly dependent upon cortical visual processing in humans. Its diffuse representation in the cerebral cortex attests to its fundamental importance to our entire perceptual-motor apparatus.

References

[1]Howard, I. P., *Human Visual Orientation*, Wiley, New York, 1982.

[2]Previc, F. H., "The Neuropsychology of 3-D Space," *Psychological Bulletin*, Vol. 124, 1998, pp. 123–164.

[3]Hughes, H., *Sensory Exotica: A World Beyond Human Experience*, MIT Press, Cambridge, MA, 1999.

[4]Previc, F. H., and Saucedo, J. C., "The Relationship Between Turning Behavior and Motoric Dominance in Humans," *Perceptual and Motor Skills*, Vol. 75, 1992, pp. 935–944.

[5]Schaeffer, A. A., "Spiral Movement in Man," *Journal of Morphology and Physiology*, Vol. 45, 1928, pp. 293–398.

[6]Mack, A., and Herman, E., "The Loss of Position Constancy During Pursuit Eye Movements," *Vision Research*, Vol. 18, 1978, pp. 55–62.

[7]Benson, A. J., and Barnes, G. R., "Vision During Angular Oscillation: The Dynamic Interaction of Visual and Vestibular Mechanisms," *Aviation, Space, and Environmental Medicine*, Vol. 49, 1978, pp. 340–345.

[8]Trevarthen, C. B., "Two Mechanisms of Vision in Primates," *Psychologische Forschung*, Vol. 31, 1968, pp. 299–337.

[9]Held, R., "Dissociation of Visual Functions by Deprivation and Rearrangement," *Psychologische Forschung*, Vol. 31, 1968, pp. 338–348.

[10]Schneider, G. E., "Two Visual Systems," *Science*, Vol. 163, 1969, pp. 895–902.

[11]Leibowitz, H. W., and Dichgans, J., "The Ambient Visual System and Spatial Orientation," *Spatial Disorientation in Flight: Current Problems*, AGARD, Neuilly sur Seine, France, pp. B4-1–B4-4.

[12]Leibowitz, H. W., Post, R. B., Brandt, T., and Dichgans, J., "Implications of Recent Developments in Dynamic Spatial Orientation and Visual Resolution for Vehicle Guidance," *Tutorials on Motion Perception*, edited by A. H. Wertheim, W. A. Wagenaar, and H. W. Leibowitz, Plenum, New York, 1982, pp. 231–260.

[13]Andersen, G. J., "The Perception of Self-Motion: Psychophysical and Computational Approaches," *Psychological Bulletin*, Vol. 99, 1986, pp. 52–65.

[14]Millidot, M., and Lamont, A., "Peripheral Visual Acuity in the Vertical Plane," *Vision Research*, Vol. 14, 1974, pp. 1497–1498.

[15]D'Avossa, G., and Kersten, D., "Evidence in Human Subjects for Independent Coding of Azimuth and Elevation for Direction of Heading from Optic Flow," *Vision Research*, Vol. 36, 1996, pp. 2915–2924.

[16]Telford, L., and Frost, B. J., "Factors Affecting the Onset and Magnitude of Linear Vection," *Perception and Psychophysics*, Vol. 53, 1993, pp. 682–692.

[17]Clark, W. C., Smith, A. H., and Rabe, A., "Retinal Gradients of Outline Distortion and Binocular Disparity as Stimuli for Slant," *Canadian Journal of Psychology*, Vol. 10, 1956, pp. 77–81.

[18]Gibson, J. J., *The Perception of the Visual World*, Houghton Mifflin, Boston, MA, 1950.

[19]Thoden, U., Dichgans, J., and Savidis, T., "Direction-Specific Optokinetic Modulation of Monosynaptic Hind Limb Reflexes in Cats," *Experimental Brain Research*, Vol. 30, 1977, pp. 155–160.

[20]Gallimore, J. J., Brannon, N. G., Patterson, F. R., and Nalepka, J. P., "Effects of FOV and Aircraft Bank on Pilot Head Movement and Reversal Errors During Simulated Flight," *Aviation, Space, and Environmental Medicine*, Vol. 70, 1999, pp. 1162–1160.

[21]Patterson, F. R., Cacioppo, A. J., Gallimore, J. J., Hinman, G. E., and Nalepka, J. P., "Aviation Spatial Orientation in Relationship to Head Position and Attitude Interpretation," *Aviation, Space, and Environmental Medicine*, Vol. 68, 1997, pp. 463–471.

[22]Cheung, B. S. K., and Howard, I. P., "Optokinetic Torsion: Dynamics and Relation to Circularvection," *Vision Research*, Vol. 31, 1991, pp. 1327–1335.

[23]Mergner, T., and Becker, W., "Perception of Horizontal Self-Rotation: Multisensory and Cognitive Aspects," *Perception and Control of Self-Motion*, edited by R. Warren and A. H. Wertheim, Erlbaum, Hillsdale, NJ, 1990, pp. 219–263.

[24]Wertheim, A. H., "Motion Perception During Self-Motion: The Direct Versus Inferential Controversy Revisited," *Behavioral and Brain Sciences*, Vol. 17, 1994, pp. 293–355.

[25]Braithwaite, M. G., Beal, K. G., Alvarez, E. A., Jones, H. D., and Estrada, A., "The Optokinetic Cervico Reflex During Simulated Helicopter Flight," *Aviation, Space, and Environmental Medicine*, Vol. 69, 1998, pp. 1166–1173.

[26]Previc, F. H., and Mullen, T. J., "A Comparison of the Latencies of Visually Induced Postural Change and Self-Motion Perception," *Journal of Vestibular Research*, Vol. 1, 1991, pp. 317–323.

[27]Zacharias, G. I., and Young, L. R., "Influence of Combined Visual and Vestibular Cues on Human Perception and Control of Horizontal Rotation," *Experimental Brain Research*, Vol. 41, 1981, pp. 159–171.

[28]Royden, C. S., Banks, M. S., and Crowell, J. A., "The Perception of Heading During Eye Movements," *Nature*, Vol. 360, 1992, pp. 583–585.

[29]Wallach, H., "Perceiving a Stable Environment When One Moves," *Annual Review of Psychology*, Vol. 38, 1987, pp. 1–27.

[30]Bridgeman, B., and Stark, L., "Ocular Proprioception and Efference Copy in Registering Visual Direction," *Vision Research*, Vol. 31, 1991, pp. 1903–1913.

[31]Irwin, D. E., McConkie, G. W., Carlson-Radvansky, L. A., and Currie, C., "A Localist Evaluation Solution for Visual Stability Across Saccades," *Behavioral and Brain Sciences*, Vol. 17, 1994, pp. 265–266.

[32]Reschke, M. F., Bloomberg, J. J., Harm, D. L., and Paloski, W. H., "Space Flight and Neurovestibular Adaptation," *Journal of Clinical Pharmacology*, Vol. 34, 1994, pp. 609–617.

[33]Graybiel, A., "Oculogravic Illusion," *Archives of Ophthalmology*, Vol. 48, 1952, pp. 605–615.

[34]Howard, I. P., Jenkin, H. L., and Hu, G., "Visually-Induced Reorientation Illusions as a Function of Age," *Aviation, Space, and Environmental Medicine*, Vol. 71, 2000, pp. A87–A91.

[35]Bles, W., and Roos, J. P., "The Tilting Room and Posturography," *Acta Otorhinolaryngologica*, Vol. 45, 1991, pp. 387–391.

[36]Ittelson, W. H., *The Ames Demonstrations in Perception*, Princeton Univ. Press, Princeton, NJ, 1952.

[37]Philbeck, J. W., and Loomis, J. M., "Comparison of Two Indicators of Perceived Egocentric Distance Under Full-Cue and Reduced-Cue Conditions," *Journal of Experimental Psychology: Human Perception and Performance*, Vol. 23, 1997, pp. 72–85.

[38]Previc, F. H., unpublished study.

[39]Gibson, J. J., *The Senses Considered as Perceptual Systems*, Houghton Mifflin, Boston, MA, 1966.

[40]Koenderink, J. J., "Optic flow," *Vision Research*, Vol. 26, 1986, pp. 161–180.

[41]Warren, R., "Preliminary Questions for the Study of Egomotion," *Perception and Control of Self-Motion*, edited by R. Warren and A. H. Wertheim, Erlbaum, Hillsdale, NJ, 1990, pp. 3–32.

[42]Rogers, B., and Graham, M., "Motion Parallax as an Independent Cue for Depth Perception," *Perception*, Vol. 8, 1979, pp. 125–134.

[43]Vishton, P. M., and Cutting, J. E., "Wayfinding, Displacements, and Mental Maps: Velocity Fields Are Not Typically Used to Determine One's Aimpoint," *Journal of Experimental Psychology: Human Perception and Performance*, Vol. 21, 1995, pp. 978–995.

[44]Amblard, B., Cremieux, J., Marchand, A. R., and Carblanc, A., "Lateral Orientation and Stabilization of Human Stance: Static Versus Dynamic Cues," *Experimental Brain Research*, Vol. 61, 1985, pp. 21–37.

[45]Dykes, J., *Spatial and Visual Effects of Stroboscopic Illumination*, Air Force Research Lab., AFRL-HE-BR-TR-2001-0145, Brooks AFB, TX, 2001.

[46]Rogowitz, B., "The Breakdown of Size Constancy Under Stroboscopic Illumination," *Festschrift for Ivo Kohler*, edited by L. Spillman and B. Wooten, Erlbaum, Hillsdale, NJ, 1984, pp. 201–213.

[47]Kruk, R., and Regan, D., "Visual Test Results Compared with Flying Performance in Telemetry-Tracked Aircraft," *Aviation, Space, and Environmental Medicine*, Vol. 54, 1983, pp. 906–911.

[48]Gibson, J. J., Olum, P., and Rosenblatt, F., "Parallax and Perspective During Aircraft Landings," *American Journal of Psychology*, Vol. 68, 1955, pp. 372–385.

[49]Beall, A. C., and Loomis, J. M., "Optic Flow and Visual Analysis of the Base-to-Final Turn," *International Journal of Aviation Psychology*, Vol. 7, 1997, pp. 201–233.

[50]Lintern, G., and Liu, Y.-T., "Explicit and Implicit Horizons for Simulated Landing Approaches," *Human Factors*, Vol. 33, 1991, pp. 401–417.

[51]Mertens, H. W., "Comparison of the Visual Perception of a Runway Model in Pilots and Nonpilots During Simulated Night Landing Approaches," *Aviation, Space and Environmental Medicine*, Vol. 49, 1978, pp. 1043–1055.

[52]Henn, V., and Young, L. R., "Ernst Mach on the Vestibular Organ 100 Years Ago," *ORL Journal of Otorhinolaryngology and Related Specialities*, Vol. 37, 1975, pp. 138–148.

[53]Gillingham, K. K., and Previc, F. H., *"Spatial Orientation in Flight,"* U.S. Air Force Armstrong Lab., AL-TR-1993-0022, Brooks Air Force Base, TX, 1993.

[54]Held, R., Dichgans, J., and Bauer, J., "Characteristics of Moving Visual Scenes Influencing Spatial Orientation," *Vision Research*, Vol. 15, 1975, pp. 357–365.

[55]Denton, G. G., "The Influence of Visual Pattern on Perceived Speed," *Perception*, Vol. 9, 1980, pp. 393–402.

[56]Larish, J. F., and Flach, J. M., "Sources of Optical Information Useful for Perception of Speed of Rectilinear Self-Motion," *Journal of Experimental Psychology: Human Perception and Performance*, Vol. 16, 1990, pp. 295–302.

[57]Hu, S., Davis, M. S., Klose, A. H., Zabinsky, E. M., Meux, S. P., Jacobsen, H. A., Westfall, J. M., and Gruber, M. B., "Effect of Spatial Frequency of a Vertically Striped Rotating Drum on Vection-Induced Motion Sickness," *Aviation, Space, and Environmental Medicine*, Vol. 68, 1997, pp. 306–311.

[58]Palmisano, S., and Gillam, B., "Stimulus Eccentricity and Spatial Frequency Interact to Determine Circular Vection," *Perception*, Vol. 27, 1998, pp. 1067–1077.

[59]Schiff, W., and Detwiler, M. L., "Information Used in Judging Impending Collision," *Perception*, Vol. 8, 1979, pp. 647–658.

[60]Andersen, G. J., Cisneros, J., Atchley, P., and Saidpour, A., "Speed, Size, and Edge-Rate Information for the Detection of Collision Events," *Journal of Experimental Psychology: Human Perception and Performance*, Vol. 25, 1999, pp. 256–269.

[61]DeLucia, P. R., "Pictorial and Motion-Based Information for Depth Perception," *Journal of Experimental Psychology: Human Perception and Performance*, Vol. 17, 1991, pp. 738–748.

[62]Howard, I. P., and Heckmann, T., "Circular Vection as a Function of the Relative Sizes, Distances, and Positions of Two Competing Visual Displays," *Perception*, Vol. 18, 1989, pp. 657–665.

[63]Post, R. B., "Circular Vection Is Independent of Stimulus Eccentricity," *Perception*, Vol. 17, 1998, pp. 737–744.

[64]Previc, F. H., and Neel, R. L., "The Effects of Visual Surround Eccentricity and Size on Manual and Postural Control," *Journal of Vestibular Research*, Vol. 5, 1995, pp. 399–404.

[65]Brandt, T., Dichgans, J., and Koenig, E., "Differential Effects of Central Versus Peripheral Vision on Egocentric and Exocentric Motion Perception," *Experimental Brain Research*, Vol. 16, 1973, pp. 476–491.

[66]Dichgans, J., and Brandt, T., "Visual-Vestibular Interaction: Effects on Self-Motion Perception and Postural Control," *Handbook of Sensory Physiology*, Vol. 8: *Perception*, edited by R. Held, H. Leibowitz and H.-L. Teuber, Springer-Verlag, New York, 1978, pp. 755–804.

[67]Andersen, G. J., "Segregation of Optic Flow into Object and Self-Motion Components: Foundations for a General Model," *Perception and Control of Self-Motion*, edited by R. Warren and A. H. Wertheim, Erlbaum, Hillsdale, NJ, 1990, pp. 127–141.

[68]Andersen, G. J., and Braunstein, M. L., "Induced Self-Motion in Central Vision," *Journal of Experimental Psychology: Human Perception and Performance*, Vol. 11, 1985, pp. 122–132.

[69]Stoffregen, T. A., "Flow Structure Versus Retinal Location in the Optical Control of Stance," *Journal of Experimental Psychology: Human Perception and Performance*, Vol. 11, 1985, pp. 554–565.

[70]Post, R. B., and Johnson, C. A., "Motion Sensitivity in Central and Peripheral Vision," *American Journal of Optometry and Physiological Optics*, Vol. 63, 1986, pp. 104–107.

[71]Wolpert, L., "Field-of-View Information for Self-Motion Perception," *Perception and Control of Self-Motion*, edited by R. Warrren and A. H. Wertheim, Erlbaum, Hillsdale, NJ, 1990, pp. 101–126.

[72]Brandt, T., Wist, E. R., and Dichgans, J., "Foreground and Background in Dynamic Spatial Orientaiton," *Perception and Psychophysics*, Vol. 17, 1975, pp. 497–503.

[73]Delorme, A., and Martin, C., "Roles of Retinal Periphery and Depth Periphery in Linear Vection and Visual Control of Standing in Humans," *Canadian Journal of Psychology*, Vol. 40, 1986, pp. 176–187.

[74]Heckmann, T., and Howard, I. P., "Induced Motion: Isolation and Dissociation of Egocentric and Vection-Entrained Components," *Perception*, Vol. 20, 1991, pp. 285–305.

[75]Ohmi, M., Howard, I. P., and Landolt, J. P., "Circular Vection as a Function of Foreground-Background Relationships," *Perception*, Vol. 16, 1987, pp. 17–22.

[76]Wist, E. R., Diener, H. C., Dichgans, J., and Brandt, T., "Perceived Distance and the Perceived Speed of Self-Motion: Linear vs. Angular Velocity?" *Perception and Psychophysics*, Vol. 17, 1975, pp. 549–554.

[77]Ohmi, M., and Howard, I. P., "Effect of Stationary Objects on Illusory Forward Self-Motion Induced by a Looming Display," *Perception*, Vol. 17, 1988, pp. 5–12.

[78]Berthoz, A., and Droulez, J., "Linear Self Motion Perception," *Tutorials on Motion Perception*, edited by A. H. Wertheim, W. A. Wagenaar, and H. W. Leibowitz, Plenum, New York, 1982, pp. 157–198.

[79]Berthoz, A., Pavard, B., and Young, L. R., "Perception of Linear Horizontal Self-Motion Induced by Peripheral Vision (Linearvection)," *Experimental Brain Research*, Vol. 23, 1975, pp. 471–489.

[80]Kennedy, R. S., Hettinger, L. J., Harm, D. L., Ordy, J. M., and Dunlap, W. P., "Psychophysical Scaling of Circular Vection (CV) Produced by Optokinetic (OKN) Motion: Individual Differences and Effects of Practice," *Journal of Vestibular Research*, Vol. 6, 1996, pp. 331–341.

[81]Leibowitz, H. W., Shupert Rodemer, C., and Dichgans, J., "The Independence of Dynamic Spatial Orientation from Luminance and Refractive Error," *Perception and Psychophysics*, Vol. 25, 1979, pp. 75–79.

[82]Brecher, G. A., Brecher, M. H., Kommerell, G., Sauter, F. A., and Sellerbeck, J., "Relation of Optical and Labyrinthean Orientation," *Optica Acta*, Vol. 19, 1972, pp. 467–471.

[83]Amblard, B., and Carblanc, A., "Role of Foveal and Peripheral Visual Information in Maintenance of Postural Equilibrium in Man," *Perceptual and Motor Skills*, Vol. 51, 1980, pp. 903–912.

[84]Lestienne, F., Soechting, J., and Berthoz, A., "Postural Readjustments Induced by Linear Motion of Visual Scenes," *Experimental Brain Research*, Vol. 28, 1977, pp. 363–384.

[85]van Asten, W. N. J. C., Gielen, C. C. A. M., and Denier van der Gon, J. J., "Postural Adjustments Induced by Simulated Motion of Differently Structured Environments," *Experimental Brain Research*, Vol. 73, 1988, pp. 371–383.

[86]Paulus, W. M., Straube, A., and Brandt, T., "Visual Stabilization of Posture. Physiological Stimulus Characteristics and Clinical Aspects," *Brain*, Vol. 107, 1984, pp. 1143–1163.

[87]Dichgans, J., Mauritz, K. H., Allum, J. H. J., and Brandt, T., "Postural Sway in Normals and Atactic Patients: Analysis of the Stabilizing Effects of Vision," *Aggressologie*, Vol. 17C, 1976, pp. 15–24.

[88] Previc, F. H., Kenyon, R. V., Johnson, B. H., and Boer, E. R., "The Effects of Background Visual Roll Stimulation on Postural and Manual Control and Self-Motion Perception," *Perception and Psychophysics*, Vol. 54, 1993, pp. 93–107.

[89] Kenyon, R. V., and Kneller, E. W., "The Effects of Field of-View Size on the Control of Roll Motion," *IEEE Transactions on Systems, Man, and Cybernetics*, Vol. 23, 1993, pp. 183–193.

[90] Howard, I. P., Sun, L., and Shen, X., "Cycloversion and Cyclovergence: The Effects of the Area and Position of the Visual Display," *Experimental Brain Research*, Vol. 100, 1994, pp. 509–514.

[91] Cheng, M., and Outerbridge, J. S., "Optokinetic Nystagmus During Selective Retinal Stimulation," *Experimental Brain Research*, Vol. 23, 1975, pp. 129–139.

[92] Howard, I. P., and Gonzalez, E. S., "Human Optokinetic Nystagmus in Response to Moving Binocularly Disparate Stimuli," *Vision Research*, Vol. 27, 1987, pp. 1807–1816.

[93] Howard, I. P., Cheung, B., and Landolt, J., "Influence of Vection Axis and Body Posture on Visually-Perceived Self-Rotation and Tilt," AGARD CP-463: in *Motion Cues in Flight Simulation and Simulator Induced Sickness*, AGARD, 1988, pp. 15-1–15-8.

[94] Paige, G. D., Telford, L., Seidman, S. H., and Barnes, G. R., "Human Vestibuloocular Reflex and Its Interactions with Vision and Fixation Distance During Linear and Angular Head Movement," *Journal of Neurophysiology*, Vol. 80, 1998, pp. 2391–2404.

[95] Matin, L., and Fox, C. R., "Visually Perceived Eye Level and Perceived Elevation of Objects: Linearly Additive Influences from Visual Field Pitch and from Gravity," *Vision Research*, Vol. 29, 1989, pp. 315–324.

[96] Stoper, A. E., and Cohen, M. M., "Effect of Structured Visual Environments on Apparent Eye Level," *Perception and Psychophysics*, Vol. 46, 1989, pp. 469–475.

[97] Witkin, H. A., and Asch, S. E., "Studies in Space Perception. IV. Further Experiments on the Upright with Displaced Visual Fields," *Journal of Experimental Psychology*, Vol. 38, 1948, pp. 762–782.

[98] Previc, F. H., and Donnelly, M., "The Effects of Visual Depth and Eccentricity on Manual Bias, Induced Motion, and Vection," *Perception*, Vol. 22, 1993, pp. 929–945.

[99] Zoccolotti, P., Antonucci, G., and Spinelli, D., "The Gap Between Rod and Frame Influences the Rod-and-Frame Effect with Small and Large Inducing Displays," *Perception and Psychophysics*, Vol. 54, 1993, pp. 14–19.

[100] Ebenholtz, S. M., and Benzschawel, T. L., "The Rod and Frame Effect and Induced Head Tilt as a Function of Observation Distance," *Perception and Psychophysics*, Vol. 22, 1977, pp. 491–496.

[101] Sigman, E., Goodenough, D. R., and Flannagan, M., "Instructions, Illusory Self-Tilt and the Rod-and-Frame Test," *Quarterly Journal of Experimental Psychology*, Vol. 31, 1979, pp. 155–165.

[102] Previc, F. H., Varner, D. C., and Gillingham, K. K., "Visual Scene Effects on the Somatogravic Illusion," *Aviation, Space, and Environmental Medicine*, Vol. 63, 1992, pp. 1060–1064.

[103] Goodenough, D. R., Sigman, E., Oltman, P. K., Rosso, J., and Mertz, H., "Eye Torsion in Response to a Tilted Visual Stimulus," *Vision Research*, Vol. 19, 1979, pp. 1177–1179.

[104] Howard, I. P., and Childerson, L., "The Contribution of Motion, the Visual Frame, and Visual Polarity to Sensations of Body Tilt," *Perception*, Vol. 23, 1994, pp. 753–762.

[105] Kitahara, M., and Uno, R., "Equilibrium and Vertigo in a Tilting Environment," *Annals of Otology, Rhinology, and Laryngology*, Vol. 76, 1967, pp. 166–178.

[106]Matin, L., and Li, W., "Multimodal Basis for Egocentric Spatial Localization and Orientation," *Journal of Vestibular Research*, Vol. 5, 1995, pp. 499–518.

[107]Nemire, K., and Cohen, M. M., "Visual and Somesthetic Influences on Postural Orientation in the Median Plane," *Perception and Psychophysics*, Vol. 53, 1993, pp. 106–116.

[108]Sedgwick, H. A., "Space Perception," *Handbook of Human Perception and Performance*, Vol. 1, edited by K. R. Boff, L. Kaufman, and J. P. Thomas, Wiley, New York, 1986, pp. 21-1–21-57.

[109]Cutting, J. E., and Vishton, P. M., "Perceiving Layout and Knowing Distances: The Integration, Relative Potency, and Contextual Use of Different Information About Depth," *Handbook of Perception and Cognition*, edited by W. Epstein and S. Rogers, Academic Press, New York, Vol. 5, 1995, pp. 69–117.

[110]Alderson, G. J., Sully, D. J., and Sully, H. G., "An Operational Analysis of a One-Handed Catching Task Using High-Speed Photography," *Journal of Motor Behavior*, Vol. 6, 1974, pp. 217–226.

[111]Servos, P., Goodale, M. A., and Jakobson, L. S., "The Role of Binocular Vision in Prehension: A Kinematic Analysis," *Vision Research*, Vol. 32, 1992, pp. 1513–1521.

[112]Foley, J. M., "Binocular Distance Perception," *Psychological Review*, Vol. 87, 1980, pp. 411–434.

[113]Allison, R. S., and Howard, I. P., "Temporal Dependencies in Resolving Monocular and Binocular Cue Conflict in Slant Perception," *Vision Research*, Vol. 40, 2000, pp. 1869–1886.

[114]Gray, R., and Regan, D., "Accuracy of Estimating Time to Collision Using Binocular and Monocular Information," *Vision Research*, Vol. 38, 1998, pp. 499–512.

[115]Cavallo, V., and Laurent, M., "Visual Information and Skill Level in Time-to-Collision Estimation," *Perception*, Vol. 17, 1988, pp. 623–632.

[116]Richards, W., and Miller, J. F., "Convergence as a Cue to Depth," *Perception and Psychophysics*, Vol. 5, 1969, pp. 317–320.

[117]Von Hofsten, C., "The Role of Convergence in Visual Space Perception," *Vision Research*, Vol. 16, 1976, pp. 193–198.

[118]Regan, D., Erkelens, C. J., and Collewijn, H., "Visual Field Defects for Vergence Eye Movements and for Stereomotion Perception," *Investigative Ophthalmology and Visual Science*, Vol. 27, 1986, pp. 806–819.

[119]Bradshaw, M. F., Glennerster, A., and Rogers, B. J., "The Effect of Display Size om Disparity Scaling from Differential Perspective and Vergence Cues," *Vision Research*, Vol. 36, 1996, pp. 1255–1264.

[120]Leibowitz, H., and Moore, D., "Role of Changes in Accommodation and Convergence in the Perception of Size," *Journal of the Optical Society of America*, Vol. 56, 1966, pp. 1120–1123.

[121]Iavecchia, J. H., Iavecchia, H. P., and Roscoe, S. N., "Eye Accommodation to Head-Up Virtual Images," *Human Factors*, Vol. 30, 1988, pp. 689–702.

[122]Alexander, K. R., "On the Nature of Accommodative Micropsia," *American Journal of Optometry and Physiological Optics*, Vol. 52, 1975, pp. 79–84.

[123]Marsh, J. S., and Temme, L. A., "Optical Factors in Judgments of Size Through an Aperture," *Human Factors*, Vol. 32, 1990, pp. 109–118.

[124]Mon-Williams, M., and Tresilian, J. R., "Ordinal Depth Information from Accommodation?" *Ergonomics*, Vol. 43, 2000, pp. 391–404.

[125]Roscoe, S. N., "Landing Airplanes, Detecting Traffic, and the Dark Focus," *Aviation, Space, and Environmental Medicine*, Vol. 53, 1982, pp. 970–976.

[126]Roscoe, S. N., "The Trouble with HUDs and HMDs," *Human Factors Society Bulletin*, Vol. 30, No. 7, 1987, pp. 1–3.

[127]Owens, D. A., "The Mandelbaum Effect: Evidence for an Accommodative Bias Toward Intermediate Viewing Distances," *Journal of the Optical Society of America*, Vol. 69, 1979, pp. 646–652.

[128]Howard, I. P., and Kaneko, H., "Relative Shear Disparities and the Perception of Surface Inclination," *Vision Research*, Vol. 34, 1994, pp. 2505–2517.

[129]Howard, I. P., and Zacher, J. E., "Human Cyclovergence as a Function of Stimulus Frequency and Amplitude," *Experimental Brain Research*, Vol. 85, 1991, pp. 445–450.

[130]Buckley, D., Frisby, J. P., and Blake, A., "Does the Human Visual System Implement an Ideal Observer Theory of Slant Form Texture?, *Vision Research*, Vol. 36, 1996, pp. 1163–1176.

[131]Knill, D. C., "Surface Orientation from Texture: Ideal Observers, Generic Observers and the Information Content of Texture Cues," *Vision Research*, Vol. 38, 1998, pp. 1655–1682.

[132]Flach, J. M., Hagen, B. A., and Larish, J. F., "Active Regulation of Altitude as a Function of Optical Texture," *Perception and Psychophysics*, Vol. 51, 1992, pp. 557–568.

[133]Beer, J. M. A., Ghani, N., Previc, F. H., and Campbell, J. M., "Speed Can Influence Aim-Point Judgments Even Before Illusory Depth Cues Enter the Picture," *Perception*, Vol. 27, 1998, pp. 58, 59.

[134]Blessing, W. W., Landauer, A. A., and Coltheart, M., "The Effect of False Perspective Cues on Distance and Size Judgments: An Examination of the Invariance Hypothesis," *American Journal of Psychology*, Vol. 80, 1967, pp. 250–256.

[135]Kaess, D. W., and Deregowski, J. B., "Depicted Angle of Forms and Perception of Line Drawings," *Perception*, Vol. 9, 1980, pp. 23–29.

[136]Cutting, J. E., and Millard, R. T., "Three Gradients and the Perception of Flat and Curved Surfaces," *Journal of Experimental Psychology: General*, Vol. 113, 1984, pp. 198–216.

[137]Flach, J. M., Warren, R., Garness, S. A., Kelly, L., and Stanard, T., "Perception and Control of Altitude: Splay and Depression Angles," *Journal of Experimental Psychology: Human Perception and Performance*, Vol. 23, 1997, pp. 1764–1782.

[138]Johnson, W. W., Tsang, P. S., Bennett, C. T., and Phatak, A. V., "The Visually Guided Control of Simulated Altitude," *Aviation, Space, and Environmental Medicine*, Vol. 60, 1989, pp. 152–156.

[139]Warren, R., "Visual Perception in High-Speed, Low-Altitude Flight," *Aviation, Space, and Environmental Medicine*, Vol. 59, 1988, pp. A116–124.

[140]Farne, M., "Brightness as an Indicator to Distance: Relative Brightness per se or Contrast with the Background?," *Perception*, Vol. 6, 1977, pp. 287–293.

[141]Peronne, J. A., "Visual Slant Misperception and the 'Black-Hole' Landing Situation," *Aviation, Space, and Environmental Medicine*, Vol. 55, 1984, pp. 1020–1025.

[142]Smith, A. H., "Gradients of Outline Convergence and Distortion as Stimuli for Slant," *Canadian Journal of Psychology*, Vol. 10, 1956, pp. 211–218.

[143]Hershenson, M., and Samuels, S. M., "An Airplane Illusion: Apparent Velocity Determined by Apparent Distance," *Perception*, Vol. 28, 1999, pp. 433–436.

[144]Lessard, C. S., Maidment, G., Previc, F. H., Self, B., and Beer, J., *Visual Scene Effects on the Somatogravic Illusion*, U.S. Air Force Armstrong Lab., AL/CF-TR-1997-0141, Brooks Air Force Base, TX, 1997.

[145]Lessard, C. S., Matthews, R., and Yauch, D., "Effects of Rotation on Somatogravic Illusions," *IEEE in Engineering and Biology*, Vol. 19, 2000, pp. 59–65.

[146]Previc, F. H., Ghani, N., Stevens, K. W., and Ludwig, D. A., "Effects of Background Field-of-View and Depth-Plane on the Oculogyral Illusion," *Perceptual and Motor Skills*, Vol. 93, 2001, pp. 867–878.

[147]Kennedy, R. S., Hettinger, L. J., and Lilienthal, M. G., "Simulator Sickness," *Motion and space sickness*, edited by G. H. Crampton, CRC Press, Boca Raton, FL, 1990, pp. 318.

[148]Stanney, K., Salvendy, G., Deisinger, J., DiZio, P., Ellis, S., Ellison., J., Fogleman, G., Gallimore, J., Singer, M., Hettinger, L., Kennedy, R., Lackner, J., Lawson, B., Maida, J., Mead, A., Mon-Williams, M., Newman, D., Piantanida, T., Reeves, L., Riedel, O., Stoffregan, T., Wann, J., Welch, R., Wilson, J., and Witmer, B., "Aftereffects and Sense of Presence in Virtual Environments: Formulation of a Research and Development Agenda," *International Journal of Human-Computer Interaction*, Vol. 10, 1998, pp. 135–187.

[149]Kleiss, J. A., and Hubbard, D. C., "Effects of Three Types of Flight Simulator Visual Scene Detail on Detection of Altitude Change," *Human Factors*, Vol. 35, 1993, pp. 653–671.

[150]Otakeno, S., Matthews, R. S. J., Folio, L., Previc, F. H., and Lessard, C. S., "The Effects of Visual Scenes on Roll and Pitch Thresholds in Pilots Versus Nonpilots," *Aviation, Space, and Environmental Medicine*, Vol. 73, 2002, pp. 98–101.

[151]Hettinger, L. J., Nelson, W. T., and Haas, M. W., "Target Detection Performance in Helmet-Mounted and Conventional Dome Displays," *International Journal of Aviation Psychology*, Vol. 6, 1996, pp. 321–334.

[152]Pierce, B. J., Arrington, K. F., and Moreno, M. A., "Motion and Stereoscopic Tilt Perception," *Journal of the Society for Information Display*, Vol. 7, 1999, pp. 193–206.

[153]Cohn, J. V., DiZio, P., and Lackner, J. R., "Reaching During Virtual Rotation: Context Specific Compensations for Expected Coriolis Forces," *Journal of Neurophysiology*, Vol. 83, 2000, pp. 3230–3240.

[154]"*Countering the Directed Energy Threat: Are Closed Cockpits the Ultimate Answer?*," North Atlantic Treaty Organization Research and Technology Organization, RTO-MP-30, Neuilly-sur-Seine, France, 2000.

[155]Johnson, S. L., and Roscoe, S. N., "What Moves, the Airplane or the World?," *Human Factors*, Vol. 14, 1972, pp. 107–109.

[156]Previc, F. H., and Ercoline, W. R., "The 'Outside-In' Attitude Display Concept Revisited," *International Journal of Aviation Psychology*, Vol. 9, 1999, pp. 377–401.

[157]Malcolm, R., "Pilot Disorientation and the Use of a Peripheral Vision Display," *Aviation, Space, and Environmental Medicine*, Vol. 55, 1984, pp. 231–238.

[158]Snow, M. P., Reising, J. M., Liggett, K. K., and Barry, T. P., "Flying Complex Approaches Using a Head-Up Display: Effects of Visibility and Display Type," *Proceedings of the Tenth International Symposium on Aviation Psychology*, edited by R. Jensen, Ohio State Univ., Columbus, OH, 1999.

[159]Allen, M. J., and Cholet, M. E., "Strength and Association Between Sex and Field Dependence," *Perceptual and Motor Skills*, Vol. 47, 1978, pp. 419–421.

[160]Darlington, C. L., and Smith, P. F., "Further Evidence for Gender Differences in Circularvection," *Journal of Vestibular Research*, Vol. 8, 1998, pp. 151–153.

[161]Witkin, H. A., and Wapner, S., "Visual Factors in the Maintenance of Upright Posture," *American Journal of Psychology*, Vol. 63, 1950, pp. 31–50.

[162]Previc, F. H., "A General Theory Concerning the Prenatal Origins of Cerebral Lateralization in Humans," *Psychological Review*, Vol. 98, 1991, pp. 299–334.

[163]Newland, G. A., "Left-Handedness and Field-Independence," *Neuropsychologia*, Vol. 22, 1984, pp. 617–619.

[164]Forssberg, H., and Nashner, L. M., "Ontogenetic Development of Postural Control in Man: Adaptation to Altered Support and Visual Conditions During Stance," *Journal of Neuroscience*, Vol. 2, 1982, pp. 545–552.

[165]Lord, S. R., and Webster, I. W., "Visual Field Dependence in Elderly Fallers and Non-Fallers," *International Journal of Aging and Human Development*, Vol. 31, 1990, pp. 267–277.

[166]Paige, G. D., "Senescence of Human Visual-Vestibular Interactions: Smooth Pursuit, Optokinetic, and Vestibular Control of Eye Movements with Aging," *Experimental Brain Research*, Vol. 98, 1994, pp. 355–372.

[167]Cheung, B. S., Howard, I. P., Nedzelski, J. M., and Landolt, J. P., "Circularvection About Earth-Horizontal Axes in Bilateral and Labyrinthine-Defective Subjects," *Acta Oto-laryngologica*, Vol. 108, 1989, pp. 336–344.

[168]Redfern, M. S., and Furman, J. M., "Postural Sway of Patients with Vestibular Disorders During Optic Flow," *Journal of Vestibular Research*, Vol. 4, 1994, pp. 221–230.

[169]Cheung, B. S. K., Howard, I. P., and Money, K. E., "Visually Induced Tilt During Parabolic Flights," *Experimental Brain Research*, Vol. 81, 1990, pp. 391–397.

[170]Young, L. R., Shelhamer, M., and Modestino, S., "M.I.T./Canadian Vestibular Experiments in the Spacelab-1 Mission: 2. Visual Vestibular Tilt Interaction in Weightlessness," *Experimental Brain Research*, Vol. 64, 1986, pp. 299–307.

[171]Young, L. R., Oman, C. M., and Dichgans, J. M., "Influence of Head Orientation on Visually Induced Pitch and Roll Sensation," *Aviation, Space, and Environmental Medicine*, Vol. 46, 1975, pp. 264–268.

[172]Lessard, C. S., Stevens, K., Maidment, G., and Oakley, C., "Comparison of Optokinetic Scene Effects on the Somatogravic Illusion," *SAFE Journal*, Vol. 30, 2000, pp. 140–155.

[173]Hettinger, L. J., Berbaum, K. S., Kennedy, R. S., Dunlap, W. P., and Nolan, M. D., "Vection and Simulator Sickness," *Military Psychology*, Vol. 2, 1990, pp. 171–181.

[174]Vitte, E., Diard, J. P., Freyss, M., and Freyss, G., "Dynamic Posturography—Equitest in Evaluation of Pilots Aptitudes," *Posture and Gait: Control Mechanisms*, Vol. I, edited by M. Woolacott and F. Horak, Univ. of Oregon Books, Eugene, OR, 1992, pp. 246–249.

[175]Brandt, U., Fluur, E., and Zylberstein, M. Z., "Relationship Between Flight Experience and Vestibular Function in Pilots and Nonpilots," *Aerospace Medicine*, Vol. 45, 1974, pp. 1232–1236.

[176]Kohen-Raz, R., Kohen-Raz, A., Erel, J., Davidson, B., Caine, Y., and Froom, P., "Postural Control in Pilots and Candidates for Flight Training," *Aviation, Space, and Environmental Medicine*, Vol. 65, 1994, pp. 323–326.

[177]Previc, F. H., "Functional Specialization in the Lower and Upper Visual Fields in Humans: Its Ecological Origins and Neuropsychological Implications," *Behavioral and Brain Sciences*, Vol. 13, 1990, pp. 519–575.

[178]Bronstein, A. M., Hood, J. D., Gresty, M. A., and Panagi, C., "Visual Control of Balance in Cerebellar and Parkinsonian Syndromes," *Brain*, Vol. 113, 1990, pp. 767–779.

[179]Simpson, J. I., "The Accessory Optic System," *Annual Review of Neuroscience*, Vol. 7, 1984, pp. 13–41.

[180]Beer, J., Blakemore, C., Previc, F. H., and Liotti, M., "Areas of the Human Brain Activated by Ambient Visual Motion, Indicating Three Kinds of Self-Movement," *Experimental Brain Research*, Vol. 143, 2002, pp. 78–88.

[181]Henn, V., Young, L. R., and Finley, C., "Vestibular Nuclei in Alert Monkeys Are Also Influenced by Moving Visual Fields," *Brain Research*, Vol. 71, 1974, pp. 144–149.

[182]Xerri, C., Borel, L., Barthelemy, J., and Lacour, M., "Synergistic Interactions and Functional Working Range of the Visual and Vestibular Systems in Postural Control: Neuronal Correlates," *Progress in Brain Research*, Vol. 76, 1988, pp. 193–203.

[183]Wylie, D. R. W., Bischof, W. F., and Frost, B. J., "Common Reference Frame for Neural Coding of Translational and Rotational Optic Flow," *Nature*, Vol. 392, 1998, pp. 278–282.

[184]Previc, F. H., Liotti, M., Blakemore, C., Beer, J., and Fox, P., "Functional Imaging of Brain Areas Involved in the Processing of Coherent and Incoherent Wide Field-of-View Visual Motion," *Experimental Brain Research*, Vol. 131, 2000, pp. 393–405.

[185]Diener, H. C., Dichgans, J., Bacher, M., and Gompf, B., "Quantification of Postural Sway in Normals and Patients with Cerebellar Diseases," *Electroencephalography and Clinical Neurophysiology*, Vol. 57, 1984, pp. 134–142.

[186]Buttner, U., and Henn, V., "Thalamic Unit Activity in the Alert Monkey During Natural Vestibular Stimulation," *Brain Research*, Vol. 103, 1976, pp. 127–132.

[187]Straube, A., and Brandt, T., "Importance of the Visual and Vestibular Cortex for Self-Motion Perception in Man (Circularvection)," *Human Neurobiology*, Vol. 6, 1987, pp. 211–218.

[188]Brandt, T., Dieterich, M., and Danek, A., "Vestibular Cortex Lesions Affect the Perception of Verticality," *Annals of Neurology*, Vol. 35, 1994, pp. 403–412.

[189]Gattass, R., Rosa, M. G. P., Sousa, A. P. B., Pinon, M. C. G., Fiorani, M., and Neuenschwander, S., "Cortical Streams of Visual Information Processing in Primates," *Brazilian Journal of Medical and Biological Research*, Vol. 23, 1990, pp. 375–393.

[190]Heide, W., Koenig, E., and Dichgans, J., "Optokinetic Nystagmus, Self-Motion Sensation and Their Aftereffects in Patients with Occipito-Parietal Lesions," *Clinical Vision Sciences*, Vol. 5, 1990, pp. 145–156.

[191]Cheng, K., Fujita, H., Kanno, I., Miura, S., and Tanaka, K., "Human Cortical Regions Activated by Wide-Field Visual Motion: An H_2 ^{15}O PET Study," *Journal of Neurophysiology*, Vol. 74, 1995, pp. 413–427.

[192]Brandt, T., Bartenstein, P., Janek, A., and Dieterich, M., "Reciprocal Inhibitory Visual-Vestibular Interaction: Visual Motion Stimulation Deactivates the Parieto-Insular Vestibular Cortex," *Brain*, Vol. 121, 1998, pp. 1749–1758.

[193]Bottini, G., Sterzi, R., Paulesu, E., Vallar, G., Cappa, S. F., Erminio, F., Passingham, R. E., Frith, C. D., and Frackowiak, R. S. J., "Identification of the Central Vestibular Projections in Man: A Positron Emission Tomography Activation Study," *Experimental Brain Research*, Vol. 99, 1994, pp. 164–169.

[194]Grusser, O.-J., and Guldin, W. O., "Primate Vestibular Cortices and Spatial Orientation," *Multisensory Control of Posture*, edited by T. Mergner and F. Hlavacka, Plenum, New York, pp. 51–62.

[195]Hikosaka, K., Iwai, E., Saito, H.-A., and Tanaka, K., "Polysensory Properties of Neurons in the Anterior Bank of the Caudal Superior Temporal Sulcus of the Macaque Monkey," *Journal of Neurophysiology*, Vol. 60, 1988, pp. 1615–1637.

[196]Friberg, L., Olsen, T. S., Roland, P. E., Paulson, O. B., and Lassen, N. A., "Focal Increase of Blood Flow in the Cerebral Cortex of Man During Vestibular Stimulation," *Brain*, Vol. 198, 1985, pp. 609–623.

[197]Previc, F. H., Beer, J., Liotti, M., Blakemore, C., and Fox, P., "Is 'Ambient Vision' Distributed in the Brain?," *Journal of Vestibular Research*, Vol. 10, 2000, pp. 221–225.

[198]Solms, M., Kaplan-Solms, K., Saling, M., and Miller, P., "Inverted Vision After Frontal Lobe Disease," *Cortex*, Vol. 24, 1988, pp. 499–509.

Chapter 4

Psychological Factors

Valerie Gawron*

General Dynamics Advanced Information Systems, Buffalo, New York

PSYCHOLOGY is the study of the mind and behavior and how that behavior is affected by personality, mental and physical state, experience, task, and environment. Each of these psychological factors and its relation to spatial disorientation (SD) is described in detail in this chapter.

I. Personality and Other Traits

Personality is "the complex of characteristics that distinguishes an individual."[1] Personality has been studied in relation to SD. For example, Ponomarenko et al.[2] began with a quote from Captain S. S. Ivanov, a world-class pilot: "In aviation cowards are not chided they are washed out." Certainly one of the characteristics of pilots is bravery or more specifically the ability to withstand the fear of heights and speeds, equipment failures, maintenance errors, hazardous weather, and, for military pilots, hostile enemy actions. This bravery can lead pilots into situations that induce SD, such as flying 1) into weather while carrying injured personnel, 2) while under pressure to complete a mission, or 3) while fatigued (see Sec. II.A) to develop tactics for new aircraft. Other relevant personality characteristics are succumbing to pressure to make a flight, overconfidence, love of flying, spatial ability, and lack of discipline.

A. Succumbing to Pressure to Make a Flight

Pilots increase their risk of SD by bending to pressure to make a flight. In an analysis of U.S. civil aviation helicopter spatial disorientation accidents from 1983–1996, one of the top factors reported was "pressure to make the flight" (Ref. 3, p. 16). Similarly, it was concluded from a questionnaire completed by 8800 Canadian pilots (1084 airline transport, 1969 commercial, 285 helicopter, and 5480 private) that pilots who had had accidents were more likely to have "flown in spite

---

This material is declared a work of the U.S. Government and is not subject to copyright protection in the United States.
*Fellow.

of advice from others" or "been pressured into flying under marginal conditions when they didn't want to fly" (Ref. 4, p. 43). These authors, however, made no attempt to correlate personality traits to type of aircraft accident.

In contrast, Mortimer[5] focused only on SD accidents. In a review of aircraft accidents reported by the National Transportation Safety Board (NTSB) during 1983–1991, he concluded that the following psychological factors were involved in the SD accidents that occurred during this period: pressure to complete the trip, concern about the weather combined with discounting "their own deficiencies and lack of adequate experience in such conditions and inexperience which forced the pilot to use spare cognitive capacity to the other tasks" (p. 1310).

B. Overconfidence

For military pilots other personality traits appear to be related to SD accidents. Sanders and Hoffman[6] compared the personality traits of pilots who had been involved in a pilot-error accident (SD was included in this category) and those who had not. Personality was assessed using Cattell's Sixteen Personality Factor Questionnaire. The subjects were 51 U.S. Army helicopter pilots. The pilots who had been in pilot-error accidents were more likely to be self-sufficient rather than group dependent, more imaginative than practical, and more forthright and less shrewd than pilots who had not been in a pilot-error accident. These results were extended in a later study involving 66 helicopter pilots.[7] For SD accidents Kuipers et al.[8] concluded, based on interviews with 209 Dutch F-5 and F-16 pilots, that personality characteristics played a substantial role (F-5 88%, F-16 86%). These characteristics included overconfidence, lack of vigilance and risk awareness, and false sense of safety.

C. Love of Flying

"The most intimate secret of the flying man arises from the genesis of the wings, as they are not of metal, but of Spirit, doling out in a measure which is still a great mystery, . . . a kingdom in the sky, grounded by rules, but unbounded by the love of flying" (Ref. 2, p. 35). Love of flying leads some pilots to fly beyond their capabilities, for example, in instrument meteorological conditions (IMC) without instrument-flight-rules (IFR) training and in conditions that might induce SD (e.g., whiteout).

D. Spatial Ability

"Spatial ability is a basic dimension of human intelligence, clearly separate from verbal intelligence or general reasoning ability" (Ref. 9, p. 103). In a classic study, Clark and Malone[10] measured the ability of 242 U.S. Naval Academy cadets to identify headings between cities. They reported large ranges in the estimated headings, including some that were 180 deg off. Errors were negatively correlated to the spatial visualization portion of the Guilford–Zimmerman test (-0.13), a mechanical comprehension test used routinely by the U.S. Naval Academy (-0.14), the American Council on Education Q (nonlanguage) (-0.19) and Total scores (-0.15), correctness of expression developed as part of the U.S. Armed Forces Institute tests (-0.15), mathematics developed by the Central Examining

Board of the Naval Air Training Command (−0.18), and personal estimate of orientation portion of the Guildford–Zimmerman test (−0.19). Clearly, poor spatial ability is related to visualization, mathematical, and spatial orientation (SO) abilities. Spatial ability is critical to maintaining SO especially at low altitudes. As Taylor[11] states, "There are large individual differences in the frequency with which pilots become geographically disoriented on low-altitude attack training missions" (B9-7). Likewise, Boer argued that pilots with good spatial ability are less susceptible to "disorientation" (Ref. 9, p. 103).

E. Lack of Discipline

In a study of five fatal accidents (four Indian Navy and one Royal Air Force), Dudani[12] reported a predominance of supervision and discipline factors. These factors included unauthorized low-level flying and aerobatics. Further, Green and Taylor[13] provide case studies in which personality contributed to an aircraft accident. A pilot with a "history of indiscipline" struck power lines while performing illegal low-level flight; another flew at 10 ft (3.05 m) over water, turned, and struck the water. Although low-altitude flight over water to minimize the risk of detection is a standard procedure in helicopters, because of the risk of SD, it is not performed unless directed to do so. As can be seen from the representation in Fig. 1, the margin of safety is very small for these maneuvers.

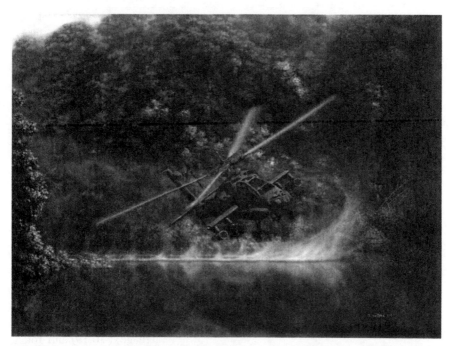

Fig. 1 Low-level flight over water showing the very small margin of safety in such operations. (Reproduced with permission of the U.S. Department of Defense.)

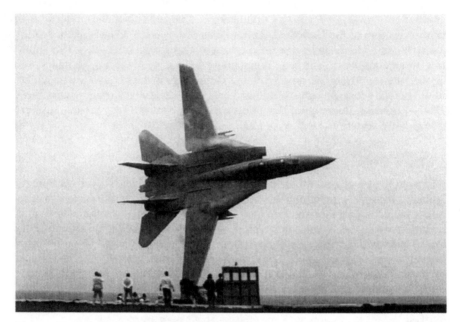

Fig. 2 Unauthorized, low-altitude flyby during deployment of the nuclear aircraft carrier *USS Stennis*. (Reproduced with permission of the U.S. Department of Defense.)

More recently another pilot flew within 10 ft (3.05 m) of an aircraft carrier (see Fig. 2). No one was injured, but the pilot was grounded for 30 days. Again, the margin of safety is very small and even slight and fleeting SD could have resulted in loss of the crew and aircraft, and damage to the aircraft carrier.

II. Mental and Physical State

The mental and physical state of pilots has been an infrequently discussed topic in SD. The reasons are many but most stem from the perceived need for pilots to be perfect, that is, pilots cannot make mistakes. They limit their perceived susceptibility to fatigue (Sec. II.A), emotion (Sec. II.B), stress (Sec. II.C), drugs (Sec. II.D), poor health (Sec. II.E), or injury (Chapter 6). Finally, they can never acknowledge a loss of situational awareness (SA) (Sec. II.F). "Few pilots like to admit susceptibility to a sensory malfunction, yet most are quick to understand when another pilot experiences the same type of problem" (Ref. 14, p. 619). Pilots, as a whole, love to fly, and anything that threatens their flight status is usually hidden—even from other pilots. This section discusses many of those hidden topics—topics that many pilots talk about only after they have retired or only to a trusted friend.

A. Fatigue

Fatigue is multifaceted and complex. The effects of fatigue not only overlap the areas of performance, physiology, cognition, and emotion, but they also combine with other states, such as boredom or drowsiness.[15] The two general types of fatigue are peripheral (physical) fatigue and central (mental) fatigue. Physical fatigue is generally defined as a reduction in capacity to perform physical work as a function of preceding physical effort. Mental fatigue is inferred from decrements in performance on tasks requiring alertness and the manipulation and retrieval of information stored in memory.[16]

Fatigue was defined as measurable decrements in performance of an activity caused by the extended time for performing the activity. This definition led to the traditional understanding that as a subject's time on task increases his or her performance decreases in a linear fashion.[15] However, other factors can also influence fatigue. For example, a 1983 study of naval aviation accidents suggested that the major contributors to fatigue might be the total time spent at work (inclusive of the task) *and* the time of day at which the work occurs.[17] Other researchers have also studied this relationship.[18] In 1996, Stoner[19] used anonymous questionnaires, physiological measurements (mean arterial pressure, pulse, and pulse pressure), the Armed Forces Vision Tester, and hematological measurements (complete blood count and sedimentation rate) to try to predict early fatigue in 42 Navy EP-3E aircrews. However, none of the physiological or hematological measurements varied between fatigue and normal states, although 14% of personnel did show increased tendencies for visual phorias that could be related to SD.[19]

Landing or takeoff under emergency conditions, dealing with in-flight emergencies, and ingress under fire are difficult circumstances for the most vigilant crews, and burdening crews with fatigue from sleep deprivation can cripple their abilities to deal with emergencies. In fact, the U.S. Air Force (USAF) Safety Center relates that of 92 Class A incidents—those that involve over one million dollars worth of damage or loss of life—between 1972 and 1995, 60% of these incidents were related to sleep deprivation.[20] Long transmeridian flights have almost three times the incident rate of shorter flights.[21] The fact that human error or loss of cockpit coordination causes as many as 75% of accidents strongly implicates fatigue and circadian disruption.[22] Dramatic deficiencies in operational performance are also easily observed in simulator tests (in commercial airline aircraft simulators, for example[23]).

In a military example SD and fatigue associated with a demanding night flying schedule and development of new tactics might have contributed to the crashes of two USAF/Lockheed F-117A fighters in 1986 and 1987 (Ref. 24, p. 22). Flying while fatigued is not unique to USAF pilots. Based on a survey of 104 naval helicopter pilots, Tormes and Guedry[25] concluded that 32% had experienced SD caused by fatigue. Recently, LeDuc et al.[26] observed eight UH-60 rated aviators while they performed missions in a desktop NUH-60 simulator after varying lengths of sleep deprivation. Hover performance was degraded, along with SD recovery. Recovery time was significantly longer when fatigued (90.5 s) than when rested (78.0 s).[26]

Repetitive missions can lead to chronic fatigue and increase the human cost of long-endurance missions. Frequently, these operations involve multiple days of sustained operations with little sleep or poor sleep between missions.[27] The impairment associated with repetitive, long-duration flights was documented during Operations Desert Shield and Desert Storm[28,29] and in a simulator study.[30]

The deterioration of physical and mental performance associated with circadian desynchrony is well documented in aviation human factors research.[23,31−33] Aircrews are at particular risk because they often must take off at night, consequently experiencing altered light and dark cycles. Light exposure can disrupt normal

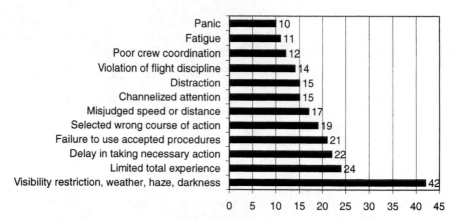

Fig. 3 Frequency of occurrence of psychophysiological and environmental factors associated with SD in U.S. Naval aviators. (Adapted from Ref. 37, p. A5-2.)

circadian cycles[34] so that recovery from mission-induced fatigue might take longer for crews exposed to unusual light cycles.

Pharmaceutical techniques have been an effective means to promote vigilance or induce sleep, and new compounds are available that are safer (better tolerated) and more efficacious. These are discussed in detail in Gawron et al.[35]

B. Emotion

Emotion is "the affective aspect of consciousness" or "a state of feeling."[1] Emotions can reduce the "pilot's ability to resist spatial disorientation" (Ref. 36, p. 65). Ninow et al.[37] studied SD in naval aviators and found many psychophysiological factors associated with SD. These factors and the frequency of their occurrence are presented in Fig. 3. Note that, although the least frequently cited, panic does occur in these highly select and highly trained pilots at a rate similar to more well known and often reported factors, such as fatigue and poor crew coordination.

Pilots often do not admit to feelings of fear, awe, reverence, serenity, anger, or grief and yet all of these affect their flying abilities. Stories are rampant of pilots physically injured off base pleading with their compatriots to get them to a civilian doctor who would not report the injury. Stories of psychological injury such as grief as a result of the loss of a loved one are almost nonexistent because psychological injury can be hidden from the flight doctor.

1. Fear

As indicated by Captain S. S. Ivanov's quote at the beginning of this chapter, the association of fear with cowardice leads some pilots to not admit to fear. But pilots are exposed to conditions that instill fear in most people: equipment failures, maintenance errors, heights, speeds, hazardous weather, and, in military pilots, hostile enemy actions. This fear can literally affect what the pilot sees, in a phenomenon called paradoxical cognition.[38] According to one researcher, "asking a subject to ignore [stimulus elements] may be as effective as asking him not to think of pink elephants" (Ref. 39, p. 8). The following anonymous quote illustrates this phenomenon in flight.

> The crew chief told me to keep an eye on the fuel level since the guy who had previously flown the airplane reported "anomalies". What the heck are anomalies? A guy in another squadron had augured in, the week before due to fuel exhaustion. Would I be next? I started out with my usual crosscheck followed by a glance at the fuel. Fifteen minutes into the flight I did my crosscheck but then stared at the darn fuel gauge. Did you know if you look at something long enough it moves? By the time I realized I was seeing the fuel load increase (and I was NOT attached to a tanker) I was spatially disoriented. I could have been on my back for all I knew.

In an early study Doppelt[40] stated that 55% of the pilots surveyed reported that vertigo did not occur in training flights but did doing the same maneuvers in operational flight due to the "scare factor" (p. 5). Further, "heightened neuropsychological arousal as in conditions of acute awareness elicited by imposed high workload or perceived threat may result in behavioral regression with a return to more primitive or infantile modes of response, like the breakdown of complex learned flying skills and higher mental functions" (Ref. 41, p. B2-6).

Based on data from Desert Storm, Durnford et al.[42] stated, "Flight over the desert and wartime were two factors linked to increased severity of SD episodes. The fact that there was no similar significant link for flight over snow (or water) suggests that wartime may be the key factor" (Ref. 42, p. 76). "In 43 percent of worst ever episodes, aircrew were not immediately aware of being disoriented" (Ref. 42, p. 76).

The fear associated with SD does not have to be related to physical danger. De Giosa[43] reported from a survey of 100 Italian pilots that over 60% attributed perceptual disturbances to economic worries. Other responses indicated that pilots were predisposed to perceptual disturbances when flying as a passenger rather than pilot, suffering from alimentary excesses, or wearing a helmet. All of these situations can be related to the fear stemming from loss of control, illness, and the threat of attack. Conversely, there is an exhilaration that comes from fear. This exhilaration comes from the adrenaline that is pumped into the blood in a primitive "fight or flight" response. For some pilots, such an adrenaline rush defies the innate fears of speed and height, as with the following anonymous pilot:

> "I always pushed the envelope—any envelope—speed, altitude, G. If the airplane didn't shake, rattle, and roll I wasn't flying at the edge. The problem with flying at the edge is falling off. Many a time I looked at my attitude gauge and realized I was plummeting to the earth when I thought I was streaking for the sky."

This phenomenon might have a neurochemical basis. Specifically, intense stimulation such as pushing the aircraft envelope can cause the brain to release dopamine. Dopamine produces a feeling of euphoria that can be very addictive. This hypothesis is further supported by work at the National Institute of Mental Health in Bethesda, Maryland, in which blood flow measurements of cocaine addicts showed an increase in the left caudate section of the brain, an area with a high density of dopamine receptors.

The relationship of neruochemical addiction and flying is supported by research conducted in the former Soviet Union. "A dangerous occupation demands . . . a sociopsychological readiness to work under extreme conditions . . . and . . . an exceptionally adaptable nervous system allowing a flexible brain function to provide creative processes, such as intuition, forecasting, and heuristics" (Ref. 2, p. 19).

These authors conclude that pilots differ from professionals who work on the ground in a number of biochemical and psychophysiological respects.

> Secretion of hormones, enzymes, sugar, and other biochemical substances of flyers are normally 3 to 4 times higher, and during flight, many even be 10 to 12 times greater; tension and concentration in the first hour on a fighter plane, is equal to 8 hours of stress for any ground transportation operator (driver); during flight, there is a constant disparity between signal perception and the actual gravitational axis of the body in space, due to changed earth gravity resulting from sustain G forces, which represents a double stress on the brain (Ref. 2, p. 25).

2. Awe

The sky has always held a fascination for humans. It has been gazed upon with wonder from the beginning of time. Pilots are unique in their ability to get up close and personal with the sky. The following anonymous quotes illustrate how the fascination with celestial events can increase the risk of SD.

> I was above the thunderclouds on a dark night and could see the lightning piercing the night. It was the best light show I had ever seen. It went on for miles and miles. Miles in which I lost track of altitude and heading. We were miles off course before I could tear my eyes away from the sight of that lightning.

> The most beautiful sight I have ever seen is a halo around the aircraft. It is formed by ice crystals and each crystal reflects the colors of the rainbow. It's like being caught inside a prism. Each time I find myself inside a halo I have to force myself to look back into the cockpit to check the attitude and often am amazed how far off straight-and-level flight I am.

Probably the most commonly reported phenomenon reported to instill awe is sunset:

> I had never seen so many colors of orange and red. The clouds looked as if they were giant sponges of color. I watched as the clouds changed shape and oranges bled to red and finally maroons. It was 100 miles (161 km) before I realized I had banked the aircraft to get a better view of the incredible sunset.

3. Reverence

Since the beginning of time, humans have imagined their god or gods as dwelling in the heavens. The separation from Earth while flying has led some pilots to experience being with God:

> When I took off that day I wasn't thinking about God—only about the mission to be flown. It wasn't a dangerous one, rather it was rather tedious and boring. I looked out the windscreen and saw the heavens stretching for eternities in all directions. I thought about life and the after life and slowly felt like I was in the presence of God. I wasn't afraid or angry, just at peace. I heard a voice inside me telling me to look at the altimeter. I had slowly climbed thousands of feet. I returned to my assigned altitude. The sense of peace left me (Anonymous).

4. Serenity

Many pilots have experienced a sense of serenity, of peace, of separation from the problems of the world. The perceived stillness can be comforting as well as a source of disorientation as attested by the following anonymous quote: "Once I reached my assigned altitude, I took a deep breadth and all the world's problems seemed to drain away. The skies were blue and here there was no war, no illness, no poverty, no ugliness. I flew for 20 minutes before I realized I was in a shallow bank and probably had been for a long time."

5. Anger

Anger affects perception and focus (see Fig. 4), as is demonstrated by the saying, "I was so angry I couldn't see straight." Although there is an outward accommodative shift that occurs with strong emotion,[44] there is a psychological component as well. Anger results in focusing attention on the object of that anger vs appropriate orientation cues, thereby precipitating SD. The following anonymous quotes illustrate this consequence:

"The dogfight lasted less than one minute and I watched as the plane I hit burst into flame and the other attacker broke off. Then I saw my wingman go after the remaining attacker. We were nearly out of fuel. I called my wingman and ordered him back. He replied, "I'm going to get that @#&&. The #$@ shot at me!" I watched as he banked wildly to catch up with the survivor. "Attitude! Attitude!" I shouted over the radio. Something in my voice finally got through and my wingman returned to straight and level. "@#$% I thought I was straight and level!" He was in fact 45° nose down."

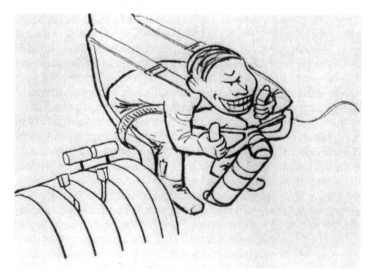

Fig. 4 Angry pilot fixated on exacting a toll with his airplane on someone or something. (Reproduced with permission of Ron Colgrove.)

"I was delivering medical supplies to a disaster area when suddenly the windscreen cracked. I realized immediately that the crack was due to a bullet. The #$@ we were trying to help were in fact shooting at us. I started a dive-bombing run but I realized I only could drop drugs and blankets on the shooter! I was 15 ft off the ground before I pulled out and began to climb."

6. Grief

Grief is another emotion that colors a pilot's perception of the world and can lead to SD:

Nine days after my son's funeral I was back flying. The folks in the mission prebrief went on as usual. No one mentioned my son or asked how I was doing. I climbed into the airplane and launched. The mission was reconnaissance and I had my hands full until I started for home. Cruising back there was a lot of white fog and I started thinking about how my son had looked in that white hospital gown lying against those white sheets. I didn't realize that I was in a dive until I heard my son's voice shouting, "Daddy, watch out!" To this day, I believe that it was truly his voice, not my imagination (Anonymous).

C. Stress

Stress is the response of the body to any demand made on it. The body's response to stress is 1) alarm, during which the pilot orients to the stressor and decides on a response; 2) resistance during which the pilot responds to eliminate or minimize the stressor; and 3) exhaustion, during which the pilot no longer has the energy to continue the response. Tepper[45] identified four categories of stressors. These are presented in Table 1.

Yanowitch listed additional chronic stressors: 1) loss of spouse through divorce, separation, death; 2) death in family; 3) illness of self or family; 4) debts; 5) number of arguments; 6) change of job; 7) change in worship; 8) change in eating habits; 9) change in sleeping; and 10) change in accident behavior (Ref. 46, p. 920).

In an early survey of military aircrew, Goorney and O'Connor reported that stressor events such as those just listed were followed by anxiety of flying. These events included disorientation and depersonalization under conditions of reduced sensory input, such as at high altitude (e.g., break-off phenomenon, see Sec. VI.A). The outcome for pilots experiencing these symptoms were permanent grounding (8%), role change or flying restriction (69%), and return to full flying (23%). Symptoms were either shown under all flight conditions (i.e., generalized anxiety) or under the conditions originally eliciting the anxiety (i.e., focal anxiety). The prognosis of returning the former group to full flying was poor.

Based on three case studies, Raymond and Moser (1995) concluded, "excess emotional stress may have an adverse effect on pilot performance and is known to increase the risk of an aircraft mishap" (p. 35). In the first case, an airline pilot crashed during low-level aerobatic maneuvers. The authors attribute the mishap to stress in the pilot's professional and personal life. However, cannabinoid metabolite (i.e., marijuana) was detected in his urine. In the second case, an Army helicopter pilot performed an unauthorized maneuver and crashed. He had contracted a sexually transmitted disease from an extramarital affair and was ejected from his home

Table 1   Aviation stressors[45]

Flying stressors	Anxiety stressors	Emergency stressors	Personal stressors
Height	Level of training	Control/trim malfunction	Hunger
Pressure changes	Level of confidence	Engine failure	Fatigue
Acceleration	Unfamiliar aircraft	In-flight fire or explosion	Loss of sleep
Motion	Unfamiliar route	Midair collision	Hangover
Turbulence	Unfamiliar airport	Bird strike	Minor illness
Low humidity	Poor runway conditions	Ditching	Self-medication
Glare	Poor weather	Loss of formation leader	Lack of family support
Vibration	Low fuel	Disorientation	Anger
Noise	Malfunctioning navigation equipment	In-flight incapacitation	Frustration
Cold	Low altitude	——	Worry
Heat	IFR and night flying	——	Oversensitivity
Inactivity	Fear of losing face	——	Guilt
Uncomfortable personal equipment	Lack of confidence in aircraft design	——	Memories of horrifying sights

and threatened with divorce. The third case involved a naval aviator who was a recovering alcoholic and had been recently divorced, denied visitation to his child, and been passed over for promotion. In addition he had impregnated a former girlfriend and was being investigated for participation in the Tailhook incident.

On the positive side, experienced pilots might be able to handle the heightened stress created by the flying environment itself better than less experienced ones. For example, Krahenbuhl et al.[47] compared catecholamine levels of pilots who had received power-on-stall and spin recovery training in a ground simulator and those who had not. The catecholamine levels were measured after their in-flight exposure to power-on stalls and spin recoveries. There were two significant differences: epinephrine level was lower, and the norepinephrine/epinephrine ratio was higher in those who had received simulator training relative to those who had not. The authors interpreted these data as indicating reduced arousal in the experienced pilots.

D. Drugs

The Federal Aviation Administration (FAA) can reexamine and revoke an aircrew's certificate when an aircrew member is "under the influence of alcohol" or taking a drug that "affects the person's faculties in any way contrary to safety." The majority of data on how drugs affecting flight safety have been from alcohol studies. These data are from accidents, laboratories, ground simulators, and actual flight. The results of each type of data are summarized next. In addition, previous discrepancies between ground simulator and flight-test results are also summarized.

1. Accident Data

In the first accident analysis to search for blood-alcohol-concentration (BAC) effects, Harper and Albers[48] reported that 35.4% of 158 fatal aircraft accidents that occurred in 1963 involved alcohol (i.e., BAC of 0.015% or above). In almost 50% of the accidents that involved alcohol, the aircraft crashed within 18 min of takeoff and/or the accident occurred at night. The pilot in about 35% of the accidents that involved alcohol had 300 hours or less flying experience. Harper and Alloy's work prompted a follow-on study by the FAA. Based on three years of autopsy data, Gibbons reported alcohol involvement in 30% of fatal accidents.[49–52] For the accidents in which the BAC was positive, 88% of the cases had BACs of 0.10% or higher.

The 1984 report of the U.S. National Transportation Board (NTSB) contained a statistical review of general aviation fatal accidents between 1975 and 1981. The major findings were that alcohol was involved in 10.5% of the general aviation accidents, 6.4% of commuter aviation accidents, and 7.4% of the on-demand air taxi accidents. In 16% of the fatal accidents, the pilot's detectable BAC was 0.04% or less. The most frequently cited cause in these accidents was "alcohol impairment of efficiency and judgment." Pilots in alcohol-related accidents were slightly more experienced than pilots in non-alcohol-related fatal accidents. In fact, in 30% of the alcohol-involved accidents the pilot had 1500 or more flight hours. Comparison of fatal and alcohol-involved fatal accidents revealed that more alcohol-involved fatal accidents occurred at night (38%) than other types of fatal accidents (22%). More recent work by Canfield et al.[53] reported alcohol at 0.04% or higher in 146 of the 1845 pilots who died in civil aviation accidents between 1989 and 1993.

In a recent study, Hordinsky and Kuhlman[54] reported that 0.04% or greater BACs were found in 8.2% of all general aviation accidents that occurred from October 1988 through September 1989. Li et al.[55] examined 337 aviation-related fatalities that occurred in North Carolina between 1985 and 1994. They found 7% of the pilots and 15% of the nonpilot occupants had BACs ranging from 0.02 to 0.14%. All four fatalities with BACs over 0.10% were pilots aged 20 to 29 years old flying nighttime general aviation aircraft. McFadden[56] reported that pilots with "driving while intoxicated" convictions have an increased accident risk. Canfield et al.[57] reported 124 out of 1683 pilots in fatal aviation accidents that occurred 1994 to 1998 had BACs above the legal 0.04% BAC level. These authors also reported incidence of controlled dangerous substances such as marijuana, cocaine, and amphetamines (89 of 1683 pilots who crashed between 1994 and 1998) and benzodiazepines (49 of 1683), prescription cardiovascular and neurological medications (240 of 1683), and over-the-counter drugs (301 of 1683) such as antihistamines. For example, Gibbons[58] suggested that positional alcohol nystagmus (PAN) might be a factor in alcohol-related accidents (see Chapter 6, Sec. VIII.B).

2. Laboratory Data

Much of the research used to test the effects of alcohol on pilot performance prior to 1970 was based on simplistic test apparatuses. For example, Jovy et al.[59] examined the effects of 0.09 and 0.11% BAC on a psychomotor performance test apparatus. This device required the subject to choose, from a pool of differently sized pellets, a suitable one to place into an opening of corresponding size in a rhythmically revolving roll. They reported an 8% performance decrement with a

0.09% BAC legal limit and a 21% decrement with a 0.11% BAC. These BACs are well above the 0.04% BAC and the test equipment was never evaluated in terms of its ability to generalize to aircraft.

Collins et al.[60] evaluated tracking performance during angular acceleration. In the presence of angular acceleration, there were decrements at 1, 2, and 4 h after ingestion (0.074, 0.073, and 0.047% BAC). Without acceleration there were significant decrements caused by alcohol only four hours after alcohol ingestion (0.047% BAC).

A number of researchers tried to evaluate the combined effects of alcohol and flight stressors such as motion and altitude. Ryback and Dowd[61] measured the response to Coriolis stimulation 7 and 34 h after drinking alcohol (0.85 to 1.7 ml of ethanol/kg of body weight). Their subjects were eight nonflying personnel and six pilots. Alcohol was also associated with both PAN and an increment in Coriolis nystagmus. Hill et al.[62] conducted similar research. During static tests, the authors reported the occurrence of Type I PAN (beating in the direction of the lower ear when lying on side or tilting the head while supine) during the first 4 h and 24–32 h after alcohol ingestion. Type II PAN (beating in direction opposite the lower ear) occurred 6–10 h after alcohol ingestion. During angular acceleration tests, fewer, shorter-duration beats of nystagmus occurred 1–2 h after alcohol ingestion. The turning sensation was shorter for the alcohol group than for the control group 1 h after ingesting alcohol or placebo. There were no Coriolis vertigo effects.

Gilson et al.[63] investigated the combined effects of alcohol (0.000, 0.027, 0.077% BAC), motion (dynamic or static vestibular stimulation), and display illumination (0.1 or 1.0 ft-L) on the performance of 24 male college students. Tracking errors increased in dynamic stimulation for each positive BAC level over baseline BAC. There were no alcohol decrements in the static motion condition. Tracking errors were also greater in dim illumination than in bright illumination. Based on these results, they concluded that alcohol would degrade pilot performance most in turbulence and at night.

In the following year Schroeder et al.[64] examined compensatory tracking performance of 24 males while stationary and while oscillating in pitch and yaw. BAC levels were 0.081, 0.075, and 0.047%, respectively, 1, 2, and 4 h after alcohol dosing. Significantly more tracking errors occurred in the yaw position with no motion for the alcohol group at 1 and 4 h after dosing than for the placebo group. Tracking performance was poorer for the alcohol group at 1 and 2 h after dosing in both planes with motion. Burton and Jaggars[65] exposed eight adult subjects to sustained $+G_z$ acceleration after alcohol doses of 0 to 3 oz (89 ml). There were significant decreases in both weapons firing time and the amount of time the target was on the screen as the alcohol dose increased. Similar decreases occurred in these measures as acceleration increased from $1-+6$ G_z. Decrements were greatest in the combined alcohol/$+G_z$ condition.

Collins[66] trained eight private pilots (flight hours ranging from 160 to 20,000 h) to perform two time-shared tasks. The first was a two-dimensional, compensatory tracking task; the second was a single-choice, visual reaction time (RT) task that occurred once every 30 s. Blood alcohol content was 0.091% immediately after alcohol dosing and 0.012% 8 h later. Reaction times were significantly longer for the alcohol group than for the placebo group 1 h after alcohol ingestion. There were no significant differences between the groups 8 h after alcohol ingestion. Nor were there any differences in reaction time between ground level and 12,000 ft (3660 m) simulated altitude. For the tracking task errors were significantly greater 1 h after alcohol ingestion than prior to alcohol ingestion or 8 h after alcohol ingestion. Just as for the RT task, there were no differences in tracking errors between ground level and 12,000 ft (3660 m) simulated altitude.

Collins and Chiles[67,68] examined the effects of alcohol (bourbon and vodka) on the performance of 11 private pilots. These pilots performed the following tasks: 1) two-dimensional, compensatory tracking, 2) 10-choice RT task, 3) 4-m vigilance task, 4) mental arithmetic task, 5) problem solving, and 6) speech comprehension. For the dynamic-tracking task the alcohol group made more errors 4 h after alcohol ingestion than the placebo group did. A trained rater reported significantly more ocular nystagmus during dynamic tracking for the alcohol group than for the placebo group. For the 10-choice RT task, performance of the vodka group was worse than that for the placebo group 4 h after ingesting alcohol. For the 4-m vigilance task performance of the vodka group was poorer than for the placebo group 4 h after alcohol ingestion. In addition, performance of both the bourbon and vodka groups was worse 4 h after ingestion than prior to or 8 h after alcohol ingestion. Collins and Chiles stated that their data did not contradict the eight-hour rule but cautioned that the combined effects of noise and altitude must also be considered. Collins et al.[69] reported decrements in performance at 0.08% BAC on reaction time, two-dimensional compensation, tracking, and pattern discrimination tasks. There were no alcohol effects on mental arithmetic, problem solving, or speech-comprehension tasks.

Stokes et al.[70] tested 13 pilots using a cognitive test battery at 0 and at 0.10% BAC. There were significant alcohol effects for the following tests: maze tracing, visual scanning, first-order tracking, dual-task tracking, and risk taking. There were no alcohol effects on the hidden figures or the visual number tests. Horne and Gibbons[71] measured the vigilance performance of eight women at 0.000, 0.035, and 0.070% BAC in the early afternoon and in the evening. Even at 0.035% BAC, there was greater decrement in the afternoon than in the evening. Neither the BAC nor the time separation between alcohol dosing and performance matched the current regulations.

More recently, the FAA has evaluated the effects of alcohol on a readiness-to-perform test.[72] Seventy-seven men were tested at breath alcohol content of 0.02, 0.04, 0.06, and 0.08%. There were significant alcohol effects on RT, percent correct, and measures of information processing that monotonically increased with breath-alcohol contents. Millar et al.[73] reported significant degradations in RT at peak BAC (0.07%).

3. Ground Simulator Data

To date, there have been 15 major evaluations of the effects of alcohol on pilot performance in ground simulators. These are summarized in Table 2. All simulator studies have shown detrimental effects of alcohol at 0.10% BAC, and significant performance deficits are observed even below 0.05% BAC.

4. Flight Data

In contrast to the 15 ground simulator studies, only one study has been performed in flight. It was conducted approximately 30 years ago in a single-engine Cessna

Table 2 Summary of alcohol research conducted in ground simulators

Reference	BACs, %	Testbed	Duration	Number of flights	Subjects	Measure	Results
74	0.000, 0.025, 0.050, 0.075	Phase II Boeing 727-232 ground simulator	1 h	8 per subject	2 air carrier captains and 2 air carrier first officers	Errors and deviations	Total errors significantly increased as a function of BAC Serious errors significantly increased from 0.000 to 0.025% BAC
75	0.000, 0.080	Flight simulator	Not stated	Not stated	Volunteers	Discomfort ratings errors	No difference Dumping fuel at 0.08% BAC Gear down at high speed at 0.08% BAC Attempting to land 10,000 ft above local field elevation at 0.08% BAC Failure to correct errors at 0.08% BAC and up to 14 h later
76	0.000, 0.011	Aerosoft 2000 fixed-based simulator	Not stated	4 simulated approaches	8 male pilots Airline Transport Pilot licensed	Vertical duration from glideslope Horizontal deviation from glideslope Deviation from optimum approach speed	No difference More in 0.04% BAC especially if not all engines operative More in 0.04% BAC
77 (also published as 78)	0.030, 0.060, 0.100	General Aviation Trainer, model 1	1 h	6 per subject	12 USAF instructor pilots	Ratings of four USAF flight examiners Combined total seconds of error (i.e., deviation in altitude, heading, turn rate, airspeed, vertical velocity, and ball angle)	Performance was significantly poorer for 0.060 and 0.100 than for the 0.000% BAC No significant difference between 0.000 and 0.030% BAC

(Continued)

Table 2 Summary of alcohol research conducted in ground simulators (continued)

Reference	BACs, %	Testbed	Duration	Number of flights	Subjects	Measure	Results
79 (also published as Henry et al.[80])	0.025, 0.055, 0.085	General Aviation Trainer, model 1	1 h	4 to 6 per subject	22 nonrated men	Total seconds of error (i.e., sum of seconds in deviation in altitude, heading, turn rate, airspeed, vertical velocity, and ball angle) Combined total seconds of error (i.e., sum of seconds in a flight segment deviation in altitude, heading, turn rate, airspeed, vertical velocity, and ball angle)	Performance was significantly poorer for 0.025 and 0.085 than for 0.000% BAC Performance was poorer for each of three segments, for the entire flight, for airspeed, and for vertical velocity Time on target and number of problems solved were significantly different from 0.000% BAC only for the two highest BACs
81	0.000, 0.040, 0.100	Frasca 141 simulator	15–20 min	28 per subject	14 private pilots	Mean absolute difference in degrees from assigned heading Mean absolute difference in feet from assigned altitude Number of communication frequency errors Number of transponder code errors Whether pilots correctly entered communication frequency at the outer marker	Older pilots (30 to 62 years old) were farther off course than younger (20 to 29 years old) For distance off course, older pilots were significantly impaired at 0.100% BAC as compared to 0.000% BAC All pilots made more radio errors at 0.100% BAC than at 0.040% BAC

81	0.000, 0.040, 0.100	Frasca 141 simulator	15–20 min	28 per subject	14 private pilots	Closest distance between subject's aircraft and target aircraft	Older pilots made more severe heading errors than younger pilots
						Number of incorrect vertical avoidances	More severe altitude errors occurred at both 0.040 and 0.100% BAC than at placebo;
						Time to detect far targets on the horizon	decrement was especially large for older pilots at 0.100% BAC
						Engine oil detection	At 2 h pilots were farther off assigned
						Carburetor ice detection	course in alcohol than in placebo condition
						Ground track distance in feet from centerline during takeoff	Pilots made more radio errors in alcohol condition at 2 h
						Absolute difference in degrees from runway heading during takeoff	No hangover effects 24 or 48 h after 0.10% BAC on course or radio errors
						Absolute difference in knots from assigned airspeed during climb out	
						Absolute difference in feet from runway centerline during approach	
						Absolute difference in feet from glideslope during approach	
						Absolute value in change of aileron in degrees during approach	
						Standard deviation of aileron movements during approach	

(Continued)

Table 2 Summary of alcohol research conducted in ground simulators (continued)

Reference	BACs, %	Testbed	Duration	Number of flights	Subjects	Measure	Results
81						Absolute value in change of elevator in degrees during approach	—
						Standard deviation of elevator movements during approach	
						Lateral distance from centerline in feet at touchdown	
						Distance in feet from the ideal touchdown spot	
						Difference in degrees from ideal heading during touchdown	
						Vertical speed during the last 0.86 s before touchdown	
82	0.04, 0.10	Frasca 141 fixed-base simulator	20–25 min	Twice each at 0.04, 0.10, then 2, 4, 8, 24, and 48 h after	7 young ($X = 25.3$) 7 old ($X = 42.1$)	Course error	Larger for older
						Radio errors	Larger for BAC
							More at 0.20 than 0.04 BAC
83	0.000, 0.010	Frasca 141 fixed-base simulator	35–40 min	12 at 0.10% BAC, 2, 4, 8, 24, and 48 h after 12 at 0.00% BAC, 2, 4, 8, 24, and 48 h after	28 male pilots aged 21–51	Perceived intoxication	More in 0.10% BAC
						Rating overall performance	Worse 0–4 h after 0.10% BAC
						Standard deviation in performance	Larger 0–8 h after 0.10% BAC

Ref	BAC	Apparatus	Duration	Sessions	Subjects	Measure	Result
84	0.000, 0.040	ATC 610 moving-base simulator	45 min	4	10 male, 2 female pilots	Threshold to detect angular motion	Higher threshold 0.04% BAC
						Altitude error	No difference
						Altitude variability	No difference
						Target detection	No difference
85	0.000, 0.040	ATC 610 ground simulator	45 min	2 per subject	12 male private pilots	Horizontal head movements	BAC decrement was greater when alcohol was received on Day 1 rather than on Day 2
						Time to detect target	Significantly poorer overall performance with alcohol
						Pitch-and-roll yoke control movements	
						Attitude indicator pitch and roll	Significantly poorer VOR tracking, collision avoidance, vertical control, vertical control limits, altitude at 0.040% BAC
						Vertical speed	
						Course deviation	
						Altimeter	
						Direction gyro	
						Airspeed	
86	0.000, 0.040	Frasca 141 fixed-based simulator	Not stated	2 per day for 2 days	12 male pilots instrument rated aged 23–49, 250–6000 h	Instrument departure procedure error	More errors 0.04% BAC
						IFR flight control error	No difference
						Error in position reports	No difference
						Failure to question erroneous clearance	No difference
						Communication error	No difference
86	0.000, 0.040	Frasca 141 fixed-based simulator	Not stated	2 per day for 2 days	8 pilots instrument rated aged 23–60, 160–2500 h	Frequency of navigation errors	More at 0.04% BAC
						Problem solving time	No difference
						Communication error	No difference
						Flight control error	No difference

(Continued)

Table 2 Summary of alcohol research conducted in ground simulators (continued)

Reference	BACs, %	Testbed	Duration	Number of flights	Subjects	Measure	Results
86	0.000, 0.040	Frasca 141 fixed-based simulator	Not stated	2 per day for 2 days	8 pilots instrument rated aged 23–58, 200–3000 h	Aircraft control error	No difference
						Checklist procedure error	No difference
						Approach chart procedures error	No difference
						ATC communication error	More at 0.04% during missed approach
86	0.000, 0.040	Frasca 141 fixed-based simulator	Not stated	2 per day for 2 days	8 pilots instrument rated aged 32–54, 170–5000 h	Number of missed approaches	No difference
						Quality of landings	More landing errors at 0.04% BAC
						Approach error	No difference
						Communication error	No difference
87	0.000, 0.020	Aerosoft 200 fixed-base simulator	40 min	1	8 male pilots instrument rated	Deviation in altitude, speed, track-keeping	No difference
						Checklist implementation	No difference
						Navigation error	No difference
						Communication error	More at 0.02% BAC
88	0.0, 0.0225, 0.045, 0.09	Illinois Micro Aviation Computer fixed-base simulator	20 min per flight	4 per session for 2 sessions	8 male general aviation pilots 21–23 years old	Altitude deviation	Significant decrement at highest BAC only
						Lateral and vertical tracking deviation	
						Sternberg RT	Significant difference in false RT but no effect on correct RT
89	0.08, 0.04, 8 h after 0.08	Frasca 141 fixed-base simulator	75 min per flight	3	11 male, 12 female licensed pilots 21–40 years old	Summary score computed as mean of general flying and communication scores	Significant decrement in performance at 0.08% BAC
							No decrement 8 h after
							No gender differences in performance
							Women had significant faster disappearance rates

						Measures	Results
90	0.000, 0.080	Frasca 141 fixed-based simulator	75 min	6: placebo or alcohol predrink, 0.08% BAC, 8 hours after	28 pilots instrument rated	Communication frequency errors Oil pressure detection Traffic avoidance Approach performance	Hangover effect for younger pilots Slower after 0.10% BAC Worse after 0.10% BAC in first than second session treatment, time, age, order interaction
91	0.000, 0.100	P-3C ground simulator	Not stated	2 per subject	10 Navy P-3C Orion pilots	Takeoff heading Landing heading Localizer deviation Glide-slope deviation Yaw on takeoff Yaw on landing	Significantly greater yaw on takeoff 14 h after attaining 0.100% BAC than in control condition Standard deviation of heading errors was greater 14 h after attaining 0.100% BAC than in control condition Variability in glide-slope error significantly greater 14 h after attaining 0.100% BAC than in control condition

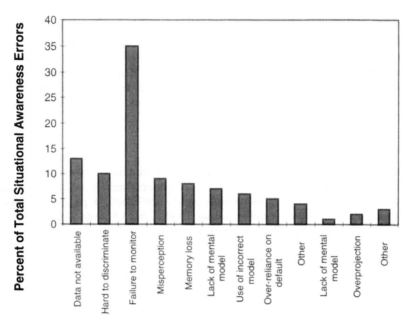

Fig. 6 Types of errors in SA reported in NASA Aviation Safety Reporting System, Jan. 1986–May 1992. (Reproduced with permission of Jones and Endsley; Ref. 99, p. 509.)

focused on the 17 human-error accidents. Of these, 15 were SA related, 4 were caused by physiological degradation associated with fatigue or drugs, and 6 stemmed from violation of existing procedures, such as omitting a task. (Accidents could be included in multiple categories.) The data from the SA-related accidents are summarized by factor in Fig. 7 and highlight task distraction as the leading contributor to SA error. Of these SA-related accidents, 72% involved problems with Level 1 SA, 22% with Level 2 SA, and 6% with Level 3 SA.

Greene[100] stated that SD is "inextricably entwined with the concept of loss of situational awareness" and that Type I SD

> ... arises when the conscious mind performs non-control related tasks and relegates control of the aircraft to the subconscious mind, which flies in accordance with inputs received from the inner ear (vestibular apparatus), ambient (peripheral) vision, and the "seat-of-the-pants". Such factors as distraction, channelized attention, and task saturation are all associated with the removal of conscious control of the aircraft and result in subconscious piloting. Temporal distortion ... appears to occur in direct proportion to the amount of stress perceived by the individual. (Ref. 100, p.1.)

Johnson stated that to avoid SD, "... situational awareness involving judgment of terrain height, aircraft attitudinal awareness, speed and distance is required" (Ref. 101, p. B2-2).

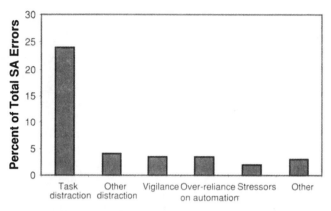

Fig. 7 SA errors associated with NTSB-reported aircraft accidents, 1989–1992. (Reproduced with permission of Jones and Endsley; Ref. 99, p. 510.)

Previc et al.[102] argued that spatial orientation is a subset of SA (see Fig. 1).

> Situational Awareness is knowledge of the aircraft's location in space (position and attitude), awareness of the environment (terrain geography and features, weather-related conditions such as turbulence and icing), understanding communication (within the cockpit and via the air traffic controller), correct reading of the instruments, and knowledge of malfunctioning controls and/or instruments (Ref. 103, p. 123).

Spatial orientation is only knowledge of the aircraft's orientation in space. Although spatial orientation is a subset of SA, they have become synonymous among many aircrews and flight surgeons.

Situational awareness requires both system SA and environmental SA. System SA includes 1) system status, 2) functioning and settings; 3) settings of radio, altimeter and transponder equipment; 4) air traffic control communications present; 5) deviations from correct settings; 6) flight modes and automation entries and settings; 7) impact of malfunctions/system degrades, and settings on system performance and flight safety; and 8) fuel, time, and distance available on fuel.[104] Environmental SA includes knowledge of weather formations (area and altitudes affected and movement); temperature, icing, ceilings, clouds, fog, sun, visibility, turbulence, winds, microbursts; instrument flight rules vs visual flight rules conditions; areas and altitudes to avoid; flight safety; and projected weather conditions.[104] For military aircraft SA also includes tactical SA. Tactical SA includes 1) the identification, tactical status, type, capabilities, location and flight dynamics of other aircraft; 2) a knowledge of one's own capabilities in relation to other aircraft; 3) aircraft detections, launch capabilities, and targeting; 4) threat prioritization, imminence and assignments; 5) current and projected threat intentions, tactics, firing and maneuvering; and 6) mission timing and status.[104]

The final types of SA include spatial/temporal SA and geographical SA. Spatial/temporal SA includes a knowledge of 1) the aircraft's attitude, altitude, heading, velocity, vertical velocity, G-loading, flight path; 2) any deviation from flight plan and clearances; 3) the aircraft capabilities; 4) projected flight path; and 5) projected landing time.[104] Geographical SA includes a knowledge of the 1) location of one's own aircraft, other aircraft, terrain features, airports, cities, waypoints, and navigation fixes; 2) position relative to designated features; 3) runway and taxiway assignments; 4) path to desired locations; and 5) climb/descent points.[104] To summarize, spatial orientation is in relation to Earth; geographical orientation in relation to topography (see Chapter 1, Sec. I).

The relationship between spatial orientation and geographical SA has been a source of some controversy. For example, Navathe and Singh[105] argue in favor of separating SD, which they attribute to receptor input error, from geographic SD, which they attribute to navigational error; and they distinguish both of these from loss of SA, which they attribute to a central error. Previc et al.[102] and Cheung[106] argue for a broader, more traditional definition of SD, but one that does not include geographical SD (see Chapter 1).

However, spatial and geographical orientations are closely related in many incidents. Based on an analysis of aviation incidents and accidents, Taylor concluded, "Geographical disorientation in flight can be insidious, compelling and as stressful as spatial disorientation. Geographical disorientation can precipitate spatial disorientation and vice versa. In severe cases, where the realization of the error is sudden, there is evidence of panic and disorganization of behaviours leading to loss of control of the aircraft" (Ref. 11, p. B9-1). Taylor provided the following accident synopsis to prove his point: "A pilot became disoriented in flight without realizing it. He was about to land at what he thought was his destination, when he suddenly realized it was the wrong airstrip. He became so shaken and confused by this sudden realization that he crash landed the aircraft" (Ref. 11, p. B9-8).

In contrast to the spatial-geographical controversy, virtually all researchers currently agree that loss of SA can lead to SD. As Montgomery et al. state, "A disorientation event is likely to be triggered when the pilot's attention to flying is drawn elsewhere. Mental processing issues (including channelized attention, task saturation, habituation, inattention, negative transfer, distraction, and temporal distortion) must be part of our spatial disorientation understanding" (Ref. 107, p. 147).

III. Experience

Spatial orientation, like other spatial behaviors, is dependent on experience. According to Howard and Templeton (1966),

> Spatially coordinated behavior is construed as the development and maintenance of a repertoire of response patters, which are molded and conditioned by the spatial characteristics of the body, and of the physical world in such a way that objectives may be rapidly and accurately achieved. Spatially coordinated behavior is only possible because there are many predictable features of the body's structure and of the structure of the world (Ref. 108, p. 7).

There are four aspects of experience that are related to SD: 1) the amount of flying hours (Sec. III.A), 2) expectation based on experiences (Sec. III.B),

3) learning that occurred (Sec. III.C) and 4) training received (see Chapter 8). One author[109] adds memory as an experience factor.

A. Number of Hours

Some researchers have found that pilots with low flight time have the greatest risk of SD. For example, Mortimer concluded from an analysis of general aviation accidents that "pilots in SD accidents lacked the flight experience necessary to recognize or cope with the stimuli that induce SD, which was compounded by fatigue, alcohol/drugs or pressure and other psychological and physical impairments" (Ref. 110, p. 25). Kuipers et al.,[8] based on interviews with 209 Dutch F-16 and F-5 pilots, concluded, that target hypnosis (see Sec. VI.B) in younger pilots is a factor in SD. One difference between novice and experienced pilots might be scanning behavior. Bellenkes et al.[111] compared the scanning performance of 24 private pilots. They compared the behavior of those with 1 h of instrument flight time (novices) with those with 80 h of instrument flight time (experts). Experts had shorter dwell time, and they more frequently checked instruments that were unchanged. The authors inferred from these data that the experts had a better mental model of patterns of aircraft response.

Situations in which the awareness of environmental elements is restricted to a single element can produce spatial disorientation. This commonly occurs in the student pilot who, under the stress of attempting to perform a demanding and unfamiliar task, allows his attention to be confined to one aspect of his task. Yet, even the experienced pilot, when presented with a high workload, when anxious, or when unduly aroused, can lose efficiency (Ref. 41, p. B2-6). Students and experienced pilots are both affected, however.

However, experienced pilots are not immune to SD. Moser reviewed Air Force accident data from 1964–1967 and concluded "the pilots involved in 91 percent of the spatial disorientation accidents had accumulated over 1,000 hours total flying time" (Ref. 112, p. 174). Braithwaite et al.[113] concluded from accident records and a survey of aircrew experience that there was no association between SD factors such as aircrew experience, flight qualification, or aircraft type rating. Similarly, Durnford et al. stated, "Experience, whether measured in terms of qualifications or flying hours, offers no protection against SD" (Ref. 42, p. 75). Jarvis also addresses the issues of currency and concluded that "the third factor noted [in F-15 SD accidents] included the level of or recency of training of the pilot: inexperience with instrument flight and a lack of recent instrument flying skills" (Ref. 93, p. 33). Baker and Lamb[114] reported that 44% of the commuter and air-taxi pilots who crashed in the Colorado Rocky Mountains had less than 100 h in type but most had over 1000 h total flight time. Thus, flight hours in type can be a better predictor of SD susceptibility.

Finally, based on analysis of 192 USAF SD fatalities, Barnum and Bonner[115] concluded:

> The average pilot who will be involved in future similar accidents ... will be around 30 years of age, have 10 years in the cockpit, and have 1,500 hours of first pilot/instructor pilot time. He will be a fighter pilot and will have flown approximately 25 times in the three months prior to his accident (Ref. 115, p. 898).

B. Expectation

If pilots pull on the stick, they expect the aircraft to climb and vice versa; if they push on the stick, they expect the aircraft to descend. Throughout a flying career pilots develop hundreds of these expectancies. Some are so highly developed that they become automated—the pilots perform the action and "see" the expected consequence even if it does not occur. Expectation is not limited to responses alone but can also occur with perceptions. "Correct sensory information may be misinterpreted by the brain—for example, causing errors of expectancy—by coning of attention (fascination), high or low arousal states, and other environmental stresses such as hypoxia and hyperthermia also affect the central nervous system" (Ref. 116, p. 1931).

Grunwald et al. note, "The observer has a priori knowledge of certain viewed objects, like size, shape, or parallelism or perpendicularity of lines or planes. These assumptions are used in a 3-D process to reconstruct a spatial layout that best matches the perceived lines-of-sight to the object coordinates" (Ref. 117, p. 425). For example, the size of objects is continually changing on the retina, but through extensive interaction with the environment humans learn the size of a given object and use the learned size to determine distance and aspect angle. This phenomenon is called size constancy and is important to visual perception (see Chapter 3, Sec. IV.C.3).

Perception in pilots depends on deploying stored knowledge rather than on responding directly to stimuli. As Monesi states, "Some general psychological concepts, like expectancy or detection theories, can be invoked as factors influencing perception and explaining perceptual errors" (Ref. 41, p. B2-6). These perceptual errors can lead to SD. "Sensory inputs may be misperceived because position and motion perception is based on past experience. Erroneous judgments of aircraft attitude, misinterpretation of lights when flying on a dark night, the so called lean on the sun are all examples of expectancy induced perceptual error" (Ref. 41, p. B2-6).

One form of expectation is based on geography because humans respond based on experiences in a particular geographical location with its characteristic stimuli and environment. A good example is provided by Navathe and Singh: "A pilot from tea plantation-covered East India, on completion of a ferry to a Western base, rounds off high for landing. Flying over tall eucalyptus trees on finals, he underestimates his height, since he is used to flying over the shorter plants of tea gardens, which give him a different perspective" (Ref. 118, p. 256).

Some behaviors are so highly trained that they become automatic. For example, experienced pilots will often subconsciously make use of the roll-angle indicator for speedy correction of extreme bank attitudes, if this indicator is immediately below the artificial horizon.[119] Eichner and Mason[120] believe that repeated practice in realistic environments is necessary to make the correct responses automated. Trumbo and Montgomery concur: "For training against Type I SD, it is necessary to establish dynamic scenarios in which the normal mental processes are disturbed by such things as temporal distortion, distraction, inattention, channelized attention, task saturation, and habituation" (Ref. 121, p.142). Further, LeDuc et al.[26] reported that a simulator could be used to produce spatial disorientation but stressed the need for real flight to train against Type I SD.

C. Learning

Learning is defined as "to gain knowledge or understanding of or skill in by study, instruction, or experience."[1] Learning includes self-study, formal training (such as described in Chapter 8), and experience. Learning is also defined as "to acquire knowledge or skill or a behavioral tendency."[1] Lack of knowledge, as well as these behavioral expectations as described in the preceding section, plays a major role in SD.

Spatial disorientation can occur not only because of erroneous or absent sensory information but because of a pilot's deficient understanding of the factors and mechanisms that result in SD.[122] Both SD training and instrument proficiency have been shown to affect the risk of SD (see Chapter 8). Further, pilots must be trained in the tricks of the trade. Benson and Burchard[122] describe how persistent disorientation in pilots can be dispelled by making a readjustment of the seat harness and the performance of routine cockpit checks, which divert attention from distracting yet clearly false sensation such as the "leans."[122] Other pilots have found that a quick shake of the head "topples the internal gyros" or more accurately provides new sensory input which is sufficient to disrupt conflict (Ref. 122, p. 21). Other learned behavior to counteract SD include the following:

> When suddenly confronted with strong illusory sensations, or where difficulties are experienced in establishing orientation and appropriate control of the aircraft, the advice to the pilot is: (1) Get on to instruments; check and cross check. (2) Stick on instruments; do not attempt to mix flight by external visual references with instrument flight references until external visual cues are unambiguous. (3) Maintain correct instrument scan; do not omit altimeter. (4) Seek help if severe disorientation persists. Hand over to co-pilot (if present), call ground controller and other aircraft, check altimeter. (5) If control cannot be regained, abandon aircraft (Ref. 122, p. 21).

IV. Task

Several task characteristics have been associated with SD. These include workload, transitions inside and outside the cockpit, distractions, and crew coordination.

A. Workload

Based on interviews with 209 Dutch F16 and F5 pilots, Kuipers et al.[8] concluded that last-minute changes in planning, unclear preflight briefings, and "hot scrambles" caused by high workload and wrong priority settings brought pilots into unexpected situations, which led to extra workload and in some cases to SD. Workload appears to be increasing in modern aircraft. In one of Gillingham's articles, he stated, "modern aircraft designs and mission requirements have substantial impact . . . the phenomenal ability of current high-performance aircraft to roll, pitch, accelerate, gain or lose altitude, and otherwise change spatial orientation parameters very quickly, presents a significant challenge to the pilot to maintain a continually accurate assessment of those parameters" (Ref. 123, p. 302).

B. Transitions

In Chapters 7 and 9 and elsewhere throughout this text, SD has been shown to be associated with disruption of visual scans, caused by transitions between weather conditions, between viewing inside and outside the cockpit, between displays, and between tasks.

1. Transitions Between Weather Conditions

SD in visual flight rules (VFR)/IFR transitions, may occur as a result of loss of perception of vection. As a pilot transitions into the clouds, optical flow cues, which normally produce a sensation of vection, may not be present. The two-dimensional primary flight displays do not generate a sensation of vection. As a result, control inputs, which were associated with vection while flying in visual meteorological conditions (VMC), are suddenly dissociated from typical visual motion cues. As the aircraft motions take it into VMC during an approach, the pilot will look out the cockpit window and his control motions will be influenced by the transformations that are taking place in the world. The gain of information in the world may be different than the gain of the primary flight displays. The pilot must adjust to differences in scale, format, and information content (Ref. 124, p. 36).

Similarly, Tormes and Guedry[25] concluded that 62% of naval helicopter pilots had experienced disorientation during transitions between IFR and VFR and 49% during transitions from hover over a flight deck to forward flight at night.

2. Transitions Between Inside and Outside the Cockpit

Collins and Harrison concluded from a survey of F-15C pilots after their return from operation Desert Storm that "visual transitions from inside to outside the cockpit (or the reciprocal) under different conditions of flight were associated with the occurrence of SD episodes" (Ref. 125, p. 405). There were 96 pilots who responded to the first section of the survey (multiple choice questions) and 56 who responded to the second section (open-ended questions). Visual transitions in weather were 3.26 times more likely to produce SD than visual transition during night. There were nearly twice as many SD episodes with visual transition than without visual transition.

3. Transitions Between Displays

Spatial disorientation related to transitions between displays is well known. In commenting on SD in the Tornado aircraft, Dell states, "In all but a few cases the disorientation has occurred on transferring from visual cues to heads-up display (HUD) and only overcome by concentration on the head-down display (HDD). Some did not dispel the feeling of disorientation until they have re-gained visual conditions." (Ref. 126, p. 7-4) As further evidence, Jarvis reported, "The second factor noted [in F-15 SD accidents] relates to a pilot procedure: waiting until the last moment to make the transition from a visual to an instrument reference and making head movements during turning maneuvers" (Ref. 93, p. 33).

4. Transitions Between Tasks

According to Jarvis,[93] of special import to SD is the transition between formation and solo flight using information on the HUD:

> Pilots should be cautioned against use of the HUD during instrument flight and during the period of transition from formation flight to solo flying during night and/or instrument conditions. Many pilots, particularly those who had not flown older operational fighter aircraft, seem to be over dependent on the HUD when flying the aircraft. The HUD is a compelling display, which draws the pilot's attention and in a situation where the pilot requires rapid recognition of his attitude, altitude, airspeed and the rates of change of each, the information is not always easy to find on the HUD. Pilots who reported less dependence on the HUD expressed a lesser problem with spatial disorientation (Ref. 93, pp. 34, 35).

C. Distracters

Distracters are often a factor in SD incidents and accidents. For example, Durnford and Crowley[127] concluded that distraction was involved in 44% of all SD accidents. Their data were from a survey completed by three experienced flight surgeons for U.S. Army helicopter accidents from May 1987–April 1992. In another aircrew survey distraction was present at the onset of the SD episode in 40% of the SD cases. Ironically, there was no link between fatigue and SD in either survey. Durnford et al. reported:

> There were few identifiable episodes of visual or vestibular illusions in this accident series. Classical causes of spatial disorientation—such as "whiteout", "brownout", and inadvertent entry into IMC' were relatively rare (accounting for 25 percent of the spatial disorientation accidents). By contrast, distraction of the aircrew from maintaining a safe flight path appears to have played a major role (Ref. 128, p. 21).

Braithwaite et al.[113] concluded from a survey of accident records that there were distracters inside the cockpit in 26% of SD accidents and outside the cockpit in 29% of SD accidents. Braithwaite et al.[129] reported distraction to be an important factor in helicopter accidents involving night-vision devices (NVD), based on U.S. Army helicopter accidents from 1987–1995. Specifically, 14.4% of the accidents involved distraction from outside the cockpit, including other aircraft operating nearby and events occurring at the place of departure or at destination. One of the most common distracters is a failed instrument. Disorientation caused by instrument failure and the unresolved conflict occurs relatively often, with 21% of pilots in the survey, Sipes and Lessard[130] experiencing this illusion between one and 10 times. Similarly, Tormes and Guedry[25] concluded that 29% had experienced spatial disorientation as a result of distraction by aircraft malfunction and 25% by a faulty instrument.

D. Crew Coordination

Multiperson crews also experience SD (Fig. 8), but there is a strong psychological benefit of being accompanied by another crew member at night or in difficult

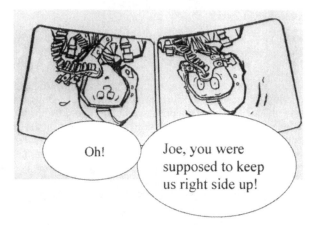

Fig. 8   Multicrew SD. (Reproduced with permission of Ron Colgrove.)

circumstances (Ref. 126, p. 703, their Fig. 9). Based on Desert Storm data, Durn-ford et al. stated, "Experience, whether measured in terms of qualifications or flying hours, offers no protection against SD. Neither is having two pilots sufficient protection; both aircrew were simultaneously disorientated in 40 percent of episodes involving NVDs. Nonetheless, good crew coordination played an important and beneficial role in many episodes" (Ref. 42, p. 75).

V.   Environment

There are many environmental factors that have been linked to SD, including unnatural sensations associated with time of day and weather. The purpose of this section is not to exhaustively review these unnatural nonvisual and visual sensations, which are reviewed in Chapters 6 and 7. Rather, a brief overview will be presented to better understand the various SD-related psychological phenomena to be presented in Sec. VI.

A.   Unnatural Sensations

The *Merriam Webster's American Dictionary* provides the following definition for sensation: "awareness (as of heat or pain) due to stimulation of a sense organ."[1] The major sense organs involved in SD are the eyes and the inner ear. However, "the sense of hearing, clearly of limited importance for spatial disorientation on earth, may prove useful during flight operations" (Ref. 41, p. B2-1). Further, sensations can be affected by inadequate cues and sensory deprivation, neither of which normally occurs on the Earth's surface.

1.   Inadequate Cues

"Inadequate cues probably account for the most important single causes of SD accidents. In fact, in accounts of SD incidents the absence of sensation is rarely reported; rather it is the unexpected vertigo or other strong illusory sensation that is described" (Ref. 41, p. B2-4).

The primary sense used by humans is vision. All major sensory systems can provide inadequate or misleading cues during flight. As Leibowitz states:

> Because vision is almost always accurate on earth, the natural tendency is to rely on the sense of vision during flight. It is clear however that in the aviation environment this can be dangerous. Vision is not always reliable in detecting the presence of other aircraft; it is essentially useless for perceiving self-motion in the absence of ground cues; it is subject to errors in the perception of velocity and height during nighttime or other degraded observation conditions; and object motion perception is unreliable at night and during other impoverished observation conditions. The essential message is that pilots must be made aware of the capabilities and limitations of their visual systems and apprised of the fundamental differences between vision while self-locomoting on the ground and when in the aircraft (Ref. 131, pp. 108, 109).

Vision of the outside world can be further degraded by glare from the sun, dazzle effects of sunlight on water or snow, or featureless terrain or water (see Chapter 7). This degradation is further compounded by poor displays within the cockpit (see Chapter 9). Rupert contends "SD mishaps occur because aircraft designers, engineers, and specifically human-factors engineers have failed to provide pilots with the information in a format that will permit them to fly as intuitively as they walk about on the earth" (Ref. 132, p. 72). This is especially true with two-dimensional displays. Recent work on viewing perspective displays suggests that "interpretive behavior associated with viewing perspective displays in which the sinusoidal pattern of azimuth errors is induced by the difference between the 3D stimulus and its 2D projection, and by the consequences of the geometric differences between the station point and the observer's actual position" (Ref. 133, p. 439).

The vestibular system also provides inadequate cues in flight. The vestibular system is well suited for routine ground operations like turning the head, walking, running, jumping, falling, etc., but for flying it is inadequate. This is because the frequency response of the semicircular canals is inappropriate under the conditions of angular acceleration prevalent in flight and because the otolith organs cannot distinguish between the force of gravity and other linear accelerations acting upon the flyer (see Chapter 6). The vestibular system thus makes errors, and these errors can result in spatial disorientation.[36]

In addition, there are conflicts between visual cues and vestibular and proprioceptive cues in flight. It is these conflicting cues that have been identified as major factors in SD accidents (see Chapters 6 and 7). Conflict situations in which visual cues contradict vestibular and other proprioceptive cues result in disorientation incidents, if the aviator is not able to disregard sensations of attitude or motion, particularly when the visual cues are reduced (Ref. 41, p. B2-5). Again, these conflicts do not normally occur on the earth's surface.

The effects of inadequate cues are best summarized by Dowd:

> In his natural environment man, by using his functioning sense organs and muscular effectors, is an almost perfect cybernetic mechanism for maintaining his position, attitude, or motion. In flight, however, man is far from perfect in this respect, especially when he is deprived of good visual contact with the earth. Of utmost importance is his ability to respond to instruments, which present him

abstracted and reduced information regarding these parameters, and upon his skill in interpreting messages from his vestibular and proprioceptive systems. Maintaining proper orientation in a high-performance aircraft in weather is one of the most complex, nonverbal, intellectual functions that a man can perform (Ref. 139, p. 758).

2. Sensory Deprivation

Pilots flying at high altitudes often complain that there is constancy in the sensory environment—no changes in light level, no vibration, no sound, and no changes in temperature. These conditions of sensory deprivation may cause visual illusions. According to Gillingham, "when sensorily deprived and adequately stressed, one will perceive what he needs to perceive in order to perform, even though it may mean supplying an illusory perception" (Ref. 36, p. 63).

The most famous sensory deprivation illusion is the Charles Bonnet Syndrome. The syndrome was named after the 18th century Swiss naturalist, who noted that his grandfather (who suffered severe vision loss as a result of cataracts) would often see visions of people, animals, and objects. Some persons exposed to sensory deprivation perceive the noise in earphones as running water or see objects as if they were in a dream, even though they are wide awake.[134] The most likely set of conditions to induce reported visual sensations (RVS) is amorphous visual stimulation (such as clouds) with moderate motility (such as five-point seat restraints in a fighter aircraft). Being on a respirator also induces RVSs—two out of 10 subjects at Boston City Hospital reported RVSs while on a mechanical respirator similar to the positive pressure-breathing mask worn by pilots of fighter aircraft. A supine position (such as the 60-deg cant of a fighter aircraft seat) is more likely than a sitting position to induce RVSs. Siatkowski et al.[135] presented case studies of patients in good physical and mental health (such as pilots), who experience RVSs during the severe visual sensory deprivation associated with the Charles Bonnet Syndrome.

Visual illusions have also been reported in normally sighted persons exposed to sensory deprivation. Iawata et al. reported that subjects in their sensory deprivation studies had stated that they were "feeling as though staying on the border between sleep and wake or dreaming while recognizing it as a dream" (Ref. 136, p. 129). Most of these subjects report visual images. In a follow-up study Iawata et al.[137] placed one man and one woman in a flotation tank for one hour. The tank reduced almost all physical stimulation. Again, the subjects experienced visual illusions similarly to dreaming. Pilots of high-altitude aircraft such as the U-2 have reported similar visual illusions. Sensory deprivation is also associated with vestibular illusions including perceived self-motion.[138] Again, this is similar to illusions described by pilots of high-altitude aircraft.

B. Time of Day

Tormes and Guedry[25] identified factors associated with disorientation in helicopters. Two of their main environmental factors included 1) night launch from forward spots on flight deck and 2) crew change with rotors engaged at night. The association of time of day with SD accidents is further described in Chapters 5 and 7.

C. Weather

In 1965 Doppelt[40] administered a questionnaire to 55 rated USAF pilots. Only two of the 55 did not report having SD episodes (vertigo). The average was 21.7 episodes per pilot or 7.5 episodes per pilot per 1000 flying hours. In other results, 90% of the SD occurred in weather, 75% at night, 50% during formation flight, and 42% during refueling.

> In particular, flying immediately beneath an overcast, in a cloud, or on top of one was particularly conducive to producing vertigo. This was more severe when flying at night. ... Many pilots described lack of confidence, a psychological factor of relevance, in their attitude display instruments and made reference to a need for a second attitude horizon (Ref. 40, p. 5).

Tredici[140] also warned about the effects of heavy rain, which reduces vision enough to render invisible such objects as aircraft, power lines, flag poles, and trees. The rain drops can act as prisms and can cause faulty distance judgment because by acting as filters lights can appear less intense and therefore give one the illusion of being at a greater distance (see Chapter 7).

VI. SD Phenomena Related to Psychological Factors

Psychological factors have been a mostly overlooked component in SD research, training, and accident investigation. However, without consideration of these factors, it is difficult if not impossible to explain the six SD phenomena described in this section. The relationship between these phenomena and the psychological factors discussed in Secs. I–V are summarized in Table 3. As can be seen from Table 3, psychological factors singly, but more often in combination, lead to SD illusions. The six illusions listed in Table 3 are described in the following sections.

A. Break-Off

Break off is a "feeling of detachment from the earth at high altitude or in poor visibility" (Ref. 130, p. 40). Symptoms are characterized by an altered awareness of the pilot's orientation and relationship to the aircraft or the Earth when flying at high altitudes or in visual conditions of flight comparable to those experienced at high altitude. Benson[141] identified four types of break-off in pilots of fixed-wing aircraft: 1) *break off without false perception of aircraft orientation*, where pilots feel overcome by a feeling of unreality and remoteness from the aircraft; 2) *break off with instability*, where pilot is suddenly overcome by a feeling of isolation and of being out of touch with the aircraft and that the aircraft is being balanced as if on a knife edge; 3) *break off with quantitative disorientation*, where pilot has a feeling of being out of touch with the aircraft, which might be accompanied by feeling of dizziness and a false perception of the aircraft's orientation; and 4) *break off with qualitative disorientation*, where pilot begins to feel out of touch with the aircraft and uneasy or experiences a qualitative error in the perception of the aircraft's altitude or motion.

Benson[142] reported that 23 of 72 pilots who had become disoriented in flight had feelings of unreality and detachment. The feelings occurred in monotonous

Table 3   Summary of SD illusions associated with psychological factors

Illusion	Personality	Mental and physical state	Experience	Task	Environment
Break off	Spatial ability	Fear Stress LSA	Learning	Transitions	Inadequate cues Sensory deprivation Time of day
Fascination	Overconfidence Love of flying Lack of discipline	Awe Reverence Serenity	Number of hours Learning	Workload	Inadequate cues
Flying carpet	Overconfidence	—	Number of hours Expectation Learning	Workload	Time of day Weather
Giant hand	Spatial ability	Fatigue Stress	Learning	Workload	Time of day Weather
Suddenly unfamiliar	Succumbing to pressure Overconfidence Spatial ability	Fatigue Fear Anger Grief Stress LSA	Expectation Learning	Transitions Distracters	Sensory deprivation Time of day Weather
Temporal distortion	Succumbing to pressure Love of flying	Fatigue Stress G Drugs LSA	Number of hours Expectation Learning	Workload Transitions Distracters Crew composition	Inadequate cues Sensory deprivation Time of day Weather

phases of light and reduced visual conditions. For fixed-wing pilots (19) these feelings occurred above 30,000 ft (9144 m). For helicopter pilots, however, they occurred between 500 and 10,000 ft (152 and 3048 m). Twenty-one of the pilots had accompanying illusions of aircraft attitude and motion. Benson[143] suggests that these were caused by vestibular asymmetry. Anxiety was reported by almost all of the affected pilots, but the frequency of occurrence was much lower among the Sipes and Lessard[130] subjects. Only 8 of 141 (6%) pilots in the survey of Sipes and Lessard[130] had experienced the phenomenon, with a mean frequency of occurrence of 17.

The break-off phenomenon might be related to the quality of light at high altitudes. There is a slight increase in the intensity of light as altitude increases to 100,000 ft (30,480 m), but its distribution is so modified at high altitude that most appears to come from below, where scattering of light by air molecules, moisture, and dust particles is greater and where clouds can create a bright visual floor. The sky above therefore appears darker at altitudes with less light falling on the cockpit interior.[116] This suggests that break off might also be related to sensory deprivation, as discussed in Sec. V.A.2.

B. Fascination

Fascination is said to occur when a pilot, for one reason or another, ignores orientation cues while his attention is focused on some other object or goal.[36] Fascination might be related to hypoxia, fatigue, drugs, and personality factors[36] as well as task novelty.[144]

Clark et al.[145] distributed a questionnaire to 226 naval aviation students asking them to describe their experiences with fascination. The students who completed the questionnaire had experienced fascination an average of 2.47 times in basic training and 3.42 times in advanced training. Two types of fascination were identified: type A, in which the pilot restricts his or her attention to a narrow area (e.g., target or landing strip) and cannot perceive other objects in view, and type B, in which the pilot perceives all of the objects in view but is blocked from responding. The researchers further broke each type of fascination into categories:

Type A fascination subclassifications:

A.1) Multitasking causes failure to perceive critical information (e.g., performing a strafing run and not maintaining altitude).

A.2) Fixation on a single object causes failure to perceive critical information (e.g., concentrating on lead's position in formation and failing to maintain straight and level flight).

A.3) Preoccupation with irrelevant objects causes failure to perceive critical information (e.g., watching smoke from rocket launch and disregarding attitude).

A.4) Concentration on a single instrument causes failure to perceive critical information (e.g., watching airspeed indicator and forgetting wing position).

A.5) Daydreaming (e.g., staring off into space and forgetting to fly the airplane).

Type B fascination subclassifications:

B.1) Clearly perceiving the situation but failing to make the proper response (e.g., flying too low over the runway and failing to initiate a wave-off in spite of runway duty officer's signals).

B.2) A magnetic attraction to the target (e.g., feeling pulled to the lead airplane).

B.3) Slow motion (e.g., seeing the target getting larger and larger and feeling that the airplane is moving slower and slower and may never reach the target).

Fascination occurred during formation flight, landings, gunnery, bombing, and rocket release. Twenty-five instructors were asked to identify the causes of fascination. They identified the following factors: tenseness, fear, difficulty in shifting attention, inexperience, mechanical flying, and mental blocks.

Type A4 fascination has been termed the "electric jet syndrome" and has been hypothesized to be caused by pilots channelizing (i.e., locking onto) a single display.[146] Type B2 fascination is especially common among student pilots. However, Kuipers et al.[8] reported that 7% of Dutch F-5 pilots had experienced target fixation. In the cognitive engineering literature, target fixation is a form of inattentional blindness.[147,148] The likelihood of this phenomena increases with shared characteristics and expected target such as size and color. An associated phenomenon, contingent orienting[149,150] occurs when the match between expectation and stimulus is high. A pilot would turn toward any stimulus matching his or her expectation. A classic example is landing at the wrong airport but one that matches the size and layout of the designated airport. This has been referred to as "believing is seeing."

C. Flying Carpet

This illusion can be characterized as an example of overconfidence. Kuipers et al.[8] reported the occurrence of flying carpet illusion in 4% of Dutch F-16 pilots. Sitting high and comfortable on top of a high-performance aircraft like the F-16, some pilots get a false sensation of safety and the feeling that nothing could happen to them. They then may cruise into bad weather with little vigilance or might fly much too low without seeing the danger.

D. Giant Hand

Gillingham and Previc[144] describe the giant-hand illusion as one in which the pilot perceives falsely that the aircraft is not responding properly to control inputs because every attempt to bring the aircraft to the desired attitude seemingly is resisted by its tendency to fly back to another, more stable attitude" (Ref. 144, p. 86). In more graphic words, giant hand is a "false banking sensation of a giant hand pushing down on one of the wings" (Ref. 130, p. 40). In the Sipes and Lessard[95] survey 35% of the pilots stated that they had experienced the giant-hand illusion, with an average occurrence of four times.

Malcolm and Money[151] reported data on three occurrences of the giant-hand phenomenon in which "the pilot has lost control because the control column has been apparently pulled forward or sideways despite all efforts on the part of the pilot to restrain it" (p. A10-2). In one instance[152] the pilot (a physician) felt the control column being pulled from him as though by a "giant hand." He tried to center the control column by pulling on it with both hands and both knees, but with no success. Realizing he was disoriented, he released his grip on the stick and watched as it floated back to the central position by itself. For several minutes thereafter, he was able to control the aircraft only by grasping the control column with thumb and forefinger. King[152] claimed to suffer from a subjective impression that the aircraft was in a steep bank to the right, and that whenever he closed his whole hand over the stick it appeared to be thrown forcibly over towards the left. The second case occurred in a fighter aircraft after the pilot turned off the afterburner. The third case occurred during a bomb-diving attack when the pilot found he could not pull out of the dive even by using both hands and his leg. The stick was firmly held well forward and to the left, and so he pushed it further forward and eventually recovered control by doing an outside roll.[151]

Lyons and Simpson[153] present a slightly different description of the first case presented. While in a left-hand climbing turn, he [Dr. King] bent his head down and to the right to find the radio compass audio switch and he experienced violent vertigo. He said "upon attempting to level the wings, I experienced extreme control stiffness and found that even using both hands and knees I could not move the control column to the right. . . . It felt as though a giant hand was thrusting the stick to the left" (Ref. 153, p. 64).

In another account a T-38 pilot reported experiencing the giant-hand illusion while flying through layered cloud decks. The instructor pilot was flying position 2 in a two-ship formation with the student situated upfront. They were vectoring for landing at about 3000 ft—just above the tops of the lower deck with another deck of clouds above them. As lead initiated a turn and descent, the pilot went to follow, and the aircraft did not respond. The pilot applied full strength to the point of getting a sore shoulder. The pilot transferred control to the student, who had no problem. The pilot tried again to make the turn but still failed, even though the student was not having a problem. The pilot stated, "The feeling the problem was mechanical was overwhelming." The pilot had remained in visual contact with the lead aircraft the entire time, but he did not experience distress.

In January 1986 a single-seat fighter pilot ejected because of the giant-hand phenomenon. The pilot was flying lead in a two-ship formation at night in instrument conditions. While in a right descending turn, he turned his head to the right to check wingman's position and had the overwhelming sensation of rolling to the left. The giant hand illusion might be linked with instrument flying conditions. For example, Lyons and Simpson[153] interviewed 97 USAF pilots and found that 15 of them had experienced the giant hand illusion, always during night or under instrument meteorological conditions. Four of the pilots mentioned its occurrence during formation flight. One pilot had multiple episodes.

According to Malcolm and Money,[151] there are four conditions that might be necessary for the giant hand effect to take place: 1) a state of anxiety or mental arousal must be prevalent for some minutes prior to the incident; 2) the control of the aircraft involves a motor task of one or both hands; 3) immediately prior to the event, the pilot is distracted from the immediate task of controlling the attitude of the aircraft; and 4) the resultant gravity vector is been rotated forward (as during deceleration), or the pilot felt that he was pitched forward, as when diving or during some types of cross-coupled head movement." Two of 20 subjects in a centrifuge experienced the giant hand phenomenon when these conditions were repeated.

A possible neurophysiological basis for the giant hand illusion, namely, the predominance of primitive vestibulospinal motor outputs over cortical ones, was presented by Lyons and Simpson[153] and is discussed in Chapter 6, Sec. VII.A. Monesi offers a similar explanation, in which cause, "Heightened neurophysiological arousal of the autonomic and peripheral nervous system may account for disorientation phenomena as the 'giant hand' because of postural hyper reflectivity or reinstatement of vestibular reflex activity by disruption of subcortical habituation" (Ref. 41, p. B2-6).

Anecdotal reports suggest that here is one effective recovery technique—use of the thumb and index finger only to control the stick. This recovery technique was tested in a laboratory, using a visual analog of the giant hand; 16 pilots performed a compensatory tracking task that presented an unstable attitude display against a large, moving background. For congruent trials the display and background moved together; for incongruent trials they moved separately. Pilots were told to recover using either the whole hand or thumb index finger. On incongruent trials Weinstein et al.[154] created a situation where pilots could not "level" the altitude display, but they did not find a significant advantage of the thumb-and-forefinger technique. Whether they created a true giant hand illusion is not clear, however.

E.   Suddenly Unfamiliar

This SD phenomenon is extremely disconcerting. One moment the pilot is confidently aviating, navigating, and communicating. The next moment, he or she is unsure which mode the aircraft is in, where the aircraft is in relation to known landmarks (geographic disorientation), and/or unsure with whom he or she is communicating. The second type of the suddenly unfamiliar phenomenon is the most common. Clark[155] distributed a flight experiences questionnaire to 336 U.S. Air Force, Army, and Navy active duty pilots. Question 11 was "I had a full view of the bay with the lights all around it. It seemed like a totally strange place, although normally it was quite familiar" (p. A1-2). The following numbers of pilots responded yes to having this experience: 23 (out of 65) during transport, 25 (out of 105) during training, 15 (out of 39) at flight altitude, 31 (out of 13) in single places, 34 (out of 99) in helicopter, and 27 (out of 137) in the 1956 sample of pilots. Kuipers et al.,[8] based on interviews with 209 Dutch military pilots, reported that many of the pilots (44% F-5 and 56% F-16) experienced this illusion and had stayed at controls but were "amazed, confused or shocked" (p. OV-E-10). The loss of match to expectation can be extremely disruptive.

F.   Temporal Distortion

One of the most common SD-related psychological phenomena is temporal distortion. Time distortions occur during many stressful events, including SD situations. According to Ponomarenko et al. (Ref. 2, p. viii), "one of the typical errors in an emergency situation is incorrect time perception." When overly stressed, the pilot's internal clock is overloaded, and time slows down to a crawl (i.e., temporal expansion). One F-16 pilot relayed that, during a near-fatal SD mishap, his time estimates were expanded approximately 10-fold. Conversely, during boredom and other underaroused states estimated time relative to actual time is reduced (i.e., time constriction).[156] Pilots have reported temporal distortion both prior to and during SD.

VII. Summary

Spatial disorientation does not occur in a vacuum. It is the result of the natural sensations that are misperceived, inaccurately processed by the brain, improperly responded to based on personality, mental and physical state, and experience, and limited by the characteristics of the tasks that must be performed and the environment in which they occur.

Six illusions have been described in Sec. VI and linked in Table 3 to psychological factors described in Secs. I–V. All but one of the illusions (giant hand) stems from a lack of and/or inadequate cues. All of the illusions involve loss of situational awareness, and some are also associated with poor spatial ability. Although pilot personality can play a large role in individual SD accidents, it had little to do with illusions with the exception of overconfidence, which is central to some illusions (e.g., flying carpet). Expectation is part of many illusions. Given the prevalence of LSA in illusions, it is not unexpected that lack of knowledge is also prevalent. Mental stress is common to most illusions. The break-off illusion is the best example of emotion affecting perception or vice versa. Clearly, the psychological factors associated with SD illusions must be either designed or trained away if SD accidents are to be reduced.

References

[1]*Merriam Webster's English Dictionary*, s.v. "personality," "emotion," "learning," and "sensation."

[2]Ponomarenko, V., Malinin, I., Boubel, T., and Ercoline, W., "Kingdom in the Sky—Earthly Fetter and Heavenly Kingdoms. The Pilot's Approach to the Military Flight Environment,"AGARD, RTO AGARDOgraph 338, July 2000.

[3]Mortimer, R. G., "Spatial Disorientation in U.S. Civil Aviation Helicopter Accidents," *Proceedings of the 9th International Symposium on Aviation Psychology*, 1997, pp. 16–20.

[4]Platenius, P. H., and Wilde, G. J. S., "Personal Characteristics Related to Accident Histories of Canadian Pilots" *Aviation, Space, and Environmental Medicine*, Vol. 60, 1989, pp. 42–45.

[5]Mortimer, R. G., "Spatial Disorientation in Fixed-Wing General Aviation Accidents,"*Proceedings of the 8th International Symposium on Aviation Psychology*, 1995, pp. 1307–1311.

[6]Sanders, M. G., and Hoffman, M. A., "Personality Aspects of Involvement in Pilot-Error Accidents," *Aviation, Space, and Environmental Medicine*, Vol. 46, 1975, pp. 186–190.

[7]Sanders, M. G., Hofmann, M. A., and Neese, T. A., "Cross-Validation Study of the Personality Aspects of Involvement in Pilot-Error Accidents," *Aviation, Space, and Environmental Medicine*, Vol. 47, 1976, pp. 177–179.

[8]Kuipers, A., Kappers, A., van Holten, C. R., van Bergen, J. H. W., and Oosterveld, W. J., "Spatial Disorientation Incidents in the R.N.L.A.F. F16 and F5 Aircraft and Suggestions for Prevention," *Situational Awareness in Aerospace Operations*, AGARD CP–478, AGARD, 1990.

[9]Boer, L. C., "Spatial Ability and Orientation of Pilots," *Handbook of Military Psychology,* edited by R. Gal and A. D. Mangelsdorff, Wiley, New York, 1991.

[10]Clark, B., and Malone, R. D., "Topographical Orientation in Naval Aviation Cadets," *Journal of Educational Psychology,* Vol. 45, 1954, pp. 91–109.

[11]Taylor, R. M., "Geographical Disorientation and Flight Safety,"*Human Factors Aspects of Aircraft Accidents and Incidents,* Technical Editing and Reproduction Ltd., London, June 1979, pp. B9-1–B9-10.

[12]Dudani, N. G., "Grouping of the Causative Factors in Investigation of Aircraft Accidents Attributed to Pilot Errors," *Aerospace Medicine,* Vol. 43, 1972, pp. 671–674.

[13]Green, R. G., and Taylor, R. M., "The Psychologist in Aircraft Accident Investigation," *Human Factors Aspects of Aircraft Accidents and Incidents,* edited by B. O. Hartman, Technical Editing and Reproduction Ltd., London, 1979, pp. B4-1–B5.

[14]Ercoline, W. R., Weinstein, L. F., and Gillingham, K. K., "An Aircraft Landing Accident Caused by Visually Induced Spatial Disorientation," *Proceedings of the Sixth International Symposium on Aviation Psychology,* 1991, pp. 619–623.

[15]McDonald, N., "Fatigue and Driving," *Alcohol, Drugs and Driving,* Vol. 5, 1989, pp. 185–191.

[16]Stern, J. A., Boyer, D., and Schroeder, D., "Blink Rate: A Possible Measure of Fatigue," *Human Factors,* Vol. 36, 1994, pp. 285–297.

[17]Borowsky, M. S., and Wall, R., "Naval Aviation Mishaps and Fatigue," *Aviation, Space, and Environmental Medicine,* Vol. 54, No. 6, 1983, pp. 535–538.

[18]Blom, D. H. J., and Pokorny, M. L. I., "*Accidents of Bus Drivers: An Epidemiological Approach,*" Nederlands Inst. voor Praeventieve Gesondheidszorg, Leyden, the Netherlands, 1985.

[19]Stoner, J. D., "Aircrew Fatigue Monitoring During Sustained Flight Operations from Souda Bay, Crete, Greece," *Aviation, Space, and Environmental Medicine,* Vol. 67, 1996, pp. 863–866.

[20]Palmer, B., Gentner, F., Schopper, A., and Sottile, A., "Review and Analysis: Scientific Review of Air Mobility Command and Crew Rest Policy and Fatigue Issues," *Fatigue Issues,* 1996, pp. 1, 2.

[21]Graeber, R. C., "Sleep in Space," *Proceedings of the 28th NATO DRG Seminar: Sleep and Its Implications for the Military,* NATO, Neuilly-sur-Seine, France, 1987, pp. 59–69.

[22]Graeber, R. C., "Aircrew Fatigue and Circadian Rhythmicity," *Human Factors in Aviation,* edited by E. L. Wiener and D. C. Nagel, Academic Press, New York, 1988, pp. 305–344.

[23]Moore-Ede, M., "Aviation Safety and Pilot Error," *The Twenty-Four Hour Society,* edited by M. Moore-Ede, Addison Wesley Langman, Reading, MA, 1993, pp. 81–95.

[24]"F-117A Crash Reports Cite Pilot Fatigue, Disorientation," *Aviation Week and Space Technology,* Vol. 130, No. 19, 1989, p. 22.

[25]Tormes, F. R., and Guedry, F. E., "Disorientation Phenomena in Naval Helicopter Pilots," *Aviation, Space, and Environmental Medicine,* Vol. 46, 1975, pp. 387–393.

[26]LeDuc, P. A., Johnson, P. A., Ruyak, P. S., Estrada, A., Jones, H. D., and Higdon, A. A., "Evaluation of a Standardized Spatial Disorientation Flight Profile," United States Army Aeromedical Research Lab., USAARL Rept. Number 99-04, Fort Rucker, AL, Feb. 1999.

[27]Neville, K. J., Bisson, R. U., French, J., Boll, P. A., and Storm, W. F., "Subjective Fatigue of C-141 Aircrews During Operation Desert Storm," *Human Factors,* Vol. 36, 1994, pp. 339–349.

[28]Bisson, R. U., Neville, K. J., Boll, P. A., French, J., Ercoline, W. R., McDaniel, R. L., and Storm, W. F., "Digital Flight Data as a Measure of Pilot Performance Associated with Fatigue from Continuous Operations During Desert Persian Gulf Conflict," *Nutrition Metabolic Disorders and Lifestyle of Aircrew*, NATO, Neuilly-sur-Seine, France, 1992, pp. 12–54.

[29]French, J., Neville, K., Boll, P., Bisson, R., Slater, T., Armstrong, S., Storm, W., Ercoline, W., and McDaniel, R., *Subjective Mood and Fatigue of C-141 Crew During Desert Storm (Nutrition Metabolic Disorders and Lifestyle of Aircrew)*, NATO-AGARD, Neuilly-sur-Seine, France, 1992.

[30]French, J., Bisson, R., Neville, K. J., Mitcha, J., and Storm, W. F., "Crew Fatigue During Simulated, Long Duration B-1B Bomber Missions," *Aviation, Space, and Environmental Medicine*, Vol. 65, 1994, pp. A1–A6.

[31]Klein, K., Wegmann, H., Athanassenas, G., Hohlweck, H., and Kuklinski, P., "Air Operations and Circadian Performance Rhythms," *Aviation, Space, and Environmental Medicine*, Vol. 47, 1976, pp. 221–229.

[32]Ribak, J., Ashkenazi, I. E., Klepfish, A., Avgar, D., Tall, J., Kallner, B., and Noyman, Y., "Diurnal Rhythmicity and Air Force Flight Accidents due to Pilot Error," *Aviation, Space, and Environmental Medicine*, Vol. 54, 1983, pp. 1096–1099.

[33]Wright, J. E., Vogel, J. A., Sampson, J. B., Knapik, J. J., and Patton, J. F., "Effects of Travel Across Time Zones (Jet Lag) on Exercise Capacity and Performance," *Aviation, Space, and Environmental Medicine,* Vol. 54, 1983, pp. 132–137.

[34]Reiter, R. J., "Pineal Melatonin: Cell Biology of Its Synthesis and of Its Physiological Interactions," *Cell Biology*, Vol. 12, 1991, pp. 151–180.

[35]Gawron, V. J., French, J., and Funke, D., "An Overview of Fatigue," *Stress, Workload, and Fatigue*, edited by P. A. Hancock and P. A. Desmond, Lawrence Erlbaum, Mahwah, NJ, 2001, pp. 581–595.

[36]Gillingham, K. K., "A Primer of Vestibular Function, Spatial Disorientation, and Motion Sickness," U.S. Air Force School of Aerospace Medicine, Review 4-66, Brooks Air Force Base, TX, June 1966.

[37]Ninow, E. H., Cunningham, W. F., and Radcliff, F. A., "Psychophysiological and Environmental Factors Affecting Disorientation in Naval Aircraft Accidents," AGARD CP–95: *The Disorientation Incident*, AGARD March 1972, pp. A5-1–A5-4.

[38]Wegner, D. M., "Pink Elephant Tramples White Bear: the Evasion of Suppression," *Psycoloquy*, Vol. 5, No. 40, 1994, paradoxical-cogniton.2.wegner.

[39]Navon, D., "The Forest Revisited: More on Global Precedence," *Psychological Research*, Vol. 43, 1981, pp. 1–32.

[40]Doppelt, F. F., "A Program for the Spatial Disorientation Demonstrator," United States Air Force School of Aerospace Medicine, SAM-TR-65-66, Brooks Air Force Base, TX, Oct. 1965.

[41]Monesi, F. H., "An Update of Findings Regarding Spatial Disorientation in Flight: A Reconstruction of Underlying Mechanisms," AGARD CP–287: *Spatial Disorientation in Flight Current Problem*, AGARD, 1980, pp. B2-1–B2-6.

[42]Durnford, S. J., De Roche, S. L., Harper, J. P., and Trudeau, L. A., "Spatial Disorientation: A Survey of U.S. Army Rotary-Wing Aircrew," U.S. Army Aeromedical Research Lab., USAARL 96-16, Fort Rucker, AL, March 1996.

[43]De Giosa, P., "Perceptual Errors in Flight—a Survey of 100 Military Pilots on Active Duty," *AGARD Conference Proceedings 287, Spatial Disorientation in Flight: Current Problems*, AGARD, Nueilly-sur-Seine, France, 1980, pp. B3-1–B3-7.

[44]Simonelli, N., "The Dark Focus of Accommodation: Its Existence, Its Measurement, Its Effects," New Mexico State Univ., Dept. of Psychology, Behavioral Engineering Lab., BEL-79-03/AFOSR-79-9, Las Cruces, NM, 1979.

[45]Tepper, M. L., "Between Incident and Accident!" *Human Factors Aspects of Aircraft Accidents and Incidents*, Technical Editing and Reproduction Ltd., London, June 1979, pp. B11-1–B11-6.

[46]Yanowitch, R. E., "Crew Behavior in Accident Causation," *Aviation, Space, and Environmental Medicine*, Vol. 48, No. 10, 1977, pp. 918–921.

[47]Krahenbuhl, G. S., Marett, J. R., and Reid, G. B., "Task-Specific Simulator Pretraining and In-Flight Stress of Student Pilots," *Aviation, Space, and Environmental Medicine*, Vol. 49, No. 9, 1978, pp. 1107–1110.

[48]Harper, C. R., and Albers, W. R., "Alcohol and General Aviation Accidents," *Aerospace Medicine*, Vol. 35, 1964, pp. 462–464.

[49]Gibbons, H. L., Ellis, J. W., and Plechus, J. L., "Medical Factors in 1964–1965 Fatal Aircraft Accidents in the Southwest, *Aerospace Medicine*, Vol. 37, 1966, pp. 1057–1060.

[50]Gibbons, H. L., Ellis, J. W., and Plechus, J. L., "Medical Factors in 1964/1965 Fatal Accidents in the Southwest," *Aerospace Medicine*, 1966.

[51]Gibbons, H. L., Ellis, J. W., and Plechus, J L., "Analysis of Medical Factors in Fatal Aircraft Incidents in 1965," *Texas Medicine*, Vol. 63, 1967, pp. 667–671.

[52]Gibbons, H. L., and Plechus, J. L., "Analysis of Medical Factors in Fatal Arcraft Accidents," *Texas State Journal of Medicine*, Vol. 61, 1965, pp. 667–671.

[53]Canfield, D., Flemig, J., Hordinsky, J., and Birky, M., "*Drugs and Alcohol Found in Civil Aviation Accidents Between 1989 and 1993*," Federal Aviation Administration Civil Aeromedical Inst., DOT/FAA/AM-95/28, Oklahoma City, OK, 1995.

[54]Hordinsky, J. R., and Kuhlman, J., "Toxicological Examination in General Aviation Accidents," *Aviation, Space, and Environmental Medicine*, 1991, p. A60.

[55]Li, G., Hooten, E. G., Baker, S. P., and Butts, J. D., "Alcohol in Aviation-Related Fatalities: North Carolina, 1985–1994," *Aviation, Space, and Environmental Medicine*, Vol. 69, No. 8, 1988, pp. 755–760.

[56]McFadden, K. L., "Driving While Intoxicated (DWI) Convictions and Job-Related Flying Performance—a Study of Commercial Air Safety," *Journal of the Operational Research Society*, Vol. 49, 1998, pp. 28–32.

[57]Canfield, D. V., Hordinsky, J., Millett, D. P., Endecott, B., and Smith, D., "Prevalence of Drugs and Alcohol in Fatal Civil Aviation Accidents Between 1994 and 1998," *Aviation, Space, and Environmental Medicine*, Vol. 72, 2001, pp. 120–124.

[58]Gibbons, H. L., "Alcohol, Aviation, and Safety Revisited: a Historical Review and Suggestion," *Aviation, Space, and Environmental Medicine*, Vol. 59, 1988, pp. 657–660.

[59]Jovy, D., Bruner, H., and Klein, K. E., "Measuring and Critical Examination of the Influence of Drugs on the Performance Ability of Aviators," *Human Problems of Supersonic and Hypersonic Flight*, Pergamon, London, 1962, pp. 410–418.

[60]Collins, W. E., Gilson, R. D., Schroeder, D. J., and Guedry, F. E., "Alcohol and Disorientation-Related Response III Effects of Alcohol Ingestion on Tracking Performance During Angular Acceleration," Federal Aviation Administration Office of Aviation Medicine, FAA-AM-71-20, Washington, D.C., 1971.

[61]Ryback, R. S., and Dowd, P. J., "Aftereffects of Various Alcoholic Beverages on Positional Nystagmus and Coriolis Acceleration," *Aerospace Medicine*, Vol. 411, 1970, pp. 429–435.

[62]Hill, R. J., Collins, W. E., and Schroeder, D. J., *"Alcohol and Disorientation-Related Responses: V. The Influence of Alcohol on Positional, Rotary, and Coriolis Vestibular Responses over 32-Hour Periods,"* Federal Aviation Administration Civil Aeromedical Inst., Rept. FAA-AM-71-39, Oklahoma City, OK, 1971.

[63]Gilson, R. D., Schroeder, D. J., Collins, W. E., and Guedry, F. E., Jr., *"Effects of Different Alcohol Dosages and Display Illumination on Tracking Performance During Vestibular Stimulation,"* U.S. Army Aeromedical Research Lab., Rept. USAARL 72-2, Fort Rucker, AL, 1971, Also published as "Alcohol and Disorientation-Related Responses. IV: *Effects of Different Alcohol Dosages and Display Illumination on Tracking Performance During Vestibular Stimulation,"* Federal Aviation Administration Civil Aeromedical Inst., Rept. FAA-AM-71-34, Oklahoma City, OK.

[64]Schroeder, D. J., Gilson, R. D., Guedry, F. E., and Collins, W. E., *"Alcohol and Disorientation-Related Responses VI. Effects of Alcohol on Eye Movements and Tracking Performance During Laboratory Angular Accelerations About the Yaw and Pitch Axes,"* Federal Aviation Administration Office of Aviation Medicine, Rept. FAA-AM-72-34, Washington, D.C., 1972.

[65]Burton, R. R., and Jaggars, J. L., "Influence of Ethyl Alcohol Ingestion on a Target Task During Sustained +Gz Centrifugation," *Aerospace Medicine*, Vol. 45, 1974, pp. 290–296.

[66]Collins, W. E., *"Performance Effects of Alcohol Intoxication and Hangover at Ground Level and at Simulated Altitude,"* Federal Aviation Administration Office of Aviation Medicine, Rept. FAA-AM-79-26, Washington, DC, 1979.

[67]Collins, W. E., and Chiles, W. D., *"Laboratory Performance During Acute Intoxication and Hangover,"* Federal Aviation Administration Office of Aviation Medicine, Rept. FAA-AM-79-7, Washington, D.C., 1978.

[68]Collins, W. E., and Chiles, W. D., "Laboratory Performance During Acute Alcohol and Intoxication and Hangover," *Human Factors*, Vol. 22, 1980, pp. 445–462.

[69]Collins, W. E., Mertens, H. W., and Higgins, E. A., "Some Effects of Alcohol and Simulated Altitude on Complex Performance Scores and Breathalyzer Readings," *Aviation, Space, and Environmental Medicine*, Vol. 58, 1987, pp. 328–332.

[70]Stokes, A. F., Belger, A., Banich, M. T., and Taylor, H., "Effects of Acute Aspartame and Acute Alcohol Ingestion upon the Cognitive Performance of Pilots," *Aviation, Space, and Environmental Medicine*, Vol. 62, 1991, pp. 648–653.

[71]Horne, J. A., and Gibbons, H., "Effects of Vigilance Performance and Sleepiness of Alcohol Given in the Early Afternoon ('Post Lunch') vs. Early Evening," *Ergonomics*, Vol. 34, 1991, pp. 67–77.

[72]NTI, Inc., *"The Effect of Alcohol and Fatigue on an FAA Readiness-to-Perform Test,"* Federal Aviation Administration, DOT/FAA/AM-95/24, Washington, DC, 1995.

[73]Millar, K., Finnigan, F., and Hammersley, R. H., "Is Residual Impairment After Alcohol an Effect of Repeated Performance?" *Aviation, Space, and Environmental Medicine*, Vol. 70, 1999, pp. 124–130.

[74]Billings, C. E., Demosthenes, T., White, T. R., and O'Hara, D. B., "Effects of Alcohol on Pilot Performance in Simulated Flight," *Aviation, Space, and Environmental Medicine*, 1991, pp. 233–235.

[75]"The Residual Effects of Alcohol," *Business Aviation Safety*, Vol. 5, 1989, pp. 54, 55.

[76]Davenport, M., and Harris, D., "The Effect of Low Blood Alcohol Levels on Pilot Performance in a Series of Simulated Approach and Landing Trials," *The International Journal of Aviation Psychology*, Vol. 2, 1992, pp. 271–280.

[77]Henry, P. H., Davis, T. Q., Engelken, E. J., Triebwasser, J. H., and Lancaster, M. C., "Alcohol-Induced Performance Decrements Assessed by Two Link Trainer Tasks Using Experienced Pilots," *Aerospace Medicine*, Vol. 45, Oct. 1974, pp. 1180–1189.

[78]Henry, P., Davis, T. Q., Engelken, E. J., McNee, R. C., Keiser, H. N., Triebwasser, J. H., and Lancaster, M. C., "*Evaluation of Two Link GAT-1 Trainer Tasks by Experienced Pilots at Three Alcohol Dose Levels*," School of Aerospace Medicine, SAM-TR-74-53, Brooks Air Force Base, TX, 1974.

[79]Henry, P. H., Flueck, J. A., Sanford, J. F., Keiser, H. N., McNee, R. C., Walter, W. H., III, Webster, K. H., Hartman, B. O., and Lancaster, M. C., "Assessment of Performance in a Link GAT-1 Flight Simulator at Three Alcohol Dose Levels," *Aerospace Medicine*, Vol. 45, 1974, pp. 33–44.

[80]Henry, P. H., Flueck, J. A., Sanford, J. F., Keiser, H. N., McNee, R. C., Walter, W. H., III, Webster, K. H., Hartman, B. O., and Lancaster, M. C., "Assessment of Performance in a Link GAT-1 Flight Simulator at Three Alcohol Dose Levels," *Aerospace Medicine*, Vol. 45, 1974, pp. 33–44.

[81]Morrow, D., Leirer, V., and Yesavage, J., "The Influence of Alcohol and Aging on Radio Communication During Flight," *Aviation, Space, and Environmental Medicine*, Vol. 61, 1990, pp. 12–20.

[82]Morrow, D., Yesavage, J., and Leirer, V., "Use of Flight Simulators to Investigate the Effects of Alcohol and Other Drugs on Performance," *Proceedings of the 5th International Symposium on Aviation Psychology*, 1989, pp. 203–208.

[83]Morrow, D., Yesavage, J., Leirer, V., Dolhert, N., Taylor, J., and Tinklenberg, J., "The Time-Course of Alcohol Impairment of General Aviation Pilot Performance in a Frasca 141 Simulator," *Aviation, Space, and Environmental Medicine*, Vol. 64, 1993, pp. 697–705.

[84]Ross, L. E., and Mundt, J. C., "Multiattribute Modeling Analysis of the Effects of a Low Blood Alcohol Level on Pilot Performance," *Human Factors*, Vol. 30, No. 3, 1988, pp. 293–304.

[85]Ross, L. E., and Mundt, J. C., "Use of Flight Simulators to Investigate the Effects of Alcohol and Other Drugs on Pilot Performance," *Proceedings of the 5th International Symposium on Aviation Psychology*, 1989, pp. 197–202.

[86]Ross, L. E., Yeazel, L. M., and Chau, A. W., "Pilot Performance with Blood Alcohol Concentrations Below 0.04%," *Aviation, Space, and Environmental Medicine*, Vol. 63, 1992, pp. 951–956.

[87]Smith, F. J., and Harris, D., "Effects of Low Blood Alcohol Levels on Pilots' Prioritization of Tasks During a Radio Navigation Task," *The International Journal of Aviation Psychology*, Vol. 4, 1994, pp. 349–358.

[88]Taylor, H. L., Dellinger, J. A., Schilling, R. F., and Richardson, B. C., "Pilot Performance Measurement Methodology for Determining the Effects of Alcohol and Other Toxic Substances," *Proceedings of the Human Factors Society 27th Annual Meeting*, 1983, pp. 334–338.

[89]Taylor, J. L., Dolhert, N., Friedman, L., Mumenthaler, M., and Yesavage, J. A., "Alcohol Eliminator and Simulator Performance of Male and Female Aviators: A Preliminary Report," *Aviation, Space, and Environmental Medicine*, Vol. 67, 1996, pp. 407–413.

[90]Taylor, J. L., Dolhert, N., Morrow, D., Friedman, L., and Yesavage, J. A., "Acute and 8-Hour Effects of Alcohol (0.08% BAC) on Younger and Older Pilots' Simulator Performance," *Aviation, Space, and Environmental Medicine*, Vol. 65, 1994, pp. 718–725.

[91]Yesavage, J. A., and Leirer, V. O., "Hangover Eeffects on Aircraft Pilots 14 Hours After Alcohol Ingestion: A Preliminary Report," *American Journal of Psychiatry*, Vol. 143, 1986, pp. 1546–1550.

[92]Billings, C. F., Wicks, R. L., Gerke, R. J., and Chase, R. C., "*The Effects of Alcohol on Pilot Performance During Instrument Flight*," Federal Aaviation Administration, Office of Aviation Medicine, Technical Rept. FAA-AM-73-4, 1972.

[93]Jarvis, D. W., "Investigation of Spatial Disorientation of F-15 Eagle Pilots," Directorate of Equipment Engineering, ASD-TR-81-5016, Wright-Patterson Air Force Base, OH, Aug. 1981.

[94]Endlsey, M. R., "Toward a Theory of Situation Awareness in Dynamic Systems," *Human Factors*, Vol. 37, 1995, pp. 32–64.

[95]Sipes, W. E., and Lessard, C. S., "Spatial Disorientation: A Survey of Incidence," *Proceedings of the Tenth International Symposium on Aviation Psychology*, 1999, pp. 910–915.

[96]Knapp, C. J., and Johnson, R., "F-16 Class A Mishaps in the U.S. Air Force, 1975–93," *Aviation, Space, and Environmental Medicine*, Vol. 67, 1996, pp. 777–783.

[97]Lyons, T. J., Ercoline, W. R., Freeman, J. E., and Gillingham, K. K., "Classification Problems of the U.S. Air Force Spatial Disorientation Accidents, 1989–91," *Aviation, Space, and Environmental Medicine*, Vol. 65, 1994, pp. 147–152.

[98]Boehme, M., "USAF Spatial Disorientation Training," *Aeromedical and Training Digest*, Vol. 4, Jan. 1990, pp. 19, 20.

[99]Jones, D. G., and Endsley, M. R., "Sources of Situation Awareness Errors in Aviation," *Aviation, Space, and Environmental Medicine*, Vol. 67, 1996, pp. 507–521.

[100]Greene, J., "Definition of Spatial Disorientation," *Aeromedical and Training Digest*, Vol. 4, Oct. 1990, p. 4.

[101]Johnson, L. W., "Medical and Operational Factors of Accidents in Advanced Fighter Aircraft," *Human Factors Aspects of Aircraft Accidents and Incidents*, edited by B. O. Hartman, Technical Editing and Reproduction Ltd., London, 1979, pp. B2-1–B4.

[102]Previc, F. H., Yauch, D. W., DeVilbiss, C. A., Ercoline, W. R., and Sipes, W. E., "In Defense of Traditional Views of Spatial Disorientation and Loss of Situational Awareness," *Aviation, Space, and Environmental Medicine*, Vol. 66, 1995, pp. 1103–1106.

[103]Jaslow, H., "Spatial Disorientation and Controlled-Flight-Into-Terrain," *Proceedings of the 1998 Advanced in Aviation Safety Conference*," Society of Automotive Engineers, Warrendale, PA, 1998, 123–129.

[104]Endsley, M. R., "Situation Awareness: Future of Aviation Systems," *Proceedings of the Human Operator in a Demanding Environment*, SAAB Aerospace, 1997.

[105]Navathe, P. D., and Singh, B., "An Operational Definition for Spatial Disorientation," *Aviation, Space, and Environmental Medicine*, Vol. 65, 1994, pp. 1153–1155.

[106]Cheung, B., "Spatial Disorientation," *Aviation, Space, and Environmental Medicine*, Vol. 66, 1995, p. 706.

[107]Montgomery, R. A. G., Patterson, J. C., and Montgomery, K. D. G., "Taking the Blinders off Spatial Disorientation," *Proceedings of the 28th Annual SAFE Symposium*, 1991, pp. 144–148.

[108]Howard, I. P., and Templeton, W. B., *Human Spatial Orientation*, Wiley, New York, 1966.

[109]Del Vecchio, R. J., *Physiological Aspects of Flight*, Dowling College Press, Oakdale, NY, 1977.

[110]Mortimer, R. G., "General Aviation Airplane Accidents Involving Spatial Disorientation," *Proceedings of the Human Factors and Ergonomics Society 39th Annual Meeting*, 1995, pp. 25–29.

[111]Bellenkes, A. H., Wickens, C. D., and Kramer, A. F., "Visual Scanning and Pilot Expertise: the Role of Attentional Flexibility and Mental Model Development," *Aviation, Space, and Environmental Medicine*, Vol. 68, 1997, pp. 569–579.

[112]Moser, R., "Spatial Disorientation as a Factor in Accidents in an Operational Command," *Aerospace Medicine*, Vol. 40, 1969, pp. 174–176.

[113]Braithwaite, M. G., Durnford, S. J., Crowley, J. S., Rosado, N. R., and Albano, J. P., "Spatial Disorientation in U.S. Army Rotary-Wing Operations," *Aviation, Space, and Environmental Medicine,* Vol. 69, 1998, pp. 1031–1037.

[114]Baker, S. P., and Lamb, M. W., "Human Factors in Crashes of Commuter Airplanes and Air Taxis," Federal Aviation Administration, Final Rept. DTFA01-90-00046, 1992.

[115]Barnum, F., and Bonner, R. H., "Epidemiology of USAF Spatial Disorientation Aircraft Accidents, 1 Jan 1958–31 Dec. 1958," *Aerospace Medicine*, Vol. 42, 1971, pp. 896–898.

[116]Harding, R. M., and Mills, F. J., "Function of the Special Senses in Flight I: Vision and Spatial Orientation," *British Medical Journal*, Vol. 286, 28 May 1983, pp. 1728–1731.

[117]Grunwald, A. J., Ellis, S. R., and Smith, S., "A Mathematical Model for Spatial Orientation from Pictorial Perspective Displays," *IEEE Transactions on Systems, Man, and Cybernetics*, Vol. 18, 1988, pp. 425–437.

[118]Singh, B., and Navathe, P. D., "Indian Air Force and World Spatial Disorientation Accident: A Comparison," *Aviation, Space, and Environmental Medicine*, Vol. 65, 1994, pp. 254–256.

[119]von Diringshofen, H., "Use of Roll-Angle Indicators for Avoiding Spatial Disorientation During Instrument Flight," *Aerospace Medicine*, Vol. 38, 1967, p. 401.

[120]Eichner, R. B., and Mason, R. P., "Refresher Naval Aviation Physiology Training Program (NAPTP) in Aircraft Simulators," *Proceedings of the 33rd Annual Safe Symposium*, 1996, pp. 20–29.

[121]Trumbo, R. B., and Montgomery, R. A., "New Dimensions in Spatial Disorientation Training," *Proceedings of the 28th Annual SAFE Symposium*, 1991, pp. 139–143.

[122]Benson, A. J., and Burchard, E., "Spatial Disorientation in Flight," AGARD, A-170, Sept. 1973.

[123]Gillingham, K. K., "The Spatial Disorientation Problem in the United States Air Force," *Journal of Vestibular Research,* Vol. 2, 1992, pp. 297–306.

[124]Bennett, C. T., "The Display of Spatial Information and Visually Guided Behavior. Visually Guided Control of Movement," NASA CP 3118, 1991, pp. 25–38.

[125]Collins, D. L., and Harrison, G., "Spatial Disorientation Episodes Among F-15C Pilots During Operation Desert Storm," *Journal of Vestibular Research,* Vol. 5, 1995, pp. 405–410.

[126]Dell, J. L., "Human Factors Aspects in High-Speed Low-Level Flight," AGARD CP 266: *Operational Roles, Aircrew Systems, and Human Factors in Future High Performance Aircraft,* AGARD, 1980, pp. 7-1–7-4.

[127]Durnford, S. J., and Crowley, J. S., "Spatial Disorientation in Rotary-Wing Aircrew: What Makes an Incident and What Makes an Accident?" *International Symposium on Aviation Psychology,* Vol. 2, 1995, pp. 1312–1317.

[128]Durnford, S. J., Crowley, J. S., Rosado, N. R., Harper, J., and DeRoche, S., "Spatial Disorientation: A Survey of U.S. Army Helicopter Accidents 1987–1992," U.S. Army Aeromedical Research Lab., USAARL 95-25, Fort Rucker, AL, June 1995.

[129]Braithwaite, M. G., Douglass, P. K., Durnford, S. J., and Lucas, G., "The Hazard of Spatial Disorientation During Helicopter Flight Using Night Vision Devices," *Aviation, Space, and Environmental Medicine*, Vol. 69, 1998, pp. 1038–1044.

[130]Sipes, W. E., and Lessard, C. S., "A Spatial Disorientation Survey of Experienced Instructor Pilots," *IEEE Engineering in Medicine and Biology*, Vol. 19, pp. 35–42.

[131]Leibowitz, H. W., "The Human Senses in Flight," *Human Factors in Aviation*, edited by E. L. Wiener and D. C. Nagel, Academic Press, New York, 1988.

[132]Rupert, A. H., "An Instrumentation Solution for Reducing Spatial Disorientation Mishaps," *IEEE Engineering in Medicine and Biology*, Vol. 19, 2000, pp. 71–80.

[133]McGreevy, M. W., and Ellis, S. R., "The Effect of Perspective Geometry on Judged Direction in Spatial Information Instruments," *Human Factors*, Vol. 28, 1986, pp. 439–456.

[134]Zuckerman, M., "Hallucinations, Reported Sensations, and Images," *Sensory Deprivation: Fifteen Years of Research*, edited by J. P. Zubek, Appleton-Century-Croft, New York, 1969, 85–125.

[135]Siatkowski, R. M., Zimmer, B., and Rosenberg, P. R., "The Charles Bonnet Syndrome—Visual Perceptive Dysfunction in Sensory Deprivation," *Journal of Clinical Neuro-Ophthalmology*, Vol. 10, 1990, pp. 215–218.

[136]Iawata, K., Yamamoto, M., Nakao, M., and Kimura, M., "A study on Polysomnographic Observations and Subjective Experiences Under Sensory Deprivation," *Psychiatry and Clinical Neurosciences*, Vol. 53, 1999, pp. 129–131.

[137]Iawata, K., Nakao, M., Yamamoto, M., and Kimura, M., "Differentiation of Physiological States Under Sensory Deprivation," *Methods of Information in Medicine*, Vol. 39, 2000, pp. 168–170.

[138]Persinger, M. A., and Richards, P. M., "Vestibular Experiences of Humans During Brief Periods of Partial Sensory Deprivation Are Enhanced When Daily Geomagnetic Activity Exceeds 15–20 nT," *Neuroscience Letters*, Vol. 194, 1995, pp. 69–72.

[139]Dowd, P. J., "Proposed Spatial Orientation Flight Training Concept," *Aerospace Medicine*, Vol. 45, 1974, pp. 758–765.

[140]Tredici, T. J., "Visual Illusions as a Probable Cause of Aircraft Accidents," AGARD CP–287: *Spatial Disorientation in Flight: Current Problems*, AGARD, Oct. 1980, pp. B5-1–B5-7.

[141]Benson, A. J., "Spatial Disorientation and the 'Break-Off' Phenomenon," *Aerospace Medicine*, Vol. 44, 1973, pp. 944–952.

[142]Benson, A. J., "Spatial Disorientation and the 'Break-Off' Phenomenon," AGARD CP–95: *The Disorientation Incident*, AGARD, 1972, pp. A11-1–11-11.

[143]Benson, A. J., "Spatial Disorientation in Flight: Scope and Limitations of Training," *Aeromedical and Training Digest*, 1990, pp. 20–23.

[144]Gillingham, K. K., and Previc, F. H., "Spatial Orientation in Flight," Crew Systems Directorate, AL-TR-1993-0022, Brooks Air Force Base, TX, Nov. 1993.

[145]Clark, B., Nicholson, M. A., and Graybiel, A., "Fascination: a Cause of Pilot Error," *Aviation Medicine*, Vol. 24, 1953, pp. 429–440.

[146]Honneger, B., "Sharing Safety Innovations," *Federal Manager*, Vol. 21, 2001 pp. 1–3.

[147]Rensink, R. A., O'Regan, J. K., and Clark, J. J., "To See or Not to See: The Need for Attention to Perceive Changes in Scenes," *Psychological Science*, Vol. 8, 1997, pp. 368–373.

[148]Theeuwes, J., "Exogenous and Endogenous Ccontrol of Attention: The Effects of Visual Onsets and Offsets," *Perception and Psychophysics*, Vol. 49, 1991, pp. 83–90.

[149]Folk, C. L., Remington, R. W., and Johnston, J. C., "Involuntary Covert Orienting is Contingent on Attentional Control Settings," *Journal of Experimental Psychology: Human Perception and Performance*, Vol. 18, 1992, pp. 1030–1044.

[150]Pashler, H., Johnston, J. C., and Ruthruff, E., "Attention and Performance," *Annual Review of Psychology*, Vol. 52, 2001, pp. 629–651.

[151]Malcolm, R., and Money, K. E., "Two Specific Kinds of Disorientation Incidents," AGARD CP–95: *The Disorientation Incident*, AGARD, March 1972, pp. A10-1–A10-4.

[152]King, P. A. H., "A Report of an Incident of Extreme Spatial Disorientation in Flight," Toronto, Canada Institute of Aviation Medicine Royal Canadian Air Force, Aeromedical Reports, Vol. 1, 1962, pp. 22–28.

[153]Lyons, T. J., and Simpson, C. G., "The Giant Hand Phenomenon," *Aviation, Space, and Environmental Medicine*, Vol. 60, 1989, pp. 64–66.

[154]Weinstein, L. F., Previc, F. H., Simpson, C. G., Lyins, T. J., and Gillingham, K. K., "A Test of Thumb and Index Finger Control in Overcoming a Visual Analogue of the Giant Hand Illusion,"*Aviation, Space, and Environmental Medicine*, Vol. 62, 1991, pp. 336–341.

[155]Clark, B., "Disorientation-Incidents Reported by Military Pilots Across 14 Years of Flight," *AGARD CP 95: The Disorientation Incident*, AGARD, 1972, pp. A1-1–A1-7.

[156]von Kirchenheim, C., and Persinger, M. A., "Time Distortion—A Comparison of Hypnotic Induction and Progressive Relaxation Procedures: A Brief Communication," *International Journal of Clinical Experimental Hypnosis*, Apr. 1991, pp. 63–66.

Suggested Reading

Cahoon, R. L., "Vigilance Performance Under Hypoxia: II. Effect of Work-Rest Cycle," *Perceptual and Motor Skills*, Vol. 31, 1970, pp. 619–626.

Fowler, B., and Prlic, H., "A Comparison of Visual and Auditory Reaction Time and P300 Latency Thresholds to Acute Hypoxia," *Aviation, Space, and Environmental Medicine*, Vol. 66, No. 7, 1995, pp. 645–650.

Fowler, B., Elcombe, D. D., Kelso, B., and Porlier, G., "The Threshold for Hypoxia Effects on Perceptual-Motor Response," *Human Factors*, Vol. 29, No. 1, 1987, pp. 61–66.

Fulco, C. S., and Cymerman, A., *Human Performance and Acute Hypoxia*, U.S. Army Research Inst. of Environmental Medicine, Natick, MA, 1987.

Guedry, F. E., and Rupert, A. H., "Steady State and Transient G-Excess Effects," *Aviation, Space, and Environmental Medicine*, Vol. 62, 1991, pp. 252–253.

Kerr, J. S., and Hindmarch, I., "The Effects of Alcohol Alone or in Combination with Other Drugs on Information Processing, Task Performance and Subjective Responses," *Human Psychopharmacology*, Vol. 13, 1998, pp. 1–9.

Kobrick, J. L., Zwick, H., Witt, C. E., and Devine, J. A., "Effects of Extended Hypoxia on Night Vision," *Aviation, Space, and Environmental Medicine*, Vol. 55, No. 3, 1984, pp. 191–195.

Lategola, M. T., Lyne, P. J., and Burr, M. J., "*Alcohol-Induced Physiological Displacements and Their Effects on Flight-Related Functions*," Federal Aviation Administration Office of Aviation Medicine, Rept. FAA-AM-82-3, Washington, D.C., 1982.

McFarland, R. A., "The Effects of Altitude on Pilot Performance," *Proceedings of the 17th International Congress on Aviation and Space Medicine*, 1968, pp. 96–108.

Molina, E. A., Guedry, F. E., and Lentz, J. M., "Initial Observations on Perceptual Responses and Disturbance Produced by the Vertifuge," Naval Aerospace Medical Research Lab. NAMRL Special Rept. 91-1, Pensacola, FL, Aug. 1991.

"Safety Study—Statistical Review of Alcohol-Involved Aviation Accidents," National Transportation Safety Board, Rept. NTSB/SS-84/03, Washington, D.C., 1984.

Nesthus, T. E., Bomar, J. B., Holden, R. D., and O'Connor, R. B., "Cognitive Workload and Symptoms of Hypoxia," *Proceedings of the 25th Annual Symposium SAFE Association*, 1987, pp. 45–47.

Rayman, R. B., and McNaughton, G. B., "Sudden Incapacitation: USAF Experience, 1970–80," *Aviation, Space, and Environmental Medicine*, Vol. 54, No. 2, 1983, pp. 161–164.

"The Residual Effects of Alcohol," *Business Aviation Safety*, Vol. 5, 1989, pp. 54, 55.

Zubek, J. P., *Sensory Deprivation: Fifteen Years of Research*, Appleton-Century-Croft, New York, 1969.

Chapter 5

Spatial Disorientation Mishap Classification, Data, and Investigation

Stephen J. H. Véronneau*

FAA Civil Aerospace Medical Institute, Oklahoma City, Oklahoma

Richard H. Evans[†]

General Dynamics Advanced Information Systems, San Antonio, Texas

I. Introduction

I NSIGHT into spatial disorientation (SD) mishaps highlights the complex interaction of human, machine, mission, and environment. That complexity is accentuated by the inadequacy of the pilot's sensory systems to provide reliable information in the flight environment. Unlike an accident stemming from medical incapacitation as a result of a disease or a physiological stressor, such as hypoxia, a spatial disorientation mishap usually involves the normal reaction of a fully functioning human. It is the challenging environment in which that healthy individual must function that often renders his or her usually effective physiological "equipment" to be inept.

The maladaption of the otoliths and semicircular canals to the flight environment, as discussed in Chapter 2, all too often leads a pilot to perform inappropriate aircraft control actions and become a part of the chain of events leading to an accident or incident. Although this natural physiological deficiency has been demonstrated to thousands of pilots with deceptively simple devices such as the Barany chair, many fail to recognize or overcome the unreliability of the vestibular-sensory inputs and subsequently fail to break the mishap chain. It is the responsibility of the accident investigator to determine at what point the chain could have been broken and to suggest an informed remedy. To do so requires astute insight into the typical sequence of an SD mishap. Accident investigators must determine if the pilots' visual and vestibular inputs contributed to an inappropriate

This material is declared a work of the U.S. Government and is not subject to copyright protection in the United States.
*Bioinformatics Research Team Leader.
[†]Member, Spatial Disorientation Countermeasures Research Team.

flight-control response. They must also determine if the subsequent aircraft orientation or performance degraded to a point from which the pilot reasonably could have recognized the flight anomaly and his or her role in causing the deviation. Finally, accident investigators must project themselves into the pilot's experience and judge the appropriateness of an intervention action taken or omitted.

Although an SD mishap sequence is not a disease process per se, with sufficient acceleration stress a debilitating medical condition can develop, that is, severe nystagmus or pilot vertigo. Also, rare medical conditions can contribute to a pilot's experiencing SD and the severity of thereof. For example, congenital (see Chapter 2, Sec. IV) anomalies, such as absence or abnormality of the vestibulo-occular reflex (VOR), can predispose a pilot to disorientation in turbulent instrument meteorological conditions (IMC). Similarly, certain medications and food supplements can increase a pilot's susceptibility to SD. The potential impact of medical issues must be considered when investigating a mishap for possible SD involvement.

The type of flight operation involved often determines the depth of understanding gained from a mishap investigation. For example, investigation of military and air carrier or other commercial mishaps is facilitated by the larger number of persons involved in the fact gathering and by the nationwide availability of expertise to assist in particular areas of complex data integration and analysis. Conversely, accident investigation for general aviation (GA), or public, not-for-hire operations, does not fair as well. Budget constraints and the relatively common occurrence of GA accidents have led to the need for some investigating agencies in countries with high per-capita GA activity to limit the extent of the investigation, finish the report, and move on to the next investigation. Some of those agencies have petitioned to eliminate GA accident investigations altogether in certain categories.

Another hindrance to thorough investigation of SD affects on GA mishaps centers on available resources with which to ascertain the presence of SD. Investigators must devote a great deal of time and energy in gaining sufficient knowledge and training to be able to examine GA accident scenes for evidence of material defects or problems in the operation, maintenance, and repair of aircraft. Consequently, less attention has been paid to becoming proficient at evaluating human factors contributions and the presence of SD in particular. To compound the problem, there is a lack of expertise to assist the GA field investigator in analyzing the human factors contribution to a mishap. In addition to the issues just mentioned are the facts that human factors evidence 1) is perishable; 2) is overlooked because of inadequate reconstruction tools, and 3) meets resistance in the review process. Resistance during review often stems from the investigator's inability to completely quantify and present the magnitude of SD effects in a particular individual, as compared to his or her adeptness at providing straightforward, traditional failure analysis of hardware items.

Overcoming these obstacles to identifying the causes of aviation mishaps is the focus of this chapter. Toward that end, the chapter will explore the role of SD in the progression of human factors events that lead to an aircraft mishap. It will identify the three types of SD as used in mishap investigation and address their relationships to specific mishap characteristics. The chapter will also present a summary analysis of SD mishap data, some investigative techniques for determining the presence and impact of SD in a mishap, and some examples of applying those techniques. The aim of this chapter is to equip operations, management, and investigative individuals with the necessary appreciation of SD as a powerful human factors element so that its prevalence in aviation mishaps may be diminished.

II. Human Factors Modeling

There have been many attempts to categorize and organize human factors components of mishaps. Civilian aviation authorities and individual military services have all developed classifications and investigator guides to meet their particular needs. Among the multitude of such efforts are several that merit particular mention here as aids to the field investigator. The following schemas provide a useful and simple underpinning to understanding human factors involvement in an accident and can be employed to extract an SD component of a mishap.

A. Man–Machine–Medium–Mission–Management Model of System Engineering

The man–machine–medium–mission–management model (also known as the 5-M risk management model) is an effective tool for examining the nature of accidents and is part of the Federal Aviation Administration (FAA) internal flight safety program. As a concept, it began with T. P. Wright, of Cornell University in the 1940s, who introduced the man–machine–environment triad into aviation safety. A fourth "M" (management) was later added in 1965 as part of the University of Southern California curriculum in system safety. E. A. Jerome added the "mission" factor in 1976 to the overall model, although it had been used in military-oriented flight safety courses before that time.[1] The components of the 5-M model are defined as 1) mission—the central purpose, function, or objectives; 2) man—the human element, which can include a multiple dimension because of multiperson interactions; 3) machine—the hardware and software components, including the regulatory aspects; 4) medium—the physical environment, both ambient and operational; and 5) management—the overarching aspects, procedures, policies, and regulations external to the flight deck. Figure 1 illustrates the various interrelationships of the individual elements and how the area of interest often lies in the interface among them. The interactions of the human operator (i.e., man) with the equipment, task, and environment (i.e., machine, mission and medium) are of particular interest to the mishap investigator.*

B. SHEL(L) Model

The elements of the SHEL (L) model are 1) software—the rules, regulations, and operating procedures, including the regulatory aspects; 2) hardware—the physical components; 3) environment—the ambient and physiological aviation environment; 4) liveware—the human element; and 5) liveware-liveware—a multiple dimension caused by multiperson interactions, such as crew resource management (CRM) and pilot–air-controller communications.†

---

*Further reading on the 5M model is available at the FAA Office of System Safety (ASY) website at the following URLs: http://nasdac.faa.gov/Risk/SSHandbook/cover.htm and http://nasdac. faa.gov/Risk/SSHandbook/contents.htm [cited Oct. 2003].

†Further reading on the SHEL model is available at the following URLs: http://www.dcs.ed.ac.uk/ home/mas/doc/icdsn2000.pdf and http://goethe.ira.uka.de/~sujan/olos/shel_model.html [cited Oct. 2003].

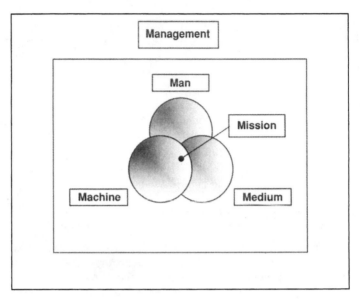

Fig. 1   Five-M model of system engineering.

Elwyn Edwards developed the original SHEL model in 1972 (Ref. 2), and Frank Hawkins modified it in 1984 (Ref. 3). The elements of the model are diagrammed in Fig. 2 to illustrate their interrelationships and are modified to show that the Liveware factor can include more than one person, hence, the second "L." The interface between each of the elements illustrates their interactions and effects on each other and suggests that assorted modifiers will produce variation in human performance in the aviation environment.

C.   Reason's Human-Error ("Swiss Cheese") Model

Professor Jim Reason's human-error model, the so-called swiss cheese model (Fig. 3), has been widely accepted into several, varied human-error investigation

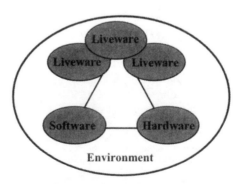

Fig. 2   SHEL(L) model of human factors interrelationships.

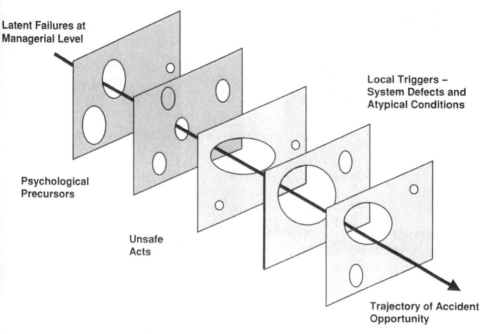

Fig. 3   Reason's (swiss-cheese) human-error model.

efforts, even recently including the investigation of medical-practice errors.[4] Aviation mishap investigation has particularly benefited from the theoretical framework that the model has provided since its introduction in 1989 (Ref. 5). Investigation of aviation mishaps has revealed that there is a sequence of actions, each seemingly unrelated to each other, but in reality linked together in a timely chain of events, which leads to the accident outcome. An interruption of any of the links in the sequence would have prevented or mitigated the accident occurrence. The model illustrates how, thankfully, aviation mishaps are rare events because of the defensive depth of the multilayered safety measures that are in place. Most potential mishap sequences are blocked, and it is the rare combination of events that gets by all of the layers. Violations, slips and lapses, and errors categorize the various elements that constitute both active and latent failures of the system being studied in a mishap sequence. Although the forms and expressions of human error, along with the interaction of humans with technology, seem to be infinite in variety, the root causes of seemingly disparate mishaps have much more in common when analyzed from this model's perspective. Because aviation accidents occur relatively infrequently, commonalities can be established only through collecting long-term, detailed human factors information from each one. Such analysis must be given emphasis equal to that traditionally placed on failure of the hardware systems.

D.   Human Factors Analysis and Classification System

The Human Factors Analysis and Classification System (HFACS), developed by Scott Shappell and Doug Wiegmann,[6] incorporates elements of the Reason

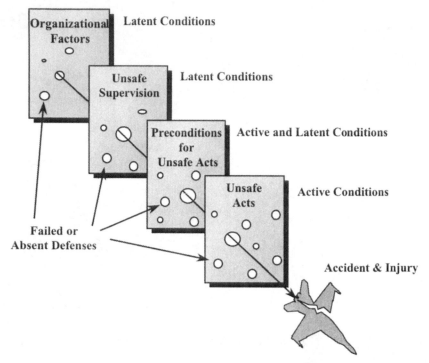

Fig. 4   HFACS modification of Reason's human-error model diagram. (Adapted from Ref. 5 and reproduced with permission of Ref. 6.)

human-error model, as well as those of other frameworks. They have categorized the layers of defense as organizational influences, unsafe supervision, preconditions for unsafe acts, and unsafe acts (Fig. 4).

Their HFACS, which is shown in detail in Fig. 5, can be used both during the field investigation and in later analysis. The system enables the investigator to spot trends in organizational influences, unsafe supervision, preconditions for unsafe acts, and in the unsafe acts themselves. It also provides a means to determine if the errors in the chain of events leading to the mishap are predominantly violations, decision based, skill based, or perceptual in nature. Remedial measures can then be targeted, allowing a multidisciplinary and comprehensive safety solution to be enacted (Ref. 6).*

These conceptual frameworks or systems for understanding aviation mishaps have been developed over the years and are complementary in many ways. Regardless of which framework is employed, it is vital to remember that the most important aspect of accident investigation is to pursue the root cause(s) as far as the evidence trail or reconstruction techniques will permit. Continuing to ask "Why?" rather than accepting the first categorization of a particular mishap

---

*More information on the HFACS can be obtained at http://www.hf.faa.gov/docs/cami/00_07.pdf and http://www.aviation.uiuc.edu/new/html/ARL/conference/shappellwiegavpsy01.pdf [cited Oct. 2003].

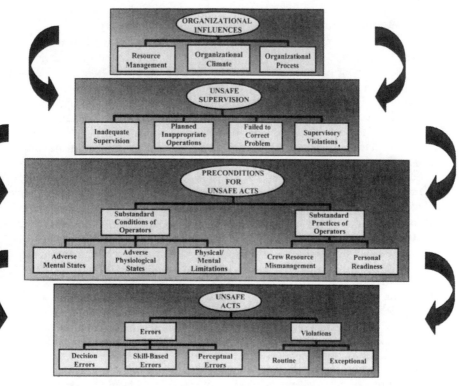

Fig. 5   HFACS model error classification system. (Reproduced with permission of Shappel and Weigman; Ref. 6.)

will advance the art and science of mishap investigation and assist in the prevention of future tragic events. In addressing the "Why?" question, it is important for the investigator to be persistent in the collection of SD indicators and patient in explaining the mechanisms of spatial orientation and disorientation to those who might have difficulty understanding the physiological and human factors constituents of SD.

III.   Spatial Disorientation Mishap Classification Issues

Determining trends and conducting other analyses of SD mishaps are affected by how one defines a SD mishap, the taxonomy used to delineate types of SD, and the relationship of a mishap classified as SD related to those of other categories. Understanding these issues is essential to appreciation of the scope of the problem and to developing appropriate prevention strategies.

A.   Spatial-Disorientation Classification Effects on Incidence

The manner by which one defines or classifies spatial disorientation is important in terms of assessing the rate at which SD occurs. Early military aviation mishap surveys (e.g., Refs. 7 and 8) typically reported SD mishaps as comprising less than 10% of the total number of Class A mishaps (mishaps in which a fatality or financial loss in excess of $1M occurred). Later military surveys, which used standard definitions adopted by leading SD researchers, found that SD mishaps either definitely or possibly contributed to 10–22% of total accidents.[9–14] A still-higher SD accident percentage was reported by Braithwaite et al.,[15] who reported an SD mishap percentage of 31% in U.S. Army rotorcraft accidents. Additionally, Neubauer[16] concluded that 27% of all U.S. Air Force (USAF) accidents could be attributed to broadly defined SD. Both of the latter two surveys included cases that involved conditions of sensory illusions in the SD category, regardless of whether or not SD was explicitly coded by the investigating flight surgeon.

Some researchers (e.g., Refs. 17 and 18) have argued for a narrow definition of SD when estimating the contribution of SD to overall aviation risk. For example, Navathe and Singh[17] argue that SD should be limited to illusions resulting only from input error, namely, visual, vestibular, and somatosensory illusions. According to Navathe and Singh,[18] common illusions involving cognitive factors such as "lean-on-sun," "breakoff," "coning of attention," and even misjudgments of height, speed, or distance should not be considered as examples of SD. Using their very conservative definition, Singh and Navathe[18] reported that only 2.1% of all Indian Air Force mishaps (and only 7.9% of those mishaps involving fatalities) were attributable to SD. Using a broader definition of SD, Navathe and Singh reported that nearly 20% of fatal mishaps were SD related. The restrictive definition proposed by Navathe and Singh[17] was rejected by leading SD researchers, including Previc et al.[19] and Cheung.[20]

Neubauer[16] similarly showed that mishap statistics might reflect very different contributions of SD, depending on the definition used by the mishap board or investigator. In a survey of USAF Class A mishaps from 1994–1998, Neubauer reported that 12.2% of all mishaps were SD related based on the specific citation of SD by the flight surgeon. However, 27% of all USAF Class A mishaps were SD related if mishaps caused by various illusions (e.g., misperception of speed/closure; misperception of distance/altitude/separation) were categorized as SD related— whether or not they were ascribed as such in the original mishap report.

Most researchers and flight surgeons today accept that such categories as misperception of distance, altitude, or separation fall within the standard definition of SD presented in Chapter 1, Sec. I. This convention is relevant now given a larger percentage of human-error-related mishaps increasing SD risk associated with all-weather and all-terrain flying, flying with night-vision devices (NVD) and other factors relating to advanced technology. In military aviation, particularly, the current definitional usage of the term "SD mishap" results in an effective SD contribution of approximately 20–30% of all Class A accidents.[16]

B. Indicators and Correlation to Types of Spatial Disorientation

The categories of Type I (Unrecognized), Type II (Recognized), and Type III (Incapacitating) SD are correlated with characteristic actions and their results in Table 1 (see also Chapter 1, Sec. I). (As noted in Chapter 1, Section I, not all flight-safety agencies use the Type III SD category.) The classifications are not perfectly exclusive, and cases can be found with elements of each mixed together.

Table 1   Correlations of mishap indicators to types of spatial disorientation

Spatial disorientation	Description	Accident correlates
Type I—Unrecognized	Unrecognized by the pilot; no conscious perception of SD	Distractions as antecedents to the accident. Crash with no distress or concern expressed. No "mayday" or other than routine communications. Unusual or inappropriate aircraft attitude, but pilot does not make any appropriate corrective action. Pilot is apparently oblivious to the situation.
Type II—Recognized	Recognized, conscious manifestation of a problem. Pilots often incorrectly refer to this experience as vertigo.	Pilot recognizes conflict between perceived and intended or expected attitude. Can assume that the instruments are operating incorrectly. Might not properly react because of difficulty accepting indicated correct control input or might just be puzzled about the situation. Confusion might persist after recovery and lead to compounding of the SD problem.
Type III—Incapacitating	Vestibulo-occular discoordination and inability to exercise manual control. Pilot experiences overwhelming physical or emotional stimuli.	Dramatic impairment or incapacitation; no stable retinal image caused by nystagmus. Vestibulo-spinal reflexes can make manipulation of the controls difficult. Could be accompanied by panic, fear, motion sickness (sopite syndrome), or helplessness. Might freeze on the controls.

Although pilots need only be familiar with a general concept of the three categories, it is very helpful for the investigator to use these specific designations in order to support clear discussion and data analysis. Application of the three types of SD when reconstructing a mishap sequence simplifies determining SD impact on the accident outcome and helps focus recommendations for corrective actions.

Rarely, one might find an orderly sequence of events in an individual mishap with Type I SD progressing to Type II and then possibly to Type III. However, it is more likely that there will either be no progression or some overlap in categorization. The majority of mishaps exhibit mostly Type I SD and then perhaps a short period of Type II SD, resulting in either recovery or a crash. It is generally agreed that Type I SD mishaps are relatively more common among helicopter pilots than among fixed-wing pilots.[9,11,15] This predominance might suggest that visual illusions are more important to Type I SD because they also are most likely to be encountered by helicopter pilots.[15] However, both visual and vestibular illusions can produce Types I or II SD or both. Type III SD is mainly related to vestibular stimulation and depends upon sufficient discoordination between the vestibular system and the extraocular muscles to produce incapacitating nystagmus or manual-control incapacitation. Only a few Type III SD mishaps have been reported.*

SD is a particularly lethal threat to solo pilots and should be immediately suspected in any unexplained mishap involving single-piloted aircraft. In multicrew aircraft it is unlikely that all flight crew members will experience the same degree or type of disorientation at the same time, which does confer some protection from an accident. However, with visual illusions and distractions that involve all cockpit crew members the possibility of concurrent impairment does arise. A chain of events that interferes with the situational awareness of all flight deck members will overcome the advantage of multicrew cockpits and should raise the suspicion of the investigating human performance expert as to the presence of SD.

The crash of Air New Zealand Flight 901 into Mount Erebus in 1979 is an excellent case study of such SD factors having a collective effect. Prior to that mishap, the company changed the aircraft's autoflight computer program without informing the flight crew of the change, and the aircraft flew a slightly different course towards the mountains of Antarctica than normal. The presumptions of the crew were of previous patterns of flight on the same route, and, thus, they did not expect any differences to arise in the mishap flight. In the reduced visibility even individuals familiar with the terrain could not detect the small change in visual perspectives from familiar landmarks, and the crew convinced themselves of being on course. Eventually, the crew felt uncomfortable with their flight but could not conceptualize or verbalize anything other than overall discomfort. The first officer suggested a 180-deg turn, but the captain was not convinced of the need to reverse course. The rising terrain was not apparent in the whiteout conditions until the alarm from the ground proximity warning system (GPWS) system sounded. The subsequent crash that resulted in loss of all life onboard was caused in part by the unknown programming change in the navigation equipment, the visual limitations of the pilots, and the visual illusions of the flight environment. All crew members succumbed to those illusions after the chain of events led to their collective loss of situational awareness.

C. Relationship Between SD and Controlled Flight into Terrain and Weather

The relationship between SD and controlled flight into terrain (CFIT) is readily apparent from considering their definitions. As illustrated in the preceding section, CFIT occurs when an airworthy aircraft, under the control of a qualified pilot, is flown into terrain (or water or obstacles) with inadequate awareness on the part of the pilot of the impending disaster. Spatial disorientation, as defined in Sec. I, of Chapter 1, is the pilot's failure "to sense correctly the position, motion or attitude of the aircraft or of him or herself within the fixed coordinate system provided by the surface of the earth and the gravitational vertical" (Ref. 21, p. 419). A "failure

---

*For an example of a Type III SD mishap, see NTSB case NYC 91FA239 at http://www.ntsb.gov/ntsb/brief.asp?ev_ id=20001212×18160&key=1 [cited Oct. 2003].

to sense correctly" is synonymous "inadequate awareness," and, assuming no suicidal intentions on the part of the pilot, one can reasonably deduce that no CFIT accident could occur without the pilot's being unaware of his or her spatial orientation.

The connection between SD and CFIT can also be made with mishap factors, most notably loss of control and weather. Accidents involving CFIT and loss of control in flight account for 17% of all commercial aviation fatalities, thereby constituting the two most prevalent causes of loss of life in worldwide passenger-jet operations.* More than half of the CFIT accidents occurred during flight in IMC. Weather is the number one causal factor cited in GA accidents and has been the greatest contributor to the fatality rate in that community. Weather-related GA accidents most often involve an unplanned or and/or sudden flight into IMC while operating under visual flight rules (VFR), which leads to CFIT or loss of control resulting from either SD or structural failure of the aircraft. Weather is also often a contributing factor in GA accidents in which improper instrument flight rules (IFR) approaches and crosswind or tailwind landings were attempted.

In light of the preceding outlined correlations, it requires only a small leap of faith to conclude that there is some overlap between SD, CFIT, and IMC/weather-related mishaps. However, SD is often not cited as a causal factor in those accidents. This omission is likely because of the already mentioned lack of research, lack of education of investigators, or a combination of factors including the difficulty of reconstructing the sequence of events in a SD mishap. The underreporting of SD factors is unfortunate, as it negatively impacts the effectiveness of many of the countermeasures developed to prevent CFIT and weather-related mishaps. Conversely, to assist in the development of effective SD countermeasures (see Chapters 8, 9, and 10) it is important for the accident investigator to intensely evaluate all related categories that might include SD components.

On a positive note, several interrelated countermeasures to CFIT accidents have already commenced. The FAA is working in partnership with industry to study and identify CFIT risk factors, develop interventions for commercial airlines and GA, and revise guidance material and regulations. The requirement for enhanced ground proximity warning systems (EGPWS), which the FAA refers to as terrain awareness and warning systems (TAWS), arose out of the plan to prevent CFIT accidents. Versions of EGPWS suitable for GA aircraft and helicopters are now on the market. Lastly, numerous FAA/industry partnership initiatives, including the National Aviation Weather Strategic Plan and the Aviation Safety Program Educational Curriculum for Pilots, are underway to ensure that more complete, accurate, and timely weather information is available to all pilots.[†]

IV. Mishap Statistics

A. Historical Background and General Issues

The effective human factors investigator must possess an appreciable knowledge of the general frequency of SD-related mishaps and how that frequency has changed over time. This section provides a foundation for such awareness by providing the

---

*Data available online at http://www.boeing.com/news/techissues/pdf/2000_Statsum.pdf [cited Oct. 2003].

[†]Further reading on GA CFIT Prevention is available at the FAA CAMI Web site at http://www.cami.jccbi.gov/aam-400A/Brochures/CFIT.htm [cited Oct. 2003].

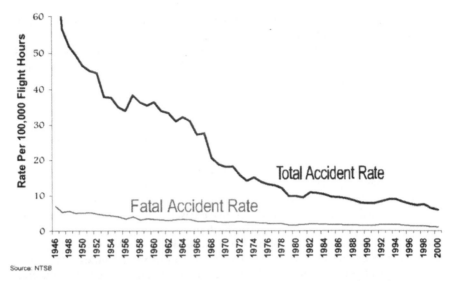

Source: NTSB

Fig. 6   General aviation total and fatal accident rate trends since 1946.

of SD and the reporting of its occurrence in a mishap. U.S. Federal Aviation Regulations (FARs) delineate the differences in the types of operation by reference to the applicable part number of the U.S. Code of Federal Regulations (CFR). The respective CFR parts will be addressed in more detail in Sec. IV.B, but let it suffice at this point to consider civil aviation as essentially consisting of the GA and commercial sectors.

Although GA total and fatal accident rates have been reported to have steadily declined over the past five decades—dramatically so between 1946 and 1978 (see Fig. 6), SD remains a notable concern, especially regarding fatalities. According to Kirkham and colleagues,[29] SD played only a small role (2.5%) in general aviation aircraft accidents in the United States. However, as in the military, it was a quite deadly factor in being the third most common cause of GA accidents with fatalities. From 1970–1975, 15.6% (627) of the 4012 fatal GA mishaps were denoted as having an SD aspect. More ominous is the fact that 90% of all GA SD mishaps were fatal. It is difficult to precisely determine the frequency at which SD has contributed to commercial accidents, but at a minimum 14 such mishaps occurred involving air carriers between 1950 and 1969. These mishaps all resulted from the pilot's succumbing to the somatogravic and visual illusions that produce the so-called dark-night takeoff accident.[30] By implication, even more SD mishaps likely occurred during the same period. Malcolm and Money[31] reported that 26 commercial airliners experienced jet-upset incidents or accidents, which might raise suspicion of their having spatial-orientation (SO) components, but those episodes were not designated as being SD related.

A word of caution is warranted at this point pertaining to the interpretation of mishap statistics. As suggested in the introduction and the preceding paragraph, there is reason for prudence in accepting mishap statistics at face value. One can safely assume that underreporting of SD occurs in all categories of accident investigation, as the investigating body often will not identify an SD factor as significantly contributing to the mishap. Unfortunately, other factors are sometimes considered as being more central to the mishap sequence for several reasons, such as holding a higher priority in an organization's operational emphasis or being more easily implemented in procedural changes. This misclassification is an example of not following a root–cause-oriented approach to mishap investigation and, rather, selecting a popular concept as the focus.

As an example, such attachment of an in-vogue categorization to mishaps might have occurred in the USAF from 1980–1989. During that time, loss of situational awareness (LSA) was assigned as a factor in 263 mishaps that resulted in 425 fatalities and together cost over two billion dollars[12] (Freeman, J. E., personal communication, 1990). Although LSA is a legitimate psychological phenomenon that began to receive great emphasis during those years, the term might have been overused in classifying mishaps. The point in question regards the relationship of situational awareness (SA) and SO. Succinctly put, one can lose SA without losing SO, but the converse is never true (see Chapter 1, Sec. I). It is quite possible for a pilot's state of awareness relative to a specific situation to be dangerously degraded while being concerned with any number of flight or mission components, e.g., geographical position or weapon status, without his or her losing their SO. However, it is illogical to assume that in most cases when LSA results in a mishap that the accident would not also be the result of the pilot's erroneous perception of aircraft orientation in relation to obstacles, terrain, water or reference aircraft (i.e., SD, as delineated in the standard definition). Therefore, one can reasonably assume that in at least the preponderance of the just-mentioned LSA mishaps the pilots were, at a critical moment, unaware of their actual aircraft attitude, altitude, or other flight parameters. They almost assuredly must have fallen victim to SD. Because of such misclassifications, the careful student of accident statistics will suspect that many more SD-related mishaps occur than are recorded. Regardless of the questionable purity of the data, analysis of it provides valuable insight into the role of SD in flight mishaps and will be addressed in more detail in Sec. IV.B and IV.C.

B. Civil Aviation

In an attempt to gain insight into the role of SD in civil mishaps, the National Transportation Safety Board (NTSB) database, covering 1983–1997 and comprising some 35,000 cases, was searched for using the following codes: spatial disorientation, aircraft control not maintained (ACNM), and visual illusions. [At the time of this writing, data from the two last years (1998 and 1999) were incomplete in terms of final accident determinations. However, the available data are included in the charts for informational purposes.] Cases were handled individually so that missing fields, such as pilot age or flight time, could be matched and reconstructed from other government databases. Then, the data were aggregated, and individual identities were stripped, producing some interesting revelations.

The first finding of note was that the NTSB rarely cited visual illusions as factors or causes in accidents (Fig. 7). This rarity is most likely a result of the already training inadequacies for accident investigators. Second, the review indicated that

Civil Accidents Coded for SD, Aircraft Control Not Maintained and Visual Illusion

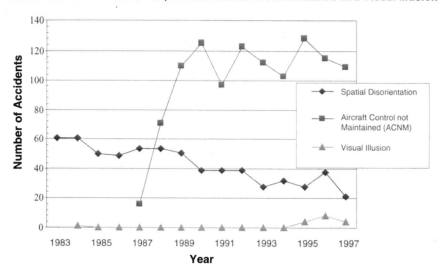

Fig. 7   SD-related civil aviation mishaps with NTSB codings of SD, aircraft control not maintained, and visual illusion. (Source: NTSB database.)

accidents coded as SD have been decreasing since 1983 (Fig. 7). Mishaps related to SD represented, on average, less than 2% of all accidents and around 10% of fatal accidents during the time period of the study. One possibility is that increases in pilot age and flight hours as well as the numbers of pilots holding instrument ratings had begun to yield a lower frequency of accidents that were caused by SD. Although the SD mishap decline—which overwhelmingly reflects the GA SD-related mishaps because they represented more than 90% of the total SD mishaps—could be interpreted as a constant improvement in system safety with respect to the reduction in SD mishaps, additional data from the NTSB suggest otherwise. In 1987 the NTSB began using a new set of codes, including aircraft control, which had the modifier of "not maintained." Because the NTSB data-coding manual included (and still does) a cross reference at the SD code entry to the "aircraft control-not maintained" codes, a direct relationship was implied. As one can see in Fig. 7, the decrease in SD-coded accidents was more than offset by the increase to a steady, high number of those coded as ACNM. One would assume that the factors which had been postulated to have aided in the supposed reduction of SD accidents—increased pilot age, flight hours, and instrument ratings—should also have applied to the ACNM accidents as well.

The conflicting SD and ACNM mishap trends can be related to incomplete training of accident investigators, but additional factors might be involved. Such issues could include the decrease in index of suspicion for SD-related mishaps, the diminished time available for GA accident investigation or a quality assurance process that does not allow for the determination of SD if the accident facts are somewhat circumstantial. With the absence of flight data and cockpit voice recorders, the investigation of human factors in GA accident investigation, in particular,

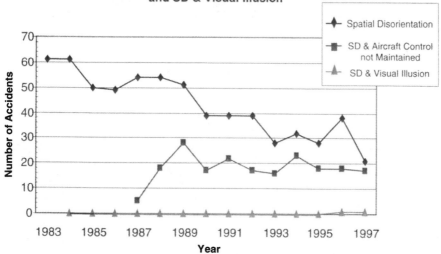

Fig. 8 SD-related civil aviation mishaps with NTSB codings of SD, SD, and aircraft control not maintained, and SD and visual illusion. (Source: NTSB database.)

can be very difficult and the facts very elusive. Thus, this inherent difficulty inevitably leads to the use of a more generic code, such as aircraft control not maintained, which by definition will include some cases of SD. These potential errors in the data notwithstanding, the NTSB review provides some enlightening information.

To permit more useful comparisons of the NTSB data, closer scrutiny of all the cases will be made to eliminate overlapping causes as well as to try to determine mishap rates for each category. Figure 8 presents NTSB mishap data of cases counted as either solely SD, a combination of SD and ACNM, or SD and visual illusion. This figure illustrates the small, known overlap between SD and ACNM codes. However, it seems clear that there are cases accumulated in the ACNM category that were likely SD mishaps or would have a large SD component as a factor. It is logical to assume that, unfortunately, the much larger number of ACNM-only cases still include some misclassified cases of SD, which are lost to analysis. Similarly, one must assume there is potential for other definition overlaps; for example, as described earlier some cases of SD can be concealed within the CFIT category. The remainder of the discussion of the NTSB data will be concerned solely with accidents that have SD coding as a cause or factor and will not address the ACNM or the visual illusion coding.

Civil mishaps involving SD occur in all phases of flight (Fig. 9); however, there is preponderance within descent, cruise, and maneuvering. There is also a sizable proportion occurring in the "not reported" category. The prolific use of this nondescript category is a data-quality issue plaguing all accident databases and again reflects the diminished time and resources available for GA investigation.

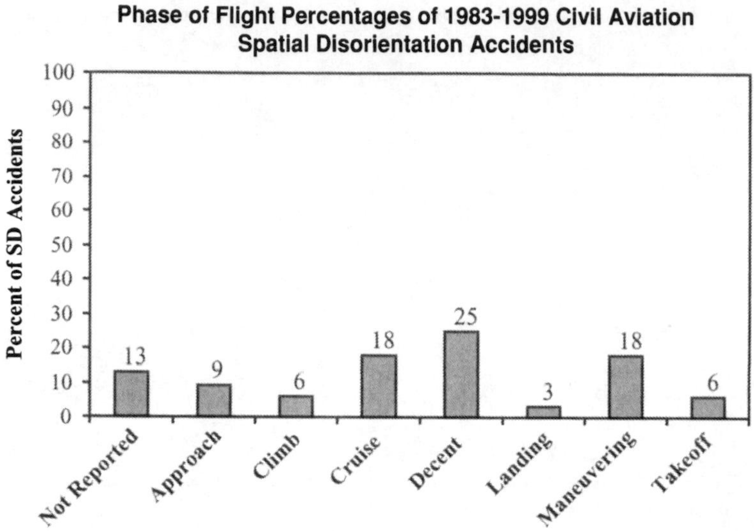

Phase of Flight Percentages of 1983-1999 Civil Aviation Spatial Disorientation Accidents

Fig. 9   Percent of civil aviation SD-related accidents by phase of flight. (Source: NTSB.)

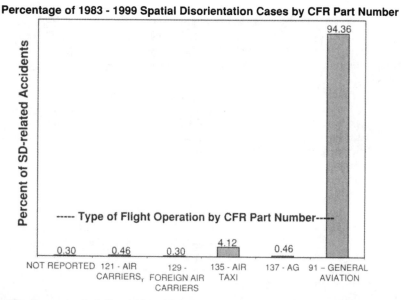

Percentage of 1983 - 1999 Spatial Disorientation Cases by CFR Part Number

Fig. 10   Percent of civil aviation SD-related accidents by type of flight operation. (Source: NTSB.)

Unfortunately, in the often-uncontrolled flight environment of GA, there is some-times no means to determine what was the phase of flight prior to the accident.

Figure 10 illustrates that the vast majority of SD mishaps (94% of the 644 cases) occur during FAR Part 91 flight operations, which is the regulatory oversight of GA activity. However, Fig. 10 also shows by the four mishaps attributed to Part 121 (domestic air carriers) the two in Part 129 (foreign air carriers), and the 27 in Part 135 (air-taxi) highlight that commercial operations are not free of risk from SD. The figure suggests that air taxi operations are the main area to target for improvement in commercial operations in order to reduce the frequency of SD mishaps.

According to the NTSB database, the percentages of SD mishaps occurring in IMC and visual meteorological conditions (VMC) were 63 and 32%, respectively, with about 5% not reported as occurring in either category. By looking more closely at the VMC and IMC datasets (Fig. 11), one can see that although the IMC SD accidents are roughly split equally between night and day, 2/3 of the VMC-associated SD mishaps occur at night, and 1/3 occur during daylight.

Figure 12 shows the average age for pilots involved in SD mishaps by year. It illustrates a gradual aging of pilots who sustain a SD mishap, consistent with the gradual overall aging of the pilot population as a whole. Figure 13 contains the average total flight time and the average flight time in the previous 90 days for pilots involved in SD mishaps, by year. The series averages for total flight time and 90-day flight time are 1650 and 55 h, respectively.

A more detailed analysis of flight hours and pilot age reveals that the greatest variation in the minimum and maximum flight hours per SD mishap pilot occurs in GA operations (ranging from 10 to 25,000 h) and commuter operations (span-ning 600 to 18,000 h). The average total flight time is the least in GA operations, but it is still impressive at 1428 hours. For other commercial operations the aver-age flight experience is quite high—10,773 hours for domestic carrier operations; 8,124 hours for foreign carrier operations; 4275 hours for air taxi operation; and

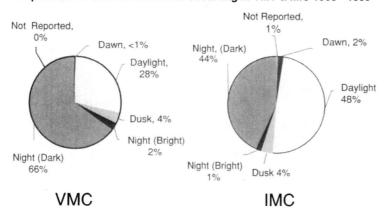

Fig. 11   Light conditions and day/night breakdown for civil aviation SD accidents in visual meteorological conditions. (Source: NTSB.)

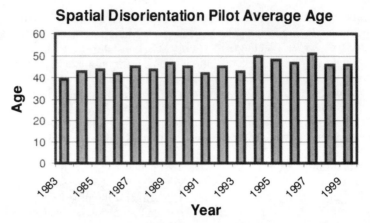

Fig. 12   Average age of civil aviation pilot experiencing SD, by year. (Source: NTSB.)

13,032 hours for agricultural flights. From these data it is evident that even experienced pilots are not immune to the risks of spatial disorientation. This reality is not surprising because there is near-universal susceptibility to SD in human pilots, and additional experience does not always make pilots immune to the typical chain of events in an SD mishap. Distractions, preoccupations, and task-management problems conspire to breach the layers of defense and result in an accident.

The average age of SD-mishap pilots, grouped by the type of flight operation, does not demonstrate much variation. The 35–45-year range captures the majority

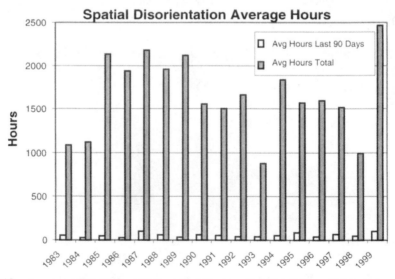

Fig. 13   Average total and last 90 days flight hours of civil aviation pilot experiencing SD, by year. (Source: NTSB.)

U.S.A. and Canadian Operators Accident Rates

Hull Loss and/or Fatal Accidents — Worldwide Commercial Jet Fleet — 1959 Through 2000

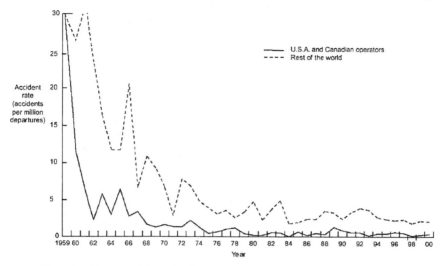

Fig. 14   Commercial worldwide jet airliner accident rates (1959–2000).

of the mishaps except for agricultural operations, in which the average age of SD-mishap pilots is 54. No reason for this age group shift has been identified, but one might suspect it could be caused by decreased motor skill reaction time in older pilots. The high-risk nature of agriculture operations—predominately crop-dusting flights—is derived from flight maneuvering in very close proximity to the ground and obstructions, where time to react to errors in orientation is severely limited.

To fully understand the significance of SD in the civil quarter, one must gain a perspective of overall civilian aviation safety and risk. First one must consider the relatively low incidence of accidents in large air carrier operations. Indeed, in spite of ever-increased utilization of the airspace and increased numbers of aircraft, flights and passengers carried, the worldwide commercial aviation accident rate has actually declined (Fig. 14). In the face of such improvement, it might be tempting to categorize the relatively infrequent losses attributed to SD as acceptable, especially because the overall accident rate is already very low and represents the lowest among all modes of commercial transportation. However, it is clear that in the public eye even the current rate is alarming in terms of lives lost, and from a business perspective it is expensive in terms of equipment and litigation. To compound those concerns, one must recognize that in spite of the cited decline the accident rate has leveled off over the past decade and has shown little tendency for further abatement.

Some efforts are underway to attain additional reductions in the incidence of commercial accidents, such as that by the U.S. Federal Aviation Administration. The stated goal of the FAA is to diminish the accident rate in commercial aviation in the United States by 80% by the year 2007. Fulfilling this broad goal will require a multiplicity of initiatives, especially because there are many, varied safety factors remaining to be targeted for improvement, and no one theme now dominates commercial aviation. However, SD presents a particularly salient target at which to aim. In addition to its known prevalence, SD's unreported presence might be an underlying factor in a large number of mishaps (see Sec. IV.A). For example, according to Boeing Corporation statistics covering 1959–2000, the largest loss of life worldwide in commercial passenger jet operation accidents occurs in two categories—CFIT and loss of-control in flight*—both of which were previously correlated with SD.

Another aspect to be considered when scrutinizing the decline in the number of worldwide commercial aviation accidents is that of equitable distribution. In certain parts of the world, a disproportionately high accident rate exists relative to the respective volumes of commercial aviation operations in each area. Removing these pockets of elevated incidence represents a challenge for safety advocates. Just as much hard work has produced the high degree of aviation safety attained in North America and much of Europe, ensuring the same level of safety throughout the world will require an international effort to promote best aviation practices. The multifactorial inputs into flight safety require that a myriad of risks be targeted for improvement, many of which might be intertwined with political-economic realities. Hopefully, SD countermeasures can be successfully employed as a universal, human factors approach in reducing overall accident rates in all parts of the world.

The frequency of SD mishaps must also be put into perspective with the distribution of all accidents. By themselves, the percentages of SD mishaps experienced in the different categories of flight operations (Fig. 10) do not necessarily indicate in which order the categories are at risk of encountering SD-related accidents. For example, the fact that GA accounts for 94% of all SD mishaps, and air carrier operations experience only 0.46%, does not indicate that SD should be considered of little risk to air carriers. On the contrary, by viewing the hierarchy of percentages relative to the rates for all accidents shown in Fig. 15, one could infer that the risk of a SD mishap is essentially the same for all categories. Each category retains the same general proportion of a mishap rate as for SD mishaps. GA operations—followed correspondingly by those for air taxi, commuter, then air carrier operations—have the highest rate of all accidents and account for the highest percentage of SD mishaps, which implies that each category experiences about the same amount of SD mishaps commensurate to its hours of operation. (In Fig. 9 air taxi and commuter operations are both contained in the FAR Part 135 category.) Nonetheless, the dramatically high number of SD mishaps experienced in GA operations implies a need to aggressively target SD in that community, even in the face of strong improvement seen in the overall accident rate in reducing the number of lives lost. Similarly, the substantial number (27 or 4.12%) of SD mishaps that occurred in the air taxi commuter group (see Fig. 10) suggests there are important benefits to be gained from directing SD research toward that subgroup of commercial aviation.

---

*Current Boeing statistics for worldwide jet fleet operations can be found at http://www.boeing.com/news/techissues/pdf/2000_statsum.pdf [cited Oct. 2003].

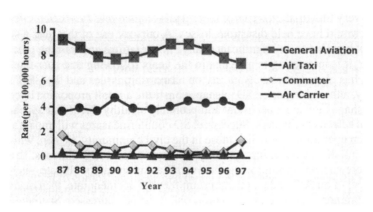

Fig. 15   Comparison of air carriers, commuters, air taxi, and GA accident rate trends. (Source: NTSB.)

In the review of the mishap rates in Fig. 15, it should be noted that in the early to mid 1990s the regulations pertaining to scheduled air carrier operations were widened in scope to include all large turboprop commuter operations, leaving only the nonscheduled and smaller commercial operations in the air taxi group. This accounting adjustment might explain the immediate decline in the commuter accident rate, but, interestingly, is not reflected in a change in the air carrier rate. One might surmise that the more stringent operating and training environment, along with 100% multicrew manning in the cockpits of the large air carriers, contributed to their retaining a low incidence of mishaps.

As illustrated in the preceding discussions, and indeed as is necessary in all statistical analyses, caution must be exercised in drawing sweeping conclusions from historical data. A particularly poignant illustration lies in the fragile separation between a great year for aviation safety and what might have happened with just one mishap. For example, in 1998 there were no passenger deaths in scheduled airline operations. In March of that year, however, a CFIT accident nearly occurred in San Francisco that would have tragically and radically altered the year's statistics. In that incident a Boeing 747 sustained a failure of the right inboard engine during a climb shortly after takeoff with 307 passengers and crew onboard, including two other pilots in the cockpit jumpseats. With great difficulty the first officer flying the plane used control wheel inputs to counter the right yaw induced by the engine failure, instead of using appropriate rudder, and he became distracted from monitoring aircraft airspeed (Type I, unrecognized SD). Additionally, the captain was also distracted from monitoring airspeed while troubleshooting the engine problem (also Type I SD). No input was noted from the two other pilots in the cockpit jumpseats. The aircraft slowed in the climb until the stick shaker (stall-warning) activated (Type II, recognized SD), whereupon the pilots lowered the nose to avert the impending stall. When the GPWS alert sounded as they approached the rising terrain of Mount San Bruno ahead of them, the crew pulled up and missed the terrain and obstructions by less than 100 ft (30.5 m). If the aircraft had crashed, it would have been the greatest accidental loss of life in United States history as a result of an aircraft mishap.

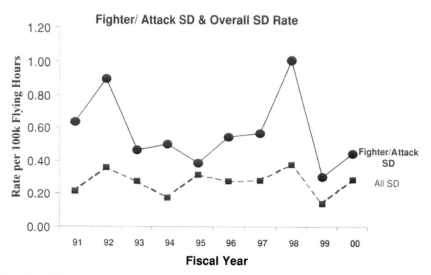

Fig. 17   USAF fighter/attack and overall SD mishap rate from 1991–2000. (Reproduced with permission of Davenport; Ref. 25.)

of multirole tasking combined with high-speed, low-altitude maneuvering; and 3) decreased training resources, especially in recent years.

Finally, the impacts of specific, associated factors in USAF SD mishaps are shown in Fig. 18, most of which are those conventionally assigned to LSA. Not surprisingly, the largest number of cases of LSA involvement in SD mishaps is attributed to attention management factors. This correlation reflects the fact that a diversion of attention from maintaining SO will naturally lead to SD, most likely Type I (unrecognized), and that it will affect the pilot's ability to recover from a Type II (recognized) SD condition. According to Davenport,[25] the most prominent attention-management factors are channelized attention, distractions, and habit-substitution/interference. The next most important category is judgment and decision making, particularly with respect to task misprioritization, course of action selected, and failure to use accepted procedures. The third largest factor affecting attention management is the category of mission demands.

2.   U.S. Army Statistics

This section focuses on U.S. Army helicopter mishaps, as rotary-wing aircraft operations comprise the bulk of Army aviation. It is recognized that the U.S. Army also suffers from a large number of fixed-wing SD accidents, but they will not be further analyzed because the Army's experience with these aircraft is similar to that addressed in preceding sections.[27,28]

The contribution of SD to U.S. Army mishaps has only recently been comprehensively compiled. Despite earlier reports from the United Kingdom concerning British Army helicopter SD accidents, the first mishap survey for the U.S. Army published in the open literature was that of Braithwaite et al.,[15] who reviewed

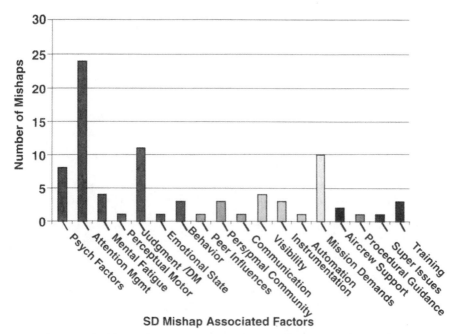

Fig. 18 Associated factors leading to USAF SD mishaps from 1991–2000. (Reproduced with permission of Davenport; Ref. 25.)

993 U.S. Army helicopter accidents from 1987–1995. Their findings are summarized in Table 4. These researchers concluded that SD contributed to 31% of all U.S. Army rotary-wing mishaps during that time span, a finding that closely mirrored the outcome of prior technical reports, which showed that SD contributed to between 15–30% of major U.S. Army rotary-wing mishaps.[15] The major new findings of Braithwaite et al.[15] were that most helicopter SD accidents were of the Type I variety, most occurred at night, most involved visual illusions, and that in 23% of the cases both front-seat crew members experienced SD. Braithwaite et al.[15] also showed that SD accidents were very expensive compared to non-SD accidents, costing over twice as much in dollars and almost three times as much in lives lost (see Table 4).

In a more recent study of U.S. Army rotary-wing accidents from 1996–2000 (Ref. 32), a total of 505 mishaps were reviewed revealing 133 SD mishaps, 355 non-SD mishaps, and 17 mishaps of unknown origin. After discarding the unknown cases, a further analysis was made on the remaining 488 that revealed that SD played a role in 27% of them. Overall and SD mishap rates for rotorcraft in the U.S. Army over the past decade are shown in Fig. 19. Although the overall trend is essentially constant, comparing 1996–1999 with 1991–1995 alone suggests that the SD accident rate is not decreasing and might, in fact, be slowly increasing. Unlike in the 1998 review by Braithwaite et al.,[15] mishaps caused by SD were equally likely to occur during night and day but more so during the night than did non-SD mishaps.

Figure 20 depicts the preponderance of SD relative to the severity of the mishap by referring to mishaps categorized as Class A (fatal or major financial loss),

Table 4   Important comparisons between U.S. Army SD and non-SD accidents (from Ref. 15)

Factor	SD accidents (categories 1 and 2)	Non-SD accidents (categories 3 and 4)
Total number of accidents	299	694
Percentage of all accidents	30.8	69.2
Percentage of class A accidents	36	18
Total cost of accidents	$46.789 million	$49.950 million
Average cost per accident[a]	$1.62 million	$0.74 million
Total lives lost	110	93
Average lives lost per accident[a]	0.38	0.14
Mean height above ground at time of the emergency[a]	65 ft	455 ft
Mean airspeed at time of the emergency[a]	28 kn	44 kn

[a]Significant difference ($p < 0.0001$ on t-testing).

Class B (nonfatal and significant financial loss), and Class C (nonfatal and moderate financial loss). The chart indicates that the greater the mishap severity, the more likely SD was involved. Specifically, the percentage of SD-related Class A mishaps was double that of non-SD Class A mishaps (see also Table 4). The percentage of Class B mishaps resulting from SD was even higher in relative terms, whereas the percentage of Class C mishaps was 12% lower than that of mishaps stemming from non-SD factors.

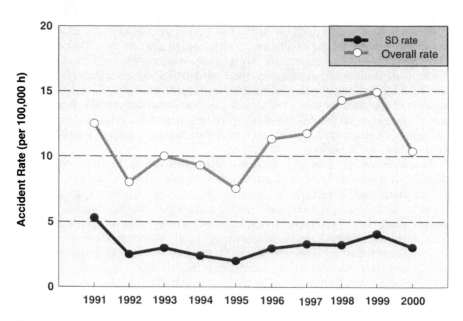

Fig. 19   U.S. Army overall and SD-specific mishap rates for rotorcraft from 1991–2000. (Reproduced with permission of Ref. 32.)

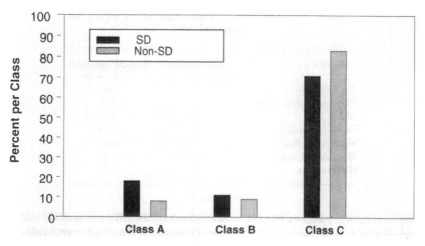

Fig. 20 Proportion of U.S. Army SD and non-SD accidents from 1996–2000, by severity. (Reproduced with permission of LeDuc; Ref. 32.)

The experience in the U.S. Army rotorcraft fleet highlights a unique SD issue for helicopter operations reported in a previous study by Braithwaite et al.,[33] namely, that classic nonvisual SD accident scenarios such as those described in Chapter 6 were uncommon (1 of 133). Instead of occurring as a result of illusions such as false pitch or the black hole, most SD accidents were caused by inadvertent drift and misjudging distances (116 of 133). These areas of special application to the rotary-wing environment might not be easily combated with conventional approaches to countering SD. Further highlighting the role of visual illusions is the finding of Braithwaite et al.[34] in a different study that the percentage of SD accidents in which NVDs were in use was double that of non-SD accidents.

3. U.S. Navy Statistics

The first major study of U.S. Navy SD mishaps was performed by Bellenkes et al.[9] and covered Class A mishaps occurring between 1980–1989. Bellenkes et al.[9] found that only 5% (33) of 660 total Class A mishaps were definitely attributable to SD, although possible, probable, or definite SD was implicated in 17% (112) of such mishaps. An equivalent number of mishaps occurred over land and sea and at various times of day. There was no effect of pilot experience, as indicated by the nearly 1500 flying hours possessed by the average SD-mishap pilot. Finally, Bellenkes et al.[9] found a similar number of Type I and Type II SD mishaps overall, but Type I mishaps predominated in helicopters, whereas Type II SD accidents were more common in fixed-wing aircraft.

Johnson[35] reviewed the USN and U.S. Marine Corps (USMC) recent experience with SD mishaps from 1990–1998.* In this review 392 (248-USN; 146-USMC) Class A flight mishaps were found for fiscal years 1990–1998 (see Table 5). The overall number of Class A mishaps per year showed a decline from 1990–1998.

---

*This study is also available at the USAF Spatial Disorientation Countermeasures Web site at www.spatiald.wpafb.af.mil/RecentTrends.aspx [cited Oct. 2003].

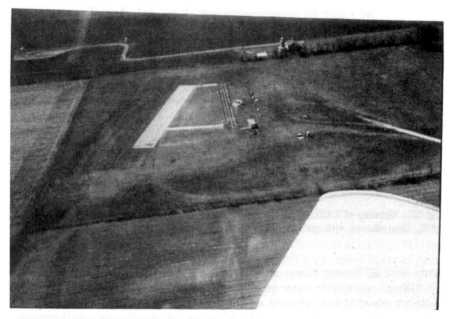

Fig. 23   Photograph of remote-controlled aircraft airstrip near Dayton, Ohio.

They then advise aborting the landing and going around in order to improve the position of the aircraft. In reality, the aircraft is low to the ground and is approaching an airstrip for *radio-controlled aircraft*. The airfield is in correct visual proportion but is very small! Such demonstrations are highly effective in making the point that a normally functioning, healthy pilot can fall victim to dangerous misperceptions.

In addition to photographs and diagrams, flight simulation can also be a most helpful tool in explaining the power of vestibular and visual illusions that confuse pilots and create false sensations of orientation. Full-motion flight simulators actually make use of linear acceleration illusions to enhance the virtual reality of the simulated flight within the constraints of their fixed bases. Because in these simulators there is no capacity to achieve sustained longitudinal acceleration, gravity is used instead (see Chapter 8, Sec. III.E). By rotating the cab without presenting a corresponding pitch alteration in the visual surround, pilots experience the sensation of forward acceleration. Conversely, by rotating the cab downward without a corresponding change in the visual presentation the force of gravity is also employed to give the pilots a sensation of deceleration in flight or of braking on taxiways and runways. This concept can be used to illustrate why during a takeoff or go-around in the real aircraft the pilot experiences both longitudinal accelerations as well as the redirection of the perceived gravity vector. Because the resulting sensation of pitching up can be quite strong, the pilot who does not make reference to the attitude indicator will underrotate the aircraft (see "Somatogravic Illusions" in Chapter 6, Sec. III.A). If the false-pitch illusion is further reinforced by a visual illusion of a false horizon, such as a shoreline or other extended cluster of lights with ocean or unlighted terrain in the distance (see Chapter 6, Sec. III.A.2), the pilot's compulsion to push the nose down can become overwhelming. It is easy to relate the preceding illustration to routine activities of every pilot who has utilized a simulator. All have trained to proficiency in acceleration and deceleration maneuvers, although most have not realized the role played by the underlying physiology of the otoliths organs. Also, familiar to many pilots is one of the most common problems seen by flight instructors—that of the training pilot's executing inadequate pitch-up during the go-around as a result of being distracted with various tasks such as reconfiguring the aircraft. Citing such standard practices and lessons learned can aid the investigator in convincing his or her audience of the presence of an SD illusion in a mishap.

The potential for even more realistic testing of an accident theory or the demonstration of acceleration, as well as visual illusions, exists with state-of-the-art equipment that is used in select research and training activities around the world. These devices are not only capable of imitating linear acceleration illusions, as just described for fixed-base simulators, they can actually replicate the forces of the illusion through their sustained rotating, or planetary motion. These machines, such as the USAF Advanced Spatial Disorientation Trainer addressed in more detail in Chapter 8, have an additional benefit of duplicating angular accelerations and offer the unique capability of generating directed gravitational forces on the pilot's physiological sensors in the same manner as occurs in flight.[36] The devices are very scarce and would not be easily obtained for investigative purposes; however, to the investigator facing a particularly puzzling accident scenario with high-level management interest, this tool might prove useful in determining the effect of acceleration on the mishap chain.

B. Reconstruction Techniques

The essence of aircraft accident investigation is the reconstruction of the sequence of events that led to the mishap. With there being a huge number of possible factors in any given case, a variety of techniques have evolved over time to assist investigators in collecting the data needed to evaluate each aspect of the flight sequence. These methods include forensic practices for examining control-surface fracture patterns, computer procedures to redisplay radar tracings, voice stress analysis, and processes to examine breakup and other deformations of the fuselage to estimate impact forces. The use of video processing techniques, even one as simple as inverting the video signal, can also be quite helpful. In one case of a civil SD mishap, an inverse image made from a handheld video camera used in the cockpit enabled visualization of the fuel flow gauge. Then, in the nonenhanced video the visible horizon was studied to determine the pitch and bank of the accident aircraft prior to its departing controlled flight and impacting the ground.

1. Animated Flight Motion

In recent years tools have been created to assist investigators in finding patterns in flight data and in-flight visualizations that help pinpoint SD factors in aircraft mishaps. Software was developed in the 1990s to use the data streams recorded on flight-data recorders (FDR) and the cockpit voice recorder to enable visualization of the flight sequence. From these data an animated model of the aircraft can be driven by the software to recreate the sequence of aircraft motions in three

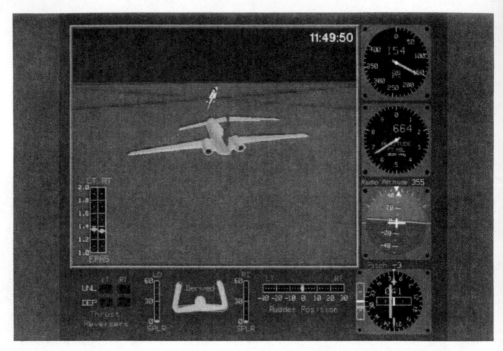

Fig. 24   Video reconstruction of flight path of an American Airlines MD-82 prior to crash in Little Rock, Arkansas, in 1999.

dimensions and to recreate the instrument readings in the cockpit. This technique allows investigators to visualize the meaning of vast amounts of data that previously had to be painstakingly examined in tabular form. The software produces an aircraft motion sequence that can be viewed from any angle, including a view from the cockpit. Limitations to these reconstructions include the paucity of data from older FDRs (inoperative or too few channels). Even on newer FDRs, not all needed data are stored, and the voice recorder only records the last 30 min of conversations in a repeating, overwriting loop. Animated reconstructions of accidents have successfully been used by the NTSB, the Australian Bureau of Air Safety Investigation (BASI), and other safety agencies. A more recent evolution of the technique was used in the investigation of an MD-82 accident at Little Rock, Arkansas (see Fig. 24).

2.   Force Calculations

The availability of acceleration data from FDRs also makes it feasible to determine the presence of patterns of aircraft motion that might have resulted in SD. In particular, one can reconstruct the G forces that the pilot experienced during the flight in order to examine the effects of acceleration on the otoliths. Using straightforward vector analysis, one can calculate the gravitoinertial force (GIF) vector to allow comparison with the actual flight path as determined from radar returns, the FDR, and eyewitness statements. Figure 25 illustrates the geometric

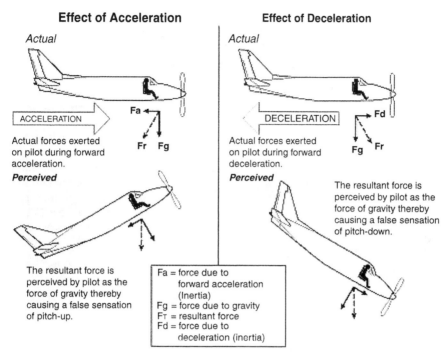

Effect of Acceleration

Actual

ACCELERATION

Fa

Fr Fg

Actual forces exerted
on pilot during forward
acceleration.

Perceived

The resultant force is
perceived by pilot as the
force of gravity thereby
causing a false sensation
of pitch-up.

Effect of Deceleration

Actual

DECELERATION

Fd

Fg Fr

Actual forces exerted
on pilot during forward
deceleration.

Perceived

The resultant force is
perceived by pilot as the
force of gravity thereby
causing a false sensation
of pitch-down.

Fa = force due to
        forward acceleration
        (Inertia)
Fg = force due to gravity
Fт = resultant force
Fd = force due to
        deceleration (inertia)

Fig. 25   Effect of acceleration on perceived pitch.

relationships between longitudinal acceleration F_a and gravity F_g—also termed normal acceleration in some aviation contexts—and the resultant GIF F_r. The GIF is the force to which the pilot's vestibular system will be exposed. Although the pilot's head position in the cockpit might not be precisely known, the GIF serves as an approximation of the perceived vertical, which determines the perception of pitch attitude (see Chapter 6, Sec. III.A).

The equation for finding the GIF magnitude is $F_r^2 = F_a^2 + F_g^2$, and the angle between the GIF and F_g can be calculated from the inverse tangent ($\tan^{-1}$) of (F_a/F_g), converted from radians to degrees. The GIF can then be plotted concurrently with the actual pitch acquired from the FDR to allow comparison of GIF vs actual aircraft pitch over time. Figure 26 shows how a comparison of the calculated GIF with FDR data leads to the conclusion that the pilots succumbed to a misperceived pitch attitude. In this example involving the crash of a U.S. Air DC-9 in Charlotte, North Carolina, the pilot's initiating a catastrophic downward pitch of the aircraft during a missed approach might have been intended to correct an erroneously perceived climbing attitude. The transfer function of the vestibular system and the interaction of the semicircular canals with the otoliths are not modeled with the preceding simple calculation, but these effects are small. Research being done by the Vestibular Research Group at the Naval Aeromedical Research Laboratory in Pensacola, Florida, addresses these latter effects. Results of that group's efforts have been incorporated into a more comprehensive model that was used in reconstructing an Airbus 320 accident involving a somatogravic

and preferred that the aircraft not do so in order to ensure that the flight remained on schedule. The pilot consulted with the copilot and was advised that one male passenger had been replaced with a female passenger, that most of the passengers would be traveling "light," and that several of them weighed less than the standard passenger weight. The pilot amended the flight plan and added fuel to complete a VFR flight to Rainbow Lake and an IFR flight to Edmonton. A copy of the original company flight plan indicated that the pilot had originally planned to leave Rainbow Lake with 504 lb (229 kg) of fuel.

Calculations completed after the accident indicated that approximately 850 lb (386 kg) of fuel were on the aircraft at the time of departure from Rainbow Lake. Weight and balance calculations using estimated baggage and standard passenger weights indicated that the aircraft was at approximately 7473 lb (3397 kg) on takeoff from Rainbow Lake and that the center of gravity was near the aft limit. Calculations using passenger self-reported weights indicated that seven of the nine passengers exceeded the standard passenger weight, that the aircraft was approximately 7683 lb (3492 kg), or about 315 lb (143 kg), above the approved gross weight at takeoff and that the center of gravity was about 0.9 cm aft of the aft limit.

The aircraft struck several trees while wings level in an approximate 3-deg descent. It came to rest upright, and the cockpit and cabin sections remained intact. The wings-level impact attitude, the shallow impact angle, the small tree size, and the presence of approximately 0.61 m of snow on the ground all contributed to maintaining the deceleration forces within the limits of human tolerance. The aircraft was reportedly equipped with a survival kit, as required by regulation, but investigators did not locate the kit in or near the aircraft.

Aircraft using Rainbow Lake airport typically take off from Runway 09 during night departures if wind conditions permit, as several lights are then visible to the east. On arrival at Rainbow Lake, the pilot had been advised by the copilot of a minor frost heave in Runway 09 near the runway threshold. To avoid the risk of damaging the nose wheel during takeoff, the pilot elected to depart on Runway 27.

The pilot selected 10 deg of flap for takeoff and rotated at 85 kn (157 km/h) indicated airspeed. He believed that the aircraft became airborne at 90 kn (167 km/h) approximately halfway down the runway and that he had established and maintained a positive rate of climb. He reported that he was waiting for the aircraft to accelerate to the blue-line speed (best single-engine rate of climb) of 107 kn (198 km/h) prior to lifting the flaps when the aircraft struck the trees. The landing gear and the flaps were in the up position at impact.

Soon after liftoff, the pilot was confronted with dark, featureless terrain. The takeoff acceleration combined with darkness and the absence of external visual cues might have led to the false-pitch illusion. However, the extent, if any, to which somatogravic illusion contributed to this accident was not determined. Rather, the TSB analysis focused on the pilot's applied IFR/night-takeoff technique, the influence of the copilot, the communications between the chartered company and the operator, the request to change the flight plan, and the effect of the overweight condition of the aircraft on the departure. Individually, these factors would likely not have been significant enough to cause an accident. When combined with dark ambient conditions and an uphill takeoff toward rising terrain, these factors collectively established a window of opportunity for an SD accident to occur.

The pilot's night departure technique is considered to be the active failure in this accident. Night departures in dark conditions require full use of the aircraft flight instruments, and it is essential that the pilot achieves and maintains a positive rate of climb. In the absence of accurate outside visual cues, the pilot must rely on the aircraft instruments to maintain airspeed and attitude and to overcome any false sensations of climb. The pilot was either relying on outside visual cues during the initial climb and/or using only a partial instrument panel scan while being influenced by the false-pitch illusion. Pilots can overcome false sensations by flying the aircraft with reference to the attitude indicator, altimeter, vertical speed indicator, and airspeed indicator, which in this case would likely have allowed the pilot to detect that the aircraft was not in a climb. The appropriate technique would have been to climb at the aircraft's best rate or best angle-of-climb speed until all obstacles had been cleared, rather than to become preoccupied with reaching the blue-line airspeed.

The role of the copilot is somewhat ambiguous, and his presence does not appear to have contributed to the safety of the flight. Because he was not familiar to the captain and because he was not delegated flight-crew responsibilities, his participation during the flight created a situation of crew resource mismanagement. The copilot's remarks regarding the weight and flight-plan changes at High Level appear to have encouraged the captain to cancel the planned fuel stop at Peace River. The copilot did not advise the captain that, if weight was a concern, he could remain in Rainbow Lake. The copilot's apparent well-intentioned advice on the frost heave near the threshold of Runway 09 influenced the captain's decision to take off on Runway 27, which was uphill toward rising terrain and had no lights visible after departure.

The estimated weight of the aircraft at takeoff ($\sim$315 lbs or 143 kg above the approved weight) and the aircraft's center of gravity (which was at or beyond the rear limit) would have increased the takeoff distance and reduced the climb performance of the aircraft. The request to the captain in High Level to add fuel in order to avoid a stop at Peace River contributed to the aircraft's being overweight on departure from Rainbow Lake.

Communication between the operator and the chartered company with regard to the duties of the copilot and the weight of the aircraft at departure from Rainbow Lake was inadequate. Both companies were familiar with Piper PA-31-350 capabilities, and the weight and balance calculations performed prior to the aircraft's leaving Edmonton indicated that the trip would have to be accomplished with a fuel stop at Peace River to accommodate the passenger load. Critical information, such as the option of dropping the copilot in the event of an overweight aircraft condition, was never provided to the chartered company. The pilot, who was the final decision maker, was put in the position of having to balance the conflicting objectives of operating the aircraft within the prescribed weight limits and satisfying the customer's demands. He was relatively inexperienced on the Piper PA-31-350 aircraft, having flown less than 100 h in it, and he was unfamiliar with its daily flight routine because he had not previously flown for the operator.

The TSB determined that the aircraft was inadvertently flown into trees and the ground in controlled flight and dark ambient conditions during a night departure because a positive rate of climb was not maintained after takeoff. Factors contributing to the accident were the pilot's concentrating on blue-line speed rather than maintaining a positive rate of climb, the dark ambient conditions, a departure profile into rising terrain, an overweight aircraft, and crew resource mismanagement.

2. Cessna 172 Dark Takeoff (1998)

On 15 December 1998, a pilot and passenger departed Shearwater, Nova Scotia, at 18:43 local time in a Cessna 172 on a night VFR flight to the Liverpool airport for a touch-and-go before a return to Shearwater. About two hours after departure, an emergency locator transmitter signal was reported, and a search was initiated. The wreckage was found the next day. The aircraft had crashed in heavily wooded terrain 2 n miles (3.7 km) west of the Liverpool airport. The two occupants were fatally injured, and the aircraft was destroyed. This synopsis is based on TSB Final Report A98A0184.

This was a time-building flight in preparation for the pilot's upcoming commercial flight test. The aircraft was equipped with an altitude reporting transponder, and a review of the radar data indicated that the aircraft approached the Liverpool airport from the east, turned south across Runway 25/07, and joined the circuit for Runway 25. The aircraft disappeared from radar at 1100 ft (336 m) above sea level while on final to Runway 25 and reappeared on radar at the same altitude just west of the airport 1 min and 27 s later. Radar coverage continued for another 47 s, during which the aircraft climbed to 1300 ft (397 m), leveled off, and then descended to 1100 ft (336 m) before disappearing from radar.

The pilot was issued his night endorsement in July 1998 and, at the time of the occurrence, had about 187 h total flight time. He had recently flown to the Liverpool airport on four occasions. Three of the flights were conducted at night with either an instructor or other pilot onboard; the accident flight was the first night flight without another pilot on board. The pilot flew with his instructor on the morning of the occurrence and slept several hours in the afternoon before returning to the Shearwater airport for the night flight.

At the time of the occurrence, the Liverpool area was under clear skies with no restrictions to visibility and no possibility of icing at lower levels. The moon was below the horizon at the time of the accident, and pilot reports indicated that dark-sky conditions existed; hence, there would have been fewer visual cues present that night than there would have been during the mishap pilot's previous flights to Liverpool. A local resident, who was using frequency-scanning equipment for recreational purposes, heard the pilot transmit his intentions and reported that there was no inflection in the pilot's voice to suggest he was experiencing difficulty.

The aircraft descended into trees about 3.7 km beyond the departure end of Runway 25, on a magnetic heading of 270 deg. The aircraft was in a wings-level, 30-deg descent angle when it struck the trees. Propeller strike marks on trees along the wreckage trail were consistent with the propeller being powered at impact. The flaps were in the retracted position. The elevator trim tab position was consistent with a slight nose-down trim setting, normal for final approach for a touch-and-go landing. The engine was examined, and there was no indication of a preimpact mechanical failure.

All undamaged light bulbs were examined by the TSB. The light bulbs for the aircraft's overhead instrument flood light, cabin dome light, compass light, and tail navigation light were retrieved from the wreckage. With the exception of those for the dome light, these bulbs would normally be illuminated during a night flight. The analysis determined that the instrument flood light bulb was illuminated at impact. The remaining lamps were either off at impact or had not received sufficient force to distort the filament.

The TSB conducted a representative night flight to the Liverpool airport in a rented Cessna 172 at a time when lighting and sky conditions were similar to those on the night of the occurrence. The purpose was to identify the visual references available to a pilot when flying a Runway 25 approach and departure/go-around. The airport is located in a sparsely populated area where there is little peripheral lighting. The runway lights were observed clearly on approach and during the go-around phase, and the aircraft passed over a road about 2.8 km west of the airport, where there was some street lighting in an area of houses. Beyond the road there were few external visual cues, and the horizon was not easily discernable. The TSB flight was recorded on radar, allowing a comparison between the radar data for the occurrence flight and the TSB flight. The TSB flight included four approaches to Runway 25, with two touch-and-go landings and two go-arounds. A comparison of elapsed time during a touch-and-go vs a go-around indicated that the mishap pilot had conducted a go-around.

When valid visual cues provided by the Earth's horizon are not present (such as when the horizon is obscured by darkness or weather), or when the pilot's attention is distracted from the primary flight instruments, the pilot's sense of orientation might be dominated by inputs from the inner ear—a very inaccurate source of attitude information during flight. In such a condition the pilot will most likely encounter SD. Knowledge and experience are the key determinants of a pilot's success in overcoming SD, and a pilot's only defense against SD is to develop the ability to override natural vestibular responses through training and practice and to always use visual information from the instruments to maintain spatial orientation and situation awareness. The environmental conditions on the night of the occurrence and the limited outside visual ground references in the vicinity of the Liverpool airport were elements conducive to SD. During the go-around, it was possible for the pilot to experience both the false horizon and false pitch illusions. At low altitude there is minimal time for a pilot to recognize an illusion and take the appropriate corrective action. The impact angle of the aircraft was consistent with the assumption of nose-down pitch attitude because of the false-pitch illusion.

The complex skill set that a pilot requires to be able to recognize and counter SD is developed through flight-instrument training, experience, and practice. In the end the TSB determined that during the climb-out following the approach to the airport, the pilot probably lost situational awareness as a result of spatial disorientation and unintentionally flew the aircraft into the ground.

VI. Summary

Spatial disorientation mishaps are a unique subset of flying accidents influenced by human factors that involve a normal physiological response to the abnormal environment of flight. To recognize the presence of SD in a mishap, the investigator must determine the level of human factors involvement, possess an understanding

of applicable physiological mechanisms and be proficient in convincingly presenting those dynamics to pilots and investigative bodies. More consideration should
be given to all human factors elements in the search for the root cause of a mishap.
Several well-established human factors models are available to aid the investigator
in focusing on the HF element, and numerous techniques have been developed to
assist in specifying the orientation misperceptions that are involved. Correlations
between types of SD and accident events can alert the investigator to the probability
of SD as a mishap factor.

It would be of great advantage to standardize the terminology and investigative
techniques used around the world so as to allow pooling of mishap data from all
sources and better scrutinize SD mishaps for possible new factors or changes in
trends. Unfortunately, methods of categorizing and evaluating mishap data across
the different flying communities are as varied as the communities themselves.
It is quite possible that the role of SD in military and civilian mishaps is vastly
underreported because of miscategorization or incomplete coding brought about
by several issues. For example, the contribution of SD to a mishap can be lost by
focusing on various attention-management factors that lead to loss of situational
awareness or controlled flight into terrain. The result could be that the mishap is
coded as LSA or CFIT, with no reference to SD whatsoever.

In spite of the limitations posed by different classification systems, code definitions, and management priorities, evaluation of reported data yields some useful
information toward understanding and preventing SD mishaps. Current data indicate that in both military and civilian operations SD continues to produce a high
percentage of fatalities, claiming nearly three times as many lives as non-SD-
related mishaps.

The incidence of SD mishaps in the military seems to be on the rise, or at best
unchanged at about 10–20% of all major mishaps and 30–40% of those involving
fatalities. The greatest threat of a military SD mishap occurs 1) during unrecognized
SD, 2) in the fighter/attack population, and 3) among experienced pilots. However,
significant losses of life and aircraft have occurred from trainer and transport SD
accidents and in VMC as well as IMC. Lighting conditions are not predictive
of the occurrence of SD mishaps, as they are generally evenly divided between
nighttime and daytime. Nonetheless, there is some indication of the probability of
a helicopter SD mishap being higher at night. Most SD mishaps in rotary-wing
operations are caused by nonstandard visual illusions involving undetected drift
and misjudged distance from obstacles.

In the civil-aviation sector the frequency of SD accidents appears to have decreased significantly since 1983, although this perceived reduction is likely a matter
of mishap coding as indicated by an offsetting rise in accidents categorized as aircraft control not maintained. General aviation suffers the highest percentage of
the civilian SD accidents (94%), of which 90% are fatal. Increased age, flight
hours, and numbers of pilots with an instrument rating all seem to have had little
or no affect in reducing the occurrence of SD mishaps. In commercial aviation
air-taxi pilots are most prone to experience a SD-related accident. SD mishaps in
air carrier operations are extremely rare, yet commercial air carriers suffer most
of their fatalities from mishaps classified as controlled flight into terrain and loss
of control inflight, both of which are directly related to SD. Of civil mishaps
coded as SD, 2/3 occur in IMC, with no prevalence (50/50) arising between

those that occur in IMC on a dark night and those in IMC on a bright day. Of the SD mishaps that occur in VMC, 2/3 take place on dark nights and 1/3 in bright daylight.

Spatial disorientation will continue to be a threat to flight safety given the underlying maladaptation of the human vestibular system to the aerospace environment even when no excessive accelerations or unusual maneuvers are present. Consequently, SD precursors should be particularly and carefully sought by investigators facing otherwise inexplicable and seemingly benign events. Modern investigative techniques can be used to uncover and document the failures of human–machine interactions and help guide development of corrective and preventive measures. Those techniques draw upon data captured by sophisticated onboard and ground-linked recording devices, as well as more crude sources of information. Straightforward calculations of the gravitoinertial force vector can effectively predict the impact of aircraft motions on the pilot's sensory mechanisms and his or her perception of aircraft attitude. Additionally, the use of visual reconstruction methods has the benefit of creating dynamic graphical materials that can be used to teach investigators and pilots about basic SD mechanisms and likely mishap scenarios. Flight simulators can provide a similar capability in recreating the effects of visual and some vestibular illusions that may have contributed to a mishap. Successfully combating SD requires a full-spectrum safety approach that contributes to and builds upon the mishap investigator's knowledge and experience.

References

[1]Wells, A. T., Chapter 4, "The Nature of Accidents," *Commercial Aviation Safety*, McGraw–Hill, New York, 2001, Chap. 4, pp. 81–98.

[2]Edwards, E., "Man and Machine: Systems for Safety," *Proceedings of British Airline Pilots Associations Technical Symposium*, British Airline Pilots Associations, London, 1972, pp. 21–36.

[3]Edwards, E., "Introductory Overview, *Human Factors in Aviation*, edited by E. L. Wiener and D. C. Nagel, Academic Press, San Diego, 1988.

[4]Reason, J., "Human Error: Models and Management," *British Medical Journal*, Vol. 320, 2000, pp. 768–770.

[5]Reason, J., *Human Error*, Cambridge Univ. Press, Cambridge, England, U.K., 1990.

[6]Shappell, S. A., and Wiegmann, D. A., "*The Human Factors Analysis and Classification System-HFACS*," Federal Aviation Administration Office of Aerospace Medicine, Civil Aerospace Medical Inst., Rep. DOT/FAA/AM-00/7, Oklahoma City, OK, 2000.

[7]Barnum, F., and Bonner, R. H., "Epidemiology of USAF Spatial Disorientation Aircraft Accidents, 1 Jan1958–31 Dec 1968," *Aerospace Medicine*, Vol. 42, 1971, pp. 896–898.

[8]Moser, R., Jr. "Spatial Disorientation as a Factor in Accidents in an Operational Command," *Aerospace Medicine*, Vol. 40, 1969, pp. 174–6.

[9]Bellenkes, A., Bason, R., and Yacavone, D. O., "Spatial Disorientation in Naval Aviation Mishaps: A Review of Class A Incidents from 1980 Through 1989," *Aviation, Space, and Environmental Medicine*, Vol. 63, 1992, pp. 128–131.

[10]Cheung, B., Money, K., Wright, H., and Bateman, W., "Spatial Disorientation-Implicated Accidents in Canadian Forces, 1982–1992," *Aviation, Space, and Environmental Medicine*, Vol. 66, 1995, pp. 579–585.

¹¹Edgington, K., and Box, C. J., "Disorientation in Army Helicopter Operations," *Journal of the Society of Occupational Medicine*, Vol. 32, 1982, pp. 128–135.

¹²Gillingham, K. K., "The Spatial Disorientation Problem in the United States Air Force," *Journal of Vestibular Research*, Vol. 2, 1992, pp. 297–306.

¹³Lyons, T. J., Ercoline, W. R., Freeman, J. E., and Gillingham, K. K., "Classification Problems of U.S. Air Force Spatial Disorientation Accidents, 1989–91," *Aviation, Space, and Environmental Medicine*, Vol. 65, 1994, pp. 147–152.

¹⁴Vyrnwy-Jones, P., "A Review of Army Air Corps Helicopter Accidents, 1971–1982," *Aviation, Space, and Environmental Medicine*, Vol. 56, 1985, pp. 403–409.

¹⁵Braithwaite, M. G., Durnford, S. J., Crowley, J. S., Rosado, N. R., and Albano, J. P., "Spatial Disorientation in U.S. Army Rotary-Wing Operations," *Aviation, Space, and Environmental Medicine*, Vol. 69, 1998, pp. 1031–1037.

¹⁶Neubauer, J. C., "Classifying Spatial Disorientation Mishaps Using Different Definitions," *IEEE Engineering in Medicine and Biology*, Vol. 19, No. 2, 2000, pp. 28–34.

¹⁷Navathe, P. D., and Singh, B., "An Operational Definition for Spatial Disorientation," *Aviation, Space, and Environmental Medicine*, Vol. 65, 1994, pp. 1153–1155.

¹⁸Navathe, P. D., and Singh, B., "Prevalence of Spatial Disorientation in Indian Air Force Aircrew," *Aviation, Space, and Environmental Medicine*, Vol. 65, 1994, pp. 1082–1085.

¹⁹Previc, F. H., Yauch, D. W., DeVilbiss, C. A., Ercoline, W. R., and Sipes, W. E., "In Defense of Traditional Views of Spatial Disorientation and Loss of Situation Awareness: A Reply to Navathe and Singh's 'An Operational Definition of Spatial Disorientation,'" *Aviation, Space, and Environmental Medicine*, Vol. 66, 1995, pp. 1103–1106.

²⁰Cheung, B., "Spatial Disorientation," *Aviation Space and Environmental Medicine*, Vol. 66, 1995, pp. 706.

²¹Benson, A. J., "Spatial Disorientation—General Aspects," *Aviation Medicine*, edited by J. Ernsting, A. N. Nicholson and D. J. Rainford, (3rd ed.), Butterworth Heinemann, Oxford, England, U.K., 1999, pp. 419–436.

²²Gillingham, K. K., and Previc, F. H., "Spatial Orientation in Flight," *Fundamentals of Aerospace Medicine*, edited by R. L. DeHart, 2nd ed., Williams and Wilkins, Baltimore, HD, 1996, pp. 309–397.

²³Nuttall, J. B., and Sanford, W. G., *Spatial Disorientation in Operational Flying*, Publication M-27-56, USAF Directorate of Flight Safety Research, Norton AFB, CA, 1956.

²⁴Kellogg, R. B., Letter report on spatial disorientation incidence statistics, The Aerospace Medical Research Laboratory, Wright-Patterson AFB, 30 March 1973.

²⁵Davenport, C. E., "USAF Spatial Disorientation Experience: Air Force Safety Center Statistical Review," *Proceedings of the Recent Trends in Spatial Disorientation Research Symposium,* 2000.

²⁶Lyons, T. J., and Freeman, J. E., "Spatial Disorientation (SD) Mishaps in the US Air Force—1988," *Aviation Space and Environmental Medicine*, Vol. 61, 1990, pp. 459.

²⁷Hixson, W. C., Niven, J. I., and Spezia, E., "Orientation-Error Accidents in Army Aviation Aircraft," *The Disorientation Incident*, edited by A. J. Benson, AGARD CP-95-Part I: AGARD, 1972.

²⁸Tyle, P. E., and Furr, P. A., "Disorientation, Fact and Fancy," AGARD CP-95, Part I: *The Disorientation Incident*, edited by A. J. Benson, NATO, 1972.

²⁹Kirkham, W. R., Collins, W. E., Grape, P. M., Simpson, J. M., and Wallace, T. F., "Spatial Disorientation in General Aviation Accidents," *Aviation, Space, and Environmental Medicine*, Vol. 49, 1978, pp. 1080–1086.

[30]Buley, L. E., and Spelina, J., "Physiological and Psychological Factors in 'the Dark-Night Takeoff Accident,'" *Aerospace Medicine* Vol. 41, 1970, pp. 553–556.

[31]Malcolm, R., and Money, K. E., "Two Specific Kinds of Disorientation Incidents: Jet Upset and Giant Hand," *The Disorientation Incident*, edited by A. J. Benson, AGARD CP-95, Part: AGARD, 1972.

[32]LeDuc, P. A., "Spatial Disorientation Accidents in U.S. Army Rotary Wing Aircraft FYs 1996–2000," Nov. 2000.

[33]Braithwaite, M. G., DeRoche, S. L., Alvarez, E. A., and Reese, M., *Proceedings of the First Triservice Conference on Rotary-Wing Spatial Disorientation: Spatial Disorientation in the Operational Rotary-Wing Environment*, U.S. Army Aeromedical Research Lab., USAARL Rept. 97-15, Fort Rucker, AL, 1997.

[34]Braithwaite, M. G., Douglass, P. K., Durnford, S. J., and Lucas, G. L., "The Hazard of Spatial Disorientation During Helicopter Flight Using Night Vision Devices," *Aviation, Space, and Environmental Medicine*, Vol. 69, 1998, pp. 1038–1044.

[35]Johnson, K., "Spatial Disorientation in Military Aviation," *Proceedings of The Recent Trends in Spatial Disorientation Research Symposium,* 2000.

[36]Holoviak, S. J., Yauch, D. W., Previc, F. H., and Ercoline, W. R., "Advanced Spatial Disorientation Demonstrator Program—A Framework for Future Spatial Orientation Training," AGARD CP–58: *Selection and Training Advances in Aviation*, 1996.

bank, they had a tendency to overbank in the opposite direction." A recent inflight study conducted by Ercoline and colleagues[8] observed that when pilots rely on their nonvisual perception of bank following the cessation of a sustained roll they inadvertently increase their bank in the direction of the previous roll (Fig. 1b). The detailed procedure involves having a pilot make, for example, a right roll to establish a desired bank, then stopping the roll at the desired bank and neutralizing the stick force to maintain the bank. Subsequently, the pilot unknowingly applies further right stick pressure as a result of the false perception of roll reversal or decrease in bank. This perception can be explained by the following mechanisms:

1) When the pilot stops the roll at the desired bank, the cupulae are initially deflected through angles equal but opposite to the original angular velocity of the roll (i.e., they generate illusory banking to the left). The pilot might succumb to the false sensation of banking to the left and apply contrary stick pressure, thereby increasing banking to the right.

2) To maintain the desired bank, the pilot would neutralize the stick by releasing pressure to the right (stick moves left, back to neutral position), which might reinforce this false sensation of rolling to the left.

3) The relatively short time constant (approximately 4 s) of postrotational decay about the roll axis can also contribute to this illusion (see Chapter 2, Sec. III.F). For example, in a roll from 80 deg left to 80 deg right in 4 s (40 deg/s), the apparent angular velocity just before stopping would have fallen to approximately 21 deg/s (using a short time constant of 4 s). On completion, it would seem to the pilot that he had only rolled through 117 deg, which would leave him or her an apparent 37 deg angle of bank further to go to the right. The pilot might succumb to this apparent bank insufficiency and resume rolling to the right, which might then put the aircraft in a dangerous attitude.

B. Coriolis Illusion

While in the procedure turn (2,500 feet), the rubber band holding my let-down chart to the knee board broke and down went the chart to the cockpit deck. I reached down to pick it up and my next look at the instruments brought a chill of horror. The needle was against the left peg, the gyro-horizon was showing an eight ball, and the altimeter was plummeting downward. I felt as though I was in a right bank and pulling G (Ref. 6, p. 68).

The Coriolis illusion, also named as the Coriolis reaction, the Coriolis phenomenon, or Coriolis effect, was named after Gustave Gaspard de Coriolis (1792–1843), who first described and quantified the Coriolis acceleration. The Coriolis acceleration is the linear acceleration a experienced by a body that moves at a linear velocity v while exposed to rotation with velocity w about an orthogonal axis such that $a = 2vw$. Analyses of the instantaneous Coriolis accelerations that occur in cross-coupled motion enable the derivation of the resulting angular acceleration. In general, Coriolis effects are used to describe the vestibular effect of tilting the head during whole-body rotation. The term Coriolis effect was introduced by Schubert[9] to describe the stimulus to the semicircular canals by integrating the components of Coriolis accelerations, acting parallel to the canal walls, around each endolymph ring. Because the stimulus can be calculated from vector algebra as the vector cross product, or cross coupling, of the ω_1 and ω_2 velocity vectors, it is also named the cross-coupled effect.[10]

The Coriolis illusion is the sensation of angular motion in response to tilting of the head (angular velocity, ω_1) while the head is undergoing passive rotation (angular velocity, ω_2) about an axis not aligned with the head tilt axis at some angle θ. With few exceptions the sensation of the apparent rotation is in the same direction as that of the precession of a wheel spinning about the ω_2 axis in response to a torque about the head tilt axis,[11] that is, about an axis approximately orthogonal to the head tilt axis and the passive rotation axis. During natural head movements and when the head motion is of short duration, angular acceleration about the head tilt axis alone yields essentially no aftereffects. The strength of the Coriolis accelerative stimulus is determined by the angular velocity of the platform ω_2 and the angle θ through which the head is moved. When the head motion is prolonged, it is the $\omega_1 \omega_2$ cosine θ component of the total angular acceleration that provokes unpleasant and nauseogenic sensations.

The illusion has been explained solely by the action of Coriolis accelerations on the semicircular canals. Comprehensive mathematical analysis can be found in a number of publications.[12–14] For ease of explanation, let us assume that the three semicircular canals (lateral, superior, and posterior) align perfectly with the Cartesian (yaw, pitch, and roll) axes (Fig. 2). Consider a subject who has been rotating clockwise as seen from above the subject's head, at ω_2 in the plane of the lateral semicircular canal (yaw) long enough (30 s or so) for the cupula to return to the neutral position and the sensation of rotation about the yaw axis to

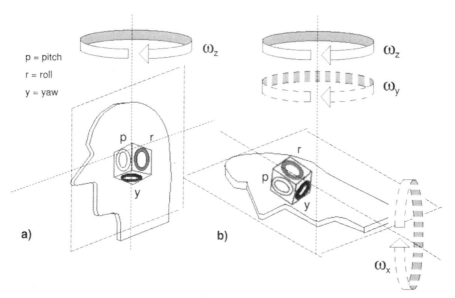

p = pitch
r = roll
y = yaw

Fig. 2   Example of Coriolis cross coupling. During passive clockwise (right) rotation, if the head is actively tilted to the right a sensation of pitch up and counterclockwise (left) yaw is experienced: curved arrows, true motion; and ---, perceived motion.

have ceased (Fig. 2a). If, in the dark, the subject's head is now passively rolled to the right to 90 deg at ω_1, the superior canal (pitch) acquires the angular momentum, since it has been brought into the plane of rotation (Fig. 2b). The torque required to impart this change in momentum causes deflection of the cupulae and a sensation of rotation, equivalent to an angular velocity of ω_2, in the pitch plane. Although the angular momentum of the subject's rotating head is forcibly transferred at once out of the old plane of rotation relative to the head, the angular momentum of the endolymph in the horizontal (yaw) plane is dissipated more slowly. The cupulae in the lateral canals are deflected by this deceleration, and they indicate counterclockwise rotation about the yaw axis of the head (Fig. 2b). Furthermore, during the lateral canal deceleration, it signals a continuous rotation, but the utricular and saccular maculae indicate that the head has not, in fact, succeeded in changing its orientation with respect to gravity. The transient cross-coupled acceleration induces a pitch-up sensation during the head roll and an unpleasant sensation of rotation in the counterclockwise direction. Similarly, in real life the combined effect of cupula deflection in all three semicircular canals is that of a suddenly imposed angular rotation in a plane in which no angular acceleration relative to the subject has occurred. The resulting Coriolis illusion experienced is one of pitching up and yawing to the left. In naïve subjects, the resulting illusion causes almost as much confusion in its discussion as in its experience.

In flight the Coriolis illusion is usually experienced when the pilot executes head movements during a constant rate turn of ω. After a certain period the cupulae in the pilot's semicircular canals (in the plane of aircraft rotation) have returned to the neutral position. When pilots move their heads about a second axis not aligned with ω, they can experience a sensation of rotation and tilt about a third axis, which is approximately orthogonal to ω and the head tilt axis. Therefore, when an aircraft is in a sharp right turn (clockwise rotation when viewed from above), if the head or body is rolled to the right shoulder relative to the aircraft, a false sensation of climb with high velocity but very little displacement is experienced. This can be extremely dangerous, especially if it occurs at low altitude. A pilot who tries to correct for this illusion by easing the pull on the control stick could very well descend into terrain.

In the preceding example, if the pilot's head is kept tilted long enough for the semicircular canals to equilibrate to the imposed angular velocities, moving the head back to the upright position would produce a diving (pitch-down) sensation with great apparent displacement but no unusual velocity.[15] In other words, an asymmetrical sensation with respect to the initial tilt and return movement of the head is experienced. The asymmetry of the sensation might be caused by the difference in orientation of the gravity vector in the two head positions. It has been shown by Benson and Bodin[16] that the threshold and rate of decay of postrotational responses are greater when the gravity vector is coplanar with the stimulated canals and least when it is normal to the plane of the canals. In the latter case, signals from the otolithic maculae indirectly modify the ampullary responses. Similarly, asymmetry with respect to tilting and righting movements of the head was also reported in the visual illusion perceived during Coriolis stimulation. Subjects reported that the velocity of a target light viewed during the Coriolis illusion was not always appropriate to the apparent displacement, that is, the target might have appeared to move fast without getting very far. The asymmetric response and the apparent discrepancy between the rate and displacement suggest the participation of nystagmus because the induced nystagmus is more intense and of longer duration when the angle between the gravity vector and the plane of the stimulated canal increases.[17]

C. Physiological Studies on the Coriolis Effect

Studies on the Coriolis effects include the symptom complex of motion sickness and autonomic responses such as heart-rate variability[18] and forearm blood-flow changes.[19] The results on heart-rate measurement are controversial. Most studies have found very small, variable, or inconsistent changes, despite substantiate symptoms of nausea and disorientation experienced by the subjects. For example, the average heart rate increases during head movements, whereas not rotating was statistically indistinguishable from that observed during Coriolis stimulation.[20] However, provocation of nausea, accompanied by an increase in forearm blood flow without changes in blood pressure or heart rate, appears to be more consistent.

The cardiovascular effects of Coriolis cross coupling were highlighted by Sunahara and colleagues.[19] They demonstrated that Coriolis cross-coupling effects caused significant increases in forearm blood flow as measured by venous occlusion strain-gauge plethysmography. In subjects with low tolerance, there was an immediate two- to three-fold increase in forearm blood flow within 2 min of head movements and concomitant reports of nausea. The increase in forearm blood flow suggests a decrease in sympathetic activity to the forearm vascular bed. However, in subjects with high tolerance there were no significant changes in forearm blood flow. This effect of forearm blood flow increase was later confirmed by Sinha,[21] who reported that the latencies to blood flow increase were 60–100 s in subjects with low tolerance. In general, the magnitude of the change in forearm blood flow correlated with the severity of motion sickness symptoms with definite nausea being the endpoint for all of these studies. Vasodilatation in the limbs impairs orthostatic tolerance, particularly if blood flow is shown to increase simultaneously in the lower limbs, which raises the possibility that G tolerance might also be impaired during subsequent increased high-G exposure.

Because the venous occlusion technique does not allow continuous data sampling, the time course of blood-flow changes might be underestimated. Recently, Cheung and Hofer[22] (2001) extended previous findings, using laser Doppler flowmetry (providing real-time monitoring of cutaneous blood flow), to investigate how the time course of the blood-flow changes correlates with the subjective reports of symptoms of motion sickness. During Coriolis cross-coupling stimulation, significant forearm and calf cutaneous blood flow were found to increase simultaneously. The temporal sequence of the peak increase in forearm and calf blood flow was consistent within subjects from trial to trial but varied across subjects. Latency to blood flow increases ranged from 14–90 s after stimulus onset, without overt symptoms of motion sickness. However, peak increase of blood flow in both forearm and calf occurred when the subject reached definite nausea. In other words humans might have different sensitivity to these Coriolis-induced vascular changes. As already mentioned, blood-flow increase in the lower limb might compromise the ability to withstand orthostatic stress. These findings might

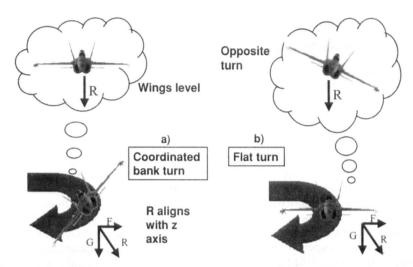

Fig. 3   False perception of attitude during turns occurs when the pilot interprets a sustained resultant vector as the earth vertical: G, gravity; F, centrifugal force; and R, resultant force.
a) During a coordinated turn, the centripetal acceleration produces F, yielding R that is aligned with the z axis of the aircraft; hence, the pilot perceives that the aircraft is wings level.
b) During a flat, uncoordinated turn, the aircraft skids, and R is no longer perpendicular to the transverse axis of the aircraft. Sensation is of turning in the opposite direction.

During a go-around or a missed approach at night, or when a high-performance aircraft accelerates down a runway and takes off into clouds, the inertial force resulting from the forward acceleration combines with the force of gravity to create a resultant gravitoinertial force directed down and aft (i.e., rotated backward). The resultant G vector is at an angle that will generate a pitch-up sensation to a nose-high attitude well beyond the angle of attack of the aircraft (Fig. 4). If visual cues are minimal, the pilot perceives down to be in the direction of the resultant gravitoinertial force and feels the aircraft is in an excessively nose-high attitude. The pilot might, therefore, attempt to correct for this pitch-up sensation by pushing the stick forward. This action will increase the forward acceleration component G_x and increase the illusion of climbing. The influence of a curved flight path (during bunting) can increase the deviation of resultant vectors (see Sec. III.A.3). If there is lag in the altimeter and vertical speed indicator (as in older aircraft), the loss of altitude might go unnoticed until it is too late to avoid ground contact. All too often, the aircraft is flown directly into the ground under fully controlled flight.

This false sensation of climb was identified by Collar[33] as a contributing factor for many accidents during World War II. More recently, two CF-18 fatal crashes involving afterburner climbs into an environment devoid of an analysis of external visual cues[4] listed somatogravic illusions as the primary contributing factor. However, this illusion also occurs in tanker/transport/bomber aircraft as indicated in the preceding example.[32] For a transport or commercial aircraft accelerating at

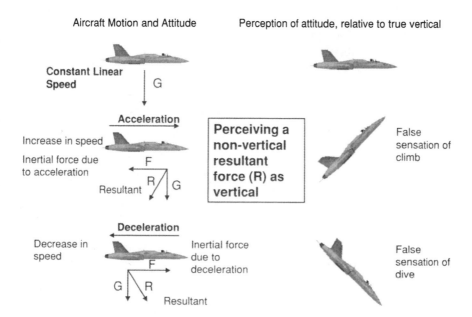

Aircraft Motion and Attitude   Perception of attitude, relative to true vertical

Constant Linear Speed   G

Acceleration

Increase in speed

Inertial force due to acceleration   F

Resultant   R / G

Perceiving a non-vertical resultant force (R) as vertical

False sensation of climb

Deceleration

Decrease in speed   Inertial force due to deceleration   F

G | \ R   Resultant

False sensation of dive

Fig. 4   False sensation of pitch during acceleration and deceleration: G, force of gravity; F, inertial force caused by acceleration or deceleration; and R, resultant force.

0.1 G, the vector angle is displaced backwards by about 6 deg. It was reported that in 27% of air transport flights that were involved in dark takeoff accidents between 1950–1965, false sensation of pitch was considered as a contributing factor.[34] Similarly, it was suggested that false sensation of climb might have been a contributing factor in 64% of Australian general aviation night takeoff mishaps.[35]

One group of pilots most susceptible to this illusion are those who take off from aircraft carriers. They can experience a 2–4-s pulse acceleration of approximately +3 to $+6G_x$ (chest to back), which results in a pitch-up sensation for 30–60 s (Ref. 28 and 36). The G_x acceleration experienced by the pilot is combined with gravity by vector addition, and the combined gravitoinertial acceleration vector is increased rapidly in length and rotated as the catapult forces are applied. The utricular otoliths detect a component of specific force in the G_x direction. Simultaneously, as the pilot is pressed against the back of the seat, pressure cues on the back also increase. In the absence of external visual cues, the pilot is normally unable to differentiate the catapult launch forces into their separate inertial and gravitational components. It has been estimated that, for an acceleration of $+4G_x$, the inertial and gravitational components of the catapult launch produce a 76-deg net rotation of the gravitoinertial vector that is increased in length by more than four times.[37] It has also been suggested that in modern fighter aircraft with 1:1 thrust: weight ratio at takeoff, the resultant acceleration vector is 1.4 G at 45 deg aft from the vertical.[38]

Furthermore, the resulting oculogravic illusion (subjective eye levels are elevated during the launch) causes the pilot's visual scene, both within and external to the cockpit, to rise (see Chapter 7, Sec. II.B.4). This can intensify the illusory perception of a pitch-up change in attitude, but the visual cues are paradoxical for objects in the external visual scene move downwards with an actual increase in pitch. It is, perhaps for this reason that the somatogravic and the concomitant oculogravic illusion are likely to influence the pilot's control of the aircraft when external visual cues are absent, as when flying in cloud or at night. In the centrifuge the change in subjective eye level was found to persist, in some cases, for as long as 3 min after the simulated launch sequence was completed.[36] When combined with the actual pitch up associated with takeoff rotation, the continued forward acceleration enhances the perceived nose-high attitude. As the landing gears are raised and the flaps are retracted, the subsequent increase in airspeed further compound the tendency to lower the nose.

When the aircraft decelerates, the pilot experiences the opposite effect; the aircraft appears to pitch down (Fig. 4). This can occur in straight-and-level flight, with the application of speed brakes or on reducing power. The resultant gravitoinertial force is at such an angle that the pilot might have a sensation of being tilted forward in a nose-down attitude. The pilot might correct for this sensation by pulling on the control stick and, depending on the pitch angle, might lead the aircraft into a stall. A pilot who is subjected to deceleration resulting from the application of the speed brake might also observe the instrument panel and the entire visual scene to move downward, which can potentiate the sensation of tilting forward. A recent survey of 141 pilots attending U.S. Air Force Advanced Instrument School revealed that the percentages of pilots experiencing a false pitch-up sensation from acceleration and a false pitch-down sensation from deceleration are 27 and 22%, respectively.[3]

The preceding discussion focuses on cases where the shearing force acts parallel to the utricular plane. A recent study reported that when subjects were tilted to 60 deg, so that a shear force was parallel to the saccular membrane and a vertical compression force was acting on the utricle, subjects also reported a pitch-down sensation.[39] However, similar illusions have not been reported in flight during coordinated turns (assuming that the pilot's head remained aligned with the vertical axis of the aircraft). The resultant shear force might be insufficient, and the paucity of the number of sensory hair cells in the saccule might have contributed to the lack of this illusion reported in flight. Further investigation into the contribution of saccular input to false perception of pitch is required. There have been a number of attempts investigating visual influences on the magnitude of somatogravic illusion (see Chapter 3, Sec. IV.D.1). The somatogravic illusion is a phenomenon that truly cannot be prevented because of the very nature of flight, but the effects can perhaps be minimized through education and awareness. Frequent reminders should serve as reinforcement to aircrew.

3.   Inversion Illusion

During an in-flight study, it was reported that transition from hypergravity (>1 G_z) to hypogravity (<1 G_z) causes disorientation; subjects had the sensation of flying in an inverted position, although no negative acceleration was present.[40] This is probably the first report of inversion illusion. More than 10 years later, while free floating during the microgravity phase of parabolic flight, Lieutenant B. C. Neider, Jr., U.S.N., also reported a reversal of personal orientation with regard to up and down.[41] He felt upside down in relation to the aircraft or that his body

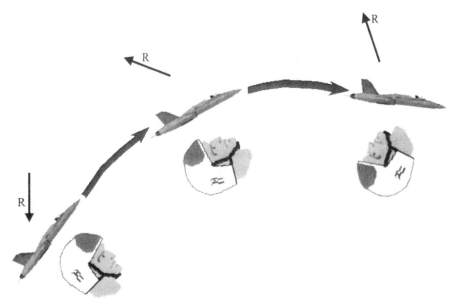

Fig. 5 Inversion illusion. When the resultant GIF (R) rotates backward pointing away from Earth, a false sensation of being upside down is experienced.

and the aircraft were inverted. Other reports were from Soviet cosmonauts who reported feelings of being inverted during orbital flight. Graybiel and Kellogg[41] indicated that while subjects with an intact vestibular apparatus experienced this inversion illusion, labyrinthine defective subjects did not, leading to the postulate that the "reversal" is of vestibular origin. A purely visual inversion illusion is also possible and is discussed in Chapter 7, Sec. II.A.3.

In high-performance aircraft, the inversion illusion can occur when the resultant gravitoinertial force vector actually rotates backwards so far as to point away from, rather than towards, the Earth's surface (Fig. 5). This maneuver gives rise to a sensation of being upside down as experienced by the pilot. A theoretical model of this mechanism was proposed by Martin and Melvill Jones.[42] Typically, this illusion can be encountered when a steeply climbing high-performance aircraft levels off, more or less abruptly, at the desired altitude. The aircraft and pilot are subjected to a $-G_z$ centrifugal force (radial acceleration) resulting from the arc flown prior to level off. As the aircraft levels off, the aircraft tends to pick up speed, adding a $+G_x$ tangential force to the overall force environment. Adding the $-G_z$ centrifugal force and the $+G_z$ tangential force results in a net gravitoinertial force vector that rotates backward and upward relative to the pilot. This stimulates the otolith in a manner similar to the way a pitch upward into an inverted position would. The otolith organs respond as if an inside loop to an inverted position had been carried out. The pilot has the sensation of tilting over backwards until nearly inverted at the apex of the climb. Pushing the control stick forward to counter the perceived pitch up typically worsens the situation by reducing the net $+G_z$ and increasing the G_x component. Money et al.[43] demonstrated the

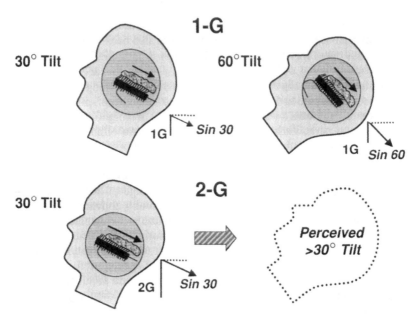

Fig. 6 G-excess effect—an exaggerated sense of body tilt occurring when G > 1. Under 1 G the pilot experiences a 0.5G (1 × sin 30 deg) pull on the utricular otolithic membranes when the head is tilted 30 deg off the vertical. At 60 deg of head tilt, the pilot experiences a 0.87G (1 × sin 60 deg) pull on the otolithic membrane. Under a 2-G environment, when the head is tilted 30 deg off the vertical, a 1-G (2 × sin 30 deg) pull occurs on the utricular otolithic membranes, causing the illusion that the head/body is tilted at greater than 30 deg from the vertical.

to 60 deg from the vertical, it will result in a 0.9-G (1 G × sin 60 deg = 0.87 G) shearing force on the otoliths. When the head is tilted to 30 deg from the vertical in a 2-G environment, the resulting shearing force on the otolithic membranes will be 1 G (2 G × sin 30 deg = 1 G). Therefore, at 2 G the perception of a 30 deg head tilt should theoretically be slightly greater than a 60-deg head tilt at 1 G. However, the preceding is a mathematical estimate. Experimental study on six subjects[50] suggested that the equation of perceived body position and shear force is not exact and could be because of nonlinearity or other factors that might have biased the postural judgment.

The G-excess effect has also been demonstrated in a number of centrifuge studies.[51,52] Pitching the head while in an excess $+G_z$ environment can cause an illusory sensation of excessive pitch if the head is forward, but head pitch translates to the roll axis as the head is turned towards the shoulder. Head tilts in the −30 to +46 deg range and with acceleration up to $+4G_z$ can cause illusionary tilts of up to approximately 10 deg (Ref. 53). However, the transient illusory perceptions produced by moving the head in hypergravity are confounded when using a ground-based centrifuge because the high angular velocity induces strong Coriolis cross-coupling effects on the semicircular canals, which is likely to mask a concomitant transient sensation engendered by the otoliths.

Using high-performance aircraft that could achieve at least $+2G_z$ while maintaining subthreshold angular acceleration, Gilson et al.[27] reported a 100% occurrence of the G-excess induced pitch illusion. The plane of the apparent attitude change was consistent, but the magnitude and direction of the apparent attitude change varied across subjects. It was also demonstrated that head movements produced transient perception of target displacement and velocity at levels as low as $+1.3 G_z$ (Ref. 54). Repeated head movements in hypergravity generate nausea by mechanisms distinct from cross-coupling Coriolis effects. Guedry and Rupert[55] suggested that a distinction between immediate transient G-excess effects and steady-state effects should be made as it has potential implications for different countermeasures. The transient component comprises confusion that might require momentary thought when head movements are voluntarily executed. The transient percept might also depend on the experience of the pilot. This speculation was based on the observation that an experienced pilot was relatively unsusceptible to the immediate G-excess effect, but was not immune to false sensation of pitch during repeated head movements.[55]

The G-excess effect is believed to cause pilots to falsely perceive that they are underbanked if they look in the direction of the turn and raise their heads. This posture causes them to experience a backward tilt sensation that is interpreted to be the aircraft rolling in the direction opposite to the actual bank attitude (Fig. 7). As a result, they might overbank and inadvertently descend.[56] Common mishap scenarios possibly related to the G-excess effect include formation flying during banked turns, which requires a pilot to maintain an upward gaze and yaw his head towards one shoulder while looking up at a lead aircraft. During a coordinated

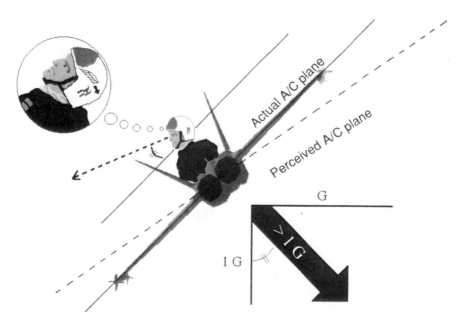

Fig. 7   G-excess effect during turns. (Reproduced from Ref. 56.)

turn (for example, left), the gravitoinertial vector remains perpendicular to the aircraft's wing line. When looking into the turn, the pilot's head is turned to the left, pitched up, and inclined to the aircraft's right (opposite the aircraft's bank). Under increased acceleration, G-induced excessive movement of the pilot's otolithic membranes causes the pilot to feel an extra amount of head and body tilt toward the back of the head and toward the right side of the aircraft. Consequently, the perceived excessive inclination of the pitched head opposite to the aircraft's bank is interpreted as being underbanked. In the absence of unambiguous visual orientation cues, the pilot might then increase the bank angle and inadvertently allow the nose to drop, resulting in a consequent loss of altitude. It is believed that the G-excess effect has contributed to low-level controlled flight into terrain,[49] although there are little flight data to support this conclusion.

IV.   Illusions Involving Semicircular Canals and Otoliths

A.   False Sensation of Banking—The Leans

The leans is one of the most common illusions that pilots experience. An early survey[57] indicated that of 24 SD items on a check list the item most frequently marked by [75% of] jet pilots was: "I thought I was in a left turn but on checking my instruments I saw that I was flying straight-and-level." In the rotary wing 91% of 104 active naval helicopter pilots reported to have experienced leans.[47] A survey of 1 Air Division of the Canadian Forces indicated that approximately 50% of pilots experienced disorientation, the majority of occurrences involving the leans.[4] Finally, a recent survey of students attending the U.S. Air Force Advanced Instrument School indicated that 94% had experienced the leans.[3]

During level flight in visually degraded conditions, a false sensation of banking can occur if pilots direct their gaze away from the instrument display. Sufficient time could pass so that one wing could drop at a subthreshold rate, which would inadvertently roll the aircraft into a bank without the conscious knowledge of the pilot. Upon checking the flight instruments, the pilot would, in most cases, simply correct the aircraft attitude by reference to the instruments. However, if the pilot returns to a wings-level attitude at a suprathreshold rate, the acceleration in the opposite direction added to the initial perception of apparent wings-level leads to the perception of a bank in the direction of the correcting roll. Pilots tend to align their head and/or trunk with the perceived vertical and consequently lean in that direction; pilots are then physically experiencing the leans (Fig. 8).

There are other causative factors for the leans. A suprathreshold change in roll followed by a subthreshold return to wings-level also induces the leans, as does recovery from a sustained coordinated turn under instrument flight rules (IFR). After a prolonged bank into a turn, the cupulae in the appropriate canals would have returned to their neutral positions. When the initial sensation of roll rotation ceases, the resultant gravitoinertial force vector is directed perpendicular to the floor of the aircraft providing a false sensation of vertical (upright). When ambiguous visual cues are present and without cross-checking instruments, a pilot can easily succumb to the sensation of flying wings level. Upon rolling out of the turn, as if the pilot adjusts the aircraft's bank angle to match the true horizon at the end of the turn, a sensation of being in an opposite bank arises. Pilots usually keep the aircraft level but tend to lean to correct their own discomfort. Another

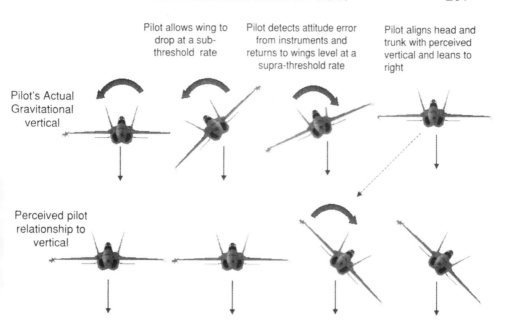

Fig. 8   Leans—pilot physically leans body in direction of perceived vertical while experiencing false sensation of bank in the opposite direction.

possible cause of the leans is the misinterpretation of a sloping false horizon (see Chapter 7, Sec. II.A). In some cases the inherent perceptual directional asymmetry in the pilot's ability to detect change in roll[58,59] might also contribute to the leans. The leans can diminish gradually or persist until unambiguous external visual references become available.

B.   Graveyard Spiral

A prominent illusion stemming from both canal and otolith inadequacies is the graveyard spiral. In this illusion, the pilot loses the sensation of turning after reaching constant velocity, as well as the sensation of banking, because the gravitoinertial force (GIF) points towards the floor of the aircraft. Graveyard spiral accidents are reported to be common in general aviation (100 deaths a year in the United States), relatively rare in military aviation (less than six a year), and rarer still in commercial airline operations.[60] However, it has been reported that a number of highly experienced airline pilots flew their aircraft into a spiral dive by moving and holding the controls to the very end in the reverse direction of that required for recovery.[61]

During a prolonged turn with a moderate amount of bank, the pilot loses the sensation of turning because the canal-cupula-endolymph system does not respond to constant angular velocity. The perception of being banked as a result of the initial rolling to the banked attitude also decays with time as determined by the relatively short effective time constant in roll rotation (see Chapter 2, Sec. III.F). In addition, the net GIF vector is directed toward the floor of the aircraft during a coordinated turn. When the pilot attempts to stop the turn by rolling back to wings level, there is a sensation of turning in the direction opposite to that of the original turn and a

V.   Visual and Audio Correlates of Somatic Illusions

There is a complement of interesting visual and audio errors related to the somatogyral and somatogravic illusions that can be demonstrated in the laboratory. Oculogyral and oculogravic illusions are the visual correlates of the somatogyral and somatogravic illusions, respectively. The oculogyral illusion usually occurs after a sudden stop from a constant rotation. Subjects sense an apparent rotation in the opposite direction, as objects in front of the test subjects appear to move in the opposite direction. The oculogravic illusion is the apparent displacement of a real target or afterimage as a result of a change in the angle between the direction of the resultant gravitational force on the observer and the longitudinal axis of the observer's body. The oculogyral and oculogravic illusions will be discussed in detail in Chapter 7, Sec. II.B.4.

Interesting errors made in auditory localization during motion stimulation have been demonstrated in the laboratory. For example, following rapid angular deceleration, subjects tend to locate the sound source as if it were displaced in the direction of the preceding rotation and in the direction opposite to rotation during acceleration. The phenomenon is termed the audiogyral illusion.[64] To localize a sound with respect to the midline of the body, a subject must take into account the position of the head with respect to the rest of the body. There is some evidence that indicates that rotatory acceleration changes the apparent position of the head with respect to a fixed reference point.[65] This implies that sound displacement that occurs during yaw rotation is caused by a change in the position of the head that is felt as straight ahead. Similarly, when a stationary subject on a human centrifuge is exposed to centrifugal force the subject will tend to reorient in conformity with the resultant of the centrifugal force and the force of gravity. It has been shown that under the preceding condition localization of a sound source in terms of Cartesian space and frontal plane of reference is influenced by the change in direction of the resultant force. This phenomenon is termed the audiogravic illusion.[66] Under static conditions and in the absence of visual cues, the subject judges the position of the auditory stimulus with reference to a point on the horizon. The estimation of the horizontal and vertical axes depends on the vestibular and somatosensory cues that orient the subject to the direction of gravity. Under conditions of acceleration, the subject orients identical sensory cues to the resultant force rather than Earth's gravity. Although the subject is stationary within the gondola of the centrifuge, there is a change in the angle between the body axes and the resultant force. The egocentric localization of the vertical and horizontal axes aligns with the direction of the resultant force but not with the true vertical. Therefore, the localization of a point source of sound within the new frame of reference causes the subject to misperceive the true position of the stimulus. It is suggested that the errors in sound localization are to be attributed to the complex interactions of sensory systems and that the resultant perception is the subject's reaction to the situation. Most recently, it has been shown that head-centric auditory localization is affected by azimuthal rotation and an increase in GIF magnitude.[67] Sound localization is shifted in the direction opposite to GIF rotation by an amount related to the magnitude of the GIF and its angular deviation relative to the median plane, thereby confirming the existence of the audiogravic illusion. Audiogravic and audiogyral phenomena might compromise the use of three-dimensional audio orientation cues in high-performance aircraft (see Chapter 11, Sec. IV.B.1).

VI.   Illusions Contributed by the Somatosensory System

With increasing gravitoinertial force, when the pilot is pressed against the back of the seat, pressure and contact cues on the back increase and become more prominent. When devoid of vision, the intense periodic touch and pressure stimulation to the body surface determines the apparent orientation of the body and can override contribution from the otolith receptors. Miller and Graybiel[68] observed that the egocentric visual localization of the horizontal, in both labyrinthine-defective (LD) and normal subjects, was found to deviate from the gravitoinertial horizontal as a function of the GIF magnitude. However, the directions of the perceived apparent rotation between the two groups were different. The interpretation of this difference is limited by the fact that there were only two LD subjects tested. Nevertheless, it appears that the somatosensory system plays a major role (perhaps even dominant) in the somatogravic illusion as postulated by Collar[33] in his analysis of night takeoff accidents. In a similar study in which five normal and five (deaf) LD subjects set a luminous line to the perceived horizontal in a rotation room, it was shown that there were no significant difference between the two groups suggesting that contact information from the feet and kinesthetic information from the legs and body were adequate for the LD group to make accurate settings.[69]

Other evidence of a somatosensory contribution to SD can be noted in the following case study:

Case 72: SH-3, night ASW, no moon or horizon. In a night dip ... (I) was trying to keep the aircraft into the wind ... became confused as to where the wind was from ... the indications of wind in windows and air speed indicator seemed to disagree ... I added rudder pedal correction ... but aircraft began to drift and whole world began to spin ... I gave the aircraft to the pilot. (Ref. 47, p. 389.)

The preceding narrative suggests that wind entering through the right cockpit window produces a subjective sensation that the aircraft is drifting right, when in fact that the aircraft might be in a stable hover. A sensation of apparent self-motion can be induced by stimulation of the somatosensory system without corresponding vestibular sensation. For example, a sensation of linear self-motion can be induced in a blindfolded stationary subject, who keeps contact with a linearly moving platform.[70] The preceding discussion provides further evidence that the interactions between the somatosensory and vestibular systems are similar to the visual-vestibular interaction.

VII.   Incapacitating Illusions

A.   Giant Hand Illusion

The giant hand illusion is the false perception by a pilot that the aircraft controls are forced into an extreme position and that they appear to be held there against the pilot's effort to direct them in the desired direction, as if by a giant hand.[71,72] A fighter pilot physician[73] first described the illusion as occurring when he was in a left climbing turn and felt that the control stick was being pulled from him as though by a "giant hand." When he tried to center the control stick by pulling with both hands and both knees, it was unsuccessful. Upon releasing his grip on the control stick, it appeared to float back to the central position by itself. For several minutes afterwards he was able to control the aircraft by grasping the control stick with thumb and forefinger. The incident occurred at night in a heavy snowstorm, and a rapid head movement precipitated the loss of control of the aircraft.

The incidence of the giant-hand illusion among fighter pilots has been estimated between 7% (Ref. 5) and 16% (Ref. 71) and 14% in rotary-wing pilots.[74] The illusion is not always overwhelming. Milder episodes of this phenomenon have occurred in which the pilot was able to recover. Malcolm and Money[72] suggested four common factors leading to the illusion: 1) the pilot is aroused or in a state of anxiety; 2) the pilot is distracted from the task of controlling the attitude of the aircraft; 3) the resultant GIF vector is rotated forward; 4) the control of the aircraft involves a motor task of one or both hands. It is proposed that the giant hand phenomenon is the result of a postural reflex response to a combination of psychological and physiological conditions affecting the pilot. Specifically, the vestibulospinal reflex was proposed as one of the potential contributing factors to the phenomenon (see Chapter 2, Sec. X). Koren and Lessard[39] reported that both flexor and extensor muscles show increased activity during G loading when the saccule is exposed to vertical acceleration and the utricles to compression forces. This rigor type of muscle activity might be part of the activation of the vestibulospinal reflex that contributes in part to the giant hand illusion.

A number of remedies for the giant hand illusion have been proposed: for example, letting go of the control stick or pushing the control in the desired direction of pull, or maneuvering with a thumb and forefinger grip.[73] The last strategy attempts to use a corticospinal motor strategy (control of fingers) to bypass the influence of the ventromedial system, including the vestibulospinal reflex pathway, which in turn mediates the control of proximal musculature (see Chapter 2, Sec. X). More recently, the thumb and forefinger grip approach was shown to be ineffective in overcoming a visual analogue of the giant hand illusion.[75] However, a visually induced giant hand illusion might not be a true representation of the illusion experienced in flight, and it might involve different neurophysiological mechanisms because the subconscious motor response of the former is driven by a visual rather than a vestibular stimulus. In addition, the laboratory environment simply cannot reproduce the emotional stress that might precipitate the giant hand phenomenon in the aircraft.

B.   Vestibulo-Ocular Disorganization

It has been reported that upon recovery from a rapid aerodynamic roll or spin, pilots became disoriented and lost control of the aircraft.[76,77] The pilots could neither fixate upon the instruments nor upon the external visual field at a higher rate of rotation (> 200 deg/s). Basic understanding of the vestibulo-ocular reflex (VOR) (Chapter 2, Sec. IV) leads to the postulate that at certain stages during, and upon recovery from aerodynamic rotation, the vestibulo-oculomotor system fails to maintain the intermittent stabilization of the retinal image that normally occurs in everyday life on the ground. In the initial stages of the rotation, compensatory eye movements driven by the VOR will be appropriate in the yaw, pitch, and roll planes for objects fixed in space outside the aircraft but not for cockpit instruments that have a fixed orientation to the pilot. As the effective canal signals decay with their respective specific time constants—16 s for yaw, 7 s for pitch, and 4 s for roll[78]—involuntary eye movements can arise with a considerably greater error in response to rotational stimuli in pitch and roll than in yaw. In addition, the optokinetic following ability of the moving visual scene is inadequate (especially in roll) when the relative angular velocities are higher than the opposing vestibular signals. On recovery to straight-and-level flight, the misleading vestibular signal invokes an inappropriate oculomotor response that cannot be suppressed by visual fixation. In other words, optokinetic stimulation predominates over the vestibular influence in the yaw plane, whereas the reverse relation holds for the roll plane where vestibular influence is dominant. These findings were subsequently verified in the laboratory.[79] Therefore, the induction of involuntary eye movements suitable to follow the outside world might have prevented the pilots from reading the instruments and might have degraded vision for instruments and the external visual scene on recovery from sustained angular motion. The rate of rotation might have been too great for compensatory eye movements to allow fixation on the outside world. As a result, vestibulo-ocular disorganization can contribute to SD induced by rapid rotation in flight.

C.   G-Vector Induced Positional Vertigo

An F-16 pilot of apparent good health experienced sudden onset of severe near-incapacitating vertigo (see Chapter 1, Sec. I) following the completion of a "check-six" (looking back over the shoulder) maneuver over his left shoulder during a $+7$–8 G_z turn (Ref. 80). Upon landing, physical examination revealed that forward head tilt and rotation produced vertigo with SD predominating. A presumptive diagnosis of benign paroxysmal positional vertigo was made. In benign paroxysmal positional vertigo, affected patients typically complain of brief episodes of vertigo precipitated by change of head posture, as in turning over in bed, looking up to a high shelf, or backing a car out of the garage. It is thought that degenerated utricular otoliths are detached and come to rest on the cupula of the posterior semicircular canal. It is speculated that the sudden onset of vertigo is precipitated by exposure to negative G and possibly off-axis $+G_z$ in flight.[80] It has also been documented that the dizziness experienced can be severe when pilots turn their head and can persist for three weeks or longer.[81] Anecdotal reports suggest that this condition has also been noted by civilian aerobatic pilots and is referred to as the "wobblies" or "vector related vertigo," which can be precipitated by high levels of $+G_z$ (Ref. 82). Although the symptoms are similar to benign paroxysmal positional vertigo, the apparent etiology is unknown. The syndrome could just as well be explained by a possible mechanism involving the brain stem, as it is near the main acceleration axis. In view of next generation of agile aircraft (see Chapter 11, Sec. III), intensive research is required to delineate this condition. In the interim the condition is best managed clinically by recognition and by allowing time for spontaneous recovery. The likely persistent symptoms after landing suggests that assisted exit from the aircraft is prudent and pilots should avoid repeated "insults."

VIII. Inner-Ear Problems Contributing to SD

A. Alternobaric Vertigo (Pressure Vertigo)

Changes in atmospheric pressure during or soon after ascent and descent have been known for a long time to cause sudden incapacitation. The initial sensations of spinning, rolling, or pitching are intense and are accompanied by nystagmus and apparent motion of the visual scene. Although this phenomenon is usually short lived and dies away in 10–16 s, some aircrew have reported less intense but persistent vertigo that lasted for minutes.[28] Melvill Jones[7] first applied the term "pressure vertigo" to the aforementioned symptom complex. He reported that approximately 10% of a group of 190 pilots interviewed had experienced vertigo immediately following changes of middle-ear pressure incurred by rapid ascent and descent. Lundgren[83] coined the term "alternobaric vertigo" in his description of a diving hazard. His surveys on aviators indicated that 17% of pilots experienced alternobaric vertigo at one time or another.[83] There are a number of case studies by Melvill Jones,[7] Enders and Rodriguez-Lopez,[84] Brown,[85] and Wicks,[86] who concluded that alternobaric vertigo is probably not as uncommon an occurrence in pilots as previously suspected. Wicks[86] further suggests that, dependent upon the cabin/ambient pressure relationship, the prevalence of alternobaric vertigo will increase as aircraft become more sophisticated and capable of significant climbing rates.

Few experimental studies of this phenomenon in humans have been published. It is generally assumed that the vertigo is caused by an overpressure (positive pressure) in the middle ear, which can affect the inner ear without requiring movements of the tympanum and the ossicles. Although the actual mechanism is unclear, it has been suggested that false sensations of movement might be precipitated by pressure changes transmitted from the middle-ear cavity to the labyrinth via the round window. As a consequence, sudden fluid flow can occur between the round window and oval window, generating eddy currents that could conceivably displace the utricular and saccular maculae and the cupulae of the semicircular canals. The ensuing vestibular stimulation then gives rise to disorienting sensations.

The increase in pressure caused by failure of ventilation of the middle ear on descent is gradual and is usually not adequate to produce any symptoms. Tjernstrom[87] made the observation that pilots usually do not clear their ears actively during descent but wait for the ear to equilibrate passively when the relative overpressure (middle-ear pressure relative to ambient pressure) has increased enough for their Eustachian tubes to be forced open. Experiments in an altitude chamber indicated that alternobaric vertigo could occur despite only moderate pressure changes. The vertigo was not induced at the moment of pressure regulation, but during the period of asymmetric middle ear pressure caused by different forcing pressures (the pressure when the Eustachian tube is passively forced open). It also occurred when the pressure in the not-cleared ear reached a certain level. In aircraft capable of rapid rates of climb, or with the sudden additional pressure created by the performance of a forceful Valsava maneuver, the increase in pressure can be sufficient to exacerbate this asymmetry. Normal subjects who seem to have high forcing pressures on one side are more susceptible to alternobaric vertigo than others. Susceptibility to pressure vertigo increases during conditions of respiratory tract infection. Mild congestion and inflammation as a result of a common cold increase the difficulty to equalize the middle ear pressure, especially when the Eustachian tubes are edematous or dysfunctional.

B.   Alcohol

Drugs and alcohol can seriously increase our susceptibility to SD (see Chapter 4, Sec. II.D). Simple prescription and over-the-counter medications are potentially lethal in the flying environment. Most antihistamines cause drowsiness and slow response times. Antibiotics such as streptomycin affect the inner ear, and cumulative dosages can be ototoxic. Many cough compounds contain alcohol and even codeine. It is well known that the aftereffects of alcohol (hangover) adversely affect an individual's general ability (see Chapter 4, Sec. II.D). After the blood alcohol concentration (BAC) has been raised high enough and the alcohol has subsequently disappeared from the blood, it continues to have measurable effects on the brain, vestibular system, and in some cases blood sugar.[88,89]

Alcohol has a physical effect on the semicircular canals as revealed by positional alcohol nystagmus (PAN) and by sensation (e.g, vertigo). An historical description of alcohol nystagmus as symptoms of alcohol intoxication is provided by Aschan et al.,[90] who indicated that alcohol nystagmus might change in its direction when the direction of the head is altered. The VOR is manifested as PAN I (positional alcohol nystagmus phase I), which persists for some time (3.6 h) after the BAC starts falling. If the head is positioned left side down, the slow phase of the horizontal nystagmus is to the left and the fast phase to the right. At approximately 6 h after ingestion, PAN II (positional alcohol nystagmus phase II) appears and lasts for another 3 h (10–11 hours after initial consumption) or until alcohol is no longer detectable in the blood. If the head is tilted left side down, the fast phase of the nystagmus is in the direction opposite to that in PAN I.[91] PAN II persists for several hours after the BAC has fallen to zero. During the period of PAN, certain orientations of the head relative to gravity, increased acceleration, or turbulence can all be expected to provoke apparent sensations of rotation. However, the otolith and somatosensory systems indicate that no motion has occurred. It has been suggested that PAN II can persist up to 34 h after drinking[92] and longer still under >1-G_z (Ref. 93).

When the BAC reaches approximately 0.04% (i.e., 40 mg of alcohol in 100 mil of blood), which can occur after a single ingestion (1 g per kg of body weight), an area of low density (a "light spot") forms on the endolymph ring in the semicircular canals.[94,95] When this light spot is present, linear acceleration or gravity causes the endolymph ring to rotate relative to the canal wall, which elicits a sensation of apparent rotation, and postural and vestibulo-ocular reflexes. Similar effects are observed after ingestion of heavy water, but in the opposite direction to those produced by alcohol.[96]

The mechanism of PAN is explained by the density differences caused by the diffusion of alcohol into the inner ear.[94] Their data suggested that alcohol does enter the perilymph and the endolymph. Alcohol appears to act in the semicircular canal to make the cupulae lighter than the endolymph until the alcohol concentration in the endolymph rises sufficiently. PAN II probably results from the presence of alcohol in the endolymph after alcohol has largely disappeared from the cupulae. Residual alcohol in the inner ear is a factor in the production of the hangover effect.

It should be obvious that pilots flying with alcohol in their semicircular canals are at increased risk of disorientation (see Chapter 4, Sec. II.D) and increased susceptibility to motion sickness.[91]

The eight-hour rule is quite inadequate for heavy drinking because there would still be significant concentrations of alcohol in the blood. (Heavy drinking is defined as having a BAC of 0.16% among occasional drinkers in a social setting.) Under some circumstances there are measurable decrements of pilot performance even at 14 h after a peak BAC of only 0.1% (equivalent to 4–6 drinks depending on the individual and speed of ingestion). Furthermore, inappropriate eye movements can degrade vision especially at night. It has been reported that at concentrations as low as 0.027% alcohol impairs the ability to employ visual fixation to suppress inappropriate vestibular nystagmus.[97,98] It has also been shown that alcohol affects the visual feedback of target position during voluntary and involuntary head movement.[99] In most cases, depending on the individual and the speed of ingestion, four to six drinks is sufficient to raise the BAC to over 0.1%, which is certainly high enough to affect visual feedback. However, the time course of the effect on visual pursuit and suppression of the vestibulo-ocular reflex follows that of BAC. There is no "post" effect as with PAN. Lastly, aircrew that are susceptible to airsickness have observed that their susceptibility to airsickness is increased by even moderate amounts of alcohol in the previous 24 h (Ref. 100). This effect of alcohol has also been observed on tolerance to cross-coupled stimulation during desensitization treatment.[101] Of course, excessive consumption of alcohol can result in vomiting even without provocative motion.

C. Pathological Predisposition to SD

Spatial disorientation in flight is a normal physiological response to altered gravitoinertial environments in the absence of any underlying pathology. However, a number of case studies have indicated that pathologic causes involving the perceptual consequences of vestibular anomalies can predispose pilots to experiencing SD. For example, individuals with vestibular directional preponderance (greater amplitude of postrotatory nystagmus in one direction over the other) on the ground suffered from strong, persistent illusions of rolling and turning to the affected side when external vision was inadequate or absent.[59,102] Another study[103] reported that, when deprived of external visual references, pilots with defective VOR sometimes experienced difficulties in maintaining aircraft control. There are other isolated cases where pilots exhibit abnormal perception under altered gravitoinertial forces, which predispose them to SD despite normal clinical findings. The range of clinical conditions with symptoms of vertigo is rarely revealed by problems in flight. Most affected individuals have symptoms on the ground.

However, unlike the visual system, the vestibular system of pilots is seldom investigated because of the lack of a practical, reliable test and the lack of normative data for comparison. Current clinical assessments of vestibular integrity are time consuming and are primarily based on the examination of eye movements induced by caloric stimulation or induced by passive rotation at frequencies below 2 Hz. However, during natural movements, head movement frequencies between 1–4 Hz are most commonly generated. In spite of considerable research, vestibular and equilibrium testing procedures are not standardized or uniformly accepted from one laboratory to another. A basic vestibular function test battery has been proposed as the fundamental group of tests required for all clinical evaluations of vestibular integrity and for selection of groups in special occupations, such as pilots.[104] This test battery includes an electrooculography calibration, a saccade test, spontaneous and gaze-evoked nystagmus tests, ocular pursuit test, positioning test, positional test, and the caloric test. Such extensive testing would be extremely costly and time consuming for the initial medical screening of all pilot candidates. What is needed is a preliminary vestibular screening test that could indicate whether a full battery of clinical evaluations is warranted. For example, the dynamic visual acuity test (oscillopsia test) is a useful screening test of visual-vestibular interaction.[105] For equilibrium testing, the tandem gait test and sharpened Romberg tests in the dark are often used. Detailed recommendations for the timing and types of vestibular assessments are listed in Appendix A.

IX. Summary

This chapter has described a number of illusions involving sensations of motion and body position, stemming from the inadequacies of the nonvisual spatial orientation systems. Among the nonvisual illusions, vestibular illusions predominate and are directly related to the limitation of these semicircular canals and the otolith systems. These illusions have been studied extensively in the laboratory and under controlled conditions during flight tests. The vestibular illusions are discussed under three broad categories, the first being illusions primarily involving the semicircular canals or somatogyral illusions about the yaw (graveyard spin) and roll axes (Gillingham illusion). The somatogyral illusion is the false sensation of rotation, or absence of rotation, which results from misperceiving the magnitude and direction of an actual rotation. The vestibular Coriolis cross-coupling illusion stems from the sensation of angular motion in response to an inclination of the head while the head is undergoing a passive rotation about an axis not aligned with the tilt axis. The second category of illusion primarily involves the otoliths and is termed somatogravic, which is the misperception of the magnitude and/or direction of a gravitoinertial force as the true vertical. These phenomena are responsible for the false sensation of bank, false sensation of pitch, and the sensation of flying inverted. In addition, an exaggerated sense of body tilt occurs when the sustained G load is greater than that experienced in a normal 1 G environment (the G-excess effect). The final category of illusion involves both the semicircular canals and the otoliths and includes the leans and graveyard spiral.

In addition, illusions contributed by the somatosensory systems and the incapacitating effects of the giant hand illusion were also discussed as to their SD impact. The contribution to SD of a number of clinical vestibular factors such as involuntary nystagmus, reduced sensitivity of the vestibulo-ocular reflex, G-vector induced positional vertigo, alternobaric vertigo and effects of alcohol on the semicircular canals were also described. Finally, a summary of practical recommendations for flight surgeons and aircrew was provided as an important spatial disorientation countermeasure.

Appendix A: Assortment of Practical Recommendations for Flight Surgeons

The interim measures to prevent SD mishaps includes improvement of ground-based and in-flight training methods for demonstrating to pilots the potential for SD and the means of coping with it. Specific SD countermeasures training for aircrew are discussed in Chapter 8. Based on the abundant scientific and accident investigation data, various investigators have suggested a number of practical SD countermeasures for providing advice to flight surgeons and aircrew over the years.[6,28,106-108] A summary of these practical measures are listed here:

1) Be well informed about the inadequacies of our sensory systems in flight. Understand that SD is a normal physiological and psychophysical response to an unnatural force environment and that it can occur to anyone regardless of skills and experience.

2) An individual should not fly unless he feels fit and well rested. Do not go flying when you are hung over, have an upset stomach, have an upper-respiratory-tract or middle-ear infection, or are mentally debilitated. Recent illness, stress, and fatigue all adversely affect an individual's general ability in the air. They also make one prone to airsickness, especially during turbulence.

3) Clinical assessment of vestibular function. As there is no "gold standard" for vestibular function test, a quick and simple screening procedure for pilots could include the dynamic acuity test, Halmagyi test, and post-head-shake nystagmus test. Abnormal results from any of these tests would not indicate that the candidate is abnormal, but would indicate that additional tests should be performed. Details of these proposed clinical tests are discussed in the next section.

4) Trainees should discuss any SD experience immediately and openly with the flight instructor, colleagues, flight surgeons, and/or flight physiologists to dispel any misinterpretation and regain confidence. Early discussion will reduce anxiety, facilitate recovery, and provide an understanding of when the effects of SD decrease an individual's performance.

5) Learn to reject bodily sensations as unreliable; do not trust or fly by the "seat-of-the-pants" sensation.

6) Avoid unnecessary interchange between flying visual meteorological condition (VMC) and instrument meteorological condition (IMC). Transfer to instrument flying well before entering cloud.

7) Be aware of conditions that are conducive to SD.

8) Pilots are often told to "believe your instruments," especially during reduced visibility. However, it is important to be sure that the pilot does not simply indulge in an attempt at changing their perception when disoriented. Pilots should be told that in case of disorientation "control the aircraft to make the instruments read correctly."

9) After a prolonged absence from flying, ensure that the first series of familiarization flights are performed using visual flight rules and then gradually regain and maintain the proficiency of flying on instruments.

10) Realize that a pilot's instructions about what to do in case of SD are useful only in dealing with recognized Type I (recognized) SD. Unrecognized SD

(Type II) should be dealt with by avoiding situations that are prone to induce disorientation. Aircrew should be taught to recognize conditions that can lead to a loss of orientation.

11) Abstain from drinking alcohol for at least 12 hours prior to flying and in no case less than eight hours prior to reporting for duty. The current recommendation for commercial airline pilots is 24 hours after a blood alcohol concentration of 0.16 % before flying. For those taking antimotion sickness medications, it is important to note the increased sedation from alcohol.

12) Pilots should be aware that often disorientation is misperceived as a failure in the flight instruments, such as in the artificial horizon, or an aircraft control system. Therefore, when a failure in a flight instrument or control system is "suspected," the pilot should be skeptical and must verify the correct diagnosis of the problem before reacting.

13) Flight surgeons should assist in implementation of a formal and standardized SD awareness training program.

14) Lastly, many problems of disorientation can be solved by using the autopilot or by passing control to another pilot (when available) who is not disoriented.

Recommendations for the pilot are summarized here.

1) Educate yourself about the mechanisms of SD.
2) Do not go flying unless you are physically and mentally fit.
3) Have a proper clinical assessment of your vestibular apparatus.
4) Be frank about your SD experience, and share this information with others.
5) Do not fly by the seat of the pants. Use your instruments.
6) Avoid unnecessary interchange between flying VMC and IMC
7) Be aware of conditions that are conducive to SD.
8) Believe your instruments but also control the aircraft to make the instruments read correctly.
9) Maintain proficiency in instrument flying.
10) Recognize conditions that precipitate SD.
11) Abstain from alcohol for at least 24 hours prior to flying.
12) Verify all instrument failure before reacting.
13) Assist in a formal and standardized SD awareness training program.
14) When in doubt, use autopilot or another pilot, if available.

A. Vestibular Screening Tests

The following tests are recommended for the Canadian Forces as initial screening for pilots who are unusually susceptible to airsickness.[109] Similarly, before entry to initial flight training, individuals with episodes of disequilibrium could benefit from the following screening tests. Abnormal findings indicate additional tests should be performed.

1. Dynamic Visual Acuity Test

a) Measure the subject's best-corrected visual acuity with an acuity chart with head still.

[16]Benson, A. J., and Bodin, M. A., "Interaction of Linear and Angular Accelerations on Vestibular Receptors in Man," *Aerospace Medicine*, Vol. 37, 1966, pp. 144–154.

[17]Lansberg, M. P., Guedry, F. E., Jr., and Graybiel, A., "The Effects of Changing the Resultant Linear Acceleration Relative to the Subject on Nnystagmus Generated by Angular Acceleration," Naval School of Aviation Medicine, Rep. 99, 1 Sept. 1964.

[18]Cowings, P. S., Naifeh, K. H., and Toscano, W. B., "The Stability of Individual Patterns of Autonomic Responses to Motion Sickness Stimulation," *Aviation, Space, and Environmental Medicine*, Vol. 61, 1990, pp. 399–405.

[19]Sunahara, F. A., Johnson, W., and Taylor, N. B. G., "Vestibular Stimulation and Forearm Blood Flow," *Canadian Journal of Physiology and Pharmacology*, Vol. 42, 1964, pp. 199–207.

[20]Lawson, B. D., and Lackner, J. R., "Physiological Responses to Head Movement," *63th Annual Aerospace Medicine Association Meeting, Proceedings*, 1992.

[21]Sinha, R., "Effects of Vestibular Coriolis Reaction on Respiration and Blood-Flow Changes in Man," *Aerospace Medicine*, Vol. 39, 1968, pp. 837–844.

[22]Cheung, B., and Hofer, K., "Coriolis-Induced Cutaneous Blood Flow Increase in the Forearm and Calf," *Brain Research Bulletin*, Vol. 54, 2001, pp. 609–618.

[23]Clark, C. C., and Hardy, J. D., "Problems in Manned Space Stations," Symposium Sponsored by the IAS with the cooperation of NASA and the Rand Corp; IAS, New York, Apr. 1960.

[24]Gray, R. F., Crosbie, R. J., Hall, R. A., Weaver, J. A. and Clark, C. C., "The Presence or Absence of Visual Coriolis Illusion at Various Combined Angular Velocities," U.S. Naval Air Development Center, Subtask MR 005 13-6002.5, Rept No. 1, Johnsville, PA, June 1961.

[25]Meda, E., "A Research on the Threshold for the Coriolis and Purkinje Phenomena of Excitation of the Semicircular Canals," Translated from *Archivio di Fisiologia*, Vol. 52, No. 2, 1952, pp. 116–134; translation by E. R. Hope, Defence Scientific Information Service, DRB, Canada, 15 Sept. 1954.

[26]Gillingham, K. K., "Training the Vestibule for Aerospace Operations Using Coriolis Effect to Assess Rotation," *Aerospace Medicine*, Vol. 37, 1966, pp. 47–51.

[27]Gilson, R. D., Guedry F. E., Hixson W. C., and Niven, J. I., "Observations on Perceived Changes in Aircraft Attitude Attending Head Movements Made in a 2-g Bank and Turn," *Aerospace Medicine*, Vol. 44, 1973, pp. 90–92.

[28]Benson, A. J., "Spatial Disorientation—General Aspects," *Aviation Medicine*, edited by J. Ernsting, A. N. Nicholson, and D. J. Rainford, Butterworth Heinemann, London, 1999, pp. 419–454.

[29]Pancratz, D. I., Bomar, J. B., and Raddin, J. H., "A New Source for Vestibular Illusions in High Agility Aircraft," *Aviation, Space, and Environmental Meidicine*, Vol. 64, 1994, pp. 1130–1133.

[30]Henn, V., and Young, L. R., "Ernst Mach on the Vestibular Organ 100 Years Ago," *Annals of the Oto-Rhino-Laryngology*, Vol. 37, 1975, pp. 138–148.

[31]Wolfe, J. W., and Cramer, R. L., "Illusions of Pitch Induced by Centripetal Acceleration," *Aerospace Medicine*, Vol. 46, 1970, pp. 1136–1139.

[32]Mortimer, R. G., "General Aviation Airplane Accidents Involving Spatial Disorientation," *Proceedings of the Human Factors and Ergonomics Society 39th Annual Meeting*, 1995, pp. 25–29.

[33]Collar, A. R., "On an Aspect of the Accident History of Aircraft Taking off at Night," Aeronautical Research Council, Reports and Memoranda No. 2277, London, 1946.

[34]Buley, L. E., and Spelina, J., "Physiological and Psychological Factors in the Dark Night Takeoff Accident," *Aerospace Medicine*, Vol. 41, 1970, pp. 553–556.

[35]O'Brien, P. A., and Lane, P. C., "The False Climb—A Fatal Illusion," Avmedia, *Journal of Australian*, New Zealand Aviation Medicine Society, 1999.

[36]Cohen, M. J., Crosbie, R. J., and Blackburn, L. H., "Disorienting Effects of Aircraft Catapult Launchings," *Aerospace Medicine*, Vol. 44, 1973, pp. 37–39.

[37]Cohen, M. M., Crosbie, R. J., and Blackburn, L. H., "Disorienting Effects of Aircraft Catapult Launchings," *The Disorientation Incident*, edited by A. J. Benson, AGARD CP-95 – Part 1: 1972.

[38]McCarthy, G. W., and Stott, J. R. R., "In Flight Verification of the Inversion Illusion," *Aviation, Space, and Environmental Medicine*, Vol. 65, 1994, pp. 341–344.

[39]Koren, I., and Lessard, C. S., "The Effect of Inertial Force Acceleration on the Otolithic Membrane," *IEEE Engineering in Medicine and Biology*, Vol. 19, 2000, pp. 48–55.

[40]von Beckh, H. J., "Experiments with Animal and Human Subjects Under Sub and Zero-Gravity Conditions During the Dive and Parabolic Flight," *Journal of Aviation Medicine*, Vol. 25, 1954, pp. 235–241.

[41]Graybiel, A., and Kellogg, R. S., "Inversion Illusion in Parabolic Flight: Its Probable Dependence on Otolith Function," *Aerospace Medicine*, Vol. 38, 1967, pp. 1099–1103.

[42]Martin, J. F., and Melvill Jones, G., "Theoretical Man-Machine Interaction Which Might Lead to Loss of Aircraft Control," *Aerospace Medicine*, Vol. 36. 1965, pp. 713–716.

[43]Money, K. E., Aitkan, J. F., Bondar, R. L., Chevrier, W. T., Garneau, M., Kereliuk, S., Maclean, S., and Thirsk, R., "Experimental Production of Pilot Disorientation in a T33 Aircraft," *Abstract of the 61st Annual Scientific Meeting*, Aerospace Medical Association, 1990, p. 182.

[44]Niven, J. J., Whiteside, T. C. D., and Graybiel, A., "The Elevator Illusion: Apparent Motion of a Visual Target During Vertical Acceleration," *Joint Rept. U.S. Naval School of Aviation Medicine*, NASA No. R-93, 1963.

[45]Roman, J. A., Warren, B. H., and Graybiel, A., "Observation of the Elevator Illusion During Subgravity Preceded by Negative Accelerations," *Aerospace Medicine*, Vol. 35, 1964, pp. 121–124.

[46]Fulgham, D., and Gillingham, K., "Inflight Assessment of Motion Sensation Thresholds and Disorienting Maneuvers," *60th Annual Aerospace Medicine Association Meeting, Proceedings*, 1989.

[47]Tormes, F. R., and Guedry, F. E., Jr., "Disorientation Phenomena in Naval Helicopter Pilots," *Aviation, Space, and Environmental Medicine*, Vol. 46, 1975, pp. 387–393.

[48]von Baumgarten, R. J., Vogel, H., and Kass, J. R., "Nauseogenic Properties of Various Dynamic and Static Force Environments," *Acta Astronautica*, Vol. 8, 1981, pp. 1005–1013.

[49]Matthews, R. S. J., "The G-Excess Effect," *IEEE Engineering in Medicine and Biology*, Vol. 19, 2000, pp. 56–58.

[50]Wade, N. J., and Schone, H., "The Influence of Force Magnitude on the Perception of Body Position. I. Effect of Head Posture," *British Journal of Psychology*, Vol. 62, 1971, pp. 157–163.

[51]Albery, W. B., Park, S., Parker, D., von Gierke, H. E., and Goodyear, C., "The G Excess Effect and Spatial Disorientation: Modifications of Attitude Perception as a Function of $+G_z$ Acceleration and Head Position," *Aviation, Space, and Environmental Medicine*, Vol. 60, 1989, p. 491.

[52]Correia, M. J., Hixson, W. C., and Niven, J. I., "On Predictive Equations for Subjective Judgements of Vertical and Horizontal in a Force Field," *Acta Otolaryngology*, (Suppl.), Vol. 230, 1968, pp. 1–20.

[53]Chelette, T. L., Martin, E. J., and Albery, W. B., (1995). "The Effect of Head Tilt on Perception of Self-Orientation While in Greater Than one G Environment," *Journal of Vestibular Research*, Vol. 5, 1995, pp. 1–17.

[54]Baylor, K. A., Reshke, M., Guedry, F. E., McGrath, B. J., and Rupert, A. H., "Dynamics of the G-Excess Illusion," *Aviation, Space, and Environmental Medicine*, Vol. 63, 1992, pp. 441.

[55]Guedry, F. E., and Rupert, A. H., "Steady State and Transient G-Excess Effects," *Aviation, Space, and Environmental Medicine*, Vol. 62, 1991, pp. 252–253.

[56]Gillingham, K. K., and Previc, F. H., "Spatial Orientation in Flight," *Fundamentals of Aerospace Medicine*, 2nd ed., edited by R. L. DeHart, Williams and Wilkins, Baltimore, MD, 1996, pp. 309–397.

[57]Clark, B., and Graybiel, A., "Vertigo as a Cause of Pilot Error in Jet Aircraft," *The Journal of Aviation Medicine*, Vol. 28, 1957, pp. 469–478.

[58]Benson, A. J., "Spatial Disorientation and the 'Break-Off' Phenomenon," *Aerospace Medicine*, Vol. 44, 1973, pp. 944–952.

[59]Rupert, A., Guedry, F. E., and Clark, J., "Medical Evaluation of Spatial Disorientation Mishaps," *AGARD Conference Proceedings 532, Aircraft Accidents: Trends in Aerospace Medical Investigation Techniques*, 1992, pp. 57-1–57-5.

[60]Roscoe, S. N., "747 Dives into Arabian Sea: Did a Design –Induced Error Cause the Deaths of 210?" *Aviation Accident Investigator*, Vol. 2, 1983, pp. 1–3.

[61]Roscoe, S. N., "Horizon Control Reversals and the Graveyard Spiral," *CSERIAC Gateway*, Vol. VII, No. 3, 1997, pp. 1–4.

[62]Winkler, A. W., "Disorientation Caused by Misinterpretation of the Gyro-Horizon," *BUMED Newsletter, Aviation Suppl.*, Vol. 5, 1945, pp. 1, 2.

[63]Roscoe, S. N., "Designed for Disaster," *Human Factors Society Bulletin*, Vol. 29, No. 9, 1986, p. 5.

[64]Clark, B., and Graybiel, A., "The Effect of Angular Acceleration on Sound Localization: The Audiogyral Illusion," *The Journal of Psychology*, Vol. 28, 1949, pp. 235–244.

[65]Lester, G., and Morant, R. B., "The Role of the Felt Position of the Head in the Audiogyral Illusion," *Acta Psychologica*, Vol. 31, 1969, pp. 375–384.

[66]Graybiel, A., and Niven, J. I., "The Effect of a Change in Direction of Resultant Force on Sound Localization: the Audiogravic Illusion," *Psychophysiological Factors in Spatial Orientation*, edited by A. Graybiel, 1950, pp. 60–66.

[67]Dizio, P., Held, R., Lackner, L. R., Shinn-Cunningham, B., and Durlach, N, "Gravitoinertial Force Magnitude and Direction Influence Head-Centric Auditory Localization," *Journal of Neurophysiology*, Vol. 85, 2001, pp. 2455–2460.

[68]Miller, E. F., II, and Graybiel, A., "Magnitude of Gravitoinertial Force, an Independent Variable in Egocentric Visual Localization of the Horizontal," *Journal of Experimental Psychology*, Vol. 71, 1966, pp. 452–460.

[69]Clark, B., and Graybiel, A., "Influence of Contact Cues on the Perception of the Oculogravic Illusion," *Acta OtoLaryngologica*, Vol. 65, 1968, pp. 373–380.

[70]Bles, W., Jelmorini, M., Bekkering, H., and de Graaaf, B., "Arthrokinetic Information Affects Linear Self-Motion Perception," *Journal of Vestibular Research*, Vol. 5, 1995, pp. 109–116.

[71]Lyons, T. J., and Simpson, C. G., "The Giant Hand Phenomenon," *Aviation, Space, and Environmental Medicine*, Vol. 60, 1989, pp. 64–66.

[72]Malcolm, R., and Money, K., "Two Specific Kinds of Disorientation Incidents: Jet Upset and Giant Hand," AGARD cp: *The Disorientation Incident*, AGARD, Vol. 95, No. 1, 1972, pp. A10-1–A-10-4.

[73]King, P. A. H., "A Report of an Incident of Extreme Spatial Disorientation in Flight," *Aeromedical Reports*, Vol. 1, Inst. of Aviation Medicine, Royal Canadian Air Force, Toronto, Canada, 1962, pp. 22–28.

[74]Braithwaite, M. G., Durnford, S. J., Crowley, J. S., Rosado, N. R., and Albano, J. P., "Spatial Disorientation in U.S. Army Rotary-Wing Operations," *Aviation, Space, and Environmental Medicine*, Vol. 69, 1998, pp. 1031–1037.

[75]Weinstein, L. F., Previc, F. H., Simpson, C. G., Lyons, T. J., and Gillingham, K. K., "A Test of Thumb and Index Finger Control in Overcoming a Visual Analogue of the Giant Hand Illusion," *Aviation, Space, and Environmental Medicine*, Vol. 62, 1991, pp. 336–341.

[76]Melvill Jones, G., "The Loss of Aircraft Control During a Single Rapid Rolling Manoeuvre," *Air Ministry Flying Personnel Research Committee, Royal Air Force, Rept.*, FPRC 933, London, 1955.

[77]Melvill Jones, G., "A Study of Human Factors in the Control of Spinning Aircraft," *Air Ministry Flying Personnel Research Committee, Royal Air Force, Rept.*, FPRC 1248, London, 1966.

[78]Melvill Jones, G., Barry, W., and Kowalsky, N., "Dynamics of the Semicircular Canals Compared in Yaw, Pitch and Roll," *Aerospace Medicine*, Vol. 35, 1964, pp. 984–989.

[79]Melvill Jones, G., "Optokinetic and Vestibulo-Ocular Responses During Simulated Two Dimensional Spinning in the Planes of Yaw and Roll and Yaw Pitch," *Air Ministry Flying Personnel Research Committee, Royal Air Force, Rept.*, FPRC 1246, London, 1966.

[80]Williams, R. S., Werchan, P. M., Fischer, J. R., and Bauer, D. H., "Adverse Effects of G_z in Civilian Aerobatic Pilots," *69th Annual Aerospace Medicine Association Meeting, Proceedings*, 1998.

[81]Anton, D., Burton, R., Flageat, J., Leger, A., and Oosterveld, W. J., "The Musculoskeletal and Vestibular Effects of Long Term Repeated Exposure to Sustained High-G," AGARD AR-317, 1994.

[82]Davis, C., Cammarota, J., Hamilton, R., and Whinnery, J., "Case Report: Benign Paroxysmal Positional Vertigo Associated with Centrifuge Acceleration Exposure," *Aerospace Medical Association*, May 1991.

[83]Lundgren, C. E. G., and Malm, L. U., "Alternobaric Vertigo Among Pilots," *Aerospace Medicine*, Vol. 37, 1966, pp. 178–180.

[84]Enders, L. J., and Rodriguez-Lopez, E., "Aeromedical Consultation Service Case Report: Alternobaric Vertigo," *Aerospace Medicine*, Vol. 41, 1970, pp. 200–202.

[85]Brown, F. M., "Vertigo due to Increased Middle Ear Pressure: Six Year Experience of the Aeromedical Consultation Service," *Aerospace Medicine*, Vol. 42, 1971, pp. 999–1001.

[86]Wicks, R. E., "Alternobaric Vertigo: an Aeromedical Review," *Aviation, Space, and Environmental Medicine*, Vol. 60, 1989, pp. 67–72.

[87]Tjernstrom, O., "On Alternobaric Vertigo—experimental studies," *Forsvarsmedicin*, Vol. 9, 1973, pp. 410–415.

[88]Wise, L. M., "Flying After the Night Before," *Approach*, Vol. 25, No. 4, 1979.

from visual illusions.[6] Because both visual mishaps and Type I SD mishaps are more common among helicopter pilots,[6,7] it might be inferred that visual illusions contribute more to Type I SD than Type II SD; however, no conclusive evidence exists for this conclusion, and certainly visual illusions can contribute to Type I SD mishaps.

Most visual illusions would be expected to occur at night or under conditions of poor visibility, when ambient vision is absent. In fact, most reports suggest that equal numbers of SD mishaps occur in the day vs night.[6,7] This is partly because there are many visual illusions that occur even in broad daylight, as will be described later in this chapter. However, it is also true that most flying, even in this age of aided night vision, is performed during the day. When equated for flying hours, the prevalence of nighttime SD mishaps is many times higher than during the day.[6] For certain maneuvers like helicopter descent to landing, the SD incidence can be up to 50 times greater at night.[8] The nighttime preponderance of SD can mostly be attributable to impoverished visual cues, but fatigue and its facilitory effect on certain visual illusions, such as the autokinetic phenomenon (see Sec. II.B.4), might also be a factor.[9]

One would likely expect most visual illusions to occur at night or under conditions of poor visibility, when ambient vision is absent. Although this supposition might seem obvious, it could be brought into question by a preponderance of reports that suggest equal numbers of SD mishaps occur in the day vs night.[6,7] Two facts bring about this parity—many visual illusions occur even in broad daylight—as will be described later in this chapter—and most flying, even in this age of aided night vision, is performed during the day, which increases the opportunity for a SD mishap to occur during those hours. However, there is not true equity between day and night SD mishaps. When equated for flying hours, the prevalence of nighttime SD mishaps is many times higher than during the day.[6] For certain maneuvers like helicopter descent to landing, the SD incidence can be up to 50 times greater at night.[8] Nonetheless, care must be taken to avoid over stating the correlation between illumination and the occurrence of visual illusions. Although the nighttime preponderance of SD is probably most attributable to impoverished visual cues, fatigue and its facilitory effect on certain visual illusions, such as the autokinetic phenomenon (see Sec. II.B.4), can also be a factor.[9]

Just as the aerial environment is notorious for the many motional illusions that derive from sustained turning and/or frequent misalignment between the gravitoinertial and gravity vectors (see Chapter 6), it is also very conducive to visual illusions. One reason visual illusions are so common in flight is that perceived optical flows and angular perspectives can hold different meanings from their presentations in the ground environment. Whereas optical flow and perspective provide rather unambiguous information on the ground as to our motion in space and the slant of the visual world relative to us, this is not the case in the aerial environment. The conflict arises from optical-flow speed and perspectival splay both being dependent on our height above ground (see Chapter 3, Sec. IV). Specifically, optical-flow speed (for a constant groundspeed) and perspectival splay are both reduced as we increase our altitude above ground and, conversely, are increased as altitude is reduced. This relationship can lead to misperception of height or speed. In the case of optical flow, we cannot tell whether we are flying low and slow or high and fast (see Fig. 1). In the case of perspectival splay, we cannot determine if

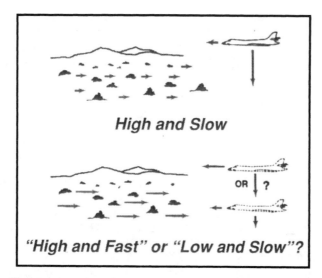

Fig. 1 Conflicting perceptions from optical flow: top panel, optical flow rate while flying slow at high altitude; bottom panel, faster optical flow rate can represent higher speed at the same altitude as above or lower altitude at the same speed as above.

we are flying high relative to a level ground plane or flying low relative to a slanted one (see Fig. 11 in Chapter 3).

Another visual problem largely confined to the aerial environment is the false horizon. There are many sources of Earth-horizontal information in the terrestrial environment (e.g., buildings, roads, etc.), and we usually do not have to worry about our altitude above ground. In the aerial environment, on the other hand, pilots tend to rely heavily on the distant horizon for roll as well as pitch and altitude information. Unfortunately, false horizons can frequently occur in the aerial environment. Sloping cloud decks are a classic example of false horizons that occur in roll, and flying straight and level over a receding shoreline at night can create the illusion of pitching upward against a stable horizon (see Sec. II.A).

An additional reason why certain visual illusions are more prevalent in the aerial environment is that the greater motional freedom allows for visual perceptions that would not be normally experienced on Earth. A prime example of these are inversion illusions, which are almost never encountered in persons without brain damage on Earth because our feet are firmly planted on the ground, and we rarely if ever experience anything more than a brief absence or reversal of our normal 1-G_z force field. During flight, however, fighter pilots know that they can roll their aircraft through 360 deg and can experience reversals of the 1-G_z force field during certain maneuvers, such as leveling off from a climb. Thus, whenever a reversal of the normal luminance gradient occurs or merely in situations where the pilot's vision is totally focused on and dominated by a lead aircraft in front of them (as during aerial refueling or formation flight), a pilot can easily begin to feel inverted. In addition, degraded visual flying environments can lead the pilot to experience visual illusions specifically linked to the abnormal acceleratory environment of flight (see Chapter 6). Prolonged acceleration and turning in one direction—neither of which frequently occurs in the terrestrial environment—are known to lead to the somatogravic and somatogyral illusions, respectively, and these illusions have visual counterparts known as the oculogravic and oculogyral illusions (see Sec. II.4).

Yet another major contributor to visual illusions in the aerial environment are the optical devices through which pilots must view the world. The most widespread of these optical garments are NVGs, whose wear is associated with a much higher rate of SD mishaps than normal daytime flying.[6] Night-vision goggles not only frequently serve to magnify visual illusions experienced with unaided vision, but they can also produce a number of NVG-specific visual illusions, as will be further described in Sec. III.C.1. Other optical devices that might, for various reasons, pose problems for the pilot include forward-looking-infrared (FLIR) displays, collimated optical devices such as head-up displays (HUD) and helmet-mounted displays (HMD), and aircraft windscreens (see Sec. III).

Finally, overall visual attentional demands are much greater in the aerial vs terrestrial environment. As noted in Chapter 4, Sec. IV.A, the workload of pilots can sometimes be so great that they can suffer from a coning ("channelization") of their attentional field,[10] also referred to as tunnel vision. (This is not to be confused by the narrowing of the functional visual field produced by the reduced blood flow at high levels of G_z.) Moreover, whereas we typically have a view of at least part of the ground plane when outdoors at all times, the pilot must often transition from out-the-window to instrument flying, as when flying through broken cloud decks. This transition process is the source of a large percentage of the SD that occurs in flight,[8,11] as vividly described by one F-16 pilot:

> After a while I suggested to break off and set up a new intercept, and when we came clear of the clouds, under a 90° angle, we were looking at the radar to find the target. Then I felt that something was wrong. The sky was rather dark and the white spots turned out to be wave tops. The sensation of climbing out of the top of the cloud layer was soon changed for the reality of a 90° dive. We pulled to 9G, to recover at an altitude of 1000 ft [305 m] (Ref. 2, p. OV-E-2).

II.   Specific Visual Illusions of Flight

This section will present the major known visual illusions of flight, with examples drawn from actual mishaps and incidents. The general subdivision of the visual illusions can be made on the basis of whether ambient vision is available but distorted vs merely inadequate, resulting in a failure of visual dominance and an overreliance on focal visual or nonvisual inputs in the latter case. In actuality, the distinction between having adequate vs inadequate ambient visual references is not clear-cut in many instances. As a general rule, an illusion is more likely to be attributed to misleading ambient visual cues under visual meteorological conditions (VMC; mostly during the day), whereas the illusion is more likely to be attributed to the lack of ambient cues under instrument meteorological conditions (IMC) and impoverished nighttime conditions. A list of the most prominent visual illusions is included in Table 1.

Table 1   Classification of SD-related visual illusions and problems

Illusions	Characteristics
Caused by distorted ambient vision	
False horizons	Polar lights
	Nighttime roadway
	Receding shoreline
	Declined horizon at high altitude
	Ground–sky confusion caused by lights or terrain features
False surface planes	Sloping cloud deck
	Rising terrain
	Foreground ridges
	Crater illusion
Inversion/luminance	Low sun angle over water
	Misperception of moon position
	Lean-on-Sun
Vertical/optical-flow	Hovering over water, snow
	Rotating lights
	Airspeed–attitude confusions
Misjudgment of terrain features	Misperception of vegetation height
	Terrain-density illusions
Caused by absent ambient vision	
Day IMC	Featureless terrain
	Whiteout
	Brownout
	Haze/fog
	Vection IMC formation flight
	Dip illusion
Nighttime landings	Approach/runway light illusions
	"Black-hole" approach
	Runway size/slope, illusions
	Surrounding terrain illusions
Illusory motion of fixed targets	Oculogyral illusion
	Oculogravic illusion
	Elevator illusion
	Autokinetic illusion
Display related	
Refractive	Windscreen magnification
	Spectacle distortions
	Color impairments caused by tinted sunglasses and visors
Collimated flight displays	Accommodative micropsia
	Mandelbaum effect
	Cognitive capture
Night-vision devices	Reduced visual acuity
	Reduced contrast
	Reduced depth perception
	False brightness cueing
	Shadowing illusions

A. Visual Illusions Caused by Distorted Ambient Vision

The illusions that are caused by distorted ambient vision include false horizons, false surface planes, inversion and other luminance-gradient illusions, vection and other optical-flow illusions, and misjudgment of terrain features. Of the preceding illusions, false horizons constitute the most serious of all sources of visual SD problems.[2,12,13] For example, 63% of the 141 experienced instructor pilots surveyed by Sipes and Lessard[13] reported SD caused by "blending of earth and sky," and 52% of them listed "sloping clouds or terrain" as a source of SD. In Matthews et al.'s survey[12] of over 2000 USAF pilots, ~67% reported having experienced SD caused by a sloping horizon and about 25% of them reported it as occurring frequently on sorties. These percentages were similar to reports of SD caused by "lost" horizons. Misjudged terrain altitude was also shown in Matthews et al.'s survey to be a major visual factor contributing to SD, being reported by about 50% of pilots.[12]

1. False Horizons

False horizons can be categorized into two main types: false bank horizons and false pitch horizons. One of the most prevalent sources of false horizons, either in pitch or bank, are nighttime ground lights, with 33% of helicopter pilots in Tormes and Guedry's 1975 survey[8] reporting a misperceived horizon as a result of such lights.

False horizons in bank are known to cause a visual form of the "leans," an illusion that is more widely associated with nonvisual factors, such as a rollout from an undetected bank (see Chapter 6). One surprisingly common false bank illusion is caused by the polar lights (auroras), which are experienced at extreme latitudes (Fig. 2a).[13] Another distortion of ambient vision is created by the lights of an isolated highway veering off into the distance (Fig. 2b), which in one pilot created a vivid sensation of being banked while breaking from a cloud layer in IMC:

> I was flying through scattered clouds at 1200 feet (366 m) during a dark night approach under Instrument Meteorological Conditions (IMC). When the plane got free of the clouds my attention was strongly attracted by an illuminated road that ran at a strange angle to the aircraft. Because I was looking through my Head-up Display, my whole peripheral visual field was filled with this line, which acted like a false horizon. The illusion that I was flying with much bank and pitch was so strong, that I got scared and broke off the approach. This happened a second time, before I managed to get hold of myself and could land safely (Ref. 2, p. OV-E-2).

False horizons in pitch are also very commonly experienced. The classic false horizon of this type is the nighttime shoreline that is mistaken for the actual horizon (Fig. 2c). When a pilot flies over the shoreline, a strong percept of climbing can occur as the shoreline recedes beneath the aircraft if it is misconstrued as the actual horizon. Perhaps the most notorious situation in this regard is taking off from Anderson Air Force Base (AFB) in Guam; even in daytime the receding cliff beyond the runway can give an illusion of climbing. The receding shoreline illusion

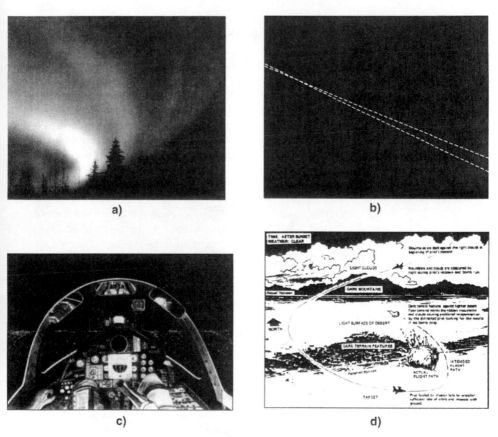

Fig. 2 Illustration of four false horizons: a) the Northern Lights (*aurora borealis*); b) a highway veering off the left; c) a nighttime shoreline (Reproduced from Ref. 14); and d) an aircraft crash into a desert floor that resembled the sky above previously flown-over mountains. (Reproduced with permission of USAF *Flying Safety* magazine; Ref. 15, pp. 12–15.)

is especially dangerous when combined with the gravitoinertial shift resulting from the forward acceleration during takeoff, which adds to the pitch-up/climbing sensation (see Chapter 6). Flying over mountains can also mislead the pilot as to the true elevation of the ground plane and horizon. During a bombing run at dusk, one pilot flew into a desert floor that contained a layer of darkened terrain sandwiched between two lighter regions of the desert floor (Fig. 2d). The pilot evidently mistook the darkened terrain for a mountain and the more distant, lighter desert floor for some clouds. His mistake was probably precipitated by his having just flown into a setting sun prior to circling for the bomb drop and perceiving a lighter sky directly above darkly shadowed mountains.[15] Misjudgment of the true elevation of the horizon and ground plane can also occur whenever a hill or mountain blocks the view of the horizon; this situation will be discussed in greater detail in conjunction with nighttime landing illusions (see Sec. II.B.3).

The same visual conditions can produce false horizons in pitch or bank, depending on the flight path of the aircraft. For example, an isolated, lit roadway can give a false sense of bank at certain angles (see preceding quote), but it also gave one squadron of F-15s the illusion of climbing into a loop as it flew over the roadway at night.[15] It is also known that, at extremely high altitudes, the actual horizon is displaced several degrees lower than it would be at a normal altitude range; for an aircraft flying level at an altitude of 15 km, the horizon appears 4 deg lower than the normal horizon.[14] From the forward view this could lead to a pitch-up sensation, but a side view could lead to an opposite wings-low bank percept. (Fortunately, the high altitudes required for a declination of the horizon also prevent the false horizon from posing as a major safety hazard.) A potentially more devastating false horizon occurring in either pitch or bank results from the confusion of star and ground lights. This illusion was the leading visual illusion reported by Vinacke[1] and the second-most prevalent visual illusion in the survey of Sipes and Lessard,[13] but it was reported by a much smaller percentage (5%) of F-16 pilots in Kuipers et al.'s survey.[2] Star-ground light confusion can occur whenever a pilot flies over a desert or otherwise thinly populated region where the density of ground lights approach that of the stars in nighttime sky. In one situation a pilot flying over a fishing fleet at night actually inverted his aircraft because of the illusion that that the fishing lights represented starlight from above.* Although a false horizon can result from this situation, another possible outcome is that no horizon can be ascertained, thereby making it more of an "absent" ambient visual illusion. Blending of Earth and sky can also occur in conditions of haze, brownout, and whiteout, as discussed in Sec. II.B.1.

2.   False Surface Planes

False surface planes can occur in either pitch or bank and tend to produce SD illusions that resemble those produced by false horizons. The most prominent surface effect that causes a bank illusion is the sloping cloud deck, which typically results from a weather front moving laterally relative to the path of the aircraft (see Fig. 3). Almost half of the pilots surveyed by Tormes and Guedry[8] reported experiencing a visual illusion caused by a sloping cloud bank. When encountering a cloud deck that slopes from left to right, it is common to level the aircraft with reference to the deck rather than the true ground plane. On the other hand, distant cloud decks that slope parallel to the flight path can lead to a pitch illusion, as might have occurred in one mishap when the pilot allegedly sensed a false sense of straight-and-level flight as he actually descended at 1160 m/min (3800 ft/min) into a large lake.[15] This example points to the fact that even though cloud deck illusions can occur at altitude, the SD they produce can linger to the point that the pilot loses too much altitude to be able to recover the aircraft.

It is more serious when a false ground plane is created. As shown in Fig. 11 of Chapter 3, an especially dangerous false ground plane occurs when the pilot misinterprets the narrower perspective information from a slanted ground plane as lying along a flat plane that is viewed from a higher altitude, thereby leading

---

* Personal communication with Dr. Alan Benson, Oct. 2000.

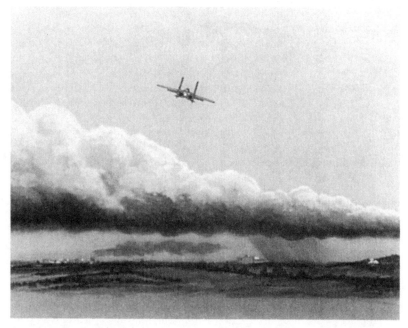

Fig. 3   Tendency to fly level to a sloping cloud deck. (Reproduced from Ref. 14.)

to an altitude misjudgment. Mishaps involving rising terrain contributed to a large proportion of the >150 USAF mishaps that occurred during low-level flight in the 1970s and 1980s (Ref. 16). One such representative mishap occurred in 1990 when a T-38 pilot flew too low over a canyon that contained rising terrain leading up to it and clipped a power cable at less than 200 ft (61 m) above the ground. The pilot, who survived the incident and flew his damaged aircraft back safely, reportedly felt his altitude was approximately double his actual one just before impact.

Rising terrain in the form of foreground ridges can pose special problems because of distance parallax and shadowing by the sun. Parallax refers to the geometrical phenomenon that nearby ground objects might be closer in altitude to the aircraft than more distant ground objects, even though the nearby objects appear at a lower angle than do the distant objects (Fig. 4a). Parallax might have been a contributing factor to the crash of a jet fighter at a training exercise in Nevada in the early 1980s (Ref. 17). The jet impacted a foreground ridge that appeared to be much lower than the distant ridge, when it was actually 6.1 m (20 ft) higher than the latter (Fig. 4b). The effects of shadowing by the sun are especially dangerous when the pilot faces the sun, in which case total shadowing of the foreground ridge occurs, and when the sun angle is directly behind the pilot, in which case no shadowing of the ridge occurs (see Fig. 5). A major contributing factor to rising terrain mishaps is the sparseness of the surrounding terrain, which removes many of the crucial size and density texture gradients normally used in judging distances (see Chapter 3, Sec. IV.C.2). Also, aerial perspective is of reduced effectiveness in dry, high-altitude locales where the air is thinner. Theoretically, the presence of a foreground ridge could be separated from a more distant one using motion

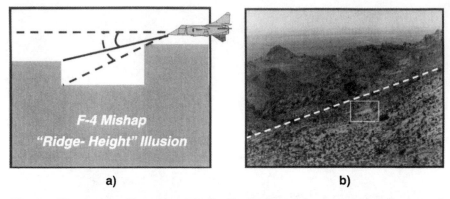

a)   b)

Fig. 4a   Illustration of how visual declination angle can be greater for a foreground ridge, despite its greater altitude.
Fig. 4b   Photo showing the impact (in box) of an F-4 aircraft against a foreground ridge (dashed line). (Photo reproduced with permission of Dr. Bob Kellogg.)

parallax cues, but the ability to detect motion discontinuities at safe distances is problematic for sparse and irregular textures.[18]

A false surface-plane illusion that occurs under nighttime conditions is the "crater" illusion, which has been reported by helicopter pilots using NVGs.[6] This illusion is caused by the position of the landing light being too far under the nose of the aircraft, rather than pointing ahead to the intended landing site. Evidently, the reflections on the surface immediately below and the sharp shadowing around it make the surface appear further away than it actually is, resulting in the increased likelihood of a hard landing.

3. Inversion and Other Luminance Illusions

An extreme distortion of ambient vision occurs whenever a pilot feels inverted while flying because of visual factors. Usually, this is caused by a reversal of the

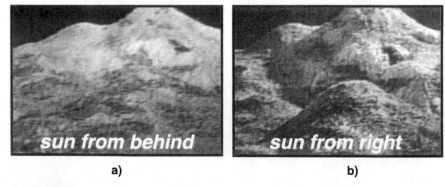

a)   b)

Fig. 5   Effects of shadowing by the sun. A simulated view of a foreground ridge when viewed with the sun a) positioned behind the aircraft and b) positioned to the right of the aircraft.

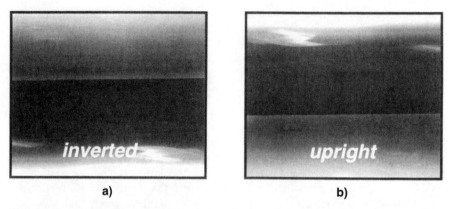

a)   b)

Fig. 6   Two simulated views of sky–water demarcation while facing a weather front at a low sun angle: a) an inverted view and b) an upright view. Either view can be interpreted as upright (or inverted).

normal luminance gradient featuring a lighter sky against a darker background. Little data exist concerning the prevalence of visual inversion illusions, but they are believed to have contributed to several SD mishaps in the past. The purely visual-inversion illusion should be differentiated from the inversion illusions experienced by pilots during level off from a climb and other maneuvers in which the G vector is reduced or even reversed in magnitude (see Chapter 6, Sec. III.A.3), as well as from inversion illusions experienced by astronauts in the 0-G environment of space. (However, there is sometimes a visual component to the latter illusion, in that astronauts might more readily experience it when looking out the window and seeing the Earth above the dark sky below it.)

Perhaps the most common type of inversion illusion occurs when a pilot flies over water while the sun is at a low angle and a weather front is approaching. In this situation, shown in Fig. 6, the water reflects the sunlight and can appear lighter than the sky as dark clouds block the sun's rays. The longer-wavelength light of the sun might additionally appear to represent a distant shoreline, thereby strengthening the illusion. Another instance in which inversion illusions can occur is at night when a full moon reflects off a low cloud deck. In this situation the cloud deck might appear so bright that the pilot of the aircraft actually perceives it to be a ceiling deck rather than a floor deck, particularly when wearing NVGs because the image intensification makes the reflection of the moon appear brighter still.* Sipes and Lessard[13] reported that 8% of their pilots experienced a false-vertical SD illusion from the position of the moon. A vivid description of one such moon-induced inversion illusions was provided by a research colleague who was also an experienced combat pilot:

> After a short period of perhaps 10 minutes of flight time, I raised up out of the cockpit again and looked out and down at what I thought should be the lights of Seoul [the capital of Korea], and lo and behold there was the moon—a bright,

---

* Personal communication with Dr. Chuck Antonio, July 2000.

full moon—below me, which immediately indicated that I was flying upside down . . . and was now looking up at the moon instead of looking down at the lights of Seoul. And, in a panic reaction believing I was upside-down, I rolled the airplane sharply 180° to put myself in the right-up position and promptly fell out of the sky. It wasn't until I had actually entered into the undercast that I realized that what I had seen was the moon reflecting off the top of the clouds!"*

The lean-on-sun illusion, reported by 10% of pilots,[13] is another example of how altered luminance gradients can disorient the pilot. When flying through clouds, the direction of the brightest portion of the visual world will vary depending on the time of day, as only during the middle of the day will the sunlight emanate from above. Hence, pilots who orient in relationship to the normal luminance gradient of our world might end up banking their aircraft when the morning or afternoon sun is at a low angle. Luminance inversions can also occur at extremely high altitudes (>30,000 m), and this has been associated with the break-off phenomenon (see Chapter 4, Sec. VI.A).

4. Vection and Other Optical-Flow Illusions

A final type of ambient visual illusion found in the aerial environment involves vection and other optical-flow illusions. Vection is not routinely perceived during most phases of fixed-wing flight for two reasons. First, most visual motion experienced by pilots occurs in the context of actual motion. More importantly, the typical optical-flow speeds are too low to experience vection at most altitudes. Below 100 m, however, optical flow is clearly experienced, and below 15 m (50 ft) a strong sense of "ground rush" occurs.[17] Vection-related illusions are perceived in certain instances and were reported by about 5% of fighter pilots in the survey of Kuipers et al.[2] By contrast, over 90% of U.S. Coast Guard helicopter pilots had experienced vection in the survey of Ungs.[19]

The most frequent situation causing vection in helicopter pilots is hovering over water, especially at night. In such a visually degraded environment, the downwash created by the rotor action of the blades creates a divergent optical flow that can actually subtend a very large visual angle (Fig. 7). Directly in front of the helicopter, the movement is perceived as forward flow that gives rise to the illusion of drifting backward[20] and a consequent tendency to move the helicopter forward. Rotor wash can also lead to vection in blowing snow conditions and during hovering over tall waving grass, particularly when wearing NVGs.[20,21]

The normal vection experience of helicopter pilots is not to be confused with the effects of rotating blades or rotating anticollision lights. Such effects are associated with a phenomenon known as flicker vertigo, which was reported by 25–30% of all pilots in the surveys of Johnson[22] and Sipes and Lessard[13] and by an even higher percentage (70%) in the survey of Tormes and Guedry.[8] Whereas vection can occur in response to such motions, the major effects of such stroboscopic motion are headaches, dizziness, and other disorientating symptoms that represent more of an annoyance or distraction to the pilot than a source of vection per se. Anticollision lights can occasionally lead to bizarre visual illusions, as when the reflection of a red rotating anticollision light off salt spray during a low-altitude

---

* Personal communication with retired USAF Col. Dan Fulgham, Sept. 1998.

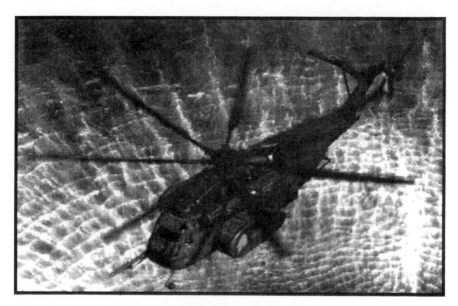

Fig. 7 Illustration of the linear motion stimulus created by the rotor wash of a helicopter. (Photo reproduced with permission of Art Estrada.)

hover led a pilot to falsely perceive a fire in one of his helicopter engines.[8] Although flickering lights can also in rare instances result in photosensitive epilepsy, there are no reports that this symptom has contributed to an actual SD incident in flight.

As noted in Sec. I, optical flow is an inherently ambiguous cue in the aerial environment because global optical-flow speed is influenced by both forward groundspeed as well as altitude (Fig. 1). Lowering one's altitude ordinarily increases the optical-flow rate by decreasing the distance to objects, but decreasing one's forward airspeed counteracts this effect. Hence, optical-flow ambiguity should be suspected whenever low-level maneuvers result in a ground impact and the aircraft's airspeed prior to impact was unusually slow. Such was the case in the aforementioned crash in Nevada, because the aircraft's airspeed was only 288 km/h (150 kn) just prior to impact.[17] A similar visual situation might have contributed to the crash of a B-1 bomber in 1997 over the Western United States.

Besides the vection and optical-flow illusions that occur in day VMC, there are other types of vection that occur primarily during formation flight in IMC, as will be discussed in Sec. II.B.2.

5. Terrain Misjudgments

Misjudgment of terrain features and a consequent overestimation or underestimation of altitude can occur even in day VMC and even with flat terrain. This problem is encountered most frequently during low-level (nap-of-Earth) flight in helicopters. Thus, these illusions are to be distinguished from the altitude illusions that occur at night and/or in IMC or the illusions associated with rising terrain described in Sec. II.A.2.

Misjudgment of terrain elevation can occur whenever the size or density of ground textures is different from what is normally encountered or expected, which requires what in pilot jargon is referred to as a "recalibration of the eyeballs." This often occurs when pilots transition to flying in a desert environment, where the terrain is sparser and the vegetation is smaller.[23,24] Sparse terrain can lead to an erroneous perception of a lower-than-actual altitude, whereas oversized and undersized vegetation can lead to an underestimation and overestimation of altitude respectively. An example of an underestimation of altitude occurred when a helicopter aircrewman almost jumped out of a plane at 9.1 m (30 ft) above ground because what he thought was a paper cup turned out to be a king-size fried-chicken carton.[16] Conversely, larger-than-expected vegetation can lead to an underestimation of altitude and too high an approach upon landing, as in the case of an Indian Air Force pilot who was used to flying over tea plantations and underestimated the height of the tall eucalyptus trees while landing in a different region of the country.[25]

Misperceived vegetation height can prove especially devastating when the vegetation is smaller than expected and the pilot unknowingly lowers the altitude of the aircraft, especially during an approach to landing (Ref. 14, Fig. 17). This can occur not only in a desert or semi-arid environment but also in extreme latitudes like Northern Norway and the Aleutian Islands, where pine and birch trees tend to be smaller on average than in the Continental U.S. and Europe.[26] Another visual situation that can give rise to an overestimation of altitude is the presence of elongated shadowing at low sun angles, which can give the impression that trees might be taller than they actually are.[16] Sometimes the misperceived height of nonliving objects, such as small rocks perceived as large boulders at a correspondingly greater distance, can also affect one's judgment of altitude.[16] Conversely, one pilot so severely overestimated his altitude that he mistook a beehive lying on the ground for a camper vehicle.*

Flying over a sparse terrain is often dangerous because of the lack of regular texture spacing, but a low texture density can also sometimes prevent a pilot from flying too low because it can lead to an underestimation of one's actual altitude, as noted in Chapter 3, Sec. IV.C.2. Conversely, flying over dense terrain can in some cases lead to an overestimation of altitude; in simulators, pockets of dense terrain often lead pilots to fly too low when asked to maintain a constant altitude.[†] As noted in Chapter 3, Sec. IV.C.2, dense vegetation on hills can even help to disguise an upsloping terrain.

To minimize the likelihood of perceiving a visual illusion during low-level flight in day VMC, pilots should be made aware through preflight planning of the terrain topography, vegetation height, and sun angle. During the sortie, pilots should 1) be alert for impending terrain changes, 2) increase their terrain-clearance altitude as their workload increases, 3) make proper use of their altitude warning and terrain-avoidance systems, and 4) never lose sight of the horizon for more than a brief instant while turning at low level and then only to quickly cross check their instruments.[27] Indeed, any turning and looking away from the horizon should always be accompanied by a slight climb of the aircraft. Finally, it has

---

* Personal communication with Wing Cdr. Roger Matthews, Oct. 2003.
† Personal communication with Dr. Rik Warren, June 1991.

been shown that extensive training at maintaining altitude under various low-level terrain conditions can improve the subsequent ability to maintain proper clearance.[28] This is especially true of low-level NVG training programs, whose emphasis on aggressive out-the-window scanning and increased attention has led to benefits even while flying at low level in daytime.*

B. Visual Illusions Caused by Absent Ambient Vision

In IMC and nighttime VMC sorties, visual illusions are caused not only by a distorted ambient visual scene but also by an absent one. A reduction in the amount and quality of ambient vision can occur when using various night-vision devices (NVD), (see Sec. III.C) as well as in four main unaided viewing situations: 1) day IMC conditions (flying over water and other featureless terrain, whiteout, brownout, and haze/fog), 2) formation flying at night or IMC, 3) nighttime (black-hole) landings, and 4) nighttime flying in which apparent movements of small spots occur even though they are actually stationary relative to the pilot (as in the oculogyral, oculogravic, and autokinetic phenomena). In predominantly fixed-wing flying communities the most serious of the preceding SD traps is the nighttime landing, in which 79% of the pilots in Sipes and Lessard's[13] survey and over 50% of pilots in Matthews et al.'s[12] survey experienced SD. This is consistent with the high prevalence of actual mishaps occurring during landing.

1. Day IMC Illusions

The day IMC illusions are very dangerous because the absence of good horizon and/or terrain information is frequently compounded by poor overall visibility in such cases as whiteout (blowing snow), brownout (blowing sand or dust), and haze or fog. The reductions in visibility tend to result in an overestimation of altitude above ground,[26] partly because loss of contrast usually occurs with increasing distance, as in aerial perspective (see Chapter 3, Sec. IV.C.2). As reported by Sipes and Lessard,[13] brownout and whiteout were experienced by 64 and 42%, respectively, of the pilots in their survey.

Featureless terrain mainly takes the form of desert, water, snow, or tundra. As with loss of visibility, lack of terrain information in these cases generally results in a tendency to fly too low, unless flying on instruments.[29] Although horizon information might be available, it is not attended to always. Close to the ground, the aircraft might appear to fall below the horizon, and a feeling of engulfment can occur.[16] A well-known near mishap caused by flying over water occurred in 1985, when an F-15 plunged nearly 4570 m (15,000 ft) in less than 10 s when the pilot did not realize he was flying straight toward the ocean. Only the sound of his rapidly diving aircraft alerted the pilot that he was in a steep descent, and he managed to recover his aircraft less than 100 m above the ocean. In a UH-60 helicopter simulator, flying over water was associated with a greater misjudgment of altitude and more frequent crashes than flying over land.[28] However, rough seas with waves and whitecaps can create sufficient texture for judging altitude, as can a helicopter's rotor wash in some cases.

---

* Personal communication with Dr. Chuck Antonio.

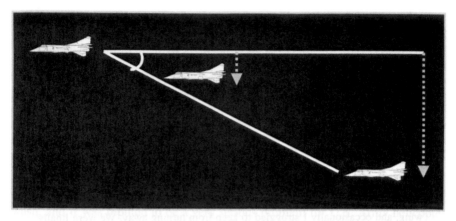

Fig. 8 Illustration of the dip illusion, in which a trailing aircraft that maintains a constant viewing angle to the leader lowers its altitude as separation distance from lead increases.

altitude.] As the trailing aircraft increases its separation distance, maintaining the same visual angle on the windscreen will require a drop in altitude because of the increased distance to lead (Fig. 8). For example, an aircraft must drop almost 100 ft (30 m) in altitude for every additional mile of separation distance to preserve a 1 deg angular relationship to lead. In this respect the dip illusion bears similarity to the Nevada fighter crash described earlier in Sec. II.A.2. Both are affected by monocular parallax. The problem of maintaining orientation relative to a small fixation target is not limited to formation flight, and some of the general aspects of target-fixation SD illusions will be discussed in the next section.

In many respects a disoriented pilot in formation can be more dangerous than a disoriented pilot flying alone because the latter can focus all of his efforts in regaining his or her spatial orientation. The issue of what procedures to follow when spatially disoriented in a flying formation—such as the lost-wingman procedure—is discussed in Chapter 8, Sec. II.E.1.

3. Nighttime Landings

A large percentage of SD incidents and mishaps occur during the landing phase of flight. In commercial aviation 70% of all controlled-flight-into-terrain (CFIT) accidents occur during the landing phase.[31] In USAF[4] and U.S. Navy[7] studies, approximately 12 and 25%, respectively, of all SD mishaps occurred during landing, with most occurring at night. As already noted, the majority of pilots have experienced SD illusions while landing at night.[12,13]

There are many reasons why landing at night is conducive to visual illusions, above and beyond the problem of nonvisible terrain surrounding the runway. Many SD incidents have occurred because of nonstandard or malfunctioning approach lights.[26,32,33] Problems in clearly demarcating the approach and runway lights can lead to landing short,[26,32] strobing lights can lead to vection sensations,[15] overly bright lights allegedly cause afterimages in helicopter landings,[33] and unevenly lit runway lights (i.e., one side brighter than the other) can cause bank illusions.[26] Nonstandard runway width and slope can produce illusions or height and distance, as will be discussed later in this section. Fog or haze can render nighttime landings still more dangerous, usually by reducing runway-light intensity and creating an illusion of approaching too high,[26] but sometimes by producing the opposite result if the fog is very low and the runway lights appear larger than normal.[15] The preceding factors are more likely to cause an SD illusion if a pilot is flying into an unfamiliar runway.[34]

Even when flying into a standard runway at night, pilots tend to make too low an approach (also known as a "duck-under" approach).[34-37] The lack of terrain information surrounding to runway—which produces the illusion of landing in a black hole—is mainly responsible for the low-approach tendency because the latter also occurs when landing over water or featureless terrain.[26,34] Indeed, 40% of all commercial CFIT landing accidents occur when the surrounding terrain is not highly textured.[31]

Most theories of the black-hole illusion have focused on the pilot's perceived form of the runway and the misjudgment of perspective that results therefrom. Runway form, with its perspective and compression cues, can reliably signal approach angle. Indeed, runway size and shape are the two most important cues used by pilots in landing their aircraft.[38] Changes in approach angle result in an increase in form ratio (FR), using the equation

$$FR = \tan\theta \times L/W \qquad (1)$$

where θ equals the approach angle and L and W represent the length and width of the runway, respectively. It has been shown that perceived FR corresponds very closely to simulated approach angle in laboratory simulations.[39] This high correlation is to be expected if size and shape constancy were to hold (see Chapter 3, Sec. IV.C.3) and changes in the projective image of the runway are interpreted as changes in our orientation and distance relative to it. Thus, misjudgment of runway form clearly contributes to the tendency to fly a low approach in the black-hole situation.

One leading theory of the black-hole illusion is that pilots base their visual approach angles on the width of the runway while landing at night, whereas during the day they base their judgments on the true perspective angle (which extends beyond the lateral edge of the runway). This relationship is shown in Fig. 9, for daytime (left) and nightime (right) landing situations. Perrone[37] argues that by using the runway half-width (x_1) at night, rather than the correct distance Y, results in a FR (in essence, perspectival splay) that conveys a steeper approach than is actually the case. Using the formula:

$$\tan\beta = 2DL\sin\theta\tan\theta/W(D + L\cos\theta) \qquad (2)$$

where $\tan\beta$ is the perceived approach angle, D is the distance of the pilot's eye to the aimpoint, θ is the actual approach path, and W and L are the width and length (from aimpoint to endline) of a normal sized runway [$W = 61$ m (200 ft); $D = 1830$ m (6000 ft), Perrone[37] calculates that the perceived approach angle for an actual 3-deg slope will be approximately doubled at night. To perceive a normal 3-deg glide slope, Perrone predicts that pilots would have to fly an actual 2 deg slope, which matches data from Mertens and Lewis.[40] Interestingly, Perrone[37] predicts that no black-hole illusion should occur for runways with a $D:W$ ratio

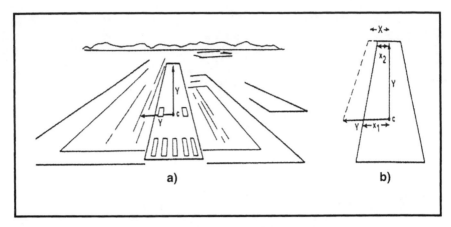

Fig. 9   Calculation of approach (slant) angle during a) daytime landing and b) night-time landing. (Reproduced with permission of Perrone; Ref. 37.)

of 16:1. Hence, if the runway width in Eq. (2) were doubled to 122 m (400 ft) the low-approach tendency would disappear.

Perrone's theory predicts the glide slope within a few miles of the runway, but does not hold for larger distances and might not be capable of explaining the black-hole illusion in its entirety. For example, we have specific distance tendencies, particularly in terms of spatial memory, that might place the ground farther away than is actually the case when it is no longer visible (Fig. 3 in Chapter 3).

Because the form ratio increases (and perspectival splay decreases) with narrower, slanted runways, a stronger illusion would be predicted (and is, in fact, obtained) from such runways.[26,35,40] In Eq. (2) a narrow runway decreases the denominator, and an increasing approach angle θ, caused by an up-sloping runway, would increase the numerator. An illustration of how narrow runways can yield a higher perceived approach angle (and, therefore, greater elevation) is shown in Fig. 10. The left photo (Fig. 10a) shows a view of a runway at Shaw AFB, South

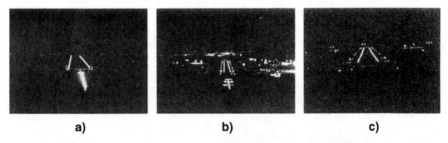

Fig. 10   Effect of runway size on perceived runway distance: a) view of a runway at Shaw AFB, South Carolina, from a mile out and 350 ft above touchdown; b) view of a runway at Ramstein AFB, Germany, from the same distance and height; and c) view of the same runway at Ramstein AFB from 1000 ft out and 120 ft above touchdown. (Photos reproduced with permission of Lt. Col. Robert Johnson.) Note the essentially same visual perspectives of a) and c).

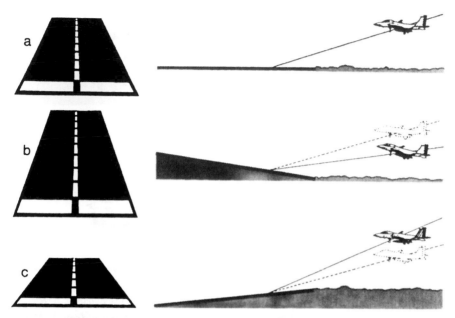

Fig. 11   Effect of different runway slopes on runway perspective on the pilot's actual approach (——) and perceived approach (---). (Reproduced from Ref. 14.)

Carolina, from approximately 1 mile (1.61 km) out and 350 ft (107 m) above touchdown, while the middle photo (Fig. 10b) shows a view of a much narrower runway at Ramstein AFB in Germany from the same altitude and distance. To achieve the same perspective angle as in Fig. 10a when flying into Ramstein AFB, a pilot must be 1000 ft (305 m) from, and 120 ft (37 m) above, touchdown (Fig. 10c)—a dangerous situation if the pilot assumes the aircraft position to be at the higher altitude.

In contrast to up-sloping and narrow runways, wider and down-sloping runways increase perspectival splay and result in a tendency to make too high an approach. The effects of runway slope on approach tendency are illustrated in Fig. 11. Even the slope of terrain leading up to flat runways can affect approach angle, with up-sloping foreground terrain resulting in a lower than desired approach, and downsloping foreground terrain producing a high approach.[26] Both of these tendencies are shown in Fig. 12.

The effects of up-sloping terrain are even more pronounced when the up-slope occurs beyond the runway. This feature, often in the form of city lights on a hillside, occurs at many commercial and military airports and tends to increase the low-approach tendency associated with normal nighttime landings. One explanation for this effect is that the decreased perspectival splay associated with the up-sloping hillside increases the distance of all elements of the scene, including the runway. However, the effect of up-sloping terrain appears to lower the position of the runway even more than the hillside lights. Hence, another explanation for this effect is that pilots erroneously move the unseen or implicit horizon in the same direction as the top of the surrounding rise, that is, toward the top of the

pattern of landing lights that effectively fused the overrun and landing light patterns. All three aircraft landed short of the runway, with the last pilot landing almost 1500 m short of the runway and causing major damage to his aircraft.

4. Illusory Visual Motion of Small Targets Resulting from Aircraft or Self-Motion

One of the most common SD incidents pilots experience while flying at night involves the illusory perception of aircraft or Earth stationary visual spots (whether they be distant stars, reflections from cockpit lights onto the windscreen, or fixed ground lights) as moving. Reflections on a windscreen tend to be the most disorientating, as reported by 36% of helicopter pilots surveyed by Tormes and Guedry.[8] Vinacke[1] reported the autokinetic phenomenon (to be described later in this section) as accounting for almost one-quarter of the visual illusions experienced by pilots in his survey, and Sipes and Lessard[13] reported that 54% of their pilots experienced illusions broadly defined as autokinetic. (One of the pilots in the Sipes and Lessard[13] survey reported over 100 instances of autokinetic illusions while flying.) In some aircraft such as the F-16—which has a large bubble canopy that at night contains prominent reflections from inside the cockpit—entire fields of reflected light might appear to move, in what has been termed the "Star Wars" effect.[2] All of these illusions pose a big danger for pilots if they mistake the movement of these fixated lights as movement relative to other aircraft, which they then follow. One of the more dramatic examples of such confusion was a case where the pilot nearly tracked a train light (which he thought to be a lead aircraft, and which was probably actually moving at the time) into the ground. Fortunately, most of the "target-motion" illusions are categorized as Type II SD, from which the pilot eventually recovers.

There are three major situations in which small, stationary lights that are fixated appear to move (Fig. 15). Two of these situations occur while the pilot is experiencing angular motion or linear acceleration, along with their aftereffects, and produce what are termed the oculogyral and oculogravic illusions, respectively (Figs. 15a and 15b). In these illusions any lights that are fixed with respect to the aircraft will appear to move in conjunction with the pilot's motion percept. The other major illusory situation occurs after a prolonged fixation lasting at least 10 s, in a phenomenon known as the autokinetic illusion (Figure 15c). One related SD trap that has proven dangerous in the past is the prolonged fixation and orientation to a moving flare dropped from an aircraft while attempting to keep the flare in sight (i.e., the "moth" effect). Although rotary-winged pilots continue to use aerial flares for marking targets and other points of interest on the ground, laser illuminators have largely supplanted aerial flares in fixed-wing aircraft; consequently, this illusion was rarely mentioned in recent surveys of predominantly fixed-wing pilots.[12,13]

The oculogyral illusion, which was first described by Graybiel and Hupp,[42] refers to the illusory movement of an observer-fixed visual field or objects lying within the field during stimulation of the semicircular canals (Fig. 15a). This illusion has both a static component (i.e., target displacement in the same direction as the perceived angular rotation) as well as a dynamic one (i.e., target rotation in the same direction as the perceived rotation). It can occur for both a structured scene,

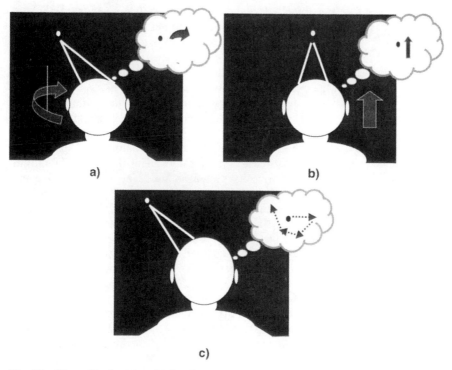

Fig. 15 Three illusions in which a fixated target appears to move: a) *oculogryal* **illusion during perceived right rotation; b)** *oculogravic* **illusion during perceived pitching upward; and c)** *autokinetic* **illusion with head stationary. (Arrows in thought balloon represent motion percept.)**

as well as for a small target light, but the oculogyral illusion is much stronger and lasts much longer when viewing a small target.[43,44] Essentially, the oculogyral illusion represents, like the various oculogravic illusions, a failure of the static visual image to achieve visual dominance over the motion percept.

The oculogyral illusion can occur during both the acceleratory (perrotatory) and deceleratory (postrotatory) phases of a turn. The threshold for the oculogyral illusion—as little as 0.3 deg/s^2 (Refs. 26 and 45)—has been shown in many studies to be less than the threshold for the perception of bodily rotation (see Chapter 2, Sec. III.E); hence, during the perrotatory phase, this illusion might actually help to detect the initial turning motion.[46] Because of their inertial lag, however, the semicircular canals no longer sense a sustained turn and can actually signal rotation in the opposite direction once the original turn is stopped. In this postrotatory situation, known as the somatogyral illusion (see Chapter 6, Sec. II.A), a pilot can fly straight and level but feel the aircraft to be turning and banked. Any lights that are fixed relative to the pilot (or aircraft) will usually appear to move in the same direction as the illusory turning. This is certainly true of cockpit lights, and even images of stars can appear to move because they are so distant that they ordinarily remain stationary with respect to the pilot in space, at least during pure linear motion of the aircraft. Although the movement of lights in the oculogyral illusion is paradoxical in that the lights appear to move without substantial displacement, the illusion is sufficient for the pilot to begin to track the lights or fly the aircraft in relation to them. Because the illusion continues, even as the pilot flies toward the lights, the pilot thereby can enter a prolonged, descending spiral without being aware of the fact that the tracked light is not actually moving in space.

The oculogravic illusion, first studied by Graybiel,[47] refers to the illusory movement of a visual target that occurs when the resultant gravitoinertial force vector deviates from the direction of gravity (Fig. 15b). As such, the oculogravic illusion represents a visual analogue of the already described somatogravic illusion (see Chapter 6, Sec. III.A). It is related to, but not dependent upon, normal otolith functioning because the somatosensory system is also capable of signaling the direction of the gravitoinertial force. It can occur in response to gravitoinertial shifts caused by either G_x (longitudinal) or G_y (lateral) forces. However, the G_y situation is less relevant in the aerial environment because pilots usually maintain their aircraft in alignment with the resultant force vector during coordinated turning, which otherwise would produce substantial G_y from the inside of the turn and lead to a perceived "skidding" of the aircraft. The threshold for experiencing the oculogravic illusion in the upright position is about 1.5 deg, which is comparable to the threshold for perceiving actual body tilt.[48]

When exposed to $+G_x$ forces during the acceleration accompanying takeoff, or $-G_x$ forces during the deceleration accompanying landing, target lights that are fixed relative to the aircraft will appear to pitch in the same direction as the pilot's whole-body somatogravic sensation. This is especially true of objects lying within the subject's frame of motion, such as cockpit instrument lights. The pitching movement of cockpit lights can confirm the subject's illusory pitch sensation, and the pilot might also attempt to orient his or her aircraft relative to the illusory movement of lights that lie outside of the cockpit. A related illusion is the elevator illusion, which results in the upward displacement of a small light as a result of excessive shearing of the otolith organs even when the resultant gravitoinertial direction does not markedly differ from vertical,[49] as can occur in a level off from a descent. (The reverse can also occur when a person is exposed to a < 1 G force; (see Chapter 6, Sec. III.A.4). The upward target movements occur partly because exposure to a >1 G_z force in the upright position is similar to a backward head tilt in that both increase the shearing of the otolith organs. [The utricle does not lie perpendicular to gravity but is rather upwardly sloped at its anterior end by about 25 deg (see Chapter 2, Sec. III.G.1). Because of this slope, a certain amount of shearing of the otolith occurs even in the upright, 1-G position, which is increased still further beyond 1 G_z and is decreased as G_z falls below 1 G_z.]

There are two major explanations as to why the oculogyral and oculogravic illusions occur. One explanation is that in order to fixate a small target subjects attempt to suppress the nystagmus resulting from either the canals (in the case of the oculogyral illusion) or the otoliths (in the case of the oculogravic illusion).[50,51] During the oculogyral illusion, the illusory turning is accompanied by a slow-phase nystagmus in the opposite direction; hence, an efferent voluntary-pursuit command in the direction of the turn must be added to suppress that nystagmus and maintain fixation on a target. This pursuit drive leads to the perception of target movement in the same direction as the turning sensation. In the case of the oculogravic and elevator illusions, $+G_x$ inertial forces and excess $+G_z$ forces, respectively, both produce a downward slow-phase nystagmus of the eyes, as would occur during a backward head tilt. This rotation, known as the "doll's eye" reflex, must be suppressed by an upward pursuit drive, which, in turn, gives rise to a perceived upward movement of a fixated target. Unfortunately, the nystagmus-suppression hypothesis is contradicted by a number of pieces of evidence, especially in the case of the oculogyral illusion. For example, the perrotatory oculogyral illusion dissipates long before nystagmus ceases during prolonged turning,[26,45] and the oculogyral illusion ends before nystagmus ceases in the postrotatory period.[44] Also, the oculogyral illusion occurs even in individuals whose eye muscles are damaged and cannot produce nystagmus.[52] Finally, an afterimage that remains stationary on the retina—thereby eliminating the need for a pursuit drive—also appears to move in the same direction as the movement of the outside scene in the oculogyral and oculogravic illusions.[45,47]

An alternative hypothesis to the nystagmus-suppression one is that the oculo-gyral, oculogravic, and elevator illusions are all related to what is perceived to lie within the pilot's frame of motion. If a pilot feels himself or herself to be rotating or tilting, it would seem only natural that objects lying within the pilot's frame of motion (i.e., that are fixed relative to his or her body) would also appear to move in the same direction. This would include cockpit lights and anything else that appears fixed relative to aircraft; indeed, when one experiences the oculogravic illusion from the cabin during takeoff in a commercial airplane, even the bulkhead of the aircraft appears to pitch up. On the other hand, apparent motion of visual images that appear to be part of Earth-fixed space (e.g., the runway and surrounding terrain, as viewed from inside the aircraft) is less likely to occur. Small lights that appear to lie outside of the pilot's frame of motion but are not perceived as Earth-fixed—such as the lights of another aircraft—might also appear to move.

The final illusion to be considered in this section is the autokinetic illusion (Fig. 15c). This illusion, which was first reported by Von Humbolt in 1850 (see Refs. 26 and 45), is caused by prolonged fixation (>10 s) of a small, dim light in a darkened environment. The velocity of the illusory target motion has been estimated as high as 10 deg/s, and the total distance "traversed" by the target can range from a few centimeters in central vision to several meters when the target is viewed peripherally.[26,45] The role of eye movements in the generation of the autokinetic illusion is somewhat more supported than in the case of the oculogyral and oculogravic illusions. Although eye movements are not of sufficient magnitude to account for the entire distance traversed by the spot, involuntary ocular drifts begin to occur with a similar latency range, and in opposite direction to, the movement of the target.[51] It is believed, therefore, that the attempt to suppress this drift—by imparting an efferent visual pursuit command opposite to the drift—produces the illusion of target motion.[26,45]

Although the autokinetic phenomenon was cited as a leading visual illusion in the surveys of Vinacke[1] and Sipes and Lessard,[13] it is likely that many illusory target motions attributed to the autokinetic illusion actually occur during aircraft motions and should be classified as oculogyral or oculogravic illusions. If, in fact, a pilot stares at a distant star or other aircraft for longer than 10 s, the autokinetic illusion can prove extremely dangerous if the pilot starts to track the illusory movement with the aircraft. Thus, pilots should be careful to avoid prolonged out-the-window fixation by cross checking appropriate spatial orientation displays at least once every 9 s and preferably more often.

III. Optical-Device Distortions and Illusions

Many visual illusions in the aerial environment are attributable primarily to the effects of optical devices. Included among such devices are 1) transparent refractive surfaces such as aircraft windscreens, 2) spectacles and visors worn by pilots, and 3) collimated viewing displays that contain primary flight information such as HUDs, HMDs, and NVDs.

A. Refractive and Other Effects of Transparencies and Spectacles

There are several transparent surfaces in an aircraft, including windscreens, canopies, and windows. Because of their thickness (typically a couple of centimeters), an aircraft windscreen can be considered a refractive surface for light passing through it at an oblique angle. Thus, most objects will appear to be magnified when viewed through a windscreen. Fortunately, the typical effects of high-quality windscreens are very small—less than 0.5 deg of magnification for objects beyond 5 m (Ref. 26). For irregular windscreens and other transparent surfaces, however, the optical distortions can be much greater. As noted earlier, windscreen visibility is considerably degraded by the prismatic effects of rain, which when it sweeps across the windscreen can result in a more distant appearance of the outside world.[26] Optical distortions can also be caused by windscreen heating devices. Finally, coatings on windscreens and canopies (particularly older ones) can create special problems for pilots wearing NVG by blocking much of the infrared light required for optimal NVG performance.

Spectacles worn by pilots can also alter the perceived size and distance of objects on the ground. This is a problem even in military aviation, where about 40% of all active-duty USAF pilots use corrective lenses, about half of which are multifocal.[53] Tredici[29] lists several incidents in which a change in the optical correction of an aviator's spectacles, the improper use of bifocal lenses, or a failure to wear properly prescribed lenses might all have contributed to a landing or other low-altitude mishap. Even worse is the unauthorized use of wide-angle camera lenses, which can distort the projective geometry of the terrain and has been implicated in at least one USAF mishap. The use of wavelength-selective sunglasses poses a different visual problem for pilots: loss of color vision. Many sunglasses and visors with short-wavelength absorbing filters—worn by at least 25% of all USAF pilots[53]— diminish the amount of transmitted blue light, which severely distorts color vision[54] and can impair the visibility of aircraft against the sky, the demarcation of the sky–water horizon, and runway markings. For example, one aircraft almost crash landed on a blocked runway because the pilots were wearing blue-bocking visors and could not see the yellow X against the whiter runway.[55] Laser-eye-protective devices that are being fielded in various flying communities can also distort color space somewhat, although none has yet been associated with an SD incident.

The best advice to aviator is to only use prescribed, officially sanctioned glasses and other optical devices in the aircraft and, even in these cases, to be aware of their optical properties.

B. Collimated Flight Displays

The advent of collimated flight displays in the 1950s (see Chapter 10) ushered in a long debate about their effects on visual perception of the world outside of the cockpit. The main concern has been whether collimated devices (specifically head-up displays or HUDs) alter distance perception through a change in accommodation. This concern has been most forcefully expressed by Roscoe and colleagues,[56-58] who claim that an inward shift of accommodation produces a minification of objects (accommodative micropsia) (see Chapter 3, Sec. IV.C.1) and an illusion that the pilot is at a higher altitude than is actually the case. Although other researchers have dismissed many of Roscoe and colleagues' specific tenets,[59,60] viewing the world through the HUD has long been accepted as a source of SD in pilots.[56,61]

It is generally agreed that, despite their infinity optics, collimated HUD and other virtual flight displays do not actually pull the pilot's accommodation outward to infinity. Generally, pilots' accommodation distance will lie beyond that of their resting accommodation, that is, slightly >1 m in the dark and closer to 2 m in clouds.[56,62] In viewing outside terrain in the daytime, pilots tend to redirect their accommodation inward to a few meters when viewing through a HUD.[56] This inward accommodation shift might be even greater in the case of monocular viewing through a helmet-mounted display.[63] The most likely causes of the inward shift in accommodation are the proximity of the viewing frame surrounding the collimated display and the mere cognitive association of the HUD as lying within the space of the pilot or cockpit. (For instance, the same auditory target appears closer if fixed with respect to the pilot or the aircraft than if it is fixed relative to the distant terrain.*)

Subject to more disputes are the *consequences* of the inward shift of accommodation. Roscoe and colleagues argue,[56-58] based upon data from studies by Hull et al.[64] and Iavecchia et al.,[56] that inward accommodative shifts result in micropsia and a tendency to overestimate the distance to the ground. Roscoe[57] argues that the discrepancy between these measurements and those of other studies that have not found a significant accommodative micropsia relate to the smaller distances used in laboratory studies. However, Marsh and Temme[59] disputed Roscoe's analysis based on both mathematical and empirical grounds and instead claim that size judgments are distorted by at most 1–2% as a result of accommodation. Moreover, Newman[60] argues that Roscoe's findings are not applicable to the actual aircraft landing situation, where many other cues are available to pilots. Indeed, he reports that there is improved landing consistency when flying with HUDs, counter to the assertion of Roscoe that long, hard landings result from HUD viewing (see also Chapter 10, Sec. III.A.3).

Although the amount of size distortion caused by HUDs and HMDs is debatable, it is generally agreed that it might be more difficult to detect runway objects and other small targets through such displays. This effect is caused by two major (and possibly interrelated) factors. One of these is a blurring of distant objects caused by the inward focus shift, known as the Mandelbaum Effect; this has been shown to produce increased detection latencies and errors for more distant targets.[62]

---

* Personal communication with R. McKinley, Nov. 1997.

The other source of the problem in detecting distant targets might be caused by a proximal attentional focus because the deficit extends to even reasonably sized out-the-window targets that would be less affected by blurring.[65] This phenomenon, known as cognitive capture (see Chapter 10, Sec. III.A.5), is tied to accommodative distance by the general linkage of eye position and attention but it might even occur when accommodation remains distant.[66] A converse phenomenon can sometimes occur when night-vision goggles are worn while viewing a HUD—the reduced acuity through the NVG can affect the visibility of the HUD against the background terrain.* This is not true of HUD symbologies that are overlaid directly over the NVG and can essentially be considered HMD symbologies (see Sec. III.C).

Because primary flight symbologies on HMDs are currently fixed with respect to the head, they can pull the pilot's attentional distance still closer into the cockpit. On the other hand, HMD symbologies and visual images that remain fixed relative to the aircraft can introduce other serious visual problems, such as temporal lags and relative motion effects (see Chapter 10, Sec. IV.A.2). This is a particular problem for forward-looking infrared images on HMDs, whose narrow field of view forces pilots to make frequent head movements to achieve a full angle of regard.[67] Despite these and other problems, collimated flight displays are undeniably successful in allowing pilots to maintain an out-the-window vantage, thereby reducing the amount of costly visual transitioning into and out of the cockpit.[66]

C. Night-Vision Devices

NVDs have revolutionized military aviation. According to one expert, "The total impact of NVDs has probably been greater than that of any technological advance since the development of the jet engine."[68] The two major types of NVDs are FLIR images from aircraft sensors and NVGs. The two differ considerably in their transmission characteristics. An illustration of FLIR and NVG views of the same scene is shown in Fig. 16.

Despite their advantages, NVDs are also a source of many visually based SD incidents and presumed SD mishaps. Approximately 3% of USAF pilots who have flown with NVGs have had an inflight accident or serious incident that was reportedly caused by the operational limitations of NVGs.[53] According to Braithwaite et al.,[6] the rate of SD accidents in helicopters when pilots are using NVDs is 9.0 per 100,000 flight hours as compared to 1.66 with unaided daytime vision and 3.87 with unaided night vision. Although a comparison of unaided and NVD-aided night flying is misleading because the missions flown are more dangerous in the latter case, the high number of NVD-related SD accidents can be traced to many visual factors, some of which do not necessarily involve visual illusions. Most NVD-related SD incidents in the U.S. Army occur during clear night conditions, especially during a new or quarter-moon.[20] The most dangerous static visual illusions involve erroneous judgments of height above ground, while the leading dynamic visual illusion (at least in rotary-winged pilots) is undetected or illusory drift.[20] There does not appear to be much of a difference between NVGs and FLIR images in terms of the likelihood of suffering from visual illusions and other problems.[20]

---

* Personal communication with Dr. Chuck Antonio, July 2000.

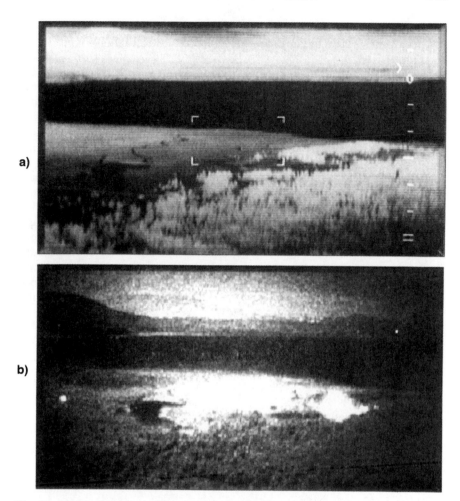

Fig. 16   View of the same scene as seen in a) a FLIR image and b) through NVGs. (Photos reproduced with permission of Dr. Chuck Antonio.) Note the differences in transmission characteristics, and the strengths and weaknesses of each view.

Several general NVD visual problems have been described by Antonio,[23,69] Berkley,[68] and Crowley,[20] among others. Visual problems caused by both NVGs and FLIR images include 1) a relatively narrow (20–40 deg) field of view (FOV), which leads to a loss of ambient vision and a greater-than-normal amount of head-scanning; 2) reduced contrast sensitivity, which increases the likelihood of Earth–sky blending and distorts the normal contrast (aerial perspective) information used in monocular depth judgments; 3) reduced visual acuity (no better than 20/40 under operational flying conditions), which can impair the visibility of power lines and other man-made objects and alter monocular depth perception; 4) aberrant color vision in the form of a monochromatic appearance of the image, an altered spectral transmission that distorts the relative brightness of objects, and color adaptation;

and 5) problems in judging depth binocularly at near distances because of the displaced camera view in the FLIR image and the optical-infinity focus of the NVG tubes.

The result of most of these general NVD problems is an exacerbation of the visual illusions commonly experienced in unaided vision. In addition to the general problems associates with NVDs, there are specific visual problems and illusions associated with each major type of NVD, as discussed in the following sections.

1. Night-Vision Goggles

NVGs intensify the image through phosphors contained in tubes covering each eye, which transmit in the 600–900 nm range. They are designed to adjust their transmission (gain) based on the brightness of the background image and offer the advantage of presenting the image from the same viewpoint as unaided vision and of being relatively insensitive to thermal effects.

Because of their intensification process, gain control, and spectral transmissivity range, NVGs can produce a number of specific visual illusions. For one, NVGs transmit well through humidity and light rain, so that pilots might not be aware that they are entering a cloud or thick fog until they have proceeded deep into it. Second, because NVGs respond to red and near-infrared light selective image intensification of red beacons on aircraft can produce an illusion that another aircraft is closer than it actually is, whereas shorter-wavelength lights can appear dimmer and farther away. Third, NVGs can only respond when a certain amount of light is already present to intensify, and they respond poorly under extremely dim (new moon) conditions. Fourth, spatially uneven or transient gain changes can occur, which can reduce the visibility of large areas of the image. For example, point sources of light such as are found in urban areas might appear to have halos, which effectively enlarge their size and might even lead them to be mistakenly combined with other lights to appear still larger (and closer in distance). In addition, the brightness of a large object in the scene, such as a full moon just over the horizon, can lower the overall NVG gain and wash out the rest of the scene or create extremely dark shadows. Conversely, flying into a shadowed area can produce an abrupt increase in NVG gain and, consequently, tend to reduce image quality through a honeycomb scintillation pattern. The general loss of detail in NVG images, especially when there is a large amount of particulates in the air (e.g., as during brownout) can prove especially dangerous by obscuring the terrain or making it appear further away than normal. Even under night VMC, pilots tend to overestimate distance and make too steep or low an approach on landing while wearing NVGs.[20,21] (One somewhat rare problem occurs when the gains of the NVG tubes in front of each eye are unequal; this can lead to the classic Pulfrich illusion of elliptical motion in depth for objects actually moving normal to the direction of aircraft motion and at a constant depth.[20])

The issue of how much NVGs affect depth perception, particularly those mediated by binocular cues, is a complicated one. In a recent USAF survey, approximately 29% of the NVG complaints involved reduced depth perception,[53] and Crowley[20] reported depth perception impairments among 11% of U.S. Army helicopter pilots. Clearly, the direction of the optical focus of NVGs toward infinity impairs depth perception at less than 8 m and could be a factor in some aerial refueling mishaps with NVGs.[21] Laboratory studies suggest that little stereopsis is present with NVGs and that subjects tend to underestimate the depth of objects in sparse environments.[70,71] However, the strength of binocular depth cues declines with distance and is of little value beyond 50 m (see Chapter 3, Sec. IV.C.1), and it has been shown that performance in avoiding obstacles at large distances (>70 m) while driving along the ground is similar using NVGs or unaided vision.[70] Thus, the misjudgment of terrain and ground-object distances reported by pilots wearing NVGs is more likely to be caused by distorted monocular luminance and contrast cues rather than distorted stereopsis per se.[21] There might also be long-term (after) effects of NVG viewing on depth perception, as prolonged NVG use in at least one study has shown to lead to a lateral phoria (horizontal deviation of one eye relative to the other).[72]

2. Forward-Looking Infrared

This technique involves thermal imaging with a camera typically attached to the front of the airframe. Thermal imaging transmits information in the 3–5 μm or 8–12 μm (infrared) ranges. Because of the weight of the camera and its need for maximal slewability, the FLIR view is from outside the cockpit and does not depict the world from either the pilot's viewpoint or even the heading of the aircraft. Despite its relatively narrow FOV (20–30 deg at a maximum), the FLIR image has the advantage of a 360-deg field of regard because the camera can be slewed in all directions. However, FLIR images are always viewed by the pilot with a certain amount of parallax, which can be very disorienting. Because the camera can be zoomed, FLIRs can process more details than NVGs but do not possess the unity magnification that NVGs do. There are two major types of FLIRs: targeting and navigational. Targeting FLIRs are usually controllable by the pilot and present a high-resolution image of a relatively small region (1 deg) surrounding or approaching a target, usually on a head-down display. By contrast, navigational FLIRs are presented on HUDs or even as head-slaved images on HMDs.

Some of the specific visual problems and illusions associated with FLIR images derive from their lack of registration with the pilot's line of sight, delays in slaving the image to the pilot's head (when they presented in an HMD), and distortions caused by the infrared transmission band.[69] Because they measure thermal transmission, FLIR images are much better than NVG images at low illumination, but they are much more easily disrupted by high humidity and moisture (e.g., rain or snow), more so using an 8–12-μm bandwidth than a 3–5-μm bandwidth. Infrared images are also affected more by diurnal crossover effects, involving the relative cooling and heating of objects caused by the rising and setting of the sun, or the presence of clouds. For example, many objects whose temperature is determined by the sunlight reach the same temperature as the background because of cooling at dusk, thereby reducing their contrast. Other thermal aberrations include the presence of exhaust or other heat long after a vehicle has moved on and the effects of thermal winds, which can create large shadows. Relative to NVGs, however, FLIR images have the advantage of being less disrupted by dust and other particulates in the air as well as by cultural lighting.[69]

A major issue involving NVG and FLIR images is their integration, both with each other and with other cockpit instruments. As noted earlier, NVG use can affect the ability to attend to and read HUD symbols, and cockpit instruments must be designed to be compatible with NVGs. Pilots must be trained to scan aggressively to utilize fully the NVG field of regard and thereby update their mental model of the outside world, while returning to their head-down instruments at regular intervals. Pilots must also learn to coordinate NVG and FLIR images and to rely more on one than the other, depending on the particular environmental conditions (e.g., FLIR at higher altitudes and under low-illumination conditions). Registration of FLIR targeting information with NVG navigational information also requires extensive training. The reader is referred to Antonio[69] for a detailed discussion of these and other NVD integration issues.

To counteract the visual decrements associated with NVDs, various training programs have been established (see Chapter 8, Sec. II.E.3). Meanwhile, technological advancement continues to improve the capabilities of NVDs. For example, a prototype panoramic NVG (PNVG) has been developed by the U.S. Air Force Research Laboratory to expand the 40-deg FOV of current NVGs to almost 100 deg

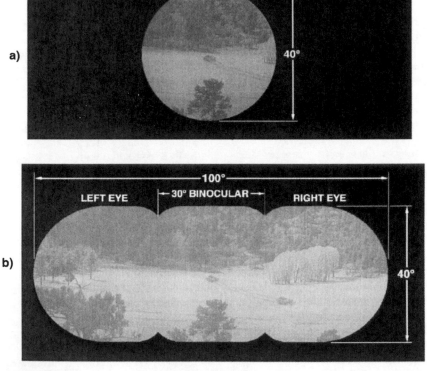

Fig. 17   Representative view through a) a current 40 deg × 40 deg NVG and b) a prototype panoramic NVG with a near (38 deg × 95 deg) FOV. (Photos reproduced with permission of Col. William Berkley.)

(Fig. 17), and the addition of primary flight symbology to NVDs might eventually ease many of the problems in transitioning between the imagery and flight instrumentation.

IV. Summary

This chapter has attempted to show that visual illusions in flight are a natural consequence of the reductions and distortions in the ambient visual cues that are crucial to our perception of self-motion and position relative to the terrain and other aircraft. Although the nighttime visual environment is statistically the most dangerous, particularly wearing NVDs, daytime SD illusions are also quite prevalent and can be traced to specific visibility and terrain factors. It is no longer justified to relegate SD to IMC or night flying, as was formally done by the USAF prior to the mid-1980s and is informally done by many flight surgeons even today. Because of the comparable rates of visual and nonvisual SD mishaps, SD visual training should be made an integral part of a well-designed SD training curriculum (see Chapter 8). Moreover, designers of primary flight displays should be on the alert for any SD traps that might increase the risk of visual illusions or otherwise compromise the pilot's view of the outside world.

References

[1] Vinacke, W. E., "Aviator's Vertigo," *Journal of Aviation Medicine*, Vol. 19, 1948, pp. 158–170.

[2] Kuipers, A., Kappers, A., van Holten, C. R., van Bergen, J. H. W., and Oosterveld, W. J., "Spatial Disorientation Incidents in the R.N.L.A.F. F16 and F5 Aircraft and Suggestions for Prevention," AGARD CP-478: *Situational Awareness in Aerospace Operations*, AGARD, 1990, pp. OV-E-1–OV-E-16.

[3] Braithwaite, M. G., Durnford, S. J., Crowley, J. S., Rosado, N. R., and Albano, J. P., "Spatial Disorientation in U.S. Army Rotary-Wing Operations," *Aviation, Space, and Environmental Medicine*, Vol. 69, 1998, pp. 1031–1037.

[4] Lyons, T. J., Ercoline, W. R., Freeman, J. E., and Gillingham, K. K., "Classification Problems of U.S. Air Force Spatial Disorientation Accidents, 1989–91," *Aviation, Space, and Environmental Medicine*, Vol. 65, 1994, pp. 147–152.

[5] Gillingham, K. K., "The Spatial Disorientation Problem in the United States Air Force," *Journal of Vestibular Research*, Vol. 2, 1992, pp. 297–306.

[6] Braithwaite, M. G., Douglass, P. K., Durnford, S. J., and Lucas, G., "The Hazard of Spatial Disorientation During Helicopter Flight Using Night Vision Devices," *Aviation, Space, and Environmental Medicine*, Vol. 69, 1998, pp. 1038–1044.

[7] Bellenkes, A., Bason, R., and Yacavone, D. O., "Spatial Disorientation in Naval Aviation Mishaps: A Review of Class A Incidents from 1980 Through 1989," *Aviation, Space, and Environmental Medicine*, Vol. 63, 1992, pp. 128–131.

[8] Tormes, F. R., and Guedry, F. E., Jr., "Disorientation Phenomena in Naval Helicopter Pilots," *Aviation, Space, and Environmental Medicine*, Vol. 46, 1975, pp. 387–393.

[9] Jain, S., "Autokinesis and Some Conditions of Fatigue," *Perceptual and Motor Skills*, Vol. 56, 1983, pp. 147–154.

[10]Williams, L. J., "Cognitive Load and the Functional Field of View," *Human Factors*, Vol. 24, 1982, pp. 683–692.

[11]Collins, D. L., and Harrison, G., "Spatial Disorientation Episodes Among F-15C Pilots During Operation Desert Storm," *Journal of Vestibular Research*, Vol. 5, 1995, pp. 405–410.

[12]Matthews, R. S. J., Previc, F., and Bunting, A., "USAF Spatial Disorientation Survey," RTO MP-086: *Spatial Disorientation in Military Vehicles: Causes, Consequences and Cures*," Research and Technology Organisation, NATO, 2002, pp. 7-1–7-3.

[13]Sipes, W. E., and Lessard, C. S., "A Spatial Disorientation Survey of Experienced Instructor Pilots," *IEEE Engineering in Medicine and Biology*, Vol. 19, 2000, pp. 35–42.

[14]Gillingham, K. K., and Previc, F. H., "Spatial Orientation in Flight," *Fundamentals of Aerospace Medicine*, 2nd ed., edited by R. L. DeHart, Williams and Wilkins, Baltimore, MD, 1996, pp. 309–397.

[15]McNaughton, G. B., "False Horizons," *Flying Safety*, Vol. 43, No. 7, 1987, pp. 12–15.

[16]McNaughton, G. B., "Hazards of Flying Low-Level," *Approach*, Vol. 33, No. 9, 1988, pp. 2–5.

[17]Haber, R. N., "Why Low-Flying Fighter Planes Crash: Perceptual and Attentional Factors in Collisions with the Ground," *Human Factors*, Vol. 29, 1987, pp. 519–532.

[18]Previc, F. H., "Detection of Optical Flow Patterns During Low-Altitude Flight," *Proceedings of the Fifth International Symposium on Aviation Psychology*, edited by R. A. Jensen, Ohio State Univ., Columbus, OH, 1989, pp. 708–713.

[19]Ungs, T. J., "The Occurrence of the Vection Illusion Among Helicopter Pilots While Flying over Water," *Aviation, Space, and Environmental Medicine*, Vol. 60, 1989, pp. 1099–1101.

[20]Crowley, J. S., "Human Factors of Night Vision Devices: Anecdotes from the Field Concerning Visual Illusions and Other Effects," U.S. Army Aeromedical Research Lab., USAARL Rept. No. 91-15, Fort Rucker, AL, 1991.

[21]Berkley, W. E., "Night Vision Goggle Illusions and Visual Training," *Visual Problems in Night Operations*, AGARD, Neuilly sur Seine, France, 1992, pp. 9-1–9-6.

[22]Johnson, L. C., "Flicker as a Helicopter Pilot Problem," *Aerospace Medicine*, Vol. 34, 1964, pp. 306–310.

[23]Antonio, J. C., "Fixed Wing NVG Class A Mishaps: Lessons Learned," *Night Vision 1998: Conference Proceedings*, 1998.

[24]Harker, G. S., and Jones, P. D., "Depth Perception in Visual Simulation," Air Force Systems Command, AFHRL-TR-80-19, Brooks Air Force Base, TX, 1980.

[25]Singh, B., and Navathe, P. D., "Indian Air Force and World Spatial Disorientation Accidents: A Comparison," *Aviation, Space, and Environmental Medicine*, Vol. 65, 1994, pp. 254–256.

[26]Pitts, D. G., "Visual Illusions and Aircraft Accidents," U.S. Air Force School of Aerospace Medicine, SAM-TR-67-28, Brooks Air Force Base, TX, 1967.

[27]Preble, C., "How Low Can a Pilot Get?" *Flying Safety*, Vol. 39, No. 1, 1983, pp. 18–24.

[28]Crowley, J. S., Caldwell, J. L., Sessions, M., and Tibbetts, C. R., "*Altitude Estimation in the UH-60 Flight Simulator*," U.S. Army Aeromedical Research Lab., USAARL Rept. No. 96-27, Fort Rucker, AL, 1996.

[29]Tredici, T. J., "Visual Illusions as a Probable Cause of Aircraft Mishaps," AGARD CP-287: *Spatial Orientation in Flight: Current Problems*, AGARD, 1980, pp. B5-1–B5-5.

[30]Gallimore, J. J., Patterson, F. R., Brannon, N. G., and Nalepka, J. P., "The Opto-Kinetic Cervical Reflex During Formation Flight," *Aviation, Space, and Environmental Medicine*, Vol. 71, 2000, pp. 812–821.

[31]Scott, W. B., "New Research Identifies Causes of CFIT," *Aviation Week and Space Technology*, Vol. 144, No. 25, 1996, pp. 40–71.

[32]Ercoline, W. R., Weinstein, L. F., and Gillingham, K. K., "An Aircraft Landing Accident Caused by Visually Induced Disorientation," *Proceedings of the Sixth International Symposium on Aviation Psychology*, 1991, pp. 619–623.

[33]Schmidt, R. T., "Reduce Risk of Inducing Spatial Disorientation Using Physiologically Compatible Ground Lighting," *Aviation, Space, and Environmental Medicine*, Vol. 70, 1999, pp. 598–603.

[34]Hartman, B. O., and Cantrell, G. K., "Psychological Factors in Landing-Short Accidents," *Flight Safety*, Vol. 2, 1968, pp. 26–32.

[35]Kraft, C. L., "A Psychophysical Contribution to Air Safety: Simulation Studies of Visual Illusions in Night Visual Approaches," *Psychology: From Research to Practice*, edited by H. A. Pick, Jr., H. W. Leibowitz, J. E. Singer, A. Steinschneider, and H. W. Stevenson, Plenum, New York, 1978, pp. 363–385.

[36]Mertens, H. W., "Comparison of the Visual Perception of a Runway Model in Pilots and Nonpilots During Simulated Night Landing Approaches," *Aviation, Space, and Environmental Medicine*, Vol. 49, 1978, pp. 1043–1055.

[37]Perrone, J. A., "Visual Slant Misperception and the Black-Hole Landing Situation," *Aviation, Space, and Environmental Medicine*, Vol. 55, 1984, pp. 1020–1025.

[38]Riordan, R. H., "Monocular Visual Cues and Space Perception During the Approach to Landing," *Aerospace Medicine*, Vol. 45, 1974, pp. 766–771.

[39]Mertens, H. W., "Perception of Runway Image Shape and Approach Angle Magnitude by Pilots in Simulated Night Landing Approaches," *Aviation, Space, and Environmental Medicine*, Vol. 52, 1981, pp. 373–386.

[40]Mertens, H. W., and Lewis, M. F., "Effect of Different Runway Sizes on Pilot Performance During Simulated Night Landing Approaches," *Aviation, Space, and Environmental Medicine*, Vol. 53, 1982, pp. 463–471.

[41]Lintern, G., and Liu, Y.-T., "Explicit and Implicit Horizons for Simulated Landing Approaches," *Human Factors*, Vol. 33, 1991, pp. 401–417.

[42]Graybiel, A., and Hupp, D. I., "The Oculo-Gyral Illusion: A Form of Apparent Motion Which May Be Observed Following Stimulation of the Semicircular Canals," *Journal of Aviation Medicine*, Vol. 17, 1946, pp. 3–27.

[43]Keller, G., and Henn, V., "Self-Motion Sensation Influenced by Visual Fixation," *Perception and Psychophysics*, Vol. 35, 1984, pp. 279–285.

[44]Previc, F. H., Ghani, N., Stevens, K. W., and Ludwig, D. A., "Effects of Background Field-of-View and Depth-Plane on the Oculogyral Illusion," *Perceptual and Motor Skills*, Vol. 93, 2001, pp. 867–878.

[45]Pitts, D. G., "Visual Illusions Associated with Acceleration," *Amercian Journal of Optometry and Physiological Optics*, Vol. 44, 1967, pp. 21–33.

[46]Benson, A. J., and Brown, S. F., "Visual Display Lowers Detection Threshold of Angular, but not Linear, Whole-Body Motion Stimuli," *Aviation, Space, and Environmental Medicine*, Vol. 60, 1989, pp. 629–633.

[47]Graybiel, A., "Oculogravic Illusion," *A.M.A. Archives of Ophthalmology*, Vol. 48, 1952, pp. 605–615.

[48]Otakeno, S., Matthews, R. S. J., Folio, L., Previc, F. H., and Lessard, M. S., "The Effects of Visual Scenes on Roll and Pitch Thresholds in Pilots Versus Nonpilots," *Aviation, Space, and Enviromental Medicine*, Vol. 73, 2002, pp. 98–101.

[49]Welch, R. B., Cohen, M. M., and DeRoshia, C. W., "Reduction of the Elevator Illusion

from Continued Hypergravity Exposure and Visual Error-Corrective Feedback," *Perception and Psychophysics*, Vol. 58, 1996, pp. 22–30.

[50]Evanoff, J. N., and Lackner, J. R., "Influence of Maintained Ocular Deviation on the Spatial Displacement Component of the Oculogyral Illusion," *Perception and Psychophysics*, Vol. 42, 1987, pp. 25–28.

[51]Whiteside, T. C. D., Graybiel, A., and Niven, J. I., "Visual Illusions of Movement," *Brain*, Vol. 88, 1965, pp. 193–210.

[52]Byford, G. H., "Eye Movements and the Optogyral Illusion," *Aerospace Medicine*, Vol. 33, 1963, pp. 119–123.

[53]Baldwin, J. B., Dennis, R. J., Ivan, D. J., Miller, R. E., III, Belihar, R. P., Jackson, W. G., Jr., Tredici, T. J., Datko, L. M., and Hiers, P. L., "The 1995 Aircrew Operational Vision Survey: Results, Analysis, and Recommendations," USAF School of Aerospace Medicine, SAM-AF-BR-TR-1999-0003, Brooks Air Force Base, Texas, 1999.

[54]Kuyk, T. K., and Thomas, S. R., "Effect of Short Wavelength Absorbing Filters on Farnsworth-Munsell 100 Hue Test and Hue Identification Task Performance," *Optometry and Vision Science*, Vol. 67, 1990, pp. 522–531.

[55]Yacavone, D. W., and Erickson, R. T., "Yellow Lens Effects upon Visual Acquisition Performance (Comment)," *Aviation, Space, and Environmental Medicine*, Vol. 63, 1992, p. 1122.

[56]Iavecchia, J. H., Iavecchia, H. P., and Roscoe, S. N., "Eye Accommodation to Head-Up Virtual Images," *Human Factors*, Vol. 30, 1988, pp. 689–702.

[57]Roscoe, S. N., "Landing Airplanes, Detecting Traffic, and the Dark Focus," *Aviation, Space, and Environmental Medicine*, Vol. 53, 1982, pp. 970–976.

[58]Roscoe, S. N., "The Trouble with HUDs and HMDs," *Human Factors Society Bulletin*, Vol. 30, No. 7, 1987, pp. 1–3.

[59]Marsh, J. S., and Temme, L. A., "Optical Factors in Judgments of Size Through an Aperture," *Human Factors*, Vol. 32, 1990, pp. 109–118.

[60]Newman, R. L., "Responses to Roscoe, The Trouble with HUDs and HMDs," *Human Factors Society Bulletin*, Vol. 30, No. 10, 1987, pp. 3–5.

[61]Ercoline, W., "The Good, the Bad, and the Ugly of Head-Up Displays," *IEEE Engineering in Medicine and Biology*, Vol. 19, 2000, pp. 66–70.

[62]Norman, J., and Ehrlich, S., "Visual Accommodation and Virtual Image Displays: Target Detection and Recognition," *Human Factors*, Vol. 28, 1986, pp. 135–151.

[63]Hale, S., "Visual Accommodation and Virtual Images: A Review of the Issues," U.S. Army Human Engineering Lab., Technical Note 3-90, Aberdeen Proving Ground, MD, 1990.

[64]Hull, J. C., Gill, R. T., and Roscoe, S. N., "Locus of the Stimulus to Visual Accommodation: Where in the World, or Where in the Eye? *Human Factors*, Vol. 24, 1982, pp. 311–319.

[65]Fischer, E., Haines, R. F., and Price, T. A., "Cognitive Issues in Head-Up Displays," NASA-TP-7111, 1980.

[66]Weintraub, D. J., "HUDs, HMDs, and Common Sense: Polishing Virtual Images," *Human Factors Society Bulletin*, Vol. 30, No. 10, 1987, pp. 1–3.

[67]Grunwald, A. J., and Kohn, S., "Visual Field Information in Low-Altitude Visual Flight by Line-of-Sight Slaved Helmet-Mounted Displays," *IEEE Transactions on Systems, Man, and Cybernetics*, Vol. 24, 1994, pp. 120–134.

[68]Berkley, W. E., "Night Operations," AGARD LS-187: *Visual Problems in Night Operations*, AGARD, 1992, pp. 1-1–1-4.

[69] Antonio, J. C., *NVG/FLIR Sensory Integration: Instructor's Guide*, 2001 (unpublished).

[70] DeLucia, P. R., and Task, H. L., "Depth and Collision Judgment Using Night Vision Goggles," *International Journal of Aviation Pscyhology*, Vol. 5, 1995, pp. 371–386.

[71] Wiley, R. W., "Visual Acuity and Stereopsis with Night Vision Goggles," U.S. Army Aeromedical Research Lab., USAARL-TR-89-9, F.t Rucker, AL, 1989.

[72] Sheehey, J. B., and Wilkinson, M., "Depth Perception After Prolonged Usage of Night Vision Goggles," *Aviation, Space, and Environmental Medicine*, Vol. 60, 1989, pp. 573–579.

Chapter 8

Spatial Disorientation Instruction, Demonstration, and Training

Malcolm G. Braithwaite*
British Army, Hampshire, United Kingdom

William R. Ercoline[†]
General Dynamics Advanced Information Systems, San Antonio, Texas

Lex Brown[‡]
*U.S. Air Force School of Aerospace Medicine,
Brooks City-Base, Texas*

"Physiological training is the main weapon against spatial disorientation at the disposal of the flight surgeon and aerospace physiologist."[1]

"Strong aeromedical and aviation training programs remain the most important defensive measure for spatial disorientation."[2]

I. Introduction

ONE of the generic aims of those with a responsibility for flight safety and operational effectiveness is to impart newfound knowledge to the user, the aviator, and commanders. Without an understanding of the nature and effects of spatial disorientation (SD), the aviator is poorly equipped to deal with the problem when it is encountered. Previous chapters have discussed the significant impact of SD on all types of flying. This chapter and those that follow are concerned with what can be done about it. It is hoped that this chapter in particular will be of value not only to those involved in aviation medicine and physiology but also to those

---

This material is declared a work of the U.S. Government and is not subject to copyright protection in the United States.
*Consultant Adviser in Aviation Medicine.
[†]Senior Scientist.
[‡]Chief, Human Performance Division.

responsible for training aircrew for their operational task, be it military or civilian. The objectives of this chapter are as follows:

1) Describe the variety of methods and apparatuses employed in instructing aircrew that range from educational material to behavior-modifying techniques.
2) Provide practical advice to aircrew flying modern aircraft whether they are military or civilian, or fixed or rotary-wing.
3) Discuss the requirement to demonstrate the effectiveness of training.

A. Instruction, Demonstration, and Training

These three terms are often used interchangeably. However, we feel that there are important distinctions among these terms, and we offer the following definitions so that readers can consider which of the methods they are currently applying. The Oxford English Reference Dictionary[3] defines "instruction" (synonymous with "teaching" and "education") as "the provision of systematic (methodological— according to a plan) information about a subject or skill." The same reference defines "demonstration" as "showing evidence of, or proving the working of," and "training" as "to bring or come to a desired state of efficiency or condition of behavior by instruction and practice."

Although all of the SD countermeasures that are being discussed in this chapter fall within the *instruction* definition, we suggest that *training* comprises didactic instruction and the learning and subsequent demonstration of competence in handling inflight disorientating circumstances and illusions, for example, recovery from unusual attitudes and/or inadvertent entry to instrument meteorological conditions. *Demonstration* of SD essentially consists of the demonstration of the limitations of the orientation senses both on the ground and in flight. Studies of the outcome of demonstration and training will be required to determine if training is actually accomplished. These issues are explored further in Sec. V.

B. Need for Training

Countermeasures to SD primarily fall into two categories: technology and training. Although training countermeasures might not necessarily be applicable to all situations, they are probably more readily applied than technological initiatives. Training is, therefore, the first prerequisite in the control of SD. Because it is relatively low tech, it might not attract the sort of attention that it deserves. Despite the acknowledgement[1,4,5] that training in SD is an essential part of the prevention of this ubiquitous hazard in aviation, there is little evidence from the peer-reviewed literature that best or even common practices have been achieved. Several publications[4,6,7] have attempted to collate the recommended practices, but their audience has been heretofore limited. This chapter aims to bring the previous work up to date and to impart the lessons learned to the public domain.

"Spatial Disorientation Indoctrination" courses for aviators have been in place at least since the late 1920s,[8] and their value in controlling the SD hazard has since been emphasized by Bending.[9] A comprehensive review of orientation/ disorientation training of flying personnel was undertaken in 1974 (Ref. 4), and it included many recommendations for the enhancement of all aspects of training. Since then, and mainly following accident analyses in both military and civilian aviation, both general and specific recommendations have been made. Similarly, surveys of the aviator's SD experience are important so that the data can be used to direct resources to the appropriate areas of SD training. Salient points from these sources and collated symposia and general reviews are summarized next, and further discussion of specific recommendations will be made in following sections. Studies that have assessed the effectiveness of training programs will be discussed in Sec. V.

Kirkham et al.[10] highlighted the inadequacy of the SD training program for general aviation pilots. They made a comprehensive series of recommendations that covered the range of training options from lectures through demonstrations to requiring flight-test examiners to assure themselves that pilot applicants have a good awareness of SD and that their students demonstrate their competence to cope with SD conditions. Although SD training is still not mandatory for general aviation, it is heartening that general aviation pilots are now strongly encouraged to participate in SD training.

U.S. Naval aviation SD accidents were reviewed in 1992 (Ref. 11). The knowledge gained from this analysis assisted in the development of SD type-specific training regimes with the aim of ultimately reducing the number of mishaps. Holland and Freeman[12] reviewed 10-year accident data from the U.S. Air Force (USAF) and recommended implementation of enhanced loss of situational awareness (LSA) and SD awareness programs for aircrew. Cheung et al.,[13] observed that remarkably little rigorous research exists concerning the optimal ways in which to prepare aircrew against SD. Durnford et al.[14] provided a review of U.S. Army helicopter accidents, which was followed by three associated reviews.[15–17] All four papers recommended that both aircrew training and crew coordination training should be targets for improvement and that a coordinated effort by the research, training, and safety organizations to consider potential solutions would be of great benefit. Although training to recover from unusual attitudes, ground-based demonstrations, and periodic refresher training are all intuitively appealing, more research must be devoted to defining the role of each training element in a holistic SD training strategy.

Other periodic reviews of accidents that have focused on training countermeasures as part of their recommendations to reduce the SD accident rate are Steele-Perkins and Evans,[18] Edgington and Box,[19] Vyrnwy-Jones,[20,21] and Braithwaite.[22] Even investigations into single-aircraft accidents have produced recommendations for enhanced training. An excellent example is the report by the National Transportation Safety Board[23] on the loss of a McDonnell-Douglas DC-8, in which unusual attitude training for flight crews was emphasized.

A survey of F-15C pilots who had flown during Operation Desert Storm[24] provided invaluable SD knowledge from which USAF research, training, and operational communities were able to reap significant benefit. Following a review of the SD incident experience of pilots attending the USAF Advanced Instrument School, Sipes[25] recommended that training programs for SD countermeasures be developed. In particular, the recommendation was made that a prior knowledge and anticipation of SD illusions and how to counter them can save lives.

C. Prior SD Training Symposia and Working Groups

Part 3 of the *AGARD Conference Proceedings on Spatial Disorientation in flight*[26] reiterated the recommendations made in the 1974 AGARD publication.[4] This conference stimulated the development of training devices by the U.S. Navy and Royal Air Force and initiated the production of training videos. It is perhaps disappointing that little progress appears to have been made in the intervening six years. In 1993 a combined Aviation Medicine—Safety Center Symposium on Spatial Disorientation was held at Pensacola Naval Air Station (proceedings unpublished). Many recommendations about training and cooperation among the three U.S. military services were made. However, although matters progressed in the research field, standardization of military aircrew training in SD was not immediately forthcoming.

Following some local training initiatives by the U.S. Army Aeromedical Research Laboratory (USAARL) and the U.S. Army School of Aviation Medicine (USASAM), the first Triservice Symposium on Spatial Disorientation in Rotary-Wing Operations was held in September 1996. This symposium sought to address three main areas: 1) the seriousness of the SD hazard; 2) current methods to control the hazard; 3) and associated safety and risk management concerns. The proceedings of the symposium are reported in Braithwaite et al.[27] The symposium was considered to be a success in raising the awareness of the impact of SD on rotary-wing flying operations in the military aeromedical and safety communities. It was made clear that SD imposes a particular hazard to rotary-wing operations that differs in many respects from that experienced by fixed-wing operators. There was unanimous agreement that initiatives to overcome the problem must be made. Further work was recommended in education, training, research, and equipment procurement, and these are summarized in Murdock[28] and Murdock and Braithwaite.[29]

Under the auspices of the U.S. Military Triservice Aeromedical Research Panel, a Technical Working Group for Spatial Orientation and Situational Awareness coordinates interaction and information exchange between the services. This group realized that technological initiatives that address SD require a great deal of effort and money to implement. However, it concluded that training enhancements, where appropriate, could be more readily achieved and therefore addressed immediately. Therefore, in January 1997 a subgroup was established to review and make recommendations on SD training. The charter of the subgroup was to review current procedures for training aviators and associated aviation personnel concerning SD and to make recommendations for improvement. Much of the information in later sections of this chapter is based on the subgroups' initiatives.[30,31]

At the 69th meeting of the Aerospace Medical Association in 1998, a panel entitled "Countermeasures to Spatial Disorientation—International Initiatives"[32] included a triservice review of SD training requirements for military aviators.[31] All aspects of training were addressed. The NATO Research and Technology Organization (RTO) also included a comprehensive discussion of the recent advances in all types of SD training[33] and specifically those rotary-wing aircraft.[34]

Since 1996, the Air Standardization Coordinating Committee (ASCC) has produced several documents on SD training within the ASCC nations: Australia, Canada, New Zealand, United Kingdom, and the United States. These documents are authorized for general release through military flight agencies.

II. Didactic Instruction

There can be little argument that classroom presentation to aviators of didactic material on SD is the prerequisite first step in their awareness training. Although many publications, films, and more recently computer presentations that provide information on SD are to be commended, in the past there has been a tendency for these to concentrate upon the mechanisms and effects of SD without giving much practical advice on how to deal with it.[1]

The specific objectives of this information-dissemination type of SD training are as follow[4]:

1) Familiarize the aviator with those factors that contribute to effective spatial orientation in the flight environment.

2) Familiarize the aviator with the various conditions and flight operations that can lead to SD.

3) Inform the aviator about different manifestations of SD and how to detect the onset or existence of SD.

4) Explain the mechanisms by which SD is produced, and discuss the normal limitations of sensory functions

5) Inform the aviator how disorientation can be overcome, and develop the necessary skills to cope with SD when it occurs in flight, even when the pilot is subjected to mental and physical stress.

A. SD Mechanisms

Benson[4] described a comprehensive academic syllabus of the orientation and disorientation mechanisms, prominent SD illusions, and the factors associated with SD. There is no better original source, and so, in order to disseminate the advice to a wider audience, it is reproduced in Appendix A. This is augmented from more contemporary publications with additional topics that have become important in the intervening quarter of a century.[7,30,35] The syllabus should be regarded as a guide and should be amended according to the experience of the audience and reviewed periodically as new advances (and data) become available. An ASCC Advisory Publication[36] provides a compendium of training curricula of the ASCC nations.

B. Practical Advice to Aircrew and Procedures to Prevent and Overcome Disorientation

Over the years, those involved in the operational aspects of SD have made various recommendations to prevent and overcome SD in flight.[1,4,5] To a certain extent, this advice has concentrated upon ways to dispel conflicting sensations (Type II and Type III SD). However, some of the recent literature[13,16,17,30] suggests that Type I SD (unawareness of an erroneous sensory input) is probably a more important cause of loss of aircraft, lives, and mission effectiveness (see Chapter 1, Sec. III for definitions of Type I, II, and III SD). This section attempts to advise aircrew on analyzing and preparing for the risk of SD as well as coping with it when it occurs. Some of the validated strategies from existing publications are reproduced verbatim. In addition, analyses of SD accidents and incidents over recent years— particularly since the advent of flight with night-vision devices (NVD)—provide specific recommendations for the types and phases of flight most associated with the hazard of SD.

Gillingham and Previc's[1] overriding principles for preventing and coping with SD are as follows: 1) minimize the likelihood of SD by frequent and systematic monitoring of the flight instruments or primary flight reference, 2) expect to become disoriented, 3) when it does occur, recognize it, and act to 4) *make the instruments read right.* The last principle has evolved over the years from the rather less instructive statement of "believe your instruments." Money[38] and Cheung[39] expand the principle as follows: it is important to be sure that the pilot does not simply indulge in an attempt at belief of perception when disoriented. Pilots should be told that, when disorientation threatens, "*control the aircraft* to make the instruments read right." Cheung[39] also emphasizes the important difference between unrecognized and recognized SD and notes that a pilot's instructions about what to do when disorientated are useful only if the disorientation is recognized. Unrecognized disorientation can be dealt with by avoiding situations that are prone to induce disorientation, and aircrew should be taught to recognize conditions that can be traps to a loss of orientation. Some examples, provided by Cheung,[39] are to 1) avoid approaches over nonilluminated terrain or over smooth surfaces; 2) avoid head movements under conditions greater than 1 G (when feasible); 3) avoid removing the gaze from flight instruments when in clouds and maintain a good instrument cross-check; and 4) avoid alcohol for 24 hours before flying.

Cheung[39] also stresses that pilots should be aware that SD can sometimes be due to the unrecognized failure of the flight instruments, such as the artificial horizon, or a failure in an aircraft control system. Therefore, when a failure in a flight instrument or control system is suspected the pilot must verify the correct diagnosis of the problem before reacting. This often means confirming the instrument reading with another independent instrument reading, for example, comparing the turn rate indicator with the attitude indicator if a false bank is suspected.

Spatial disorientation can often be resolved by using the autopilot or passing control to another pilot (when available) who is not disoriented. Abandonment of the aircraft (if possible) is the final course of action. Although in some respects this last point is an admission of defeat, any attempt to regain control of the aircraft should not be prolonged to an extent that safe escape becomes impossible. It is for this reason that due attention should always be paid to the altimeter in those situations where difficulties are experienced as a result of SD.[40]

Some additional general principles based on recent advances of aviation training may be added as follows[7]: 1) conduct an appropriate analysis of the risk of SD before flight and periodically throughout the flight as circumstances dictate; 2) be aware of your personal skill limitations especially with respect to currency and competency at that particular task; 3) maintain good crew-resource-management (CRM) procedures; and 4) avoid becoming distracted from the task of flying the aircraft.

It is important to realize that the foregoing are **general** principles. There are many factors unique to the type and model of aircraft and the way in which they are used. Spatial Disorientation Countermeasures (SDCM) instructors are therefore encouraged to apply these principles to their **specific** requirement. Of utmost importance is the development of an awareness of the potential for SD during flight briefings prior to flight involving night, weather, or conditions where visibility is significantly reduced. When SD does occur, aircrew should be encouraged to recognize the SD problem early and to initiate corrective actions before aircraft control is compromised. To illustrate how official publications regarding in-flight procedures are disseminated to pilots in an effort to prevent SD mishaps, an excerpt from a U.S. Army Field Manual (FM 3-04) is reproduced at Appendix B. The advantage of disseminating educational material in this way is that it reassures pilots (particularly in military air forces) that the "executive" realizes the limitations of human performance.

C. Instructional Materials

Didactic material for SD training is available in many types of media from textbooks through video films to interactive computerized lessons. The choice of material is dependent upon the instructor's preference and its availability. Many contemporaneous information and teaching aids are currently available on the coordinated Web site.* The incorporation of SD training during CRM training is discussed in Sec. II.E.4. Examples of SD actually experienced by aviators who have lived to tell the tale are of considerable importance in emphasizing the vulnerability of all who fly. These can be either prepared in advance or solicited from the audience, especially during refresher training.

D. Timing of Training

The timing of initial didactic SD training within the overall flight-training syllabus varies considerably among military air forces,[6] and there remains an absence of mandatory training for general aviation pilots in many countries. However, various civilian aviation authorities do strongly encourage pilots—especially instructor pilots and those seeking an instrument rating—to attend training courses on physiological topics.[41] There are clearly constraints upon instructors when such training can be programmed within flight training programs, but authorities generally agree on the following principles of SDCM training[6]:

1) A basic course in aviation medicine/physiology (including SDCM training) should be programmed early in the flying course.
2) If there is a significant period (> eight weeks) between the initial course and the commencement of instrument-flying training, a short refresher period on SD should be incorporated.
3) Prior to the commencement of flying training with NVDs, the limitations of these devices on spatial orientation should be stressed.
4) Special-to-type SDCM training should be included when a pilot starts flying a significantly different aircraft (especially if converting from fixed to rotary-wing and vice versa).
5) Refresher didactic training, with the emphasis on case-based experiences, should be conducted periodically (at least every 4 to 5 years) and should be a "currency" requirement.
6) If there is a significant SD event involving a particular type of aircraft, the lessons learned from this individual occurrence should be rapidly disseminated.

---

* Data available online at http://www.spatiald.wpafb.af.mil [cited Oct. 2003].

E. Specialized Didactic Instruction

In their technical report Gillingham and Previc[1] provide details of conditions conducive to SD. Many environmental and behavioral circumstances (e.g., confusion of light sources and target fixation) are common to all forms of flight and have been covered in preceding chapters. The particular types and phases of flight associated with an increased risk of SD have been noted in these chapters and other publications (Refs. 7, 13, 42, and many others referenced in this section). These specialized circumstances, which should be emphasized during didactic instruction, are summarized in the following paragraphs.

1. Formation Flying

Formation flying and air-to-air refueling, particularly at night, have been associated with an increased risk of SD. The leans are readily experienced when flying with reference to a leader's wing, and breaking in and out of clouds can be particularly disorientating. The following general advice is extracted from a report by Gillingham and Previc[1]:

> Separate aircraft from the formation under controlled conditions if the weather encountered is either too dense or turbulent to ensure safe flight; A flight lead with SD will tell the wingmen that he/she has SD and to comply with single-ship procedures. If possible, wingmen should confirm straight-and-level attitude and provide verbal feedback to lead. If symptoms do not abate in a reasonable time, terminate the mission and recover the flight by the simplest and safest means possible.

In specific reference to a two-ship formation, Gillingham and Previc[1] recommend the following steps: 1) wingman will advise lead when he or she experience significant SD symptoms; 2) lead will advise wingman of aircraft attitude, altitude, heading, and airspeed; 3) the wingman will advise lead if problems persist, and then if so, lead will establish straight-and-level flight for at least 30 to 60 s; 4) if the preceding procedures are not effective, lead should transfer the flight lead position to the wingman while in straight-and-level flight, and once assuming lead, maintain straight-and-level flight for 60 s; and 5) if necessary, terminate the mission and recover by the simplest and safest means possible. If there is a large formation, Gillingham and Previc[1] argue that the leader should separate the flight into elements to more effectively handle a wingman with persistent SD symptoms and establish straight-and-level flight. The element with the pilot with SD should remain straight-and-level while other elements separate from the flight. When a disoriented pilot separates from the formation, this is known as a lost wingman. Gillingham and Previc[1] offer the following specific advice and caution during the lost wingman procedure.

> The lost wingman procedure must be made as uncomplicated as possible while still allowing safe separation from the other elements of the flight. Maintaining a specified altitude and heading away from the flight until further notice is an ideal lost wingman procedure in that it avoids frequent or prolonged disorientation-inducing turns and minimizes cognitive workload. Often, a pilot flying wing in bad weather does not lose sight of the lead aircraft but suffers so much

disorientation stress as to make the option of going lost wingman seem safer than that of continuing in the formation. A common practice in this situation is for the wingman to take the lead position in the formation, at least until the disorientation disappears. This procedure avoids the necessity of having the disoriented pilot make a turn away from the flight to go lost wingman, a turn that could be especially difficult and dangerous because of the disorientation. One should question the wisdom of having a disoriented pilot leading the flight, however, and some experts in the field of SD are adamantly opposed to this practice, with good reason (Ref. 1, p. 96).

2. Low-Visibility Helicopter Flight

Pilots of helicopters (and tilt-rotor aircraft) are particularly susceptible to disorientation because of the ability of their aircraft to move along, as well as about, lateral and vertical axes. Recent research in rotary-wing operations[14,16,17,37] has shown that SD caused by the misperception of motion in a low-G environment in conditions where good visual cues are absent is very common. These SD illusions primarily comprise subthreshold drift and, to a lesser extent, subthreshold rotation in the hover and low-speed maneuvers. Specific advice on coping with SD in rotary-wing flight (particularly during low speed and hover operations) is given next.

a. Recirculation of dust and snow. In all but the safest and most familiar surroundings, rotary-wing pilots must always expect their visual reference with the ground to be obscured in the final stages of the approach to land. The maintenance of some forward ground speed during the approach, followed by a run-on landing (should terrain conditions allow) or a "zero-zero" (speed and altitude) landing, will keep a recirculating dust or snow cloud behind the aircraft and mitigate against the loss of visual reference of the landing point. If visual references are lost, the previously planned overshoot must be initiated without delay. This disorientating hazard is no longer restricted to helicopter flight. A vectored thrust or tilt-rotor aircraft such as the V-22 Osprey is just as capable of obliterating all visual cues close to the landing point.

b. Inadvertent entry to instrument meteorological procedures. Most helicopters have significantly less power available, and they fly much nearer to the ground than high-performance fixed-wing aircraft. Therefore, the time to correct a control error and the ability to clear unseen terrain is less. Consequently, rotary-wing aircrew should be prepared to more quickly initiate inadvertent instrument meteorological condition (IMC) procedures when visual references are lost.

c. Geographical aspects. Unfamiliarity with the terrain over which a pilot flies, particularly during low-level or nap-of-Earth (NOE) flights, can often impose an increased risk of SD. Pilots tend to become familiar with the visual perceptual contrasts in their own training areas, especially during flight with NVDs, in which the significance of altered cues must be learned. If they are then deployed to an area of operations that is radically different to their normal experience, for example, from a flat, dry desert training environment to a mountainous, temperate area, they are at risk of misinterpreting the orientation information provided by the terrain.[43] In particular, thermal-imaging devices can provide them with diametrically opposite information in these two extremes as the thermal crossover phenomenon occurs (see Chapter 7, Sec. III.C).

3. Flight with NVDs and Helmet-Mounted Devices

Flight with image-intensifying night-vision goggles (NVG) has significantly enhanced the capability of military flight operations. Although compared with unaided vision they significantly improve a pilot's visual capability, they do not turn night into day, and they have many limitations to orientation of which the pilot must be aware. When compared with normal day vision, these include a reduced visual acuity, the absence of color and other depth perception cues, and a severe restriction of the visual fields (see Chapter 7, Sec. III.C.1). The image intensification process also tends to intensify normal daylight illusions, for example, illusory motion.[44] The limitations of both NVGs and thermal imaging aids have been shown to be a significant contributor to SD accidents and incidents.[16,17,37,45] Awareness of the limitations and proficiency in their use is the key to successful completion of a NVD mission; consequently, the increased risk of SD during flight with NVDs should be stressed during both training and operations. Examples of NVG-specific course materials are contained in Antonio.[46,47]

a. Fixed-wing flight with NVGs. Prevention of SD when using NVGs begins with adequate mission planning, emphasizing weather, terrain, illumination levels, and the high risk of task saturation.

Awareness of the limitations of NVGs and demonstrations by instructor pilots of both the degraded perception of visual cues and visual illusions is of paramount importance in the prevention of SD. Compensation for the narrow field of view (FOV) of NVGs is achieved by employing a constant, aggressive scan to enlarge the total field of regard. An effective scanning technique is essential for maintenance of good situational awareness and spatial orientation, including altitude awareness. For example, a dramatic loss of altitude awareness can occur if the scan is interrupted (e.g., if the neck is "splinted" during a high-G maneuver). Experience has also shown that improving scan technique is one of the most effective methods for overcoming a misperception or illusion that has already occurred.[44,46]

Additionally, proper preflight adjustment of the NVG is critical. Personal factors that could contribute to SD are low experience and inadequate currency in NVG flying, fatigue, and other stressors. One must be prepared to transition to instrument flight at any time, and one, therefore, must maintain an aggressive instrument cross check complementary to the NVG scan. Aside from the potential SD traps common to anyone using NVGs, such as misperception of motion and distance cues, terrain contour, or elevation, there are two SD traps that might be more important to aircrew in fast jets. Because of their operating airspeeds, changes in perception of scene flow can prove illusory. For example, transitioning from a cultural landscape to water, such as crossing a coastline, could give a sensation of a sudden deceleration in ground speed or change in altitude. Another SD problem is unperceived flight into IMC, with concurrent loss of horizon signaled by only subtle cues in the NVG image such as a decrease in scene detail or increased scintillation (Brown, D. L., "Preventing and Avoiding Spatial Disorientation During Fast Jet Flight," personal communication, Royal Air Force Centre of Aviation Medicine, Henlow, England, U.K., 2001).

Overcoming SD while using NVGs is no different than any other instance of SD. First, one must recognize the SD, with the immediate need to ascertain aircraft orientation by reference to the appropriate flight instruments. At the same time the aviator must overcome the urge to maintain visual orientation using NVGs—the reason why SD occurred in the first place. The phase of flight is important, with more urgency at a very low altitude or during a rendezvous with another aircraft than when operating as a single ship at a medium-altitude level. A prepared pilot will rehearse reactions to SD by knowing exactly what instruments to use for spatial orientation, how to coordinate with other crewmembers, and by practicing different scenarios in a simulator. Safe execution of the mission is enhanced by knowledge and preparation and tempered by practice.[48]

   b.   Helicopter low-level and NOE flight with NVGs.   This subsection concentrates on NOE operations, including ground cushion maneuvers. It is strongly recommended that only helicopters equipped with a functional radar altimeter (preferably one with an audio low-altitude warning alarm) be flown during NVG operations. An audio warning on the radar altimeter was the most frequently cited technological requirement to control the hazard of SD during military flight operations[16,17,37] and is considered by the authors to be a prerequisite for the effective maintenance of height awareness during rotary-wing NVG flight. Standard operating procedures should be developed and practiced using this device. A constant aggressive scanning technique[44,47] and good CRM are perhaps even more important for rotary-wing operations than they are for fixed-wing flight because operations are conducted much closer to the ground, and the margin for error is therefore less. An inadequate scanning technique and poor CRM were attributed to the genesis of 79.7 and 68.6% of U.S. Army helicopter accidents, respectively.[16,17,37]

   The following recommended strategies are primarily preventive, but suggestions on dealing with SD once it has been recognized are also given. Just as with daytime flight, flight with NVG requires aircrew to perceive adequate visual cues in order to be safe and effective. Spatial disorientation occurring during rotary-wing NOE flight with NVG is essentially caused by a failure to acquire or recognize the visual cues that are essential to the maintenance of spatial orientation in the NOE environment.

   Generally, the closer one is to the ground the better are the available visual cues, as long as they exist in the first place. Anticipation of a visually degraded environment, and thus the techniques that will be required to maintain orientation, is essential. A common problem is the failure to appreciate when there is little or no contrast or ground texture, two of the most reliable depth cues during NVG flight when close to the ground given that many of the three-dimensional visual cues are lost during NVG flight (see Chapter 7, Sec. III.C). Therefore, the best advantage of the resulting two-dimensional environment must be taken to prevent SD. For example, it would be reckless to plan an approach to a single visual reference point in a snowfield while wearing NVGs. The crew should plan to follow known "solid" line features such as hedgerows rather than transit across open spaces with little or no orientation information available. In these circumstances it is also advisable in side-by-side helicopters for the pilot who is immediately adjacent to the feature to take control. Flying with NVGs is a skill that is easily lost, and therefore currency and competency are significant factors affecting orientation. The more skilled pilot should therefore undertake the more difficult task.

   Although many NVG standard operating procedures allocate flight instrument monitoring duties (particularly speed and altitude) to the nonhandling pilot, two pairs of eyes directed "outside" the cockpit are strongly advised in the final stages of the approach to land and during hovering maneuvers. The specific characteristics of an individual pair of NVGs and the external illumination conditions also contribute to SD. If the NVGs are not functioning properly, or if flight is planned for a particularly dark night, the pilot is already placing himself or herself at a disadvantage. The fixed-wing lost wingman procedure can be adopted during helicopter NVG flight at transit altitude. However, transit flights in helicopters are usually at a significantly lower altitude than fixed-wing flights, and so, as the visual scene is more likely to be "cluttered" by terrain features, the technique of sky-lining the lead aircraft by slightly reducing altitude is a useful way for the wingman to maintain or regain his/her orientation within the formation.

When in NOE flight, military helicopters tend to operate as a single ship in a group, and so the strategies for overcoming SD need only concern that particular aircraft (providing the pilot has a good situational awareness of the location of the other aircraft in the mission). As far as coping strategies are concerned, a handling pilot who loses visual reference should immediately inform the nonhandling pilot. If the nonhandling pilot has maintained visual references, he or she should take control immediately. If both pilots have lost visual references, the previously planned overshoot must be initiated. If solo, the pilot must initiate the previously planned overshoot without delay, based on a lower threshold of uncertainty than in a two-seat aircraft. The majority of rotary-wing accidents and serious incidents that have arisen suggest that aircrew did not appreciate the particular environmental and equipment limitations and subsequently failed to modify their visual scanning technique. The importance of maintaining excellent visual reference with the ground and neighboring obstacles at all times cannot be overstressed.

c. Helicopter flight with monocular helmet-mounted devices. The Apache helicopter's integrated helmet and display sighting system (IHADSS) presents peculiar circumstances in that it incorporates a monocular display in which a visual image from a forward-looking infrared (FLIR) sensor is combined with flight and target-acquisition symbology and presented to the pilot's right eye during night flight while vision in the left eye remains unaided. Once again, the emphasis must be upon avoidance of SD, and most of the recommendations made in the NVG section are pertinent to flight using FLIR.[47] The primary advantage of the Apache IHADSS over the NVG is the inclusion of flight reference symbology (although projecting symbology into NVGs has recently been introduced in some military aircraft). However, the scanning technique is both within the HMD—moving the eye(s) around the display—as well as moving the eyes and head around the cockpit and external environment. Recovery from SD can therefore be assisted by this technology, and it is possible (with appropriate training) to control the aircraft to make the instruments read right even during NOE and hovering flight. When HMDs are used in the modern Apache helicopters (U.S. Army AH-64D and the British Army's Apache AH Mk 1), recognized SD coping strategies once visual cues are lost at any stage of flight are as follows:

1) Use the aircraft visible light source (landing lamp).

2) Use the secondary FLIR sensor. There is both a FLIR pilot's night-vision system (PNVS) and a target-acquisition and designation system (TADS), although the latter's resolution and lateral slew rate is not as good as the former.

3) Hand over control to the other pilot.

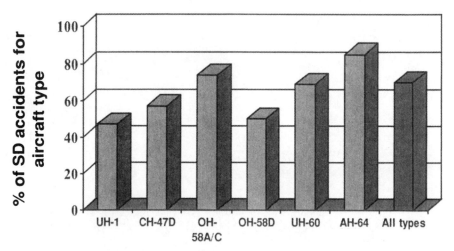

Fig. 1   Percentage of U.S. Army SD accidents in which poor CRM was considered to be a factor. (Reproduced with permission of Braithwaite et al.; Refs. 16, 17, and 37.)

4) If both aircrew have lost references, execute the vertical helicopter instrument recovery procedure (VHIRP). This is summarized as follows: 1) apply collective power to initiate a vertical climb using the HMD's instrument reference; 2) declare to the other pilot that one is executing VHIRP; 3) ensure that the climb is vertical and when clear of obstacles, transition into forward flight; 4) select the flight page on the left-hand multipurpose display so that the unaided left eye now has an instrument reference, while still using the HMD's instrument reference; and 5) change instrument reference from the HMD to the multipurpose display flight page and continue as a traditional instrument recovery.

4.   SD and Crew Resource Management Instruction

Poor CRM has been cited as an important factor leading to an increased risk of SD in many aircraft accidents and incidents.[16,17,37,48] Figure 1 shows the percentage of episodes in which poor CRM was considered to be a factor in a series of U.S. Army rotary-wing accidents. The results of an aircrew survey[49] showed that there was a significantly increased severity of the worst-ever SD episode if poor CRM had either contributed to the generation of the incident or had hampered recovery. In many accidents better allocation of crew duties, for example, one pilot attending inside and the other attending outside the cockpit, might have meant that at least one crew member would have escaped SD. Conversely, results from the same survey suggested that good CRM attenuates the severity of the SD incident (see Fig. 2). In the accident studies one of the most frequently cited enhancements to controlling the SD hazard was improved CRM. Allied to better crew coordination was another frequently identified potential solution: improved scanning both inside and outside the cockpit.

In a study of loss of situational awareness and SD in the USAF from 1980–1999 (Ref. 12), it was demonstrated that the introduction of CRM programs resulted in a dramatic decrease in the loss of aircraft from these causes.

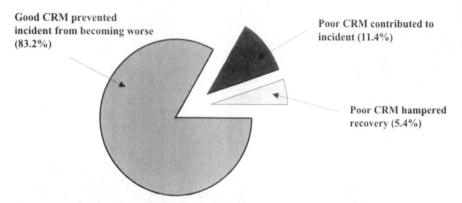

Good CRM prevented
incident from becoming worse
(83.2%)

Poor CRM contributed to
incident (11.4%)

Poor CRM hampered
recovery (5.4%)

Fig. 2   Relationship between CRM and outcome of U.S. Army SD incidents, according to aircrew survey. (Reproduced with permission of Durnford et al.; Ref. 49.)

According to a review of the CRM syllabi of U.S. forces,[30] SD appears to be mentioned in CRM courses, but there is no standardized syllabus, and training is very dependent on the instructor and the type of airframe. The recommendation was made that each service should examine its own greatest SD threats, list them, and provide the information to CRM trainers and mission planners for inclusion in these processes. There is anecdotal evidence that this initiative is helping to raise the awareness of SD as a continuing significant aviation hazard, but definitive analyses are yet to be published.

5.   Instruction Directed at Instructors and Nonaircrew

It must be remembered that the problem of SD is not just the pilot's concern. Most military flights are authorized, and the authorizing officer has a responsibility to ensure that the crew are best prepared for their mission. This fact is also pertinent to civilian agencies. In their review of general aviation accidents, Kirkham et al.[10] recommended that it is important for examiners (and authorizing) officers to satisfy themselves that the pilot has a good awareness of the SD hazard and risk and is competent at the strategies to prevent and overcome SD. Training in SD should not be confined to aircrew. Air traffic controllers have also contributed to SD mishaps (see Chapter 4, Sec. II.F) and require a basic awareness of SD in order to appreciate the physiological limitations that are experienced by the pilots they control, especially because most of them are not pilots themselves.

III.   Ground-Based Devices

Because SD-related aircraft mishaps continue on their steady pace, perhaps even increasing,[50] it makes sense for all program managers to review current ground-based training practices and to determine if something can be done to reduce the number of SD accidents. Studies have shown the potential positive impact if ground-based devices are used to teach certain aspects of SD.[1,51,52] This section aims to provide the reader with an overall understanding of issues to consider when selecting a ground-based device for SD countermeasures training, some of the different types of devices available, their capabilities, and where more detailed information can be found. The selection of a particular device should be considered in the context of the overall flight training program goals and budgets, and we do not advocate one device over another. Regardless of the type of device one considers, we feel strongly that all flight-training programs should incorporate a device designed to safely expose pilots (or pilot trainees) to the vestibular and visual conflicts associated with SD inflight.

A. Past Devices for SD Demonstration/Training

Previc and Ercoline[53] summarize an historical account of past spatial disorientation devices developed for the sole purpose of demonstrating SD illusions. They found that over the past 70 years these devices evolved from simple rotational-only chairs, like the Barany chair, to complex machines with wide FOV; collimated visual systems; reprogrammable glass cockpits; cockpit motion in pitch, roll, yaw, and planetary orbit (each axis is associated with a degree of freedom); and pilot-in-the-loop controls (see Fig. 3).

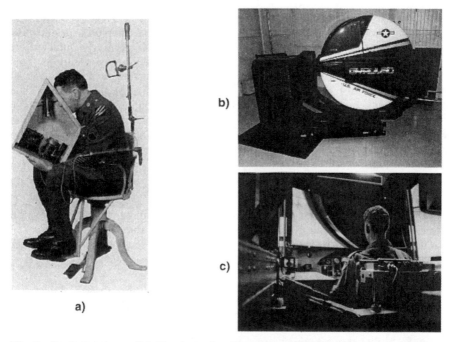

Fig. 3   Evolution in spatial disorientation demonstrators/trainers from the 1920s to the 1990s: a) Barany chair c. 1920, with Ocker box containing rudimentary instrumentation, rotates only in yaw; b) flight simulator—caliber USAF Advanced Spatial Disorientation Trainer (ASDT) capable of producing variable gravitoinertial force and 360-deg motion in pitch, roll yaw and planetary rotation; c) ASDT reconfigurable cockpit with wide FOV visual scene, allowing pilot-in-the-loop control. (Photos reproduced with permission of USAFSAM, Brooks City-Base, Texas.)

The Ruggles Orientator, a device well rooted in the history of flight simulators, seems to have been an exception to these early devices (see Fig. 3 in Chapter 1). It was developed in the very early part of the last century and provided full motion (360 deg) about the pitch, roll, and yaw axes, while the subject in the seat could control the response with a type of aircraft control stick. Actually designed and first used for the selection of candidates for pilot training, it never reached its designed intent and was soon abandoned.[8] However, as far as motion for a ground-based trainer goes, it was ahead of its time. When eventually modified, it provided the workings of the first known pilot-in-the-loop flight procedures trainer—the beginning of the flight simulator business. [Carl Crane, who collaborated with Co. Ocker in research and training in SD and instrument flight during the 1920s and 1930s (see Chapter 1), claimed to have patented a modified Ruggles Orientator as the first flight simulator. Because of restrictions placed upon military personnel regarding owning patents, Crane gave his patent rights to Edwin Link, who eventually developed the Blue Box, the first flight simulator used in training throughout the world.*

Previc and Ercoline[53] also found that devices developed for teaching SD countermeasures were usually used as demonstrators. Measuring the effectiveness of the training rarely seemed to be an issue, mainly because the devices never realistically had the capability of a flight simulator. This changed with the advent of the Gyrolab 2000 around 1993. The device, first known as the USAF Advanced Spatial Disorientation Demonstrator (ASDD) during its development and now as the Advanced Spatial Disorientation Trainer (ASDT), set a new standard for combining presentation of SD illusions and flight simulation (see Fig. 3). This device was built to provide the pilot with the capability to fly into and out of SD illusions—profiles were actually developed that could be integrated into the simulator's dynamic model of the aircraft. The pilot could now conduct realistic flight tasks in the flight simulator, respond to flight situations or illusions via the aircraft controls, and experience Type I and Type II SD. Basic SD profiles were developed and tested in 1995, and the results were very much in support of this type of training.[54]

B. Issues to Consider for Selecting a Device

Dowd[55] summarizes six issues to consider when defining a spatial orientation trainer: similarity, reproducibility, recovery capabilities, training, safety, and costs. Although we agree with the intent of these six criteria, we prefer a set of five similar factors or issues for consideration when trying to decide on a device.

1. Ability to Demonstrate Common Illusions

The primary goal of any SD countermeasures program should be the ability to safely demonstrate many of the illusions associated with SD related-mishaps. Because this is almost impossible to do in flight, the next best thing is a ground-based device. So, the primary feature of any ground-based device is to demonstrate the most common illusions, assuming that those illusions are ultimately responsible for most SD-related aircraft accidents. Based on the responses of more than 2500 USAF pilots when asked about the SD illusions they experienced, the leans was

---

*Personal communication with Carl Crane, 1975.

by far the most common in-flight SD illusion.[48] In addition, pilots reported experiencing a wide variety of the other known illusions, but most did not consider these to be as threatening as the leans. Almost all pilots reported experiencing the leans at one time or another, and demonstration of this illusion should be a basic requirement for any acceptable ground-based device.

In addition, the device should have the flexibility to be programmed to reproduce other SD illusions when an illusion is found causal in a mishap. It is recommended that a thorough review of the SD-related mishaps be studied before selecting a device. This will also help in deciding the fidelity of the device needed to generate the illusions. Exactly how the illusion is produced (an issue discussed next) can be a point of contention, but the idea of being able to at least demonstrate most of the most common illusions remains a desirable quality in ground-based SD devices.

2. Reproducibility and Consistency of an Illusion

Reproducibility is another way of determining how well the feel of an illusion on the ground simulates the sensation as it occurs in the aircraft. This is often difficult to quantify because of the many psychological factors that influence SD and the individual variability found across subjects. However, knowing a rough approximation of the range of sensory responses, and most of the conditions used to generate the sensations, will help define the specifications for the range of motion and quality of visuals needed in the ground-based device of choice. One must consider the pilot population for which the device is being used to train. It is likely that more experienced pilots will require a higher fidelity. There are two major ways to reproduce motion-related SD illusions.

The first approach requires at least a four degree-of-freedom (DOF) motion platform (one DOF being the planetary arm movment) and a fundamental understanding of how to control the direction of the net force vector, also known as the net gravitoinertial force. It also requires a simplified model of the vestibular system, or at least an understanding of the vestibular responses of the semicircular canals and otoliths (see Chapter 2). The philosophy is to match the movement of the device's attitude indicator with the actual movement of the cab. Control of the net force vector is fundamental in accomplishing this relationship—termed a "true-reading" attitude display. Ercoline et al.[56] applied this philosophy when developing the five basic SD demonstrations introduced with the ASDD. Even when using this philosophy with the most sophisticated SD ground-based motion system of its type at that time, slight deviations from this procedure were still required to generate robust SD illusions. Exactly how far ground-based devices can go before overcoming these limitations has yet to be determined.

The second approach is much less expensive. In this case the pilot experiences the illusion by tilting the cab to generate the somatosensory perception (e.g., body-seat pressure). This philosophy uses gravity to make the pilot feel the illusion as if in flight, although the actual display of the attitude indicator might not reflect the true orientation of the cab. As long as the pilot feels the force consistent with the illusion, and the attitude indicator is not required to reflect the actual attitude of the cab, then a form of reproducibility has been achieved. Because a planetary arm is not required, this approach might be adequate for the demonstration of an illusion, and it might very well turn out to be all that one can afford. It is yet to be shown whether there are any learning differences between the two approaches.[57]

3. Instructor–Pilot Interaction

The control station should provide the instructor with the capability to change instrument readings and orientations of the cab. As mentioned earlier in this chapter, modern technology and the development of training devices have made it possible to allow pilots to practice the skill of making the instruments read right, but the instructor must have some control to keep the pilot unaware of the next SD event. This capability will allow pilots to practice Type I SD (usually accomplished with the use of visual traps like channelized attention or task saturation; see Chapter 4), as well as experience a recognized conflict (for the practice of Type II SD) while applying flight procedures to maintain safe control of the aircraft. This feature also allows the instructor to vary the level of difficulty associated with each SD illusion.

4. Training Capability

Currently, this can be considered the weakest link in judging existing devices. No one really knows how well these devices train (see Sec. I.A and V). Training capability implies a capacity to change pilot behavior through a positive transfer of training between the SD device and the aircraft. There are a few reports where the quality of training experienced by the pilot in an SD motion demonstrator has been perceived as valuable, but this is only a subjective measure.[52,56] Because of this, there are those who feel that nonmotion devices are adequate trainers for learning of skills to cope with SD illusions. It is hard for the authors to imagine a device for the demonstration or training of SD countermeasures without a motion base in at least pitch, roll, and yaw. A fourth DOF, planetary movement is encouraged if it can be afforded.

5. Costs of Devices

Costs of SD countermeasures trainers with reasonable motion and visuals can range from ~$100K to the more advanced systems that exceed several million U.S. dollars. The differences in the costs are usually associated with the following factors: 1) the level of fidelity and range of motion, 2) the level of resolution and FOV of the visuals, 3) the level of flexibility and interaction required by the pilot and operator, and 4) the level of support to maintain the device.

One should consider two types of costs when deciding on the appropriate training device, that is, initial costs and recurring costs. Initial costs, those costs associated with the actual purchase and installation of a device, are best found by direct communications with the manufacturers listed in Table 1. Recurring costs, those costs associated with the maintenance of the device, are difficult to predict, but

Table 1   List of known SDCM demonstrator/trainer
manufacturers

Company name	Web site	Phone
AMST (Austria)	www.amst.co.at	43 7722 892-0
ETC (USA)	www.etcusa.com	215-355-9100
Wyle Laboratories (USA)	www.wylelabs.com	310-322-1763

they must take into account the costs of computer upgrades, general maintenance of the device, and visual scene modifications. This is usually driven by how fast technology changes and by how many new features come on the market.

In summary, the issues to consider for selecting a device should include number of demonstrations, reproducibility of illusion, instructor–student interaction, training capability, and costs. Each of these five aspects can vary in the level of sophistication, but it is appropriate for a flight-training manager to be aware of each. The devices now on the market can satisfy most of these needs with a wide variety of flexibility. Each program should look at its training objectives and its budget when trying to decide which device is most appropriate for its needs. Consideration should also be given to the relative merits of a ground-based device vs the development of a worthwhile in-flight demonstration sortie (see Sec. IV).

C.   SD Illusions and Ground-Based Requirements

When discussing the types of SD illusions that can be generated with ground-based devices, one should remember the fundamentals of spatial orientation. As described in Chapter 1, Sec. III, there are three types of SD: Type I (unrecognized), Type II (recognized), and Type III (incapacitating). Type I is usually associated with a breakdown in the instrument scan, whereas Types II and III are associated with actual recognized conflicts between two or more sensory systems.[1] Type III SD, an overwhelming breakdown in aircraft control, has yet to be adequately demonstrated or consistently induced in any ground-based device (e.g., Ref. 58). Any ground-based device capable of making a positive influence on preventing Type I SD will need a realistic instrument panel and a visual system to generate a significant amount of workload to distract the pilot away from the instrument crosscheck. For preventing Type II SD, a motion base is needed, in addition to the requirements for preventing Type I SD. Table 2 provides the user with a listing of several named SD illusions and the motion and visual systems considered necessary for their demonstration. SD terms like somatogyral, somatogravic, oculogyral, and oculogravic are not included because these terms are not widely used in the operational world. We consider a wide-FOV visual essential for a high-quality display ground-based training device (i.e., at least 100 deg horizontal and 50 deg vertical). It is desirable to have wraparound visual scenes, but the current cost to support this requirement is very high. For current systems high resolution is important within the central 40 deg of FOV and becomes less important as information is displayed further into the periphery.

As mentioned in Sec. III.B, there are two motion philosophies to apply when trying to produce many of the SD illusions. The difference between philosophies will dictate what is required of the motion base. Let us use the dark-takeoff illusion, which involves the somatogravic illusion, to apply both procedures.

Under the philosophy of not requiring the attitude indicator to match the orientation of the cab, tilting the cab backwards produces the feeling of being pitched up. The minimal motion needed is pitch. Here the sensation felt by the pilot in the cab is one that can be interpreted as accelerating down the runway. The force of gravity acting on the pilot's back produces the feedback (i.e., pressure from the cab against the back of the body), informing the pilot of an acceleration or climb. In this approach the pilot is usually shown a visual scene that depicts the pilot in a level attitude while translating down a runway, but verbal instructions can produce

Table 2 Types of SD illusions and the generalized motion and/or visual requirements

Illusion	Motion	Visual
Coriolis	Continuous yaw	——
Autokinesis		Point light source
Graveyard spin	Continuous yaw	——
Graveyard spiral	Limited pitch and roll and planetary motion	——
Gillingham illusion	Continuous pitch and yaw	——
Leans (visual)		Wide FOV (>40 degrees)
Leans (vestibular)	Continuous yaw and limited pitch; Limited pitch and planetary motion	——
Black-hole approach	——	Wide FOV
Dark-takeoff illusion	Pitch	Wide FOV
	Planetary motion	
False horizon	——	Wide FOV
Giant hand	Unknown	Unknown
Elevator illusion	Continuous yaw, limited pitch, and planetary motion	——
G-excess illusion	Limited pitch, limited roll, and planetary motion	Wide FOV
Subthreshold motion	Pitch, roll, yaw, and/or planetary motion	——
DIP	——	Narrow FOV
Runway height misperception—high flare	——	Wide FOV
Inversion illusion	Continuous yaw, limited pitch, and planetary motion	——

a similar mental state. This visual flow will look as if the pilot is accelerating in a level attitude while in actuality the cab is tilted in pitch. If the attitude indicator were shown to the pilot, it would have to be scaled (i.e., not a true representation of the cab) to reflect the visual depiction of level pitch. The pilot's sensory conflict would be generated by the difference between the pitch of the cab as shown on the level attitude indicator (a false reading) and the sense of being pitched up by the tilt of the cab (a true perception). This approach requires the attitude indicator to be incorrectly oriented when compared to the cab's actual orientation. (Use of this technique is commonly exploited throughout the flight simulator community. Actually the subject does not perceive a pitch up in a simulator, but rather acceleration.)

Under the desired outcome of the second motion philosophy, the attitude indicator must be true reading; therefore, the demonstration of the pitch-up illusion must be generated in a way similar to that encountered in flight. The attitude display must indicate level (a true situation) while the cab matches the attitude indicator (also true). In this case planetary motion (i.e., radial acceleration, see Chapter 1, Sec. IV.A.2) is needed to generate an inertial force on the back of the pilot. The pitch-up sensation comes from centripetal force generated by the angular velocity of the cab and the force of gravity. The net gravitoinertial force produces a perceived pitch approximately equal to the inverse tangent of the ratio of the radial force to the gravitational force. There is no requirement to scale the pitch of the attitude indicator because it reflects the true pitch of the cab. The pilot not only sees an accurate display of pitch but also can apply forces to the control stick to make the attitude instrument behave as in flight. The negative side of this approach are the costs needed to generate these radial forces (planetary arm), the presence of suprathreshold angular motion, and Coriolis stimulation of the semicircular canals when head movements are made.

D. Types of SD Demonstrators/Trainers

Devices for demonstrating SD, or training to counter SD, come in several shapes and sizes. The three major types of devices are listed next. The taxonomy used is the authors' way of organizing the variability across the devices. As mentioned in the preceding section, the level of fidelity, objectives of the training program, and amount of money available for purchasing a device will ultimately determine the machine to be deployed.

1. Nonplanetary Devices

These devices are the least expensive and the most plentiful. They are relatively easy to move because they are lightweight and their motion platform does not require a permanent fixture in the floor. They range from a simple, single-DOF (yaw) motion base attached to a cockpit that incorporates a virtual helmet to a more sophisticated, three-DOF device (limited pitch and roll, and continuous yaw) used by Oklahoma State University. Examples of a three-DOF device are shown in Fig. 4. Some recently developed devices have included another DOF—vertical heave. Costs of nonplanetary devices range from less than $100K to slightly more than $500K, depending upon the number of DOFs and the fidelity of the visuals incorporated within the cab.

Collimated visual scenes can be found on devices that transmit the outside scene to the pilot via a curved mirror or collimating lens. Although the use of multiple monitors could increase the FOV to more than 40 deg, we have not found any device currently on the market that uses more than one visual display monitor.

2. Constant-Radius, Planetary Arm Devices

These devices are much less common than the nonplanetary systems, probably because they are more expensive to purchase and maintain, and they require facility modification or construction to house the device. They usually contain a four-DOF motion base (see Fig. 5), with some devices capable of adding heave (vertical

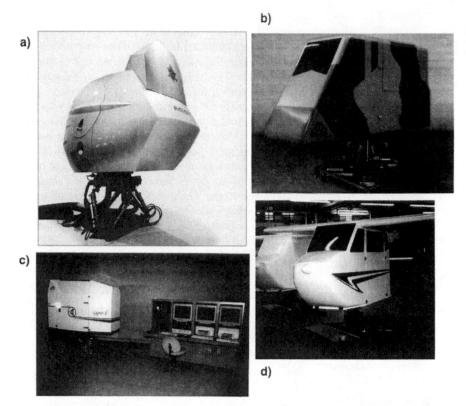

Fig. 4   Four examples of three-degree-of-freedom (limited pitch and roll, continuous yaw), nonplanetary devices: a) DISO by AMST, b) GAT II by ETC, c) GYROFLIGHT by ETC, and d) GYRO IPT I by ETC. (Photos reproduced with permission of manufacturers.)

motion) as a fifth DOF. Depending on the length and speed of the arm and the fidelity of the visual scene requirement, these devices can cost several million U.S. dollars. The authors feel that simple devices with planetary motion and no other DOF do have utility in demonstrating somato/oculogravic illusions.

3. Variable-Radius, Planetary Arm Devices

Although the concept of moving the cab along the planetary arm has been successfully used for acceleration training and research, it is a relatively new feature for SDCM training devices. It was applied to this application to reduce some of the vestibular cross-coupling sensations produced by the planetary motion devices. The illustration in Fig. 6 of the Desdemona, under development by AMST, shows the integration of vertical (heave) and variable-radius planetary motion, along with pitch, roll and yaw (six DOF).

4. Summary of Types of Training Devices

Any of the ground-based devices can enhance the capabilities of a flight-training program. Their full use might be dependent upon the knowledge of the profile

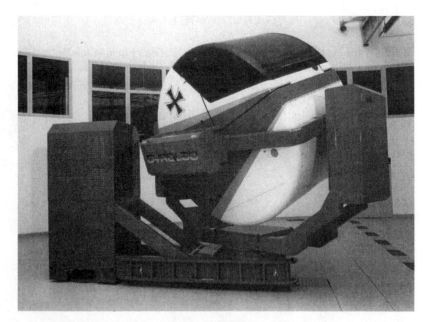

Fig. 5 Example of a constant-radius planetary device: the GyroLab 2000 by ETC, shown here as the German Air Force Flight Orientation Trainer (FOT). The Gyrolab 2000 has four degrees of freedom: pitch, roll, yaw, and planetary orbit. (Photo reproduced with permission of manufacturer.)

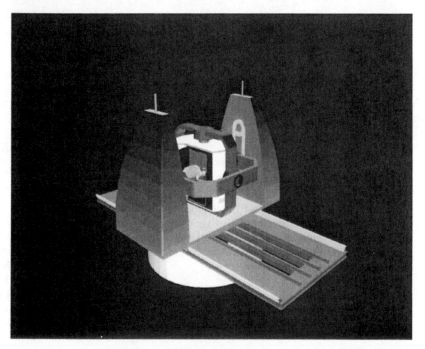

Fig. 6 Illustration of an example of a variable-radius planetary device: the Desdemona, under development by AMST. (Illustration reproduced with permission of manufacturer.)

Table 3 **List of some current SD demonstrators. The planetary arm of the Desdemona device can vary with the radius of the cab (+)**

Device	Yaw	Pitch/ roll	Plane -tary	Heave	CGI visuals[a]	HDD[b]	Pilot in the loop	Flight simulator
Vertifuge (Wyle)	X	X	X	——	——	X	X	——
GAT II (ETC)	X	X	——	——	X	X	X	X
DISO (AMST)	X	X	——	——	X+[c]	X	X	X
Gyro IPT II (ETC)	X	X	——	X	X	X	X	X
Gyrolab 2000 (ETC)[d]	X	X	X	——	X+[c]	X+	X	X
Desdemona (AMST)[e]	X	X	X+[f]	X	X	X	X	X

[a]CGI = computer-generated imagery for external visuals.
[b]HDD = head-down displays (might or might not be computer generated).
[c]CGI external visual scene of DISO and Gyro 2000 are collimated (+).
[d]Gyrolab 2000 visual system can provide a separate head-up display (+).
[e]Device not completed at time of publication.
[f]Planetary arm of Desdemona device can vary with radius of cab (+).

designer, and not just the available technology. Several features to consider when looking into the use of such a device should include the following: 1) full 360 deg of yaw movement; 2) limited pitch and bank motion (continuous 360 deg is not required for these axes); 3) flight simulator movement features (washout, washback, and scaling in pitch and bank), with the capability to enter and exit when specified; and 4) computer-generated out-the-window visuals (the wider the FOV the better), linked to motion response times of less than 150 ms (a time-delay response required of most flight simulators); 5) head-down cockpit instruments (and possibly head-up and helmet-mounted displays); 6) planetary motion and heave; 7) pilot-in-the-loop control in both flight simulation and SD illusion modes; and 8) control station instructor operation over instruments, visuals, and sound.

A device with these features will be capable of producing most SD illusions, and, at the same time, produce realistic flight simulation and situation awareness. Table 3 provides a simple comparison of capabilities across the SD devices in use and under development. A preference of one over another will depend on the desired level of training for the program.

E. Flight Simulators as Ground-Based Training Devices

The use of a flight simulator to provide SDCM training in place of a device designed specifically for SD demonstrations is always a topic for discussion. Flight simulators have already been successfully used for the demonstration of certain rotary-wing SD illusions.[16,17,37] With the exception of some of the motion-related illusions, the flight simulator presents an excellent opportunity to capitalize on this training device to enhance awareness and coping strategies for helicopter operations. A synopsis of the U.S. Army experience and further enhancements to this type of training is included in Appendix C. There are a few SD illusions that are not possible in a traditional flight simulator.[59] These illusions, usually of the somatogravic or somatogyral type, require special motion platforms and an understanding of the causes of SD.

An FAA approved flight simulator is a device that is a full-size aircraft cockpit replica of a specific type of aircraft. It includes the hardware and software necessary to mimic the aircraft both on the ground and in the air, and it typically uses a six-DOF motion system. It also uses a visual system for each pilot that provides at least a 45-deg horizontal FOV and a 30-deg vertical FOV. Finally, the system must be evaluated and approved by the FAA.[60] Each simulator is then further characterized by fidelity, as defined by visual characteristics or range and speed of motion.

The FAA requires a flight simulator to have a motion base. This is not the case for many military flight simulators—a point of debate that has yet to be fully resolved.[61] The fighter-type simulators do not use motion systems, whereas the large cargo and passenger-type simulators do. Unfortunately, the regulations do not define a SD demonstrator or SDCM simulator. The most exposure to SD required of USAF pilot trainees is to experience a motion-related vestibular illusion with either the Barany chair or the Vista-Vertigon, if available.[62] It can only be assumed from this requirement that most flight-training program directors feel the training received via the current devices is adequate. If an organization does not have access to a SD demonstrator, we then encourage them to evaluate the possibility of using flight-training simulators to demonstrate SD illusions.

F. Organizations Performing Ground-Based Demonstrations/Training

Within the past several years a few flight-training programs around the globe have taken an interest in SD demonstrators. In 1974 the United Kingdom Royal Air Force (RAF) flight physiology program began using a spatial-disorientation familiarization device (SDFD) that provided planetary rotation and enabled the demonstration of the somatogravic illusion.[26] The SDFD has since been replaced by two Gyro IPT 1 systems. The German Air Force uses a flight orientation trainer (FOT) as a spatial orientation trainer for a select group of pilots. The German FOT is basically the same device as the USAF's ASDT, which are both versions of the ETC Gyrolab 2000. The USAF ASDT is presently being used to train instrument flying instructor pilots at the USAF Advanced Instrument School. Several Middle and Far East countries use various versions of the Gyrolab 2000. The Royal Netherlands Air Force physiology refresher program currently incorporates the AMST DISO for spatial orientation training, and this organization is playing a significant part in the development of the Desdemona. The FAA recently purchased two portable spatial disorientation demonstrators and plans to use these devices to reach general aviation pilots with a SD awareness program. Oklahoma State University has just purchased a new GAT II (spatial orientation and flight trainer) device. The U.S. Navy operates a unique system, the Multistation Disorientation Demonstrator (MSDD) at the Navy Aeromedical Research Laboratory, Pensacola, Florida. This device has been used to simultaneously demonstrate a variety of SD illusions to as many as 10 people.[63] The U.S. Navy is currently pursuing acquisition of a more advanced SDCM trainer.

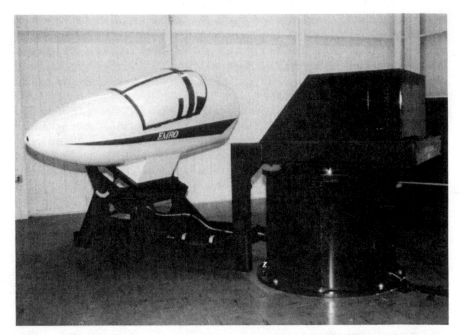

Fig. 7   Vertifuge by Emro (now Wyle): an example of a constant-radius, planetary arm device. (Photo reproduced with permission of USAFSAM, Brooks City-Base, Texas.)

Over the past three or four decades, the U.S. Navy and Air Force successfully used a constant-arm planetary device called the Vertifuge (see Fig. 7) for research and limited training. The USAF School of Aerospace Medicine used one of these devices for research as recently as 1993 when it was replaced by the ASDD. Although we do not know of anyone still using a Vertifuge, we feel it appropriate to mention that lessons learned from it have good application to any SD countermeasures training program. Those who used of the Vertifuge set the stage for advancing the concept of more sophisticated SD demonstrators.[64]

IV.   In-Flight Demonstration and Training

One of the most important SD countermeasures is the aviator's awareness of his or her physiological vulnerability to SD and the operational circumstances and phases of flight in which SD is most likely to occur. There are many distinct advantages to conducting SD demonstrations in the environment in which aviators operate (see Sec. V), not the least of which is to allow the aviators to discover personally that their sensory system is inadequate to maintain orientation when deprived of visual cues.[4] After all, the aircraft is the perfect dynamic flight simulator!

A.   Historical Perspective

Crawford and Davis[65] and Henning[66] developed a series of flight maneuvers for the induction and demonstration of SD for the U.S. Navy and USAF, but there was only minimal follow-through of this initiative, and the procedures were discontinued. However, a specific rotary-wing SD demonstration sortie was developed by the British Army and has been conducted since 1982 (Refs. 19 and 67). Student pilots experience the demonstration during their initial flying training course and every five years thereafter. The rotary-wing SD demonstration sortie has since been adopted by the U.S. Army[37] and the Canadian Forces, and it is hoped that it will be standardized across the ASCC nations.[68] Furthermore, following an ASCC initiative, a high-performance fixed-wing version of the demonstration has been redeveloped[69] (Brown, D. L., "The Fixed Wing in Flight Spatial Disorientation Demonstration," Royal Air Force Centre of Aviation Medicine, personal communication, Henlow, England, U.K., 2000). The fundamental procedures of both demonstrations are summarized next and described in detail in Appendices D and E.

B. Rotary-Wing Demonstration

In the ideal version of this demonstration, three students are flown on each sortie. Each experiences one or more forward flight maneuvers and a hover maneuver. The sortie should not be flown with less than two students, as there are distinct benefits from observing the reaction of peers as well as experiencing the maneuvers themselves. During the transit to the demonstration area, the physiology of the orientation senses is briefly reviewed. A series of forward flight and hover maneuvers are then conducted. In turn, students are instructed to sit free of airframe structures other than the seat, note the aircraft's initial flight parameters, close their eyes and lower their dark visor, and, as the "subject" for that maneuver, to give a running commentary on their perception of the aircraft's flight path. In this way the subject is deprived of vision, so that the unreliability of the nonvisual orientation senses can be demonstrated. The other two students (observers) are asked to observe but not comment until after the maneuver is complete. A verbal debrief is conducted immediately after each maneuver.

1. Illusions Demonstrated

The following illusions are demonstrated: somatogyral illusion, the contribution of suprathreshold and subthreshold vestibular and kinesthetic stimuli to SD, and the absence of veridical information on altitude and airspeed in conditions of poor visibility. Full details are described in Appendix D.

2. Conduct of the Demonstration

The option of who is to conduct the sortie and the type of helicopter must be determined. These are addressed next, enabling trainers to choose the situation which best suits their needs and resources. Three standards are presented, and their advantages and disadvantages are presented in Table 4. The gold standard, in which the pilot is an expert on SD, must be regarded as the preferred solution. The bronze solution, in which only an instructor pilot and students are present, is the absolutely acceptable minimum and should only be accepted if a higher standard is not possible. The British Army is the only service to have had comprehensive experience of this demonstration over the last 20 years. Their flight surgeons are

Table 4 Rotary-wing demonstration standards

Standard	Pilot	SME[a]	Advantages	Disadvantages
Gold	Flight surgeon (FS)	FS is also the pilot.	The pilot-FS intimately knows the "desired" response to each demonstration. FS is available to explain/debrief any nuances that might arise. FS can make immediate minor modifications to the demonstration. As an IP is not present, for ab initio students, this appears as a nonthreatening demonstration and not a "check-ride." Three (the optimum number) students can be flown in most small helicopters and is therefore also cost effective.	FS must also be a pilot. Helicopter must be qualified for single pilot operations.
Silver	Instructor pilot (IP)	FS	Is acceptable for nations/services whose FS are not pilots. FS is available to brief/debrief each demonstration. Could be just acceptable when the aircraft passenger load is limited to 3 (IP plus 2 students).	Both IPs and FS require training. FS must train IP in the conduct of each demonstration. Not as "flexible" as Gold standard. IP must be trained in the conduct of each demonstration and in the correct briefing/debriefing procedures.
Bronze	Instructor pilot	Nil		The least desired and flexible option. As only the IP is present, might be perceived by students as a further check-ride.

[a]SME = subject matter expert.

also pilots who both fly and conduct the sortie, and the demonstration has been fully validated when conducted in this manner. Many other organizations have flight surgeons who are not rated aviators. As an alternative, an instructor pilot could therefore fly the sorties—the silver standard. However, it is highly desirable that a flight surgeon should conduct the sortie, preferably from the other front crew seat. The flight surgeon will have performed the ground-based training and should, therefore, be on hand to explain the mechanics of SD. This is possible as evidenced by the introduction of the SD demonstration sortie to U.S. Army Aviation in 1995 (Ref. 37).

The type of helicopter used to conduct this sortie should be capable of carrying seated, forward-facing passengers in the rear cabin and enable them to have a reasonable view of both the instrument panel and the outside terrain. Those experiencing the sortie should not face backwards or sideways because they would not be exposed to the same direction of accelerative forces with which they are familiar as front-seat crew members. Ideally, the aircraft should be qualified for single-pilot operations.

Flight surgeons experienced in this demonstration can readily train their colleagues as well as instructor pilots. Experience from introducing the sortie to U. S. Army Aviation,[16,37] in which the flight surgeons were not rated pilots, was that training and practice sessions for each instructor pilot were performed individually and took approximately 1.5 h. This training time could be reduced if several instructor pilots were shown the sortie simultaneously. The core of aeromedical training expertise should continue to be at an aeromedical training center, with new flight surgeons being trained as they attend the flight surgeon course.

There is good evidence from the British Army Air Corps' experience[70] that the initial SD sortie is best flown just before students learn instrument flying in helicopters. To aid understanding and awareness, the period since students last attended aeromedical lectures on SD should not be too long (less than eight weeks is suggested). The sortie should also be flown every 4–5 years as part of refresher training in SD.

Although inclusion of this demonstration sortie in a rotary-wing flight syllabus entails an additional flight to be programmed (for every three students), the authors believe that there is a positive cost–benefit relationship.[67] Both internal and external validation of this demonstration is discussed in Sec. V.

C.   High-Performance Fixed-Wing Demonstration

To date, this demonstration has only been flown in the Hawk T Mk 1 training aircraft of the United Kingdom's Royal Air Force (Brown, D. L., "The Fixed Wing in Flight Spatial Disorientation Demonstration," Royal Air Force Centre of Aviation Medicine, personal communication, Henlow, England, U.K., 2000), but it is being assessed by other air forces and in other airframes. A combination of somatogravic and somatogyral illusions convincingly illustrates how inaccurately the human senses predict orientation relative to the Earth's surface. Each illusion is outlined in Appendix E, followed by a description that can be used by the instructor pilot to explain the illusion, where in flight it can occur, and the consequences of succumbing to the illusion.

1. Illusions Demonstrated

The following eight illusions are demonstrated (full details are described in Appendix E): pitch misperception, elevator illusion, false climb in a turn, diving during turn recovery, the leans, postroll effect (Gillingham illusion), tilt with skid, and Coriolis.

2. Conduct of the Demonstration

High-performance fixed-wing aircraft have a maximum of two seats. In contrast to the rotary-wing demonstration, this demonstration must therefore be performed one-to-one and implicitly must be conducted by either a flight surgeon-pilot or an enlightened instructor pilot. Hopefully, once a knowledge base is established within the training organization, the proper instructor training can be readily prepared.

Contrary to the rotary-wing demonstration, it is suggested that no extra training sortie be required to perform this demonstration. The eight illusions can be flown in a total time of about 20 min either en route to a training area or returning to base. Alternatively, a few can be demonstrated on several sorties. However, it is essential that the training objectives be established.

D. In-Flight Training Procedures

Having experienced a formal demonstration of the limitations of the orientation senses in flight, it is imperative that the student pilot be trained in both the prevention of SD in flight and the strategies to overcome SD when it occurs. Specific didactic instructions for coping with SD during various forms of flight and circumstances were provided in Sec. II.E. This subsection will cover the general principles of inflight training, in particular the importance of setting training objectives.

Cheung[39] emphasized that the practical understanding of SD is best attained through exposure to visual and vestibular illusions in an actual flight environment in a well-planned and controlled manner. In-flight training ideally leads to an enhanced SD awareness and a behavior modification through personal experiences gained during actual flight. These experiences, in turn, encourage avoidance of future SD situations and enable the pilot to recover from SD. In-flight training in SD has generally been restricted to instrument flying training, including procedures to be taken upon inadvertent entry into IMC, and to recovery from unusual attitudes. Whereas it cannot be refuted that these skills are important, there is an apparent lack of consistency in the way that procedures are taught.[1,6] Furthermore, there is increasing evidence that the traditional methods are not as effective as they should be in overcoming SD in flight.[4] The establishment of training objectives can improve both.

1. Instrument Flight Training

Currency and competency at flying with reference to flight instruments has long been the recommended mainstay of coping with SD.[1] Military aviation authorities have recognized this fact since shortly after World War I, and procedural instrument flight is the normal method employed by commercial aviation. There is also now a much greater emphasis on encouraging the general aviation pilot to achieve and maintain an instrument flying rating.[10] However, there appears to be a tendency for a large proportion of instrument flight training to be conducted in flight simulators rather than in the actual aircraft. Although it is realized that this decision is resource-driven, flying-training authorities should question whether a positive transfer of training is really being achieved. Flying by instruments is a more difficult psychomotor task than flying by external visual reference and is thus more susceptible to impairment by task load, anxiety or other stresses that might raise the level of behavioral arousal above the optimum.[4,71]

Therefore, to become more proficient when actual IMC conditions are encountered it is most important that instrument-flying training should include as many additional stressors as are compatible with flight safety. A graduated syllabus of increasing imposed difficulty as the students progress through flying training is recommended, as is frequent refresher training and testing.

2. Inadvertent Entry into IMC

Although training objectives to achieve competency in general instrument flight will be aircraft type and model specific (because of differences in flight-control and management systems), it is possible to define a generic training objective for inadvertent entry to IMC. The following is extracted from an ASCC publication[72] to provide a common training base for aircrew on joint and combined operations.

Training is to be conducted during both elementary and advanced (including operational conversion) flight training, and also during conversion to each specific aircraft type. An assessment of skills should also be made during revalidation of an instrument flying rating. The following are the MINIMUM requirements for which a training objective is to be stated. During a training flight in visual meteorological conditions (VMC), the instructor will announce a simulated inadvertent entry to IMC. If the aircraft is appropriately rated, the procedure is to be performed during both day and night flight. It will also be performed during flight with NVDs if the aircraft is appropriately equipped and the student is rated on NVDs. The student will correctly perform the procedures for inadvertent entry to IMC, i.e. immediate reversion to flight by reference to the primary flight instruments. Indicated airspeed and vertical speed are to be appropriate to the aircraft type. A climb to the safety altitude is to be achieved. Flight Instructors are to be taught to perform and assess these procedures during their own instructor training.

3. Recovery from Unusual Attitudes (Positions)

If pilots fail to maintain their desired orientation in flight but recognize that they have become disoriented, they must be able to effectively recover the aircraft to within safe operating limits. This is a rare, but not unknown event in commercial flying,[23] yet is common in both high-performance and helicopter operations in military flying,[48,49] and is extremely common in general aviation flying, particularly among those pilots who do not have an instrument rating.[10] It is, therefore, an essential proficiency at which the pilot must become and remain skilled.

Most military air forces include unusual attitude recovery in their training syllabi, but there is evidence that the standards and periodicity with which they are performed is extremely variable.[6,73] By definition, pilots are required to recover from a circumstance in which they have recognized that they are disorientated and therefore, more emphasis on Type II SDCM training is required. A suggestion is to routinely allow the student pilot to enter an unusual attitude by flying with his/her eyes closed for a period of time and then recover from it with eyes open, in addition to the more traditional method in which the instructor places the student into an unusual attitude.

Although flight instruction manuals are aircraft specific in the execution of these exercises, a generic training objective is possible. Appendix F contains an extract from an ASCC publication[72] to provide a common training base for aircrew on joint and combined operations. A more detailed description of specific unusual attitude recognition and recovery procedures is described in Chapters 9 and 10.

Attitude recovery training is rare in general aviation, but there is an increasing trend in commercial aviation to include the teaching and practice of recovery from unusual attitudes ("airplane upsets") during both initial pilot training and during refresher sessions. Programs range from classroom lectures complemented with ground-based demonstration through demonstration and training in flight simulators to employing small aerobatic aircraft to train novice pilots in handling extreme attitudes. Despite the appeal of such training among pilots who have received it,[74,75] there is some concern that the ground-based simulation might provide false or improper cues and lead to negative transfer of training[76] and that the aerobatic experience might not equate to that of a large commercial aircraft. To date, no formal evaluation of the effectiveness of existing airplane-upset training programs has been conducted, although NASA and the Airplane Upset Training Aid Consortium are currently planning such a test. Nevertheless, major commercial airlines (e.g., American, SAS, US Airways) appear committed to enhancing the competence of their crews through this enhanced training.

V. Efficacy of Demonstration and Training

The systems approach to training (SAT) requires organizations to monitor the efficacy and validity of training. This section examines the available evidence for the benefits of existing SD training programs and initiatives and provides the reader with some suggestions as to how to monitor the effectiveness of SD training.

Validation of SD training effectiveness is the process of determining 1) whether training has achieved the specified training objectives (internal validation) and 2) whether the training objectives reflect the operational flying requirements (external validation). Continuous and systematic validation of training is necessary to establish that training is effective and to ensure that it is adjusted to meet changes in flying requirements. Such changes might be caused by the introduction of new or modified equipment, by new techniques, or by the restructuring of the flying demands to include new tasks or exclude old ones.

Once the decision to perform SD training has been taken, consideration of the most cost-effective means of carrying out the training is necessary (i.e., efficiency). Assessment of SD training *effectiveness* is a principal concern of instructors. Measures of SD training *efficiency*, on the other hand, are the concern of others besides the instructor and are likely to involve consideration of budgetary and other factors beyond the competence of those immediately concerned with training. It must be stressed that these processes are particularly important in the prevailing climate of fiscal constraint and limited resources.

Validation allows training programs to meet changes in the job requirements. This is extremely important in aviation. General aviation aircraft are becoming more diverse—some more sophisticated, whereas others arguably simpler than before (e.g., microlights or ultralights). In the military field, despite advances in control and instrument technology, aircrew certainly do not have a lesser number of tasks, but these tasks have significantly changed in nature over the years. As far as training in SD is concerned, it is reasonable to make the following statements with respect to the SAT process: 1) the job can be generally defined as the optimal performance of the pilot in his/her duties, and specifically as the prevention and/or control of the hazard of SD; 2) training objectives must be established for SDCM training; 3) where they have been set, the training objectives must be designed to result in an improvement in flight safety and an enhancement in mission effectiveness. That is, training must prepare the pilot to be more aware of the SD hazard to prevent himself/herself from becoming disoriented and to recognize and to overcome SD.

The metrics that should be used to determine the effectiveness of SD demonstration and training are difficult to define, and different studies have used different outcomes. The extremes range from user satisfaction to training at the "soft" end of the effectiveness continuum to a demonstrated reduction in the SD accident rate at the "hard" end. The former can really only be regarded as a measure of internal validation, whereas the latter goes much of the way to being an external validation assessment. However, even the latter is fraught with problems because of the differences in both the analysis and subsequent classification of the SD accident. It is even more difficult to measure the effectiveness of SD training in preventing the SD incident that compromises mission effectiveness. It is well established that SD incidents that "just frighten" the pilot are grossly underreported, possibly because some pilots still feel that they should be invulnerable to SD. Unless open reporting procedures can be encouraged and instituted, incident reports can only be useful as training aids and not as an appropriate measure for the effectiveness of SD training.

Despite previous recommendations that ground-based and inflight training methods should require validation to ensure that the implemented training is likely to be effective,[77] there have been few formal reports addressing this issue, and most of these have only been concerned with internal validation. The following paragraphs summarize the available evidence.

Collins et al.[78] analyzed the responses of 674 students attending Federal Aviation Administration (FAA)-certified and ground schools concerning the conduct of SD training. More than 1/3 evaluated the training as inadequate, primarily from a lack of appropriate training materials. Recommendations were made for improvements and are summarized in a review of SD in general aviation pilots.[10] This is a good example of external validation, albeit in the user-satisfaction category, leading to an enhancement of the training. Although a follow-up study could not be found in the open literature, the SDCM training of general aviation pilots has since been significantly enhanced as a result of the earlier survey.[41]

Walsh[73] surveyed 131 USAF undergraduate pilots by means of a questionnaire that requested details of their in-flight SD training experience and opinions on its efficacy. In particular, the extent and degree of success of in flight training was analyzed. Alarmingly, over 53% had received neither inflight demonstrations nor classroom discussions. Although the effectiveness of the inflight demonstration of

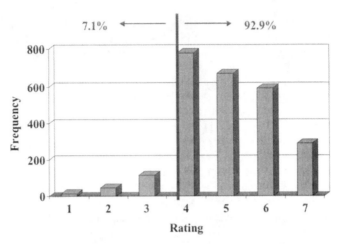

**Fig. 8   Distribution of USAF aircrew responses on the value of SD training: 1 = no
value, 4 = satisfactory, 7 = excellent in all respects. (Reproduced with permission of
Matthews; Ref. 48.)**

the leans was regarded as satisfactory by 91%, only 31% considered the graveyard
spiral demonstration to be effective. The survey concluded that there was a need for
a well-defined, validated set of demonstration procedures to elicit specific illusions
in flight. This study clearly identified a lack of training objectives resulting in either
the omission of demonstrations to a large proportion of students or an ineffective
execution of the training.

In the largest-ever survey of USAF aircrew concerning their experiences of SD,
in which over 2500 responses were received, Matthews[48] asked specifically about
satisfaction with SD training. The distribution of responses is shown in Fig. 8.

Generally, aircrew were happy with the training they had received as shown
by the 92.9% who rated their training as satisfactory or better. The satisfaction
level was higher among pilots who had received training from a variety of sources
(lectures, ground-based training devices, and in-flight training) as compared with
pilots who had received limited training opportunities. S. R. Holmes ("A Spatial
Disorientation Survey of UK Aircrew," Defence and Evaluation Research Agency,
personal communication, Farnborough, England, U.K., 2001) has performed an
identical survey in the United Kingdom, and the preliminary responses are similar
to Matthew's findings. These surveys demonstrate that from an operator's viewpoint, SD training is generally regarded as being satisfactory. However, there is
little *direct* evidence that the training is proving effective in reducing the incidence
or severity of SD in flight. Until this can be proven, the existing data provide a
good argument that further training enhancements are still required.

There have been several recent user surveys of the more sophisticated ground-
based demonstration devices. An evaluation of the ASDD demonstration profiles
was performed[54] which assessed the illusion effectiveness (for Type I SD) and
the ability to generate visual-vestibular conflicts (Type II SD). Thirty-four of 40
subjects provided overall comments of their ASDD experience on the postsession
survey. Representative comments (edited and condensed) included: "excellent at

showing the affects of SD"; "just experiencing the symptoms in a controlled environment will place most aviators in a position of realizing they aren't perfect and that it can happen to them"; "a great improvement over other means of demonstrating SD"; "SD training should be incorporated in both undergraduate pilot training as well as periodic (annual) simulator rides throughout career"; "I derived the biggest benefit from the visual illusions which I have experienced routinely in operational flying."[54] The study concluded that the ASDD is feasible to demonstrate to aircrew how to recognize and manage SD, thereby providing internal validation of its training. However, the capability of the ASDD (now ASDT) to conduct SDCM training has yet to be fully evaluated.

Winfield et al.[79] questioned RAF aircrew undergoing aviation medicine training about their in-flight SD experiences, with the aim of improving the demonstration profiles in a Gyro IPT 1® demonstrator. Their data enabled them to develop the software and training programs to match the illusions and provocative conditions that were being experienced in flight. Consequently, the quality of SD ground-based training was improved, although as yet there has not been a concomitant reduction in the RAF SD accident rate. Again, internal validation measures are required to fine-tune the SD profiles and demonstrate their acceptability to the user community.[79]

The introduction of SD flight simulator scenarios has been mentioned in Section III.E and Appendix C to this chapter (see also Ref. 80.). Their potential benefit to increasing pilot awareness of the SD hazard was assessed by questionnaire following demonstrations to 30 experienced volunteer aviators.[81] For 15 of the 18 scenarios, the mean scores based on a scale of 1 (extremely poor) to 5 (excellent) were 4.5 or above for the question, "How do you rate the effectiveness of the scenario for training aviators." Of particular note was that the highest ratings came from the instructor pilot subgroup. The ability to convince these particular personnel that this enhancement to training was worthy was a most significant achievement and assisted considerably in the program's implementation not only as SD training but also as continuation training for CRM.

An assessment of the rotary-wing SD demonstration sortie as part of the U.S. Army's Initial Entry Rotary-Wing (IERW) course was assessed in a similar fashion to the simulator scenarios. Forty-five aviators and training personnel experienced the sortie and gave their opinion in questionnaires. The maneuvers performed in the SD demonstration sortie, as well as the sortie overall, were extremely effective at demonstrating the limitations of the orientation senses. Indeed, when the subjects were asked to compare the SD sortie with their previous SD instruction, demonstration, and training experiences, it attracted a significantly higher rating in its effectiveness (see Table 5). The survey demonstrated that introduction of the sortie into the IERW training syllabus would distinctly enhance the SD training of aviators and associated personnel and that the introduction of the sortie into refresher training in field units would also be desirable.

The majority of the studies already mentioned have been concerned with internal validation. What is lacking in most cases is the external validation: Has the training prepared them for the mission they perform? The only known type of specific SD instruction for which this process has been applied is the rotary-wing SD demonstration sortie in the British Army. Its value was assessed by a questionnaire administered to all Army aircrew, most of whom had flown for some time after they

Table 5   Rating of the effectiveness of previously experienced types of SD instruction, demonstration and training, and the SD demonstration sortie[16,37]

Type of instruction[a]	Number of responses	Median rating[b]	25–75 percentile range
Classroom instruction	43	7.0	6.0–10.0
Discussion of SD accidents/incidents	33	7.0	6.0–10.0
Barany chair	33	8.0	6.0–10.0
Other SD demonstration devices	16	10.0	5.0–12.0
Recovery from unusual attitudes in an aircraft	31	10.0	7.0–11.0
Recovery from unusual attitudes in a flight simulator	33	10.0	9.0–12.0
SD demonstration sortie[c]	45	13.0	12.0–13.0

[a]Not all subjects had experienced all of the types of SD instruction, demonstration, and training.
[b]Rating range: 0 = extremely poor, 7 = adequate, 13 = excellent.
[c]Significantly higher rating score than all of the other forms of instruction (by Wilcoxon matched pairs signed ranks test, $p = 0.001$).

had been trained by this method.[70] A total of 347 questionnaires were received, reflecting a response rate of 79%. The results, based on a five-point scale, are shown in Fig. 9. The wholehearted support of the aircrew for this demonstration was most reassuring and confirms that they at least *thought* that they had been adequately trained for their jobs.

An *objective* analysis of the rotary-wing SD demonstration sortie assessed the benefits in terms of operational outcome—its effect on the SD accident rate in

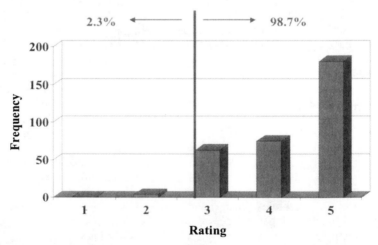

Fig. 9   Distribution of British Army helicopter aircrew responses on the value of the SD demonstration sortie: 1 = no value, 3 = satisfactory, 5 = beneficial in all respects. (Reproduced with permission of Durnford; Ref. 70.)

the British Army.[67] The SD accident rate for the 10 years (1971–1982) before the demonstration was introduced (2.04 accidents per 100,000 flying hours) was compared with a similar period (1983–1993) following its introduction (0.57 accidents per 100,000 flying hours). A Poisson regression analysis revealed a significant difference between both the two accident rates [chi-square $(df = 1) = 5.86$; $p = 0.02$] and the type of accident in the two periods [chi-square $(df = 1) = 73.97$; $p = 0.0001$]. Thus the data show a highly significant reduction in the SD accident rate after the SD demonstration sortie was introduced.

However, there are several confounding factors in this analysis. Some factors have tended to reduce the orientation error accident rate, including 1) the introduction of aircraft with automatic flight control systems and stability augmentation in the late 1970s; 2) the installation of additional aircraft flight instruments (e.g., radar altimeters) in the early 1980s; and 3) the phasing out of predominantly single-pilot operations in the mid-1980s. On the other hand, a counterbalancing factor that has tended to increase the SD accident rate is the much greater use of NVGs since the mid-1980s. Although it might be reasonable to assert that the SD demonstration sortie, through raising aviator's awareness of the limitations of the orientation senses, has contributed to reducing the accident rate in which SD is involved, there is yet no proof that this is so. It is hoped that other services that have introduced this method of demonstration will conduct similar analyses in the future. Perhaps future studies should focus on the enhancement of mission effectiveness (albeit a no less "noisy" statistic than accident rates), as this is an area that gets the attention of those who control training and technology resources.

VI. Improvements in SD Education

A recurring theme during reviews of SD training is that the quality of training varies considerably and is, in part, dependent upon the competence and knowledge of the trainer. Some suggestions on how the quality of teaching and professional knowledge of the instructor can be enhanced, are given here:

1) A coordinated Internet Web site for SD,* which includes up-to-date educational information, should be consulted regularly.

2) Regular promulgation of "lessons learned" from individual SD accidents and incidents should be disseminated at the earliest opportunity. Information to enhance awareness is most often derived from periodic reviews of accidents or aircrew opinion, by which time it has lost a significant amount of its educational impact. Although it is realized that information on an accident or incident cannot be released until the enquiry is complete, safety centers can play a major role by succinctly summarizing the salient points as soon as possible thereafter. A vehicle for promulgation of information of this type exists in some air forces (e.g., Israeli) and has been proposed within the NATO Research and Technology Agency forum.[82]

3) Aircrew should be encouraged to share their personal SD experiences during refresher training sessions. These case-based vignettes are most powerful educational tools and serve to reinforce the fact that all aviators are vulnerable to SD and

---

*Data available online at http://www.spatiald.wpafb.af.mil [cited Oct. 2003].

to demystify some of the problems. If this effective benefit to training is employed, it is implicit that aircrew must be assured by their authorities that no blame will be attributed to them.

4) If some of the in-flight demonstration and training is to be performed by instructor pilots, it is most important that they are trained in the execution of the SD maneuvers, the psychophysiological response of the student, and what the student must do to both recognize and rectify the situation. As most instructor pilots are, by definition, experienced pilots, there has often been a long period since they were trained in aviation physiology. Therefore, a physiological training session is required in instructor pilot courses both as a refresher and as an aid to what the instructor pilot will tell his/her students. The instructor is then better able to provide a flexible approach to the individual student whose susceptibility to SD is extremely variable. If this is not done, there is a real danger that in-flight demonstration and training will become too impersonal, and so the intended enhancement of awareness and skills to recognize and deal with SD will not be achieved.

5) A feedback relationship should be established between the research and training communities, particularly as new and technologically advanced ground-based flying training devices are introduced. Examples of cooperation include avoiding the designation of a particular device solely for training or research and including trainers and researchers in device planning meetings. Miller[83] states that, "it is of utmost importance that the leaders of the research community 'connect' with the leaders of operating forces as well as aviation's resource sponsors to focus development and deploy the common solutions to SD." A forum for discussion has been established at the SD Web site mentioned earlier.

VII. Summary

This chapter has attempted to be comprehensive in its approach to education as a useful countermeasure to the hazard of SD and has emphasized many of the recent initiatives. In summary, the following conclusions are highlighted:

1) Pilots that have experienced SD in flight are better able to appreciate its significance.
2) Ground-based and inflight instruction, demonstration, and training are vitally important, and all should be incorporated into a flight-training program.
   a) Instruction must comprehensively cover the physiological and psychological aspects of SD and be specific to both the aircraft and types of mission that the aviator flies.
   b) As a minimum, ground-based demonstration of SD illusions should be conducted at least in a basic rotary device.
   c) Consideration should be given to the use of flight simulators for ground-based training.
   d) In-flight demonstration is valuable and need not require additional flight time as it can be readily incorporated during the transit time from base to training areas.
   e) In-flight training in coping with inadvertent entry to IMC and recovery from unusual attitudes should be mandatory.

f) Training objectives for all types of instruction must be set.

3) In the military there is an increase in the amount of night flying. This trend will eventually filter into general aviation. Therefore the increased hazard of SD that occurs with night-vision devices must be seriously considered.

4) There have been recent initiatives in the private and commercial sectors to encourage general aviation pilots to undertake SD training and demonstration. However, although some SD scenarios are discussed during line-oriented flight training it is still not mandatory for commercial aviation pilots to attend additional SD training.

5) Training in SD should not be confined to aircrew. Air traffic controllers also require a basic awareness of SD.

6) The relatively small additional cost of procuring and maintaining demonstration and training equipment and instituting effective training programs must be weighed against the cost incurred from mishaps and loss of mission effectiveness.

7) When selecting a SD demonstration/training device or program, flying-training authorities should always question whether a positive transfer of training is being achieved.

8) Finally, training countermeasures might not necessarily be the ideal solution to the SD hazard or appropriate to every circumstance, but they are the most readily applied once the authorities are convinced to implement them.

Appendix A: Didactic Syllabus of the SD Mechanisms

This is a syllabus based on Benson[4] with additional topics (*in italics*) that have become important in the intervening quarter of a century.

I. Introduction
   A. Definition of spatial orientation in flight, hence spatial disorientation (SD)
      1. *The ASCC agreed definition of SD is based upon Benson[4] as follows: A term used to describe a variety of incidents occurring in flight where the pilot fails to sense correctly the position, motion, or attitude of the aircraft or of himself within the fixed coordinate system provided by the surface of the Earth and the gravitational vertical. In addition, errors in perception by the pilot of his position, motion, or attitude with respect to his aircraft, or of his own aircraft relative to other aircraft, can also be embraced within a broader definition of spatial disorientation in flight.*
   B. Importance of correct perception of orientation in aircraft control
   C. *Operational* and flight safety importance of orientation. SD jeopardizes flight safety (*and mission effectiveness*) because of the following:
      1. Control based on false perception leads to loss of control and the orientation-error accident.
      2. Conflicting orientation cues or abnormal sensations can heighten arousal and performance might be impaired.

D. Aircrew need to know the following:
   1. Types of illusory perceptions occurring in flight
   2. Flight conditions and maneuvers likely to induce SD
   3. How to cope with disorientation if and when it occurs
II. Mechanism of Orientation in Flight
   A. Dependent upon correct integration and interpretation (perception) of sensory information from the following:
      1. Eyes. *Anatomy and physiology of the eye. Psychophysiology of vision. Focal and ambient vision. Depth perception.*
      2. Inner ear, especially vestibular part. *Anatomy and physiology of the vestibular apparatus.*
      3. Other receptors in skin, capsules, or joints and supporting tissues responding to the force environment.
   B. *In the absence of veridical information provided by technological enhancements,* vision is the only reliable channel of information using either:
      1. External visual cues, when flying in visual meteorological conditions (VMC)
      2. Internal visual cues from instruments, when flying in instrument meteorological conditions (IMC)
   C. The aviator has to learn how to interpret cues. Interpretation of instrument cues is a more recently learned and more difficult task than interpreting external cues; proficiency has to be maintained by practice. Nonvisual cues are frequently either inadequate or erroneous and do not allow the aviator to maintain a correct perception of aircraft orientation. They do, however, assist the pilot in sensing transient changes in aircraft attitude and motion and hence with visual cues can contribute to correct orientation in flight.
III. Mechanism of Disorientation in Flight
   A. Caused either by:
      1. Erroneous or inadequate sensory information transmitted to the brain
      2. Erroneous or inadequate perception of sensory signals transmitted to the brain
   B. Input error
      1. External visual
         a. Cues inadequate as when flying at high altitude, at night, in cloud or other poor visibility conditions
         b. Cues erroneous (i.e., departing from expectancy), e.g., sloping edge of a cloud bank or auroral display
      2. Instruments
         a. Inadequate sensitivity to displayed variable
         b. Erroneous signal caused by malfunction or dynamic limitations
         c. Vision impaired by nystagmus, glare, flash, etc.
      3. Vestibular and other receptors:
         a. Fail to indicate change in angular velocity or direction of gravity when stimulus below threshold
         b. Semicircular canals do not signal sustained rotation.

      c. Erroneous signals are generated by linear and angular acceleration stimuli that differ in time course and/or intensity from those to which the body is normally exposed on the ground, e.g., postrotatory phenomena, somatogravic illusion, stimulation of semicircular canals by pressure change, etc.

C. Central error
  1. Limitation of span of attention—coning of attention or fascination
  2. False perception of cues because of the following:
    a. Error in expectancy (e.g., cloud leans, somatic autokinesis)
    b. Disturbed cerebral function consequent to the following:

- High arousal (anxiety)
- Low arousal
- Alcohol and other drugs
- Hypoxia and hypercapnia
- Illness
- Fatigue

  3. Dissociative sensations, e.g., break-off phenomenon

IV. Commonly Described Illusions
  A. False perception of attitude:
    1. Leans (subthreshold acceleration)
    2. Somatogravic illusions—pitch-up on acceleration, pitch-down on deceleration, inversion during bunt ("jet-upset" incidents)
    3. Misinterpretation of visual cues—false-horizon reference, ground–sky confusion, "lean-on-the-sun" illusion
    4. Cross-coupled and G-excess illusions
  B. False perception of motion
    1. Somatogyral illusion—on recovery from prolonged angular motion
    2. Subthreshold accelerations
    3. Cross-coupled (Coriolis) stimulation
    4. Pressure (alternobaric) vertigo
    5. Flicker vertigo and other illusory sensations induced by moving visual stimuli (waterfall effect in helicopters)
  C. Dissociative sensations
    1. Break-off phenomenon
    2. Magic-carpet illusion (flying)

V. Causal Factors
  A. Flight environment
    1. IMC—in particular on transfer from external visual to instrument cues.
    2. Night—isolated light sources enhance probability of oculogravic, oculogyral, and autokinetic illusions–ground–sky confusion.
    3. High altitude—dissociative sensations; false horizontal reference; Also break off in helicopters at lower altitudes or on crossing escarpment
    4. Flight over featureless terrain—false perception of height

    5. Hazard of SD during flight with night-vision devices (NVDs)—image-intensifying night-vision goggles (NVG) and infrared systems

B. Flight maneuvers

    1. Prolonged acceleration and deceleration in line of flight and catapult launches—somatogravic and oculogravic illusions.

    2. Prolonged angular motion—sustained motion not sensed, somatogyral illusions on recovery, no sensation of bank during coordinated turn, cross-coupled, and G-excess illusions if head movement made while turning

    3. Subthreshold changes in attitude—the leans induced on recovery

    4. Workload of flight maneuver—high arousal enhances disorientation and reduces the ability to resolve perceptual conflict

    5. Ascent or descent—pressure vertigo.

    6. Cloud penetration—VMC/IMC transfer and attendant problems, especially when flying in formation or on breaking formation; Lean-on-the-sun illusion

    7. Low-altitude hover—dust, *snow,* or water can obscure external cues (VMC/IMC transfer)—waterfall illusion

C. Aircraft factors

    1. Inadequate instruments

    2. Inoperative instruments

    3. Visibility of instruments

    4. Badly positioned displays and controls—head movement required to see and operate

    5. High rates of angular and linear acceleration, high maneuverability

    6. View from cockpit—lack of visible aircraft structures enhances Break off, poor visual frame of reference

D. Aircrew factors

    1. Flight experience

    2. Training, experience, and proficiency in instrument flight

    3. Currency and competency of flying practice

    4. Mental health—high arousal and anxiety increases susceptibility to disorientation

    5. Physical health—upper-respiratory-tract infection and pressure vertigo

    6. Alcohol and drugs—impair mental function and ability to suppress nystagmus

Appendix B: Example of Disseminated Advice on Managing SD

ACTION: Identify the measures that help **prevent** spatial disorientation.
CONDITION: While serving as an aircrew member.
STANDARD: In accordance with FM 3-04 (2000).

1) Develop the aviator through the following:
    a) Training: Training is the most important measure to reduce the possibility of spatial disorientation. Through training, an aircrew member learns

the hows and whys of spatial disorientation. An aircrew member must understand the limitations of the sensory mechanisms, the particular flight maneuvers that can lead to spatial disorientation, and the conditions where errors in perception are most likely to occur.

    b) Instrument proficiency: Instrument training must be performed on a regular basis in order to maintain proficiency. It also reinforces the skills necessary for a good instrument cross-check.

2) Fly the aircraft:

    a) Never try to fly both VMC and IMC at the same time. If you lose sight of the ground or significant objects, transition to the instruments, and perform the emergency IMC procedures.

    b) Never fly without visual reference points (either an actual horizon or an artificial horizon). Always have a way of confirming the horizon position with other instruments.

    c) Utilize continuous scanning techniques during the day and during night operations. Never stare (either at lights or objects).

3) Instrumentation:

    a) Trust your instruments.

    b) Cockpit design: Position new equipment within the cockpit in areas that reduce the necessity for head movements. Ideally, instruments should be as easy to interpret as external cues.

4) Avoid self-imposed stressors. They irritate sensory illusions.

ACTION: Identify the corrective actions to treat spatial disorientation.
CONDITION: While serving as an aircrew member.
STANDARD: In accordance with (IAW) FM 3-04 (2000).

1) Transfer control of the aircraft if there are two pilots. (Seldom will both pilots experience disorientation at the same time.)

2) Delay intuitive reactions.

3) Refer to the instruments immediately upon losing the horizon as reference.

4) Develop and maintain an instrument cross-check.

MAKE THE INSTRUMENTS READ RIGHT!

Appendix C: Use of Flight Simulators for SD Training

1) At the U.S. Army Aeromedical Research Laboratory (USAARL), flight scenarios were developed in the UH-60 simulator.[80] Actual SD accident summaries from the U.S. Army Safety Center (USASC) were reviewed, and those that could reasonably be replicated in a visual simulator were selected. The research data collected following comprehensive demonstrations indicated a very favorable response to this method of training. The result was that aviators receiving SD scenario training increased their situational awareness of the conditions and events that lead to SD. In addition, the scenarios provided training to assist aviators in **overcoming** SD once it was encountered.

Additional benefits from this method of training were found to be the reinforcement of crew resource management elements and the development of decision making, risk assessment, and judgement skills. Once the scenario had been recorded and the simulator programmed to its initial condition, the outline procedure was as follows:

a) The student flies the scenario and gets disoriented.
b) The IP debriefs student, explaining that this was a SD situation.
c) The IP then instructs "how to prevent SD."
d) The IP then instructs " how to overcome SD."

An example of one of the scenario "scripts" is given here:

a) *The Instructor sets the simulator initial conditions (type of flight—NVG in this case, location—an airfield in this case, weather conditions, visibility, etc.).*
b) *The student is assigned the role of pilot in command, and the instructor pilot (IP) plays the role of the scenario IP.*
c) *After takeoff from the airfield, the IP turns to a heading of 090 and flies at 70 knots at 100 ft above ground level (AGL). The IP simulates a local area orientation flight and points out different geographical points to keep the student's focus outside the aircraft. Approximately 1 min after takeoff, the IP allows the aircraft to ascend to 140 ft. After another minute or so, over terrain with limited contrast and visibility, the IP places the aircraft in an undetected 200-ft/min descent and allows it to descend. As the aircraft descends through 30 ft, the IP asks, "Where's the ground? You have the controls!"*
d) *Debriefing points: Tell the student, "That was spatial disorientation. The situation we just experienced actually occurred and resulted in an aircraft mishap. The following is a summary of the actual SD accident." (READ TO STUDENT): While in cruise flight, on an NVG local-area orientation training flight late in the duty day, the IP, who was on the controls, noted that he was 140 ft AGL. The IP began a descent to return to an altitude of 100 ft AGL as planned for the flight. The IP failed to arrest his descent and impacted a 22-ft high sand dune approximately 5 ft from the crest. The aircraft impacted the ground at 69 kn and at approximately 200 ft/min rate of descent in a near-level attitude. None of the crewmembers noticed the descent or saw the sand dune prior to impact. All crewmembers sustained injuries, and the aircraft was totally destroyed.*
e) *Ask the student:*
"Why did this happen?" (Solicit feedback from student.)
"What factors made the likelihood of SD worse in this situation?" (The following list is not exhaustive):
    Lack of or poor visual cues
    Crew resource management failure
    Perception of linear motion below threshold (rate of descent too low to perceive)
    Probable visual illusion (underestimating height above ground)
    Poor awareness of the risk of SD in flight conditions
    Fatigue

"How could this be prevented?" Suggestions are as follows:

> *Perform proper crew resource management. (The nonhandling pilot should assist the handling pilot by monitoring the radar altimeter.)*
> *Perform tasks and maneuvers in accordance with the Standard Operating Procedures applying appropriate environmental considerations.*
> *Follow published guidance and regulations, to include crew rest/duty day restrictions.*
> *Maintain situational awareness.*
> *Be familiar with potential visual illusions.*
> *"How could this be overcome?"*
> *By performing proper aircrew coordination*

   f) *Demonstrate the preventive action by performing proper aircrew coordination.*

   g) *Demonstrate the corrective action by increasing altitude (collective) as soon as a descent is detected by any crewmember.*

   h) *The student completes the internal validation questionnaire.*

2) USAARL concluded that these scenarios provided valuable training material that will have a positive impact on reducing SD mishaps.[81] USAARL's liaison with the U.S. Army Safety Center (USASC) has ensured that the scenarios reflected the actual accident as much as possible and that the scientific background to the scenarios and the associated debrief were sound. Eighteen scenarios have been validated in the UH-60 simulator and the majority adapted for the AH-64 Combat Mission Simulator.[84] USAARL continues to monitor the training package to assess the impact on attitudes and practice after distribution. It is vital that the scenarios are not viewed in isolation, but as the central part of a complete training package that is part of the larger training process. The intention is that the scenarios will be reviewed periodically in consultation with the USASC and other agencies. USAARL will continue to produce new scenarios and scripts in response to the Army's accident trends, ongoing research, and evaluation of the training package's practical use in the field.

3) Organizations that are responsible for SD training, and do not have access to a SD demonstrator/trainer, are encouraged to evaluate the usefulness of flight-training simulators to demonstrate SD situations. If further training by this method were employed, an economy of resources would soon be realized. Scenarios should be weapon-system specific, including components of previous accidents, high-risk phases of flight, or system anomalies. They should also be multitask, high workload with a console operator capable of instructing in the maintenance of ongoing orientation. Examples of potential scenarios (Brown, D. L., "Preventing and Avoiding Spatial Disorientation During Fast Jet Flight," Royal Air Force Centre of Aviation Medicine, Personal Communication, Henlow, England, U.K., 2001) are as follows: a) low-level abort into weather, b) maneuvering over water with a hazy horizon, c) tanker rendezvous/rejoin at night with reduced visibility, and d) cockpit distraction or novel situation such as CRT and mission data computer failure while on NVGs.

4) The primary purpose is to place aircrew in a situation where there is a high risk to becoming disoriented and then train them to always know where they

are in space, while operating the weapon system. In essence, the concept is to rehearse high-risk profiles to amplify the mental model and free up short-term memory during real flight. Such a syllabus should be required at the following points: a) advanced flying training, b) operational flying training units, c) upgrade to flight lead or instructor pilot, d) conversion to a new aircraft, e) standardization/evaluation check rides, and f) annually.

5) Finally, research initiatives such as simulator eye tracker systems can be utilized during training to provide feedback to the student aviator. An efficient and effective scan pattern is critical to the maintenance of spatial orientation, and it is known that the scan can be affected by experience, skill, workload, and fatigue. Eye tracking provides real-time objective evidence of missed cues in maintaining spatial orientation or situational awareness. Such feedback is invaluable as a training aid, especially early in a training course on a new weapon system (Brown, D. L., "Preventing and Avoiding Spatial Disorientation During Fast Jet Flight," Royal Air Force Centre of Aviation Medicine, Personal Communication, Henlow, England, U.K., 2001).

Appendix D: Rotary Wing In-Flight SD Demonstration

A. Level Turn

Straight-and-level flight is established at 90–100 kn. After a few seconds, a gently increasing (suprathreshold) roll to 30-deg angle of bank is commenced while maintaining airspeed and altitude. This is stabilized, and, on completion of a turn between 180 and 360 deg, the aircraft is rolled wings level again at a suprathreshold rate. Subjects are told to open his eyes once they perceive themselves again flying straight and level.

Debriefing points: The onset of the roll is normally detected, but as the semicircular canal response decays a false sensation of a return to straight-and-level flight is perceived. As the roll to level flight is made, a sensation of turning in the opposite direction is perceived. The limitations of semicircular canal physiology are discussed.

B. Straight and Level

Straight-and-level flight is established at 90–100 kn, and one of the other students is asked to close his/her eyes. The aircraft is flown with no alteration of altitude, heading, or airspeed.

Debriefing points: Because of small aircraft movements from turbulence and the aerodynamic response of the helicopter that stimulate the vestibular apparatus and/or the kinesthetic receptors above their threshold, students perceive climb, descents, or turns in unpredictable and varying amounts. The erroneous sensations produced by brief stimulation of the kinesthetic receptors and vestibular apparatus are discussed.

C. Straight-and-Level Deceleration

Straight-and-level flight is established at 90–100 kn into wind, and once the subject has closed his eyes the helicopter is slowed within 30–40 s to below 30 kn (55.5 km/h) (preferably a free-air hover) with no change of heading or altitude.

Debriefing points: The deceleration is rarely perceived to the extent to which it has occurred. The nose-up pitch associated with the attitude change in the final stages of slowing the aircraft usually convinces the subject that a climb is taking place. In addition, a turn is often falsely perceived when balance variations are made to keep straight. The absence of accurate physiological perception of airspeed is discussed.

D. Inadvertent Descent

This maneuver is commenced from about 500 ft (152.5 m) above ground level. Straight-and-level flight is established at 90–100 kn, and the student closes his eyes. While initiating a descent at below 500 ft (152.5 m) per minute, a series of turns is commenced. When the aircraft is established in flight below 50 ft (152.5 m) AGL, the subject is asked to report his heading, height, and airspeed and then open his/her eyes.

Debriefing points: The descent is not usually perceived, and because of the proximity of the ground at the end of the maneuver this demonstration forcibly and convincingly demonstrates the danger of inadvertent descent.

E. Hover Maneuvers

As the helicopter has a unique ability to accelerate about, as well as along, orthogonal axes, the final series of demonstrations started from a 5- or 6-ft hover. In turn, the students are exposed to a variety of linear and rotational movements while maintaining hover height. The students are prompted to continue a running commentary (to occupy channels of attention) and so exacerbate the onset of SD. Within these exercises various maneuvers are "hidden" so that when the student opens his eyes, a dramatic end point is evident, for example, climbing backwards at 10–15 kn, landing without the subject realizing it, and a gentle transition to forward flight.

Debriefing points: Most aircrew are able to maintain their orientation for 10–15 s before losing it. These exercises have a most educational effect upon the subject and observing students. The poor ability to detect subthreshold linear and angular accelerations is discussed, and the relevance of physiological orientation limitations in the context of snow, sand, and night operations is emphasized.

Appendix E: Fixed Wing In-Flight SD Demonstration

A. Pitch Misperception

The student is instructed to close his/her eyes. The instructor pilot (IP) accelerates the aircraft from 150 kn (277.5 km/h). The student is then asked to estimate the perceived pitch change. Alternatively he/she is given control of the aircraft (with eyes still closed) and instructed to maintain level flight. The result is either a perceived pitch-up sensation, or the student pushes the nose over if he/she has been given control.

Debriefing points: This illusion results from the linear acceleration acting on the otoliths of the inner ear. The resultant vector from the linear acceleration and normal gravity gives the sensation of an increase in pitch. Such an illusion can occur in a phase of flight of sustained acceleration, such as on takeoff, particularly in afterburner or catapult launches. To overcome the sensation of an increasing pitch attitude, the pilot will pitch the nose down and, if not attentive to the actual aircraft attitude, will result in controlled flight into the terrain (CFIT).

B.   Elevator Illusion

The student is instructed to close his eyes. The IP establishes a constant rate climb/descent and then levels off. The student is given control of the aircraft (with his/her eyes still closed) and instructed to maintain level flight. The result is that the student reenters a climb or descent.

Debriefing points: This illusion can occur during a constant rate climb on a standard instrument departure (SID) with an intermediate level-off, or during descent on an instrument approach with an intermediate level-off. The pilot misperceives the resultant G vector associated with the pitch angle and, if not attending to the attitude indicator upon level off, will tend to resume the climb or descent to achieve the same "seat-of-the-pants" feeling. At best, the pilot will be violated for busting a hard altitude; at worst, a stall or CFIT will happen.

C.   False Climb in a Turn

The student is instructed to close his eyes. The IP slowly (< 2 deg/s) achieves 45-deg bank angle. The student is asked what attitude he/she perceives and is given control of the aircraft (with eyes still closed) and instructed to maintain level flight. The result is that the student perceives a climb, lowers the nose, and descends.

Debriefing points: This is another somatogravic illusion that can subtly occur anytime during flight, in VMC or IMC, if the pilot is not attending to the actual aircraft attitude. If one unknowingly allows a subthreshold turn to occur, especially in level flight, the pilot will sense the increased G and, thinking that the aircraft is still wings level, will sense that the aircraft is climbing. The natural corrective control input would be to lower the nose. If operating at low altitude, the result would be disastrous.

D.   Diving During Turn Recovery

The student is instructed to close his eyes. The IP sustains a 1.5-G turn and then recovers to straight-and-level flight. The student is asked for his/her perception of the aircraft's attitude during recovery. The result is that the student perceives a nose-down pitch change with recovery to the 1-G environment.

Debriefing points: This somatogravic illusion is opposite to the preceding one. In this case the pilot is in a known sustained turn with the associated increase G level. If not attending to attitude and performance instruments, the pilot will sense the lesser 1-G environment upon rollout and feel like the aircraft is descending. The tendency will be to raise the nose of the aircraft. This often occurs, for instance, when a student practicing steep turns climbs during turn reversal because of the decreased G passing through level flight.

E. Leans

Students are instructed to close their eyes. The IP conducts a 270–360 deg of turn at a 30-deg bank and then recovers to straight-and-level flight (at a suprathreshold rate). The students are then asked to describe the aircraft's attitude. The result is that the student perceives a turn in the opposite direction.

Debriefing points: Every instrument rated pilot has experienced this somatogyral illusion. During IMC flight, a suprathreshold roll in the opposite direction from an established turn (which feels like level flight) sets up the appropriate rotatory stimulus in the semicircular canals. Now the pilot feels the aircraft is in a turn in the opposite direction, even though the attitude indicator shows straight and level flight, hence, the leans.

F. Postroll Effect

The student is instructed to close his/her eyes. The IP establishes 45-deg bank, and then rolls 90 deg in the opposite direction. The student is given control of the aircraft (with eyes still closed) and instructed to maintain the aircraft attitude. The result is that the student increases the roll and allows the nose to drop.

Debriefing points: This illusion, possibly prominent in several low-level CFIT accidents, is primarily somatogyral in origin, although there could be a somatogravic component. During roll reversal, the pilot can sense a roll in the opposite direction and compensate by increasing the roll in the direction of turn. If not attending to the real aircraft attitude while attempting to maintain the same seat-of-the-pants sensation, the pilot simultaneously allows the nose of the aircraft to drop. The increasing roll rate and decreasing pitch attitude will result in an unusual attitude at cruising altitudes and possible impact with terrain at low level.

G. Tilt with Skid

The student is instructed to close his eyes. The IP puts in full rudder trim, and then the student is asked to describe the aircraft's attitude. The result is that the student perceives a sensation of tilt.

Debriefing points: When cross-controlling an aircraft (admittedly rare in modern fast jets), a pilot could get a somatogyral input about the yaw axis that is interpreted as a tilt or perhaps a roll. The reaction would be to input controls to counter the perceived aircraft motion. This can happen when applying rudder to counter a crosswind condition. If in IMC, the pilot could enter an unusual attitude.

H. Coriolis

With the student's eyes open, the IP performs at least four continuous aileron rolls. The student is then instructed to move his/her head out of the rotating plane (forward or to one side). The result is that the student perceives a tumbling sensation.

Debriefing points: From the time that we entered pilot training, we have all been cautioned about moving our heads in the cockpit because of the Coriolis effect. Although a rare occurrence during flight, continuous aileron rolls effectively induce somatogyral motion about the longitudinal axis. Once the pilot places his/her head out of plane, a tumbling sensation ensues, which is short lived.

Appendix F: Training Objective for Recovery from Unusual Attitudes[72]

During a training flight in simulated IMC conditions (blackout screens/visors fitted to the aircraft/student) and with the instructor acting as safety pilot, the student is to be instructed to close his or her eyes while still on the controls (see note 1). When the aircraft has significantly departed from stable flight (see note 2), the student is to be instructed to open his or her eyes and return to the original flight parameters (altitude, heading, and airspeed). If this procedure fails to induce an unusual attitude (UA), or significant departure from the original flight parameters, the instructor is to fly the aircraft into a UA while the student sits free of the controls with his or her eyes closed. The instructor will then hand control back to the student who is to recover the aircraft to the original flight parameters

Notes:

1) Automatic flight control system and stability/trim control can be released to assist departure from the stable flight parameters.

2) Significant departure will be dependent upon aircraft type. Suggestions are a change of heading of at least 30 deg.

Objective: Both the techniques to regain both proper control of the aircraft and a return to the original flight parameters are to be performed correctly. Although the precise procedures are aircraft dependent, the general principles are as follows: wings level, pitch level, apply appropriate power setting, return to original airspeed, altitude, and heading.

The unusual attitudes to be achieved can be specified in the Instrument Rating Test documents. An example for helicopters is 1) an autorotative turn at low indicated airspeed and not more than 30-deg angle of bank and 2) a descending turn at high-indicated airspeed and not more than 30-deg angle of bank. Flight instructors are to be taught to perform and assess these procedures during their own instructor training.

References

[1]Gillingham, K. K., and Previc, F. H., *"Spatial Orientation in Flight,"* Air Force Materiel Command, AL-TR-1993-0022, Brooks Air Force Base, TX, 1993.

[2]Chase, N. B., and Kreutzmann, R. J., "Army Aviation Medicine," *Fundamentals of Aerospace Medicine*, edited by R. L. DeHart, Lea and Febiger, Philadelphia, PA, 1985, pp. 632–650.

[3]Pearsall, J., and Trumble, B. (eds.), *The Oxford English Reference Dictionary*, 2nd ed., Oxford Univ. Press, Oxford, England, U.K., 1996.

[4]Benson, A. J., *"Orientation/Disorientation Training of Flying Personnel: A Working Group Report,"* AGARD, Rep. 625, 1974.

[5]Benson, A. J., "Spatial disorientation—Common Illusions," *Aviation Medicine*, 3rd ed., edited by J. Ernsting, A. N. Nicholson, and D. J. Rainford, Butterworth-Heinemann, Oxford, England, U.K., 1999, pp. 437–453.

[6]Braithwaite, M. G., "Towards Standardization in Spatial Disorientation," *Position Paper to Working Party 61 of the Air Standardization Coordination Committee*, 1994.

[7]Lawson, B., Braithwaite, M. G., and Yauch, D., "Training in Spatial Disorientation," *The Proceedings of the Second Meeting of a Subgroup of the Triservice Technical Working Group for Spatial Orientation and Situation Awareness,"* Armstrong Lab. Brooks Air Force Base, San Antonio, TX, Sept. 1997.

[8]Ocker, W. C., and Crane, C. J., *Blind Flight in Theory and Practice,* Naylor Printing Co., San Antonio, TX, 1932.

[9]Bending, G. C., "Spatial Disorientation in Jet Aircrews," *Journal of Aviation Medicine,* Vol. 30, 1959, pp. 107–112.

[10]Kirkham, W. R., Collins, W. E., Grape, P. M., Simpson, J. M., and Wallace, T. F., "Spatial Disorientation in General Aviation Accidents," *Aviation, Space, and Environmental Medicine,* Vol. 49, 1978, pp. 1080–1086.

[11]Bellenkes, A., Bason, R., and Yacavone, D. W., "Spatial Disorientation in Naval Aviation Mishaps: A Review of Class A Incidents from 1980 Through 1989," *Aviation, Space, and Environmental Medicine,* Vol. 63, 1992, pp. 72–74.

[12]Holland, D., and Freeman, J., "Loss of Situational Awareness and Spatial Disorientation in the USAF, 1980–1989," *Proceedings of the 63rd Aerospace Medical Association Annual Meeting,* 1992.

[13]Cheung, B., Money K., Wright, H., and Bateman, W., "Spatial Disorientation-Implicated Accidents in Canadian Forces, 1982–92," *Aviation, Space, and Environmental Medicine,* Vol. 66, 1995, pp. 579–585.

[14]Durnford, S., Crowley, J. S., Rosado, N. R., Harper, J., and DeRoche, S., *"Spatial Disorientation: A Survey of U.S. Army Helicopter Accidents 1987–92,"* U.S. Army Aeromedical Research Lab., USAARL Rept. 95-25, Fort Rucker, AL, 1995.

[15]Braithwaite, M. G., Groh, S., and Alvarez, E. A., *"Spatial Disorientation in U.S. Army Helicopter Accidents: An Update of the 1987–92 Survey to Include 1993–95,"* U.S. Army Aeromedical Research Lab., USAARL Rept. 97-13, Fort Rucker, AL, 1997.

[16]Braithwaite, M. G., Durnford, S. J., Crowley, J. S., Rosado, N. R., and Albano, J. P., "Spatial Disorientation in U.S. Army Rotary-Wing Operations," *Aviation, Space, and Environmental Medicine,* Vol. 69, 1998, pp. 1031–1037.

[17]Braithwaite, M. G., Douglass, P. K., Durnford, S. J., and Lucas, G. L., "The Hazard of Spatial Disorientation During Helicopter Flight Using Night Vision Devices," *Aviation, Space, and Environmental Medicine,* Vol. 69, 1998, pp. 1038–1044.

[18]Steele-Perkins, A. P., and Evans, D. A., "Disorientation in Royal Navy Helicopter Pilots," AGARD CP–255: *Operational Helicopter Aviation Medicine,* 1978, pp. 48-1–48-5.

[19]Edgington, K., and Box, C. J., "Disorientation in Army Helicopter Operations." *Journal of the Society of Occupational Medicine,* Vol. 32, 1982, pp. 128–135.

[20]Vyrnwy-Jones, P., "A Review of Army Air Corps Helicopter Accidents 1971–1982," *Aviation, Space, and Environmental Medicine,* Vol. 56, 1985, pp. 403–409.

[21]Vyrnwy-Jones, P., *"Disorientation Accidents and Incidents in US Army Helicopters, 1 Jan, 1980 - 30 Apr, 1987,"* U.S. Army Aeromedical Research Lab., USAARL Rept. 88-3, Fort Rucker, AL, 1998.

[22]Braithwaite, M. G., *"An Aviation Medicine Review of Army Air Corps Helicopter Accidents, 1983–1993,"* Defence Research Agency Centre for Human Sciences, Rept. TR 94016, Farnborough, U.K., 1994.

[23]National Transportation Safety Board, Aircraft Accident Report, Air Transport International, IN, Flight 805, Douglas DC-8-63, N794AL, *Loss of Control and Crash,* Swanton, OH, 15 Feb. 1992.

[24]Collins, D. L., and Harrison, G. H., "Spatial Disorientation Episodes Among F-15C Pilots During Operation Desert Storm," *Journal of Vestibular Research, Equilibrium and Orientation*, Vol. 5, No. 6, 1995, pp. 405–410.

[25]Sipes, W. E., "Spatial Disorientation—What Kinds and How Often?," *Proceedings of SAFE Association 36th Annual Symposium*, 1998, pp. 164–172.

[26]Perdriel, G., and Benson, A. J., (eds.), "Spatial Orientation in Flight: Current Problems," AGARD CP–287, 1980.

[27]Braithwaite, M. G., DeRoche, S. L., Alvarez, E. A., and Reese, M., *Proceedings of the First Triservice Conference on Rotary-Wing Spatial Disorientation: Spatial Disorientation in the Operational Rotary-Wing Environment*, U.S. Army Aeromedical Research Lab., USAARL Rept. 97-15, Fort Rucker, AL, 1997.

[28]Murdock, E. A., "*Spatial Disorientation: Tracking Down a Killer,*" *Flight Fax*, Vol. 25, No. 5, 1997, pp. 2–4.

[29]Murdock, E. A., and Braithwaite, M. G., "*Spatial Disorientation: Reining in a Hazard,*" *Flight Fax*, Vol. 25, No. 7, 1999, pp. 1–4.

[30]Lawson, B., and Braithwaite, M. G., "Training in Spatial Disorientation," *The Proceedings of the First Meeting of a Subgroup of the Triservice Technical Working Group for Spatial Orientation and Situation Awareness*, 1997.

[31]Lawson, B., Braithwaite, M. G., and Yauch, D., "A Triservice Review of Spatial Disorientation Training Requirements for Military Aviators," *Proceedings of the 69th Aerospace Medical Association Annual Meeting*, 1998.

[32]Braithwaite, M. G., and Gaffney, C. L., "Countermeasures to Spatial Disorientation— International Issues," *Proceedings of the 69th Aerospace Medical Association Annual Meeting*, 1998.

[33]*RTO Meeting Proceedings 21: Aeromedical Aspects of Aircrew Training*, NATO Research and Technology Organization, 1999.

[34]*RTO Meeting Proceedings 19: Current Aeromedical Issues in Rotary Wing Operations*, NATO Research and Technology Organization, 1999.

[35]"*Aviation Medicine/Physiological Training of Aircrew in Spatial Disorientation,*" Air Standardization Coordinating Committee, ASCC Air Standard 61/117/1, Arlington, VA, 1997.

[36]"*Spatial Disorientation Training Curricula,*" Air Standardization Coordinating Committee, ASCC Advisory Publication (draft), Arlington, VA, 2000.

[37]Braithwaite, M. G., Hudgens, J. J., Estrada, A., and Alvarez, E. A., "An Evaluation of the British Army Spatial Disorientation Sortie in U.S. Army Aviation," *Aviation, Space, and Environmental Medicine*, Vol. 69, 1998, pp. 727–732.

[38]Money, K. E., "Disorientation," *Nouvelle Revue D'Aeronautique et D'Astonautique*, Vol. 4, 1997, pp. 40–43.

[39]Cheung, B., "*Recommendations to Enhance Spatial Disorientation Training for the Canadian Forces,*" Defence and Civil Inst. of Environmental Medicine, DCIEM Rept. 98-R-32, North York, Ontario, Canada, 1998.

[40]Benson, A. J., and Burchard, E., "*Spatial Disorientation in Flight: A Handbook for Aircrew,*" AGARD, AGARDOGRAPH 170, 1973.

[41]Antunano, M. J., "Practical Application of Virtual Reality Technology in Spatial Disorientation Training of Civil Aviation Pilots," *Proceedings of the 48th Annual Meeting of the International Academy of Aviation and Space Medicine*, 2000.

[42]Navathe, P. D., and Singh, B., "Prevalence of Spatial Disorientation in Indian Air Force Aircrew," *Aviation, Space, and Environmental Medicine*, Vol. 65, 1994, pp. 1082–1085.

[43]Cheung, B., Money, K., and Sarkar, P., "Loss of Situation Awareness in the Canadian Forces," AGARD CP–575: *Situation Awareness: Limitations and Enhancement in the Aviation Environment*, AGARD, 1996, pp. A1-1–1-8.

[44]Berkley, W. E. "Night Vision Goggle Illusions and Visual Training," AGARD LS-187: *Visual Problems in Night Operations*, AGARD, 1992, pp. 9-1–9-6.

[45]Crowley, J. S., *"Human Factors of Night Vision Devices: Anecdotes from the Field Concerning Visual Illusions and Other Effects,"* U.S. Army Aeromedical Research Lab., USAARL Rept. 91-15, Fort Rucker, AL, 1991.

[46]Antonio, J. C., *"Instructor Guide: Night Vision Goggle Training Course,"* MCAS, and AFRL/HEA, MAWTS-1, Yuma and Mesa, AZ, 1994.

[47]Antonio, J. C., *"Instructor Guide: NVG/FLIR Sensor Integration,"* MCAS and AFRL/HEA, MAWTS-1, Yuma and Mesa, AZ, 1999.

[48]Matthews, R. S. J., "Spatial Disorientation—A Continuing Threat in Air Operations," *Proceedings of the Threats, Countermeasures and Situational Awareness Symposium*, 2000.

[49]Durnford, S. J., DeRoche, S. L, Harper, J. P., and Trudeau, L. A., *"Spatial Disorientation: A Survey of U.S. Army Rotary Wing Aircrew,"* U.S. Army Aeromedical Research Lab., USAARL Rept. 96-16, Fort Rucker, AL, 1996.

[50]Davenport, C., "USAF Spatial Disorientation Experience: Air Force Safety Center Statistical Review," *Proceedings of the Recent Trends in Spatial Disorientation Research Symposium*, 2000.

[51]Albery, W. B., "Ground-Based Spatial Disorientation Training in the USAF," *Proceedings of the Recent Trends in Spatial Disorientation Research Symposium*, 2000.

[52]Dowd, P. J., *"A Critical Assessment of Ground-Based Devices for Spatial Orientation Training,"* Air Force Systems Command, USAFSAM-TR-73-23, Brooks AFB, TX, 1973.

[53]Previc, F. H., and Ercoline, W. R., "Ground-Based Spatial Disorientation Training in the United States Air Force: Past and Current Devices, *Proceedings of the Eighth International Symposium on Aviation Psychology,* edited by R. A. Jensen, 1995, pp. 1318–1322.

[54]Yauch, D. W., Ercoline, W. R., Previc, F. H., and Holoviak, S. J., "The Advanced Spatial Disorientation Demonstrator: Component, Profile, and Training Evaluation, AGARD CP–588: *Selection and Training Advances in Aviation*, AGARD, 1996, pp. 28-1–28-5.

[55]Dowd, P. J., *"The USAF Spatial Orientation Trainer: Background and Apparatus,"* Air Force Systems Command, USAFSAM-TR-73-46, Brooks AFB, TX, 1973.

[56]Ercoline, W. R., Yauch, D. W., Previc, F. H., and Holoviak, S. J., "Advanced Spatial Disorientation Demonstrator—Troop Trial Results (SD Illusions)," *AGARD* CP–588: *Selection and Training Advances in Aviation,* AGARD, 1996.

[57]Berkley, W. E., "Spatial Disorientation in Night Vision Goggles Operations," *Proceedings of the Recent Trends in Spatial Disorientation Research Symposium*, 2000.

[58]Weinstein, L. F., Previc, F. H., Simpson, C. G., Lyons, T. J., and Gillingham, K. K., "A Test of Thumb and Index Finger Control in Overcoming a Visual Analogue of the Giant Hand Illusion," *Aviation, Space, and Environmental Medicine*, Vol. 62, 1991, pp. 336–341.

[59]Gillingham, K. K., *"Advanced Spatial Disorientation Training Concepts,"* USAF School of Aerospace Medicine, Technical Review 11-74, Brooks Air Force Base, TX, 1974.

[60]Spanitz, J., "Medical Standards and Certification," *Federal Aviation Regulations*, U. S. Dept. of Transportation, ASA-98-FR-AM-BK, Aviation Supplies and Academics, Inc., Newcastle, WA, 1998.

[61]Nash, T., "Shaken or Stirred," *Military Training Technology Magazine*, Oct./Nov. 1997, pp. 20–22.

[62]Grohosky, E. A., *"Syllabus of Instruction, 19th AF Syllabus P-V4A-A/J (T-37), T-37 Joint Specialized Undergraduate Pilot Training,"* Headquarters 19th AF, Randolph AFB, TX, 1995.

[63]Rupert, A. H., and Gadolin, R. E., *"Motion and Spatial Disorientation Systems: Special Research Capabilities,"* NAMRL Special Rept. 93-1, 1993.

[64]Ross, G. D., "The Versatile Vertifuge," *Airman Magazine*, March 1986, pp. 45–48.

[65]Crawford, W. R., and Davis, H. F., *"Orientation/Disorientation Training of Flying Personnel: A Working Group Report (1974),"* AGARD, Rept. 625, AGARD, France, Annex F.1, 1967.

[66]Henning, C., *"Orientation/Disorientation Training of Flying Personnel: A Working Group Report,"* AGARD, Rept. 625, Annex F.3, 1974.

[67]Braithwaite, M. G., "The British Army Air Corps in Flight Spatial Disorientation Demonstration Sortie," *Aviation, Space, and Environmental Medicine*, Vol. 68, 1997, pp. 342–345.

[68]*"In-Flight Demonstration of Spatial Disorientation in Rotary-Wing Aircraft,"* Air Standardization Coordinating Committee, ASCC Air Standard (draft), Arlington, VA, 2000.

[69]*"In-Flight Demonstration of Spatial Disorientation in Fixed Wing Aircraft,"* Air Standardization Coordinating Committee, ASCC Air Standard (draft), Arlington, VA, 2001.

[70]Durnford, S., "Disorientation and Flight Safety—A Survey of UK Army Aircrew," AGARD CP–532: *Aircraft Accidents: Trends in Aerospace Medical Investigation Techniques,"* AGARD, 1992, pp. 32-1–32-14.

[71]Dobie, T. G., "The Disorientation Accident—Philosophy of Instrument Flying Training," *Conference Proceedings of The Disorientation Incident*, AGARD CP-95, AGARD, 1971, pp. A 15-1–A 15-4.

[72]*"In-Flight Training in Spatial Disorientation,"* Air Standardization Coordinating Committee, ASCC Air Standard (draft), Arlington, VA, 2000.

[73]Walsh, P. T., *"A Survey of Spatial Disorientation Training Experience in USAF Flying Personnel,"* Residency in Aerospace Medicine (USAF) Academic Project, Brooks Air Force Base, TX, 1990.

[74]Davisson, B., "What Can Aerobatics Do For You?," *Air Progress*, Vol. 42, 1980, pp. 20–72.

[75]Ethell, J., "Upside Down is Rightside Up," *Air Progress*, Vol. 48, 1986, pp. 51–77.

[76]Gawron, V. J., and Reynolds, P. A., "When in-Flight Simulation Is Necessary," *Journal of Aircraft*, Vol. 32, 1995, pp. 411–415.

[77]Gillingham, K. K., "The Spatial Disorientation Problem in the United States Air Force," *Journal of Vestibular Research, Equilibrium and Orientation*, Vol. 2, No. 4, 1992, pp. 297–306.

[78]Collins, W. E., Hasbrook, A. H., Lennon, A. O., and Gay, D. J., *"Disorientation Training in FAA-Certified Flight and Ground Schools: A Survey,"* Federal Aviation Administration Office of Aviation Medicine, Rept. 77-24, 1977.

[79]Winfield, D. A., Brailsford, F. S. B., Copple, J., Daniels, S. M., Forbes, G. M., Hamilton, A. E. R., Hansford, N. G., and Morris, C. B., "A Study of Spatial Disorientation in RAF Aircrew," *Proceedings of the 69th Aerospace Medical Association Annual Meeting*, 1998.

[80]Estrada, A., Braithwaite, M. G., Gilreath, S. R., Johnson, P. A., and Manning, J. C., *"Spatial Disorientation Awareness Training Scenarios for U.S. Army Aviators in Visual Flight Simulators,"* U.S. Army Aeromedical Research Lab., USAARL Rept. 98-17, Fort Rucker, AL, 1998.

[81]Johnson, P. A., Estrada, A., Braithwaite, M. G., and Manning, J. C., "Assessment of Simulated Spatial Disorientation Scenarios in Training U.S. Army Aviators," *RTO Meeting Proceedings 19: Current Aeromedical Issues in Rotary Wing Operations*, NATO Research and Technology Organization, 1999, pp. 15-1–15-8.

[82]Braithwaite, M. G., "Aviation Medicine and Physiology Training in the British Army," *RTO Meeting Proceedings 19: Current Aeromedical Issues in Rotary Wing Operations*, NATO Research and Technology Organization, Neuilly sur Seine, France, 1999, pp. 1-1–1-6.

[83]Miller, W. F., "The SD/LOC Syndrome: Spatial Disorientation and Loss of Consciousness," *Aviation, Space, and Environmental Medicine*, Vol. 72, 2001, pp. 321.

[84]Gore, W., *Spatial Disorientation Awareness Training Scenarios for AH-64A Aviators on the Combat Mission Simulator*, Western ARNG Aviation Training Site, Silver Bell Army Heliport, Marana, AZ, 2000.

Chapter 9

Flight Displays I: Head-Down Display Topics for Spatial Orientation

William R. Ercoline*

General Dynamics Advanced Information Systems, San Antonio, Texas

Carita A. DeVilbiss[†]

Army Research Laboratory, Ft. Sam Houston, Texas

Richard H. Evans[‡]

General Dynamics Advanced Information Systems, San Antonio, Texas

I. Introduction

Aircraft displays are the pilot's window on the world of forces, commands, and information that cannot be seen as naturally occurring visual events or objects.[1]

T O the uninitiated, aircraft displays hardly look like the window referenced in the preceding quotation. The instrument panel of almost every aircraft cockpit contains knobs, switches, buttons, levers, lights, and displays of one or more functions (Fig. 1)—not quite what one would imagine being a window on the world. Nevertheless, a window is exactly what it is. It is not a transparent pane, but, rather, a variably translucent portal to perception that begins to clear after extensive training and effort. Success at the task of making sense of the information on the aircraft displays (i.e., using them as if they were a window to the world) is dependent upon the creativity of instrument designers, the ingenuity of flight training instructors, and the procedural fortitude of pilot trainees. After weeks of ground training, about 30 hours of practice in the aircraft, and a proficiency evaluation ride, an average student pilot is judged proficient in the skill of interpreting these displays for basic

---

This material is declared a work of the U.S. Government and is not subject to copyright protection in the United States.

*Senior Scientist.

[†]Human Factors Engineer.

[‡]Member, Spatial Disorientation Countermeasures Research Team.

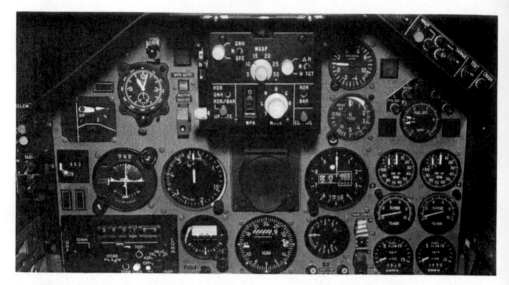

Fig. 1 Low-tech, fighter-type cockpit instrument panel comprised of many head-down displays from which the pilot contrives a mental view of the world of forces, commands, and information. A single display is used to present one particular type of flight data. (Photo courtesy of Gateway and Kaiser Electronics.)

flight. Reaching instrument-flying proficiency is more challenging still and might well be the most difficult psychomotor task a pilot trainee will ever accomplish.

In addition to demanding precision maneuvering of the aircraft, instrument flight is made difficult by its requirement to assimilate a multitude of data from a myriad of sources. All of the information on the displays is important at one time or another, and the level of priority for each changes from task to task and flight to flight. This fluid operating environment requires the pilot to perform a constant scan for the necessary information. Adding to the difficulty is the fact that, for the most part, the displays are not intuitive.[2] Specifically, they do not look like the real world as it appears when viewed on a clear day through the cockpit windscreen. Because of this abstraction, the pilot trainee does a lot of "chair flying" (i.e., imaginary mental exercises of flight) in order to better grasp just what each display is telling him or her and how to apply the displayed information to precise instrument procedures. This composite process of harmonizing concrete and abstract cognition with coordinated physical motor functions makes the skill of instrument flight both art and science. The pilot must paint the picture in his or her mind, while exercising precise manipulation of some of the world's most sophisticated machinery.

Likewise, the job of the display designer (and his or her close companion, or possibly alter ego, the researcher) is complex and, to a degree, even more difficult. The display designer must understand the task of the pilot, know how the pilot interprets the instrument information, how the display symbology behaves, and how to make instrument improvements to be cost efficient. The designer must know almost everything with which a pilot must cope and must apply this knowledge to an environment of unusual forces and motion. Consequently, he or she faces a difficult challenge in attempting to improve upon existing displays and must learn from the experience of those who have gone before. In addition, the designer must understand the science of human factors engineering and be willing to gain an understanding of the unexpected perceptions the pilot experiences when engaged in flying an aircraft.[3] (The medium upon which the symbology is presented is mostly irrelevant to this text, although some characteristics are addressed later in the chapter regarding specific design features.)

Toward the end of producing effective spatial-disorientation countermeasure displays, this chapter sets about the broad purpose of building a bridge between the needs of the pilot and the needs of the display designer. The two communities succeed in combating spatial disorientation only by working together as it requires true teamwork to provide for the pilot's demand for visually dominant, operationally relevant displays and the designer's bent toward mechanical efficiency and physical practicality. The chapter is generally directed toward enlightening the designer and researcher as to correlations between basic flight parameters and their display constituents and typical display mechanizations.

To eliminate ambiguity in the discussion, the terms cockpit instruments, aircraft displays, and instrument displays are equated. The subject of instruments or displays are those that present basic flight information to the pilot through some type of symbology (e.g., numbers, letters, lines, figures, colors, etc.) on one or more media embedded in the cockpit instrument panel. The many other cockpit instruments that impart ancillary information such as fuel state, cabin environmental conditions, etc. are not addressed. Because the pilot must look essentially downward into the cockpit to see the instruments, the term head-down display (HDD) is used to categorize them.

Although the head-down array historically has been considered the foundation for providing flight information to the pilot, in today's aircraft other options might be desirable. Additional or alternate display locations might include above the panel (head-up display or HUD), in the top portion of the panel (head-level display), on the pilot's head (head-mounted display or HMD), or anywhere else technology permits. These other types of displays have their own attributes and limitations and must be appropriately integrated with the HDD. They are discussed in more detail in Chapter 10. However, several references to studies and lessons learned regarding HUDs are included in this chapter to provide background information and perspective on the characteristics of numerous HDD features.

This chapter focuses on the pilot–machine interface factors that promote basic instrument flight skills and identifies HDD design issues that pertain to improving the displays' usefulness for spatial orientation (SO). The chapter specifically concentrates only on those HDD characteristics that relate to the prevention of Type I (unrecognized) spatial disorientation (SD) and recovery from Type II (recognized) SD.

The chapter contains two major sections: piloting topics and design topics. Piloting topics are associated with the organization and location of displays used for instrument flight, the manner in which pilots use these displays, and the impacts of the pilot's visual scan both inside and outside the cockpit during instrument flight. The HDDs used for spatial orientation are identified, and the term primary flight reference (PFR) is defined. Also, the PFR's relevance to SD is described.

Symbology modifications and design features that have been applied to those instruments crucial to the pilot's maintenance of spatial orientation are discussed in the design topics section. Those critical displays primarily include the attitude indicator, the airspeed indicator, and the altimeter. Lastly, the section reviews the performance metrics traditionally employed when evaluating various symbology modifications to these displays. The reader should keep in mind that although the performance metrics are included in this chapter on HDDs, they could also be used on any type of display, that is, HDD, HUD, HMD, or those developed in the future.

Throughout the chapter various physical dimensions are cited for perspective and context in describing a particular display or flight maneuver. They are not provided for scientific precision. Also, because of the diverse nature of the cockpit symbology and display design business some dimensions given are not consistent with those of other publications on the topic. For simplicity, the most commonly accepted dimensions are used, for example, feet, inches, etc., and the metric system (or MKS) equivalent is provided in parentheses immediately following the units for easier application to readers more accustomed to their use. For the most part this chapter addresses display issues that are relevant to both fixed- and rotary-wing aircraft. However, some explicit differences exist between the two types, and, where appropriate for perspective, the two are separately mentioned. Nonetheless, some rotary-wing issues are omitted, as it is beyond the extent of this discussion to delineate each difference. Similarly, a description of all the HDDs in the cockpit and the numerous display issues associated with each is well beyond the scope of this text.

To gain an appreciation of the function of the complete expanse of the design of all instruments for instrument flight, one should reference one or more of the leading human factors or aviation psychology texts. Examples of these texts include *Human Factors in Engineering and Design* by Sanders and McCormick,[4] *Human Factors in Aviation* by Wiener and Nagel,[5] and *Display Technology—Human Factors Concepts* by Stokes et al.[3] As one studies these texts, one will likely find it somewhat surprising to learn about the numerous ideas that have been researched (many of which have shown potential for enabling more intuitive HDDs) and then realize how few of these ideas have been actually implemented. There are many reasons for this situation, but the discussion of them is also beyond the intent of this chapter.

II. Piloting Topics

Previous chapters have established the physiological and psychological challenges presented to the person who has been thrust into the three-dimensional world of flight. When pilots move about in this three-dimensional world, they must extract artificial information from instrument displays in order to maintain a proper spatial orientation. It is impossible to adequately extract this artificial information from the world beyond the cockpit instrument panel by just looking outside the windscreen. To judge parameters such as airspeed and altitude in that manner is particularly difficult, and although judging pitch and bank by viewing the real world is much more accurate, it is made dramatically more difficult by visual limitations such as fog or darkness.[6,7] Consequently, the pilot must refer to the instrument displays in both good and bad weather conditions in order to fly the aircraft safely.

The need for displaying spatial orientation information during all phases of flight was not immediately appreciated in the early days of instrument flying. It was a lesson learned the hard way, through trial and error. Many of the early pilots, all of whom were chosen for their supposed innate ability to function in the new airborne environment, were slow to accept that an erroneous perception of spatial orientation was a normal phenomenon.[8] Learning to cope with misperceptions required trust in "artificial" information—a proposition that initially met much resistance. Also, compounding the difficulty of providing orientation information was the fact that instrument design was not deemed as important as it is today. It was considered more important just to have the information available—in any format.[9] Designing it for ease of use or interpretation was often a nonissue. While some pilots of today still believe design is not important, the apparent disregard is not as prevalent as in the early days of flying. Maybe progress has been made? Nonetheless, even with more sophisticated display mediums and technologies available in the present time (e.g., the glass cockpit) too many pilots still fail to perform the seemingly simple task of looking at and interpreting the instruments as frequently as they should. Some mishap researchers attribute this difficulty to a relationship between age and the changing technology,[10] i.e., the older the pilot, the greater the challenge in adapting to new presentations, but it might be that the task is not as simple as it seems. The aircraft mishap rate caused by human error, and in particular the mishap rate associated with SD, is the single most significant problem facing aviation safety today,[11–13] and suggests a more deep-scated issue relating to what the pilot perceives from the instruments (see Chapter 5). Let us now look at the spatial orientation (SO) terms associated with aircraft flight.

A.   Axes of Motion and Controls

Effective interpretation or designing of any SO display begins with an understanding of how an aircraft is maneuvered in flight, that is, how it moves within the planes or about the axes of motion (see Fig. 16 in Chapter 1). As an aircraft rotates about the three axes of motion (lateral, longitudinal, and vertical), it subtends a spatial angle relative to the Earth's surface. That spatial angle is termed *aircraft attitude* and is the central theme of a spatial orientation display's design and function. To cause the aircraft to assume a particular attitude, the pilot must actuate the control stick (or wheel or yoke) and the rudder pedals and produce a rotation about the various motion axes.

Moving the stick changes the positions of the ailerons and elevators relative to the airflow, and determines rotational movement of the aircraft about the lateral and longitudinal axes of the aircraft. These rotational movements are more commonly termed pitch and roll,[14] respectively. Forward and backward movement of the stick produces aircraft pitch, which is motion about the lateral axis of the aircraft. Left-to-right movement of the stick produces aircraft roll, which is rotational motion about the longitudinal axis of the aircraft. The specific attitude angles achieved from pitch-and-roll motion are most properly termed elevation and bank, respectively. However, it is common for the elevation idiom to be interchanged with the expression pitch, as will be done in this chapter. The rudder affects motion about the aircraft's vertical axis and is controlled by the pedals at the pilot's feet. That rotational movement is termed yaw. In positively stable aircraft (as virtually all are now days) yaw motion is constantly being opposed by air pressure on the rudder. That pressure attempts to return the rudder to zero deflection, which would result in zero yawing motion. Yaw angle, or yaw attitude, is the angle subtended between the two orientations of the longitudinal axis of the aircraft when yaw is introduced and when it is neutralized. If the aircraft is in level flight, a change in yaw attitude will also equate to a change in compass heading. A constant yaw angle, other than zero, can be attained only by either an asymmetric thrust or drag condition or the rudders being constantly deflected either by positioning the rudder pedal or other aerodynamic controls designed for that purpose, i.e., trim systems, which will be addressed in Sec. II.C.1.

The aircraft's yaw attitude plays an important role in preventing and recovering from spins, compensating for asymmetrical power or thrust after engine loss and in enabling smooth turns that produce neither a slipping nor sliding force vector. In-depth understanding of the use and necessity of yaw can be gained from textbooks on aerodynamics, but for the purposes of this discussion the reader is encouraged to accept that most yaw input has little effect on spatial orientation in conventional, fixed-wing aircraft. It has much more relevance to helicopter and advanced, vectored-thrust aircraft. It is included here for the sake of academic completeness, and because the slip indicator, which presents yaw angle information, is still presented on many primary instrument displays. Yaw-attitude displays are further discussed in Sec. II.B.1.a.

B. Principal Categories of Instrument Displays

The spatial precepts just described are incorporated into the displays that enable the pilot to effectively produce aircraft attitude and motion. Aircraft motion is often found grouped into three basic categories: one for aircraft control inputs, one for aircraft performance outputs, and one for aircraft navigation. The resultant information is displayed by any of several means—on many instruments, a few instruments, or, more recently, a single cockpit instrument display. This concept of control, performance, and navigation displays is familiar to any instrument-rated pilot, and display designers should also understand it. Instrument organization is taught to the pilot during the ground portion of instrument training, and it allows the pilot to mentally compartmentalize the displays into the three major areas of flight information. Grouping the displays in this manner organizes them as they relate to immediate (aircraft control) inputs and the expected, time-delayed aircraft responses resulting from those inputs (see Table 1). This taxonomy is used throughout this chapter, but an alternative method of organizing instrument information is mentioned in Sec. II.C.1.

Ocker and Crane[9] appear to have first described these three functional groups of HDDs, but they did not use the exact expression of "control, performance and navigation." Navigation at the time was called "avigation" to avoid confusion with the term used for sea or ground guidance. The specific terms of control, performance, and navigation probably evolved around World War II (WWII) when official instrument training programs were implemented to help stem the numerous SD-related mishaps occurring at the time.[15]

Table 1   Control, performance, and navigation taxonomy

Indicators	Control	Performance	Navigation
Power	X		
Attitude	X		
Angle of attack		X	
Airspeed		X	
Altimeters		X	
Turn and slip		X	
Vertical velocity		X	
Horizontal sit.		X	X
Radio magnetic		X	X
Bearing distance heading		X	X
Course			X
Range			X

1.   Control Instruments

Control instruments comprise the displays of aircraft attitude and power. They directly reflect the response of the aircraft to stick, rudder, and throttle inputs. The pitch-and-roll rotational motions resulting from stick movement are displayed via the attitude indicator (AI), which is discussed later in the chapter. Either the heading indicator or the inclinometer displays the yaw rotational motion. The inclinometer, or slip/skid indicator, registers displacement of a wooden ball in a liquid-filled tube. It is simply termed the "ball" and basically informs the pilot of the degree to which the aircraft is in coordinated flight. Aircraft power is displayed via an engine instrument, usually either a tachometer that is sometimes called the rpm gauge or a temperature gauge that reflects thrust capabilities. This display normally shows the pilot the approximate output of the engine(s) as compared to the amount of output available.

a.   Attitude displays.   During the early years of aviation, pilots tried to use external visual cues for maintaining attitude.[16] Instruments were at times present in the cockpit for altitude, airspeed, and heading, but control of the aircraft's rotational motion about its lateral and longitudinal axes was left to the pilot's perception. At night or in clouds these aviators relied on their natural instincts or gravity to keep the aircraft upright—a decision that was all too often a fatal mistake. It was not until 1926 when Ocker conceived and constructed the first demonstration of how a turn indicator could prevent misperceived bank and turn motion that pilots and designers began to realize the necessity of providing orienting instrumentation for flight.[9] Although Ocker highlighted a pilot's normal physiological shortcomings through use of a ship's turn needle (designed and built by E. Sperry[17]) in a ground-based demonstrator, it soon became apparent that actual "blind flying" required another type of instrument.

The solution to the blind-flying problem was finally realized in 1929 when the national challenge was made for someone to fly the first blind sortie from takeoff to landing, without looking outside. The term blind refers to the fact that the pilot would not be allowed to see outside of the cockpit, requiring him or her to rely

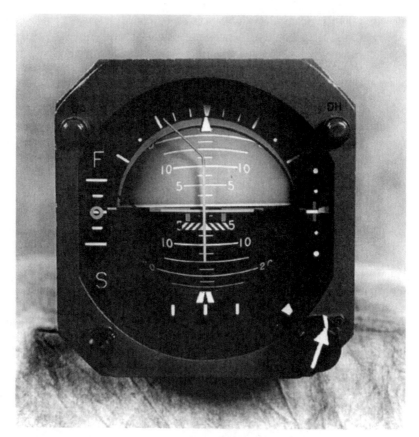

Fig. 2 Mechanical attitude indicator with flight director bars in view. Sky is represented by light color (blue or white), while ground is much darker (usually brown or black). A white sky pointer and bank scale are displayed on the case. The knob with the white arrow is for adjusting the pitch of the attitude sphere to align with level flight. (Photo courtesy of NASA Ames Research Center, Moffett Field, California.)

solely upon instrument information displayed in the cockpit. Therefore, with the exception of the artificial world displayed via the symbology in the cockpit, the pilot was flying blind.

One of the new displays used in this cockpit was the artificial horizon attitude indicator, which simultaneously presented the pitch and bank of the aircraft.[17] The basic design, as directed by project lead Jimmie Doolittle and his distinguished colleagues, contained a gyro-stabilized sphere displaying pitch and bank. It was so well accepted that this HDD attitude indicator of 1929 survived virtually unchanged for the next 70 years (see Fig. 2). Modern, digital signal-input displays have permitted the attitude information to be displayed via an electrooptical system (see Fig. 3), replacing the old mechanical device, but the mechanization of pitch and bank movement has not changed. Other methods of displaying attitude information are possible, but this basic display of pitch-and-bank information

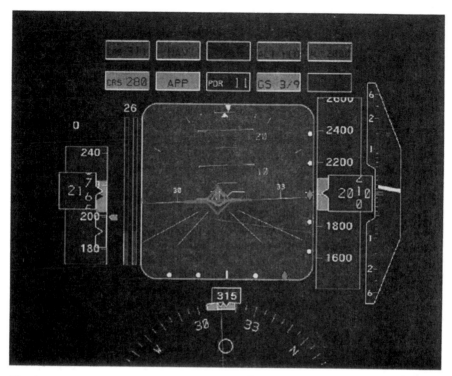

Fig. 3 Illustration of an electro-optical attitude indicator (and other instruments) as displayed with a liquid crystal display (LCD). A cockpit with these displays is commonly referred to as a "glass cockpit." (Courtesy of NASA Ames Research Center, Moffett Field, California.)

has become standard. (A notable departure from the standard mechanization as described was incorporated in Russian aircraft.) The attitude indicator was, and continues to be, the foundation of "blind flying." However, its design has not been without controversy and has been considered a cause or contributing factor in many SD-related mishaps.[18–20]

Although pitch and bank are the primary emphasis of attitude displays, the presentation of yaw or slip/skid must briefly be touched upon. As already mentioned, yaw normally is less relevant to spatial orientation than are pitch or bank, but displaying the result of rudder input can still be critical to aircraft control. Pilots of multiengine aircraft, especially those with noncenterline thrust, are required to reference the ball when an engine fails. Evaluating the amount of rudder input made in an attempt to maintain coordinated flight can make the difference between a successful vs a failed recovery. Yaw holds significant importance for helicopter and unconventional aircraft operations, such as with the vectored-thrust Harrier jump jet. It has special relevance in highly maneuverable aircraft like the Comanche Helicopter and the F-35 Joint Strike Fighter. The display of yaw/rudder/pedal input could become even more important as SD problems arise in the new flight regimes used by these latter aircraft. However, at present, yaw attitude is generally

above the Earth increases. Barometric altimeters are designed to display altitude relative to the pressure difference outlined on a standard atmospheric pressure chart. The pressure differentials on the chart correlate to pressure exerted by various heights of columns of mercury and are represented on the altimeter as a function of change from a reference setting. For example, if the barometric scale is referenced, or "set" to 29.92 in. (760 mm) of mercury (sea level, standard conditions, one atmosphere) and the instrument is supplied with a static pressure of 20.58 in. (523 mm) of mercury [pressure at 10,000 ft (3049 m) as found on an atmospheric chart under standard conditions], then the altimeter will indicate 10,000 ft. This reading results because the pressure difference on a standard day between sea level (29.92 in./760 mm) and 10,000 ft (20.58 in./523 mm) is equivalent to the pressure exerted by a 9.34-in.-high (237-mm) column of mercury. Any time the altimeter senses this pressure difference between the barometric scale setting and the actual static pressure supplied to the instrument to be 9.34 in. of mercury; it will indicate (i.e., display) 10,000 ft. A typical mechanical altimeter face is shown in Fig. 5. Again, the fixed-scale moving pointer is found in many of these displays. It is not unusual to see both the airspeed and altitude displayed in the similar formats.

Note: Because the actual height of these standard pressure levels varies slightly with atmospheric conditions, the altimeter rarely indicates true height because a

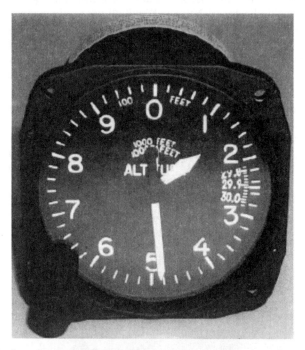

Fig. 5   Typical mechanical altimeter with barometric pressure setting window at the three o'clock position. Large white pointer indicates hundreds, and small white pointer indicates thousands. A ten-thousands pointer can be seen in some altimeters, as well as warning stripes for low altitude (usually below 10,000 ft). (Courtesy of NASA Ames Research Center, Moffett Field, California.)

standard day is not very common. Therefore, the indicated altitude of 10,000 ft might not be the actual altitude. This seemingly dangerous situation does not cause any aircraft separation problem for air-traffic-control purposes because all aircraft flying in the same area are similarly affected. However, under certain conditions, as when flying in mountainous regions, terrain clearance can be a very real problem. Ultimately, it is the pilot's responsibility to maintain terrain clearance, but an informative display, such as a good radar altimeter, will help.

Similar to airspeed, there are several types of altitude (absolute, pressure, density, indicated, calibrated, true, and a few more); and to make it even more difficult, there are several types of altimeter settings (e.g., QNH, QFE, and QNE) used throughout the flying community. Again, the pilot is responsible for knowing and applying the differences, but the display designer can help by making it clear as to which type of altitude and setting is being displayed on the altimeter. Unfortunately, there have been many tragic cases where pilots have read the wrong altimeter information correctly (an issue for pilots) and, even worse, read the correct altimeter information wrongly (an issue for display designers). Many of the altimeters used today are of the Kollsman design as used by Doolittle on the first blind sortie.[17]

   c. Vertical speed displays. Vertical speed displays present the time rate of change of altitude, usually reflected in feet per minute. They have been called vertical-velocity (vertical-speed) indicators and rate-of-climb indicators. Generally, they use the rate of change of static pressure in measuring barometric altitude changes. The display provides the pilot with an accurate depiction of both the magnitude of the change rate (displayed with reference to a moving pointer against a fixed scale) and the direction of the vertical change (indicated by the location of the pointer in either the top-half or the bottom-half of the scale); hence, the term vertical velocity. Vertical velocity, when coupled with forward motion, as is common in fixed-wing aircraft, is extremely difficult to judge by looking through the windscreen or canopy even when the visibility is good. Reasons for this difficulty can be found in Chapters 3 and 7, where explanations are presented for some of the visual illusions associated with flight, for example, estimating the landing location from the visual field.[21] It is far more effective to take a quick look at the vertical-velocity/speed indicator (VVI/VSI) to correctly interpret the rate-of-altitude change than to determine the rate from either the movement of the altimeter or the outside visual-flow pattern. Many SD-related mishaps have been attributed to pilots failing to monitor (or become aware of) a change in the altimeter reading.[22,23] See Fig. 6 for a depiction of a typical HDD vertical-speed indicator.

   d. Heading, angle of attack, turn rate displays. These performance displays are included in this discussion because they are important to consider for most flight tasks and often command a significant amount of instrument scan dwell time.[25] They are grouped together in this chapter because of their collectively lesser role in the direct maintenance of spatial orientation and relatively limited application to combating and recovering from SD. Figure 7 illustrates an arrangement of all the control and performance displays.

   Heading primarily deals with geographic orientation rather than spatial orientation, whereas the information displayed by the angle-of-attack (AoA) indicator and turn-rate indicator (turn needle) are essentially derivatives of the basic control and performance instruments already mentioned. Some pilots place great

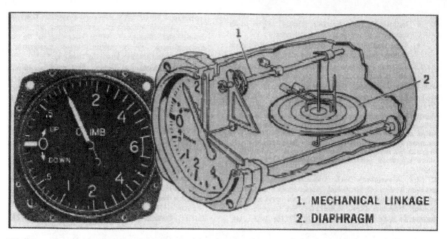

1. MECHANICAL LINKAGE
2. DIAPHRAGM

Fig. 6 Typical vertical-speed (or vertical-velocity) indicator with the neutral state index at the nine o'clock position. When the pointer is above the index, the display represents a climb, whereas a displacement below this position indicates a descent. Movement in the clockwise direction indicates either a climb or a reduction in descent and vice versa. Color is sometimes used to aid with ease of interpretation. (Courtesy of AF Flight Standards Agency; Ref. 24.)

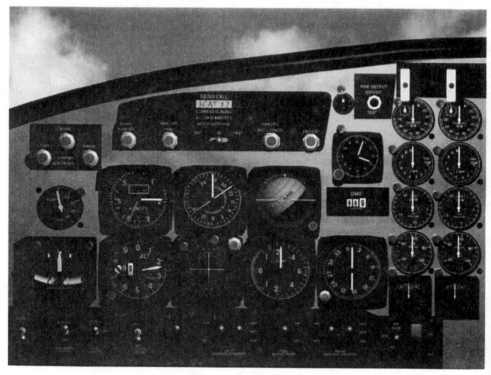

Fig. 7 Representative grouping of control and performance displays (although not the most ideal arrangement). (Courtesy of General Dynamics Advanced Information Systems.)

emphasis on the AoA and turn-rate indicators in order to help maintain situation and spatial awareness. In high-performance aircraft—military fighters, in particular— AoA can assume a critical role, and the display can actually be used as a control instrument. However, the general consensus of most basic flight training programs still considers airspeed, altitude, and vertical speed to be the primary performance displays for spatial awareness.

3. Navigation (Geographic Orientation) Instruments

The navigation instruments include various types of course, range, and glide slope indicators, bearing pointers, and waypoint depictions. These displays indicate the position of the aircraft in relation to a selected navigation facility or a physical waypoint (or fix) over the ground, sometimes with respect to a given coordinate system, such as latitude and longitude. They are primarily associated with geographic orientation. These displays are usually depicted from a plan, or overhead, view that is sometimes referred to as the "God's eye" view. However, they can be oriented from other frames of reference, as well. The navigation displays are mentioned here because many of the newer aircraft combine them with the spatial-orientation displays on the same display surface or medium, which can elicit confusion. Additionally, these displays are important to overall situation awareness.[26] Caution must be exercised when combining the two types of displays. Unless implemented and integrated with all three dimensions in mind, a single display used for both spatial and geographic orientation symbology will depict information from two different perspectives, that is, one perspective from above looking downward and another from inside the aircraft looking forward. The conflict between the two perspectives might contribute to SD.

Presenting a single perspective from a "God's eye" view (see Fig. 8) can also contribute to the pilot's being unaware of the spatial orientation situation. When a navigation display presents only geographic parameters, for example, a horizontal situation display that depicts the aircraft position relative to a desired course, the pilot receives little, if any, spatial orientation information from it. This type of single-function display has been associated with SD as a compounding factor, most notably by increasing the visual task loading needed to interpret the information, which has led to the pilot not realizing a change in spatial orientation. Symbology features for enhancing navigation, or geographic orientation displays, are discussed in detail in many of the human factors display textbooks and in several human factors publications.[27,28]

C. Instrument Cross-Check

Blind flying means just one thing: flying an airplane while unable to see the natural instrument (which is visual reference of terrestrial or astronomical objects) sufficiently in detail to establish a plane of reference that bears a known relation to the earth's surface, which is the means by which every pilot controls his craft. There are other aids to manual flight control, but there is no substitute for visual reference.[29]

The procedure for gathering information from the instrument displays has been termed the instrument cross-check or instrument scan. Exactly when the concept was first established is anyone's guess, but it was well rooted in the work of Doolittle

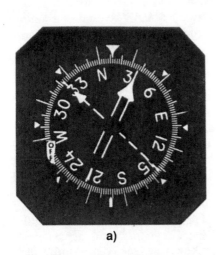 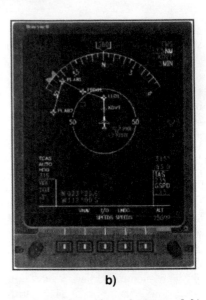

a)   b)

Fig. 8   Two navigation displays: a) the conventional, bearing pointer format and, b) the more modern "glass" horizontal situation display, showing a plan view of waypoints and course lines. This newer technology usually incorporates color along with a variety of symbols and alpha-numeric characters. (Courtesy of NASA Ames Research Center, Moffett Field, California.)

and Sperry in 1929 (Ref. 17) and that of Ocker and Crane about the same time period.[9] Because all of these early display pioneers and pilots found instrument flight to be one of the most demanding activities to perform with an aircraft, they worked diligently in arranging the instruments to ease their workload. While their efforts to establish and then improve upon the crosscheck did not eliminate SD, they did make it more manageable.

The instrument cross-check is simply the visual scan pattern the pilot employs when reading, that is, interpreting, the various displays in the cockpit for any given instrument task (see Fig. 9). From this scan the pilot pieces together information that reflects the current state of the aircraft and projects its future state—a condition also known as situation awareness.[30,31] Therefore, to satisfy the need for situation awareness, generally, and spatial orientation, specifically, the pilot is challenged to always be scanning for the critical flight parameters and to apply that data in predicting changes in the aircraft's orientation. If the pilot loses spatial orientation, the pilot also loses situation awareness (although the reverse is not always true). Developing a well-defined, standardized scan procedure to integrate and assimilate this information is a part of every instrument-rated pilot's training.

1. Procedures

There appears to be two ways to teach a novice pilot candidate how to perform an instrument cross-check. The Federal Aviation Administration (FAA) has adopted the pattern known as the primary/supporting concept, whereas military flight training programs have adopted the control/performance concept of instrument flying.

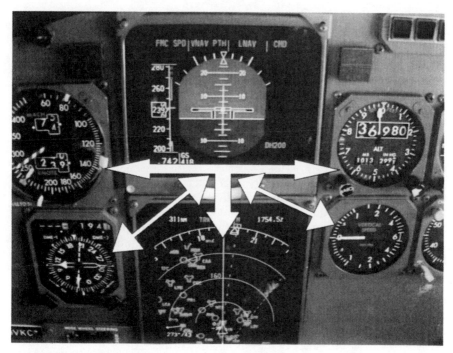

Fig. 9 Arrows illustrate the typical instrument cross-check pattern with individual instruments. Depending upon the flight task, the frequency and dwell time on each display can vary.

The control/performance concept and can be organized into four steps:

1) Establish an attitude or power setting on the control instruments that would result in the desired performance. Known or computed approximate attitude changes and approximate power settings will help to reduce the pilot workload.

2) Trim until control pressures are neutralized. [Trim refers to eliminating counterpressure on the aircraft control surfaces and thereby also on the control sticks and/or rudder pedals. Trim is not usually associated with the display of spatial orientation information, but it is essential for precise aircraft control. Also, it can indirectly contribute to SD, especially Type I (unrecognized), by causing inadvertent, subthreshold control inputs or by introducing excessive resistance to normal control inputs. See Glossary for more details about trim.] Trimming for hands-off flight is essential for smooth, precise aircraft control. It allows pilots to divert their attention to other cockpit duties with minimum deviation from the desired attitude.

3) Cross-check the performance instruments to determine if the established attitude or power setting is providing the desired performance. If a deviation is noted, determine the magnitude and direction of adjustment required to achieve the desired performance.

4) Adjust the attitude or power setting on the control instruments as necessary.

Some pilot training programs might teach slight variations of this constantly repeated sequence, but the basic four-step procedure is essentially standard training practice throughout many of the flying communities mentioned. To apply this procedure effectively, the pilot must become intimately familiar with the representations on the control and performance instruments and understand the predictable affect of the magnitude of a specific control input. Thus a display designer must consider both the resolution *and* the movement of the display. At times the design of one parameter might very well influence the design of the other.

As mentioned, the FAA mandates another scan philosophy called the primary/supporting concept.[32] This procedure focuses attention first on the most important performance parameter for a particular phase of flight and then directs that adjustments be made by reference to the applicable supporting instrument that provides confirmation of the correction. At times, the AI, for example, can be the primary or a supporting instrument, depending upon the parameter in question and might or might not receive the majority of the dwell time. In the procedure of either the control/performance or primary/supporting cross-check, it is always necessary for the pilot to realize that only the AI and power displays represent physical changes made to aircraft systems, whereas the other displays indicate the results of those changes. The difference between the two instrument cross-check philosophies relates more to the FAA's concern over low-proficiency pilots not becoming aware of deviations from assigned or desired parameters than to a disagreement over the nature of the function of a display.[32]

Regardless of the procedure used, instrument design plays an integral role in the effectiveness of the display. If the pilot is to make meaningful adjustments by reference to the instruments, then those instrument displays must contain symbology that enables him or her to correctly assess the current state of the aircraft and to make quantifiable (precise) changes that will produce the desired future state (e.g., resolution and movement). Precisely flying an aircraft is a never-ending process of interpreting symbology and making inputs, followed by a series of ever-decreasing adjustments. (The mechanization of the HDD symbology and the aerodynamic capabilities of an aircraft have a direct influence on the pilot's ability to precisely control the aircraft. This implies that the inherent characteristics of a display for one particular type of aircraft might not be the same for another aircraft with a different aerodynamic response.)

2. Cross-Check Efficiency

The physical arrangement of the displays and their individual symbology—especially the ones for spatial orientation—can have a direct bearing on the efficiency of the instrument cross-check. As the reader has undoubtedly deduced, the pilot's ability to rapidly locate and interpret the displays has a significant influence on how well he or she maintains situation awareness and spatial orientation. Cross-check efficiency also determines how quickly a pilot reaches instrument proficiency and, most importantly, how smoothly and effectively the pilot returns the aircraft to a desirable spatial orientation condition if SD is encountered.[33]

When following the control/performance concept, instructor pilots teach their students to refer to the AI for the vast majority of the time, albeit in brief segments while alternating across the other displays. The actual time a pilot spends looking at each instrument can vary significantly from the amount spent by another pilot; however, it appears that when following the control/performance convention certain instruments are scanned about the same amount by all pilots while performing a given task. The AI consumes approximately 50% of the visual time the pilot spends when employing the control/performance instrument cross-check.[34] All of the other instruments combined receive the remaining time. Individual dwell times vary slightly across these other displays, depending on the task, but the altimeter, vertical-velocity indicator, and airspeed indicator each receive about 10% of the remaining time. Even if the pilots were flying an instrument approach with course guidance present on a HDD display, then the separate course guidance indicator receives about 10% of the cross-check time. The AI still receives about the same amount of visual time as before. These results suggest that three instruments (the attitude indicator, the altimeter, and the airspeed indicator) consume the vast majority of the time a pilot spends scanning the displays during a flight in instrument conditions. Of course, the dwell times will likely change in visual conditions because of external information being readily available.[22,35] It follows then that from where the pilot elects to visually acquire the information is a function of the degree of ease in locating and interpreting it. Consequently, the arrangement and design of these three displays (or four, if one considers the vertical-velocity indicator) will have a direct impact on instrument crosscheck efficiency, situation awareness and, ultimately, spatial orientation.

Because of these fundamental requirements, the arrangement of these principal instruments, which are needed for almost all flight tasks, has been established for many years. Typically, the attitude indicator is located in the center of the instrument panel directly positioned in front of the pilot at the controls. The airspeed indicator is located to the left of the AI, while the altimeter and vertical speed indicator are situated to the right of the AI, making a level row across the middle of the head-down instrument panel. The navigation information is traditionally located directly below the AI, making a vertical column with the attitude indicator. This arrangement has been termed the T cross-check arrangement because of its resemblance to the letter T. During the development of the instrument panel for the first blind flight in 1929 (Ref. 17), Doolittle established the basic T as the easiest arrangement for integrating critical SO information, although the vertical speed indicator can be seen directly to the right of the attitude indicator (assumed more important for the task of judging height above field elevation or touchdown).

It is mentioned at this time that a relatively newly observed head response to horizon movement has been identified in the research. The response, termed the OKCR or optokinetic cervical reflex, is described both in this chapter and in several of the other chapters in this book. Its finding can have major implications to instrument design once thoroughly understood. Up until this finding, most researchers have assumed the pilot maintains a fixed-head orientation (aligned with the nose of the aircraft). It appears this is not the case when a wide horizon can be seen. A short description of the OKCR and its potential impact follows.

3. Outside Visibility

Conditions of in-flight visibility will have an impact on the pilot's workload, susceptibility to SD, and maintenance of situation awareness. It is important for the display designer, when considering symbology features that counter SD, to appreciate the various in-flight visibility conditions affecting the pilot's actions and the reflexes resulting from various in-flight visibilities.

For years pilots have been taught to maintain an upright posture when banking the aircraft. This practice maintained what was thought to be the natural head orientation, that is, aligned with the net gravitoinertial force vector. Recently, Patterson[36] has shown that when the real horizon is visible during a turn the pilot will subconsciously align his or her head with the horizon (up to 15 deg of bank), regardless of the increased G forces and bank experienced. Patterson and colleagues term this response as the OKCR. When flight is conducted by reference to the instruments, this effect does not take place, and the pilot naturally maintains an upright head position aligned with the orientation of the cockpit. Thus, when viewed in instrument meteorological conditions (IMC) the perceived orientation and movement of an artificial horizon on an AI might well be different than that which would have been perceived of the true horizon in the same orientation viewed in visual meteorological conditions (VMC). Patterson and colleagues believe this dichotomy can partially explain why many pilots report experiencing Type II (recognized) SD when flying in and out of clouds. They can become disoriented because the artificial horizon of the traditional AI does not correctly mimic the way they perceive the true horizon. Apparent horizon movement and control response to it has been a design issue since the first artificial horizon.

Because the horizon is elementary to spatial orientation and the instrument cross-check, how well the pilot can interpret its movement impacts his or her overall performance while using a particular display. (Further discussion of the importance and effect of perceiving horizon position and movement in an attitude display is contained in Appendix A of this chapter.) Consequently, when evaluating a display for its affect on spatial orientation, the researcher must take into account the degree to which the pilot can discern the horizon. This variable can be quite elusive to control during empirical studies. The pilot's ability to see the horizon is easily controlled in a laboratory, but in most in-flight studies that ability is highly variable as a function of flight conditions. Although most pilots describe their visual environment in terms of VMC, visual flight rules (VFR), IMC, and instrument flight rules (IFR), researchers must use care in applying these acronyms in order to avoid confounding study results. (Definitions of each of these acronyms are included in Appendix B in this chapter.) For example, a pilot can technically be flying in VFR conditions, or VMC, and yet might not be able to see the actual horizon. Even on some clear days, the true horizon might not be visible. Therefore, to ensure validity of comparisons during studies of pilot responses to HDDs it is important for the researcher to elicit from the pilot the exact visual conditions he or she experienced when encountering SD.

D.   Fundamental Displays for Spatial Orientation

"Spatial disorientation is an erroneous sense of any of the flight parameters displayed by the aircraft control and performance instruments" (Ref. 37, p. 297).

In the preceding definition a clear relationship is postulated involving the terms spatial disorientation, control and performance instruments, and the erroneous sense of the parameters displayed by those instruments. This operational definition of SD considers all of the control and performance instruments as important, and,

**Table 2a   Relationship between flight motion and flight
instruments: angular flight parameters**

Axis	Position	Velocity	Acceleration
X	Bank (AI)[a]	Roll rate (AI)	Change in roll rate (AI)
Y	Pitch (AI)	Pitch rate (AI)	Change in pitch rate (AI)
Z	Heading (Comp)[b]	Turn rate (Comp/needle)[c]	Change in turn rate (Comp/needle)

[a]AI = attitude indicator (pitch and bank).
[b]Comp = compass.
[c]Needle/ball = turn needle or ball on turn-and-slip indicator.

**Table 2b   Relationship between flight motion and flight
instruments: linear flight parameters**

Axis	Position	Velocity	Acceleration
X	Lat/long (Nav)[a]	Airspeed (A/S ind)[b]	Change in airspeed (A/S ind)
Y	Lat/long (Nav)	Slip/skid rate (Ball)	Change in slip/skid rate (Ball)
Z	Altitude (Alt)[c]	Vertical speed (VVI/Alt)[d]	Change in vertical speed (VVI/Alt)

[a]Nav = navigation (INS, HSI, etc. . . .).
[b]A/S ind = airspeed indicator.
[c]Alt = altimeter.
[d]VVI = vertical-velocity indicator.

indeed, they are during their respective tasks. However, to address a comprehensive countermeasure to SD these two categories of instruments must be resolved into the minimum needed to enable the pilot to construct an adequate mental model of the aircraft's spatial orientation, regardless of the task. This refinement requires a closer examination of the relationship between the motion of the aircraft (and pilot) and the taxonomy of the fundamental control and performance instruments. A more generalized, internationally accepted definition of SD identifies SD parameters as those that relate to the motions of the aircraft about the two primary rotational axes (pitch and roll) and the vertical position and motion of the aircraft relative to the Earth.[38] The instruments that traditionally display rotational position and motion and vertical translation are annotated in Tables 2a and 2b with the major axes depicted in Fig. 10.

Tables 2a and 2b reveals that the primary instruments for displaying spatial-orientation information of position and motion are the altimeter and the attitude indicator. In addition, airspeed must be included because flight would not be possible without it, and the aircraft's potential for maneuvering correlates directly to

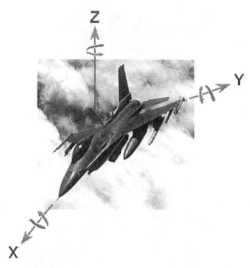

Fig. 10   Major axes between flight motion and flight instruments. (Courtesy of USAF; data available online at http://www.af.mil/photos/fighters.)

the magnitude of the airspeed. In sum, airspeed displays the longitudinal motion needed to generate lift, the altimeter displays height above the surface of the Earth, and the attitude display provides the aircraft's orientation with respect to its two major axes of movement. Therefore, the minimum, critical information the pilot needs in order to maintain spatial orientation is attitude, airspeed, and altitude. These fundamental parameters must be displayed somewhere in the cockpit on the HDDs, either separately or integrated. Studies have shown that when this information is not provided complete loss of control will occur in approximately than 2 mins.[39]

Without the critical information available to build the correct mental model, the pilot is guaranteed to experience the most dangerous type of spatial disorientation—Type I (unrecognized). Even with the fundamental spatial orientation information provided and viewed, the pilot can still experience Type II (recognized) or Type III (incapacitating) SD. To combat any type of SD, he or she must be able to recognize the situation and then apply the correct control inputs to maneuver the aircraft to a known spatial orientation in spite of other sensations experienced at the time. Therefore, the degree to which the design of an instrument display compels the pilot to appropriately respond to its information is critical to the success of the pilot–machine interface. Unfortunately, even with the advent of the advanced displays of today, SD-related mishaps continue to occur after the pilot recognizes SD and is still unable to safely recover the aircraft.[40]

E.   Primary Flight Reference

As already suggested, the term primary flight reference (PFR) could conceptually apply to one, a few, or many instruments in the cockpit. The challenge to the pilot and display designer is to understand what information is considered primary, when it is needed, and how best to display it during any given task. In the logic of the preceding discussion on fundamental displays, the assumption is made that the primary spatial orientation information must be displayed at all times. Technically speaking, any of the navigation, engine performance, or general awareness displays that have been discussed can contain information that is of prime importance at a given moment, but those displays will never be of first importance all of the time. The displays that contain fundamental spatial orientation information will always be of first importance in order to ensure constant maintenance of aircraft control.

During the mid-to-late 1980s, when the U.S. Air Force (USAF) realized a potential mismatch between the displays used in current instrument training programs and the rapid influx of new technologies into the more modern aircraft cockpits, the definition of PFR reached a high level of concern. This concern eventually spawned a research program that called for an endorsement of the head-up display (a new technology at the time) as the PFR during instrument flight. It also encouraged standardization of all displays, including HDDs, whenever possible.[41] The outcome of the USAF project established primacy of certain flight information that would be considered the basics of the PFR. Interestingly, it was found that no official endorsement process was in place for any of the military instrument displays. Because of this and other related regulatory shortcomings, the following official statement was included in the guidance document governing display symbology of military aircraft: "A primary flight reference (PFR) is any display, or suite of displays or instruments, that provide all required information for flight and complies with the requirements of this standard for information content and presentation" (Ref. 42, p. 6).

Although the process began with endorsing the HUD as a PFR, the term soon applied to HDDs as well. Consequently, PFR requirements now apply to any display or display suite considered as primary. Those requirements are specific and must, at a minimum, include the critical parameters mentioned for each task (see Table 3) identified in MIL-STD 1787C, Table 1 (Ref. 42). Not surprisingly, the terms of pitch (or flight path for a head-up display) and vertical velocity, bank, airspeed, and altitude are required to be displayed during all maneuvers. This information can be represented on separate displays (a suite of instruments) or on a single display, but the information must be displayed at all times. The primary purpose of MIL-STD 1787C is to ensure that the information *is* displayed, and less so *how* it is displayed. The display designer must determine what features and symbology to use (e.g., color, size, movement, location, arrangement, etc) and determine some of the metrics with which to measure the display's effectiveness. With the MIL-STD 1787C requirement an official link was established between the operational definition of SD and the cockpit displays needed for its prevention.

III. Design Topics

Preceding sections have established a relationship between the information a pilot must obtain in order to perform any given flight task and that which he or she needs to maintain or regain spatial orientation. The following sections will approach the topic of spatial orientation displays from the designer's view and will suggest display enhancements that hold promise in reducing the pilot's workload.

Table 3   Data required on the PFR during specific maneuvers [MIL-STD-17987C (Ref. 42), Table 1]

Required information	Instrument takeoff	Climb	Cruise	Fix to fix	Hold	Penetration	Arc	Non-precision approach	Precision approach	Flt dip approach	Cat II/III approach
Precise pitch angle	X[a]	X	X	X	X	X	X	X	X	—	X
Climb/dive angle[b,c]	X	X	R[d]	R	X	R	X	X	X	X	X
Precise bank angle	X	X	X	X	X	X	X	X	X	X	X
Approximate bank	X	X	X	X	X	X	X	X	X	X	X
Barometric altitude	X	X	X	X	X	X	X	X	X	X	X
Airspeed	X	X	X	X	X	X	X	X	X	X	X
Heading	X	X	X	X	X	X	X	X	X	X	X
Horizontal flight path[e]	S[f]	S	S	S	—	S	—	S	S	S	S
Bearing	S	S	S	S	S	S	S	S	S	S	X
Distance	S	S	X	S	X	S	S	S	X	X	X
Lateral deviation	X	—	—	—	X	X	—	X	X	X	X
Vertical deviation	—	—	—	—	—	M/G[g]	—	—	X[j]	X	X
Flight director	—	—	—	—	S	S	S	S	S	S	S
Timing	—	—	—	—	X	—	X	X	—	S	S
Absolute altitude[h]	—	—	—	—	—	—	—	—	X	—	X
Angle of attack	X	X	X	X	X	X	X	X	X	X	X
Yaw[i]	X	X	X	X	X	X	X	X	X	X	X
Longitudinal acceleration	R	R	R	R	R	R	R	R	X	X	X
Speed/AoA deviation	R	R	R	R	R	R	R	X	X	X	X
Vertical velocity	X	X	—	—	—	X	—	X	X	X	X

[a] X = always required for this maneuver.

[b] Replaced by pitch and vertical velocity when the climb/dive marker is invalid or unavailable.

[c] Vertical velocity is added to the display when the aircraft is in a high AoA, CDM-limited condition.

[d] R = strongly recommended for this maneuver.

[e] Required only on displays which are designed to conform to an outside visual scene or display (e.g., HUD, FLIR, or radar imagery overlays).

[f] S = required only if these data are not in view elsewhere in the cockpit (single-medium PFR).

[g] M/G = Required only for MLS or GPS curved path procedure.

[h] Absolute altitude generally refers to above ground level (at current location), but altitude relative to a reference (such as the end of the runway) can be used.

[i] Required only for aircraft that utilize these data caused by aircraft limitations such as asymmetric drag/thrust.

[j] Not required for PAR approaches.

Table 4 presents a comparison of the spatial-orientation information attained from observing the real world vs that derived from instrument displays. At first glance, one might wrongly deduce that the instruments present a much more precise and useful view of the world than that extracted from mere estimated parameters of the actual environment. Although the information presented on the instruments is usually more precise, its usefulness is affected by the increased mental processing time required for its interpretation.

In setting about the task of designing SD-resistant displays, one will discover a large amount of data pertaining to the human response to different types of visual information.[43] Even if a review of the literature is limited to the displays used for instrument flight, the amount of information is still almost overwhelming.[5] Narrowing this latter information to only those displays that provide spatial-orientation information is something that can be adequately addressed in the next several pages, but still contains quite a bit of information. Toward that end, this section focuses on the display designer's areas of primary responsibility in combating SD, namely, attitude, airspeed, and altitude. It does not take into account a type of "bail-out" technology known as ground-collision-avoidance automation. This technology appears to be on the horizon, and the challenging task of integrating it with the more traditional visual aircraft displays is yet to be realized.

In focusing on these three essential elements of flight information, it seems appropriate to review several time-tested human factors principles of instrument design that were established by Fitts[44] when display development was beginning to receive its first serious emphasis. Many of these tenets still apply to the spatial-orientation features mentioned in the rest of the chapter.

1) Every display should be designed for quick perception.

2) Every display should be designed so that the meaning of the indication is immediately apparent.

3) A display should provide information that is precise and complete.

4) Single displays and entire display systems should be as simple as possible.

5) Different displays and controls should be easily distinguishable.

6) Displays that provide related information, or to which are referred in rapid succession, should be grouped.

7) Controls and instruments should be designed so that they move in the "expected" direction.

8) Controls should be designed to permit the required speed, precision, timing, and/or smoothness of operation.

9) The mode of action, location, and arrangement of controls should provide for overall simplicity of operation and movement efficiency.

10) Equipment should be designed for use by operators who have only a moderate amount of training, who are less than average in skill, and who will use the equipment under adverse conditions.

11) Equipment should be designed so that continued operation for a number of hours results in minimum fatigue or loss of operator efficiency.

12) Principal aspects of design, arrangement, and location of displays and control equipment should be standardized.

Table 4   Comparison of SO information between the real world and the instrument displays

State	Extracting from the real world	Extracting from the instrument display (artificial world)
Attitude	——	——
Pitch	Estimated angle between the real horizon and the imaginary extension of the longitudinal axis of the aircraft	Fairly precise angle that can be interpreted by comparing the nose of a miniature aircraft symbol against the pitch lines displayed on the sphere of the attitude indicator
Bank	Estimated angle between the real horizon and the imaginary extension of the lateral (transverse) axis of the aircraft	Fairly precise angle that can be interpreted by comparing the sky pointer and the bank scale that is displayed around the perimeter of the attitude indicator. Markings are shown at 10-deg increments, and then in 30-deg increments after the first full 30 deg. The approximate bank angle can also be estimated by comparing the miniature aircraft symbol against the horizontal attitude pitch lines.
Airspeed	Estimated rates of relative motion of nonmoving objects on the Earth's surface or the estimated relative motion of clouds. Changes of airspeed are estimated by the change of the visual flowfield.	Precise numerical reading that can be interpreted the location of a pointer along a scale ranging from 0 to a maximum airspeed OR read directly from a digital readout.
Altitude	Estimation of apparent size, shape, and brightness of objects on the surface of the Earth	Precise numerical reading that of a pointer along a scale can be interpreted by pointer along a scale ranging from 0 to 100,000 ft; usually requires different levels of sensitivity to show all full range of vertical motion OR a digital readout
Change in altitude	Estimation of changes in the apparent size, shape, and brightness of objects on the surface of the Earth	Estimated by the rate of change of the altimeter scale OR directly by comparing a pointer against scale

A. Attitude Information

"I sketched a rough picture of the dial for an instrument which I thought would do the job and showed it to Elmer Sperry, Sr., a great engineer and inventor who had established and headed the Sperry Gyroscope Co. and who was very interested in aviation" (Ref. 17, p. 345).

The preceding quote describes how the forerunner of the modern attitude indicator was created in 1929. Along with its wide success, this attitude display also has been the most controversial display in the cockpit. The source of dispute lies in its most basic feature—how it moves.

1. Attitude Indicator Movement

Though extremely rare among instrument rated pilots, it is possible—even for airline pilots—to confuse the moving horizon bar of the gyroscopic attitude indicator and the fixed airplane symbol when they find themselves suddenly and unexpectedly in an unusual flight attitude. When this occurs, the initial reaction— to fly the horizon bar back to straight and level flight—will increase rather than reduce the bank angle (Ref. 20, p. 1).

The principal issue pertaining to AI movement has been that of the indicator's own internal movement, sometimes termed "mechanization." There also have been indications that abnormal roll maneuvering of the aircraft can cause visual distortion of the artificial horizon,[19] but this concern is minimal compared to the confusion sometimes presented by the manner in which the major components of the AI move relative to one another. It is the latter issue that will be addressed here. Because the attitude indicator is an integrated display of aircraft pitch and bank, the problems associated with its movement can be best understood by first examining the depiction of each of those two elements. Pitch *movement*, as discussed in Sec. II.A and outlined in Table 2, refers to the rotation about the aircraft's lateral axis, and pitch *attitude* is the angular displacement between the nose of the aircraft and the horizon. On a typical attitude indicator—a gyro-stabilized sphere, rigidly mounted in space, and which appears to rotate within its case—pitch is displayed by means of the relationship of the aircraft symbol to a set of moving, sequential, horizontal lines. The horizontal lines are marked on the rotating sphere and represent discrete pitch-angle values, usually in 5- and 10-deg increments. The attitude display's design represents the real world as if the pilot were looking through a small portal. For example, as the pilot pulls back on the control stick and raises the nose of the aircraft then the artificial horizon (0-deg pitch line) appears to decline in the visual field just as would the real horizon if the pilot were looking at the real world.

Bank, as presented in Sec. II.A and Table 2, is the angular displacement between the horizon and the aircraft's lateral axis, and roll is the rotational motion about the longitudinal axis. Bank is most often displayed by a "sky" pointer at the top of the instrument case against a circular bank scale that is fixed and indexed around the circumference of the attitude display. This indexed bank scale is normally graduated to reflect precise bank angles in 10-deg increments for the first 30-, 15-deg increments up to 60 deg and then 30-deg increments thereafter. On occasion, a "ground" pointer has been used in lieu of a sky pointer and is depicted in the bottom half of the display case against a scale marked in the same increments as the

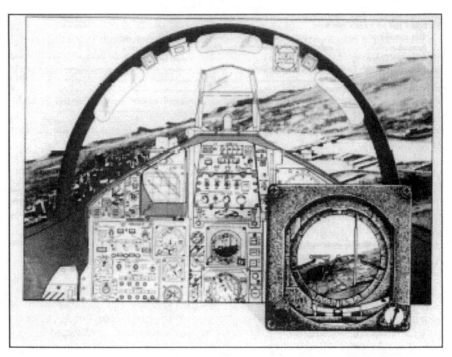

Fig. 11 Depiction of typical western-world attitude-indicator concept integrating pitch and bank. The insert in the lower right depicts the world as the designer expects the pilot to perceive the world when viewing it through the attitude indicator (inside-out concept). (Courtesy of U.S. Air Force Flight Standards Agency; Ref. 24.)

sky pointer. A pilot also obtains a general sense of bank by reference to the angle produced between the horizon line (and essentially all of the pitch lines together) and the center of the instrument case (or more technically correct, the wings of the miniature aircraft symbol). A determination of direction and rate of roll motion is made from the rotation of the pitch lines and the sky or ground pointer.

A major point of contention in depicting bank, and to a lesser degree pitch, lies in the perceptual model of how a pilot perceives the motion of the pitch-and-roll indications on the display. Figure 11 presents an example of an attitude indicator that is designed to depict an integrated model of both pitch attitude and bank and how the display designer imagines the real world to be represented on the AI. In this example, it is presumed that the pilot will interpret the representation as if looking from inside the aircraft to the outside in the same manner as if looking out the windscreen. However, as mentioned in Roscoe's preceding statement, this artificial display can sometimes produce a problem in the perceptual transfer from artificial depiction to actuality.

The conflict that arises between reality and the pilot's mental model is reflected in the question, While flying, do pilots perceive the *horizon line* to move ("inside-out" orientation), or do they perceive the *aircraft symbol* to move against a stable horizon line ("outside-in" orientation)?[45] Figure 12 illustrates these two orientation concepts.

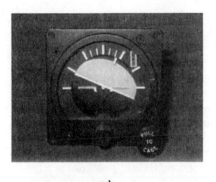
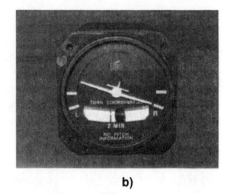

a)   b)

Fig. 12   Illustration comparing the depiction of a) left bank with an inside-out attitude indicator to b) right bank with an outside-in turn indicator. (Courtesy of NASA Ames Research Center.)

In addressing the question of which concept is most effective for recognizing attitude, one soon discovers that the dominant problem element is bank interpretation. Previc and Ercoline[46] accomplished a review of many of the research articles on the subject of bank perception and how to best display this parameter on the AI. They found that novice subjects always performed better with a moving-aircraft symbol (outside-in) attitude indicator than with a moving-horizon symbol (inside-out) attitude indicator. Experienced pilots achieved about the same results with both types of displays, presumably because of their training and experience.

A third type of motion of an attitude indicator, termed the frequency-separated attitude display, is found in the literature and is briefly mentioned here.[47] This AI was found to produce fewer errors in roll interpretation than either the inside-out or outside-in orientations. On the frequency-separated AI the artificial horizon movement is determined by the frequency of the roll rate. During the initial part of a rapid roll, the aircraft symbol moves as in an outside-in display. After this initial movement, and when the roll rate decreases, to a predetermined amount, the artificial horizon begins to move, and the aircraft symbol becomes stationary as on the inside-out display. Evaluations of these three mechanizations have tended to focus on "correctness" of the subjects' inputs, most often measured in the number of roll reversals. Roll-reversal errors are generally those that are associated with incorrect initial movements the pilot executes in responding to an attitude that requires immediate adjustment. They often occur during unusual attitude (UA) recognition and recovery tasks and are easily recorded while measuring performance of a display. (A detailed description of the UA recognition and recovery task is given in Sec. III.D.1) More importantly, roll reversals are associated with SD mishaps in that critical time to recover is lost, and an already dangerous situation is exacerbated when the pilot rolls the aircraft in the wrong direction.[20,48]

The importance of minimizing roll reversals notwithstanding, the careful display designer must consider more than just UA recognition and recovery when developing an effective AI. After resolving the correctness aspect for reacting to a UA, the designer must then preserve a display's utility for precision tracking, which will be necessary during other flight tasks. Although only the classic inside-out or outside-in concepts are currently used on AIs today, with the "inside-out" being, by far, the most prevalent throughout the world, both formats pose problems of significant concern. Interestingly, the frequency-separated display has remained only a concept, in spite of research indicating that it presents roll better than the inside-out attitude indicator and enables more precise attitude tracking than the outside-in attitude indicator.[47] Reasons are not known for the frequency-separated format having been abandoned as an enhancement to the AI, but it is in the authors' opinions that adherence to convention is a likely factor.

Despite the popularity of the inside-out AI motion concept, not all design specialists have been convinced of its benefits. Ocker and Crane[9] and Roscoe[20] felt it was at the root of many SD mishaps, and the noted Russian human factors specialist Dr. Vladimir Ponomarenko[49,50] strongly encouraged its replacement with the outside-in attitude display. During Ponomarenko's work at the former Soviet Institute of Aviation Medicine, Moscow, he and his colleagues were able to establish the outside-in display concept as the most effective for reducing SD and convinced the appropriate authorities to implement the design as the standard for the AI in Soviet-made aircraft. Russian manufacturers continue to use the outside-in AI for head-down attitude displays in the majority of their aircraft.

The Russian studies cite the superior attribute of the outside-in presentation as that of reducing the pilot's cognitive effort. They ascribe the increased mental efficiency as being a result of a direct correlation to how a pilot understands his or her spatial relationship with the actual horizon. Ponomarenko and colleagues[50-52] state that a pilot learns from early training to maneuver an aircraft in reference to a static horizon and earth's surface, rather than the reverse concept depicted on an inside-out display. He quotes a former USSR pilot, P. Bananov, as saying, "Not a single pilot thinks for a moment that during aerobatic maneuvers the earth or horizon moves." More objectively, Ponomarenko[52] demonstrated that reversals in pitch and bank were dramatically reduced with the outside-in AI for both novice *and* experienced pilots.

Roll-reversals with the inside-out AI appear to be attributable to the strength of the pilot's spatial model of the connection between stick displacement and the *perceived* resultant movement of the aircraft symbol vs the *actual* movement of the pitch-and-bank cues. That is, if a pilot intuitively makes a connection between the pitch-and/or-bank symbols while moving the stick, he or she will perceive the direction of the symbol movement as being opposite that of the stick and in conflict with the desired motion of the aircraft. For example, when pushing the stick to the left (counterclockwise, creating an aircraft left roll) the pilot might perceive the stick action as causing the horizon to rotate to the right (clockwise) rather than the aircraft symbol to rotate to the left (counterclockwise). Because the desired aircraft motion is to the left, the pilot then experiences a conflict from the perceived movement to the right. This conflict sometimes leads to reversal in the pilots' roll input. In the context of reacting to an undesirable attitude, the pilot might deduce that to return the horizon to level when it is slanted right (left bank) requires a movement of the stick to the left. That action would increase rather than decrease the bank angle. Consequently, to correctly use the inside-out display pilots must project themselves into the aircraft symbol. Referenced studies suggest that this projection is particularly difficult in high-workload scenarios.[53]

The reader might be tempted at this point to decry the inside-out AI design as contradicting the seventh of Fitts' basic design principles outlined earlier, that is, controls and instruments should be designed so that they move in the expected direction. However, one must keep in mind that if the pilot were able to assume a proper orientation inside the aircraft symbol as just described, he or she would not experience any discontinuity, and the display would indeed move in the expected direction. This appears to be supported by the results from the OKCR studies. An interesting aside to this topic is the observation that although the aforementioned incompatibility issue applies to perceived pitch movement as well as to bank, pitch-reversal errors do not appear to be as prevalent as roll-reversal errors. The reason for this is still unclear (perhaps the OKCR?). One of the authors (William Ercoline) noted while conducting unusual attitude recovery studies that pilots consistently attempted to make roll inputs prior to pitch inputs. This seemed to be the case even when the pilots were given instructions to make pitch changes first. One possible contribution to such prioritization might be standard unusual attitude training practices, which are described as a performance metric in Sec. III.D.1.

Some insight into the pilot's perception of pitch-and-bank movement can be obtained by considering the effectiveness of the attitude indicator symbology relative to the robustness of the artificial world depicted on the display. The inside-out concept appears to work well when flight symbology is superimposed over a sensor/virtual image or when it is truly conformal to the out-the-window environment, as with the HUD. It appears that in these cases the pilot is easily able to insert him or herself into the inside-out orientation and overcome the incompatibility between stick and symbology movements. Conversely, incorporating an outside-in presentation on a real-world display produces some unique challenges. For example, the depicted bank angle between the real horizon of a space- or Earth-stabilized video image and a superimposed aircraft-stabilized outside-in attitude display would be twice the actual bank of the aircraft. Regardless of this potential spatial orientation problem, the Russian approach to providing attitude information on a HUD still employs the outside-in bank concept in an effort to directly correlate head-down and head-up data.[54]

From available evidence one might deem that adopting the outside-in approach would be a foregone conclusion for other than virtual or real-world displays. However, legitimate concerns over such a proposal have been expressed. One such alarm regards the possibility of negative transfer of training. This psychological dynamic usually stems from residual effects found when a person transitions from one design philosophy to another. It supports the fear that there are too many inside-out displays already in use to permit changing to another concept. Additional unease arises over violating the principle of standardization that would result from simultaneous implementation of two concepts so diametrically opposed to each other. German Air Force (GAF) researchers expressed this apprehension during the reunification program between East Germany and West Germany because they had pilots who were uncomfortable transferring between the two concepts.[55] After a good deal of debate, the GAF decided to control their pilots by restricting any from crossing between the two displays.

Thus, although it appears that there are better ways of designing the movement of the attitude indicator than the inside-out concept and new information as to our understanding of perceptual spatial orientation, changing the current method

Table 5 Recommended color-use chart from MIL-STD 1787
(Ref. 42)

Function	Color required
Warnings, warning-level flight envelope or system limits, and dangerous military threats	Red
Cautions and other information with cautionary level of impact, such as unknown aircraft tracks, TCAS threat advisories, and scale marks indicating approach to abnormal/out of tolerance conditions	Yellow and Amber
Sky-on-attitude indicator	Blue
Earth-on-attitude indicator	Brown or Black
Advisories	Blue or Green
Selected menu options or captured modes, question marks for missing data, and status "normal"	White or Green
Pilot-selected navigational information or subsystem values (i.e., joker fuel, bingo fuel, or altimeter setting)	Magenta

of displaying bank information can present more problems than anyone wants to accept. The remaining discussion of attitude displays presents some less controversial design features of the *artificial* displays.

2. Color

The first attitude display used by Doolittle incorporated a contrasting color scheme of white in the top half of the attitude sphere and black in the bottom half. This black-and-white feature was used for many years, with some occasional and notable departures, such as the military's all-black J-8 AI. In the 1960s the Collins AI combined a brown bottom half representing the ground and a blue top that represented the sky in order to depict a perspective more in tune with the actual world. With the advent of multicolor electronic displays in the 1980s, designers recognized the advantage of using various hues to enhance attitude recognition.[54] As with many other aspects of electronic symbology, the options were restrained only by the imagination of the manufacturers and designers and a few physical limits of the technology. Ad hoc industry standards evolved, but little regulatory guidance was issued. Recommended color schemes for military application were established and are described in MIL-STD 1787C (Ref. 42). They are reproduced here as Table 5.

In addition to selective tones, changes in color intensity or density have been employed on several attitude displays, and the technique seems to improve the pilot's ability to quickly recognize the aircraft orientation during unusual attitude recoveries.[57] As the pitch either increases or decreases, the shade becomes lighter or darker, respectively, which helps to alert the pilot as to pitch magnitude. This intuitive presentation appears to reduce cognitive processing time compared to that required to read and interpret the numbers next to the pitch lines. For example, the brown shading for nose-down pitch changes from a light-brown shade for 30 deg of nose-down pitch to a much darker brown at 60 deg of nose down. The intent is to command more of the pilot's attention with a dark, more ominous shade as the pitch angle approaches a potentially dangerous value.

Although color is well established as providing added perceptual information,[58] its use is not mentioned in Fitts' design principles. However, his first two principles support the use of color in using the terms "quick perception" and "immediate recognition." Its importance is essentially uncontested in this day in time, but it can present technological challenges. For example, the use of light filters (sunglasses or laser eye protection) could cause certain colors to become difficult to see, especially in diminished illumination as when using night vision devices.[59] These situations are usually found during covert military operations. As always, it is important to consider the entire human-cockpit integration continuum when developing displays for spatial orientation.

3. Location

The location of the attitude indicator is critical in expeditiously alerting the pilot of an unexpected attitude. If placed too far from the center of the cockpit or field of view, it will be referenced too infrequently and require excessive time to visually acquire. Fortunately, the attitude indicator is usually found in the center of the instrument panel and central to the T instrument arrangement. Nevertheless, a few aircraft have the HDD AI located in a less than optimal place. This reclined seat and cockpit layout almost requires the HUD to display the spatial-orientation symbology. It is recommended that, at the very least, the attitude indicator be placed as centrally as possible in the predominant field of regard for a given flight task in order to require the least amount of head and eye movements (see Fig. 13). This tenet is important for two reasons: 1) the attitude indicator is the instrument scanned most during instrument flight, and 2) head movement can produce vestibular illusions that lead to SD. As with mechanization, little direct guidance exists for AI location within the military. However, the FAA requires central location for passenger carry, and the sound philosophy of central placement can also be found in MIL-STD 1787C, which defines the general arrangement and area to locate the primary flight reference—the display or displays that include essential attitude information.

4. Other Attitude Indicator Symbology Modifications

Because of the inflexibility of the mechanical attitude indicator, few substantive changes to it were contemplated or studied over the years other than its perceived movement by Roscoe and colleagues and the use of color by many others. However, since the advent of multifunctional displays (MFD) there have been numerous symbology design modifications that attempted to make the AI presentation reflect visual cues as seen in the real world. In addition to the already mentioned color applications for pitch, there have been many other format changes and enhancements that make the spatial orientation task of the pilot easier, such as combining all the information on to one display. Some of the more important individual symbology ideas are mentioned here.

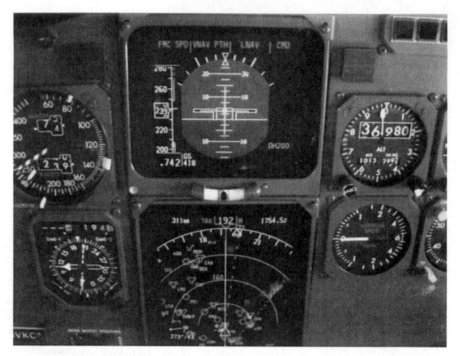

Fig. 13 Typical arrangement of the flight instruments emphasizing the central location of the attitude indicator.

a. Shape of the pitch lines on the attitude display. Most attitude displays contain a series of parallel lines at regular intervals in the center of the display to represent incremental angles of pitch. When these lines are referenced to the aircraft symbol, the pitch of the aircraft can be determined to a fairly precise degree, but that determination often requires significant mental effort, especially in dynamic, high-workload situations. Several design techniques have been used to make the job of interpreting the extent of pitch easier. Some of these enhancements have included inserting words like "climb" or "dive" between the pitch lines, or adding thickness to the lines as the pitch becomes greater. Another modification integrates symbology that flashes or blinks when bank angles exceed a predetermined amount, for example, greater than 60 deg of bank. Burns and Lovering[60] demonstrated better spatial awareness by adding arrows called "teeth" to each pitch ladder line. The teeth grew in length as the pitch became greater. All of these concepts have produced improved performance for a variety of flight tasks and have received positive feedback. One shape symbology known as articulation—involving increasing the slope or bend of the pitch lines at large nose-down attitudes—has met with mixed user acceptance (see Chapter 10).

b. Size of the bank indication. For attitude information the axiom "bigger is better" generally holds true. However, most cockpits have a limited amount of "real estate" set aside for the AI. Designers learned long ago that it is difficult to expand the display of pitch or bank without impacting on the space needed for displays of geographic orientation or other flight information. Nevertheless, creativity has sometimes overcome physical barriers.

One technique that attempted to use existing cockpit space to provide the pilot with a large visual cue for bank was the peripheral-vision horizon display, sometimes known as the Malcolm Horizon.[61] The display consisted of a laser beam, oriented to reflect the true horizon, which was projected across the instrument panel of the aircraft. The purpose of the peripheral horizon line was to take advantage of the ambient portion of the visual system (see Chapter 3). It was postulated that when the horizon line moved, pilots would sense the motion with peripheral vision, regardless of the direction of their focal gaze. In light of what is now known about response to the OKCR, it would have been interesting to note the behavior of the subject's head during these studies.

The Malcolm Horizon concept worked well in several ground-based studies, but significant technical issues arose in flight when the aircraft was at extreme pitch angles. In those severe situations the horizon line moved away from the instrument panel and became a nuisance to the pilot as it was reflected off the windscreen and canopy. Additionally, the laser line became irregular when the light reflected off instruments of varying depths.[62] In spite of the difficulties, the concept showed promise and was adopted for limited use in the SR-71, but it never garnered widespread acceptance. The authors have heard recently that the device was reevaluated in the Sea Harrier in Australia and was found to be potentially helpful. One potentially fruitful medium for peripheral attitude indicators might be the helmet-mounted display. A helmet-mounted display would allow for a wide projection of an artificial horizon line without it being affected by the physical restrictions of the instrument panel.

   c. Compression and expansion. These two concepts relate to the global facet of pitch presentation. It is well established that pilots interpret gross attitude more accurately and quickly with displays that present an overall global or "big-picture" view. Conversely, minute attitude changes are most accurately controlled with a small-scaled display. The two perspectives must be weighed against requirements for both spatial orientation and precision instrument flying; therefore, the following discussion addresses both of those aspects of displaying pitch.

The term compression refers to the space provided between the pitch lines. It directly affects the span of pitch that can be seen at any one time in the display's field of view. The amount of compression can range from none, which would reflect pitch angles conformal to the out-the-window scene as on a HUD (Fig. 14a), to a portrayal of all 180 deg at once (90 deg up and 90 deg down). Most of the current HDD pitch scales display either about ± 40 deg or about ± 20 deg (Fig. 14b). Possibly these normal ranges of scales have been historically selected in compromising between providing enough space for precise interpretation of a specific angle and the need to cover a range sufficient to provide a global picture. When large, 5-in.-diam attitude director indicators were commonly installed, for example, USAF century series fighter aircraft, the ± 40-deg range seemed to be the norm. Decreased sizing of the instrument seemed to bring decreased compression ranges, as well—again, most likely in an effort to provide maximum precision while retaining effective global perspective. Typical electronic flight instrumentation systems (EFIS) attitude displays tend to use the approximately ± 20-deg range (Fig. 14b).

Another argument against a 180-deg span (full compression) might be the resultant slower movement of the display, which can detrimentally mask the rapidity at which the pitch is changing. As compression increases, the movement of the attitude indicator's pitch lines necessarily decreases. Full compression can also

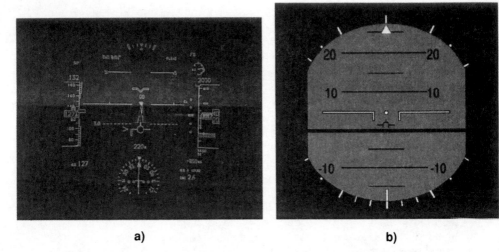

a)   b)

Fig. 14   Comparison of noncompression and compression on pitch/climb–dive-angle representations.
a) Noncompressed horizon and pitch lines on a HUD conform to the real-world scene and provide the highest level of precision. (Reproduced with permission of USAF Flight Standards Agency.)
b) Typical ± 20-deg compression on an electronic attitude director indicator (EADI) provides better global perspective from the 40-deg field of view (in pitch) vs the 18-deg range through the HUD. (Courtesy of Maj. Rick Fullmer, USAF Advanced Instrument School.)

present some drawbacks if overlaid on conformal displays, such as a forward-looking infrared (FLIR) image, in that apart from the horizon line pitch lines will not represent actual pitch angles against the real world (see Chapter 10). Nevertheless, there are no known studies that have demonstrated an advantage of either limiting or not limiting the compression of the pitch lines.

A few endeavors have been made to increase the sensitivity of the conventional ±40-deg pitch attitude scale (i.e., expanding the scale) to aid in precision flying. One attempt at a higher fidelity AI modified the pitch scale by expanding the first 5 deg of pitch over the space normally used for the 10 deg of pitch range.[63] In this case the pitch scale moved faster when in the ±5-deg window, and it provided the pilot with better sensitivity and response during instrument approaches. The remainder of the scale incorporated normal (±40 deg) compression for increased global spatial orientation. Although improved performance during instrument-landing-system (ILS) approaches was shown with this arrangement, there is no known aircraft using the technique on the HDD.

Similar modifications aimed at simultaneously improving precision and spatial orientation have been explored with HUDs and might find utility in the head-down environment. Some of these ideas, which will be discussed further in Chapter 10, include using a variable compression ratio that increases as pitch magnitude increases and variable gearing, which slows down the scale movement as the pitch-change onset rate increases.[64] As with the expanded scale, no studies are known that have addressed the application of these concepts to HDDs.

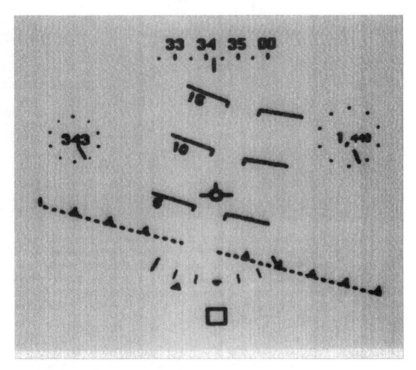

Fig. 15   Example of the ghost horizon. The dashing (ghosting) alerts the pilot that the horizon symbol is not superimposed upon the real world. When the (true) horizon line is fully in view and matches the real horizon, the horizon symbol is solid. (Courtesy of General Dynamics Advanced Information Systems.)

   d.   Ghost horizon and sliver.   Another design concept developed to aid the pilot in quickly recognizing the pitch of the aircraft was to provide a constant horizon reference when the pitch attitude exceeded the attitude indicator's field of view. Two techniques have found favor with avionics manufacturers and have been studied to various degrees. One of the techniques displays an imaginary "ghost" horizon line, and the other retains part of the pitch depiction (a small sliver of color). These two design features have been implemented to enhance the pilot's ability to accomplish unusual attitude recoveries. The ghost horizon has been shown to be effective,[65] while benefits of the "sliver" remain under investigation.
   The ghost horizon is a dashed artificial horizon line that remains in the depicted field of view of the attitude indicator when the primary horizon line departs from view (see Fig. 15). With this design the pilot is still required to read the pitch scale to determine the precise pitch angle, but it does provide a quick reference of the shortest direction toward the real horizon. This concept originated during the HUD standardization effort and is a required display element when the HUD is considered to be the PFR.[42]
   The "sliver" is similar to the ghost horizon in that it retains a small portion of the climb–dive color demarcation at the edge of the attitude indicator display when the horizon departs from the depicted field of view. The remaining color in the large

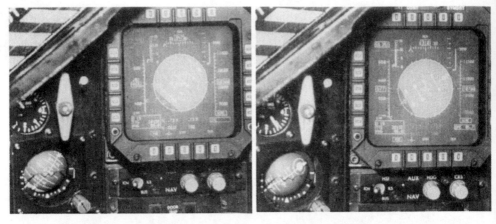

Fig. 16 Potential confusion from the sliver. This design maintains a small portion of the horizon information in the field of view, even if the proportional position of the horizon is beyond the display range. Both figures depict a bank of roughly 130 deg, but the figure on the left depicts a dive of about 25 deg, whereas the figure on the right depicts a dive of more than 70 deg. Actual dive angles can be seen with the smaller AI in the lower left of each photo. (Courtesy of Col. Lex Brown, USAF School Of Aerospace Medicine, Brooks City-Base, Texas.)

part of the display gives the impression of climbing (if blue) or diving (if black or brown) and provides an immediate reference toward the horizon. This feature has produced mixed results. Although the method seems to help in gross recognition, it might not inform the pilot as to the extent of pitch beyond the displayed amount; instead, it can lead the pilot to think the pitch angle is not as great as is actually depicted by the pitch ladder (see Fig. 16).

 e. Aircraft reference. The aircraft symbol (sometimes referred to as the miniature aircraft symbol) is central to interpreting the AI, but it is hardly standardized. It has taken on several different shapes from the conventional W to various angled bars to the "wedge" on the Collins attitude director indicator (ADI). Each has its own positive and negative characteristics, most of which were determined by physical and mechanical limitations of the instrument.

As noted earlier, the way a pilot reads the AI to determine the precise pitch angle is to reference the aircraft symbol in the center of the display against the horizontal lines of the attitude-indicator's pitch scale. Similarly, one of the quick methods of determining bank is to interpret the vertical alignment of the pitch lines relative to the aircraft reference. In both applications the effectiveness of these aspects of the pitch-and-bank displays in enabling precision flying and spatial orientation is dependent upon the interaction of their elements with the aircraft reference symbol. It follows that this symbol should be meticulously designed.

In one study Ercoline and DeVilbiss[66] compared the traditional W shape of the aircraft reference with an opened step configuration (see Fig. 17). This design technique cleared the middle of the symbol, thereby allowing the pilot to see the pitch scale's horizon-pointing attributes. The step design improved the subject pilots' abilities to recognize and recover from unusual attitudes and is indicative

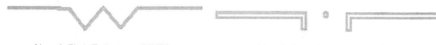

Aircraft Pitch Reference (HUD)   Aircraft Pitch Reference (HDD)

Fig. 17 Two miniature aircraft symbols commonly used for the attitude indicator pitch reference. The term "miniature aircraft symbol" has been used to identify any of the symbologies used to depict the aircraft pitch angle and is often termed the pitch reference symbol.

of how seemingly subtle alterations can produce profound improvements. The aircraft reference symbol has undergone precious little other study to optimize it with regards to countering SD.

f. Longitudinal acceleration cue and speed worm. The longitudinal acceleration symbol (LAC) and speed worm are products of HUD symbology development and depict energy available and airspeed error. As with many other HUD symbols, they hold promise for improving HDDs by increasing cross-check efficiency. The symbols are included within the attitude-indicator display and are usually found to the left side of the aircraft reference. In addition to reducing overall workload, especially during critical maneuvers such as approach and landing, they help the pilot control stick inputs when encountering unexpected windshear or turbulence. These design features have shown favorable results during HUD flight tests[67] and are being considered in new aircraft development and modifications, such as for the F-22 and T-38C.

The LAC, also termed the acceleration caret, denotes the potential energy available at any given time and represents the capability of the aircraft to change its energy state, that is, gain or lose airspeed or gain or lose altitude. This symbol moves relative to the aircraft reference and displaces upward for acceleration and downward when the aircraft is decelerating. Its index of steady-state flight (neither acceleration nor deceleration) is the wing tip of the miniature aircraft symbol.

The speed worm is a direct reflection of the difference between current and commanded (sometimes called "sct" or "bugged") airspeeds. Its desired-state index is also the wing tip of the aircraft reference symbol, and the worm "grows" out of the wing tip to roughly indicate the magnitude of the error. The worm extends above the wing tip to indicate a fast condition and below to portray being slower than commanded speed. The speed worm can be mechanized to indicate AoA relative to on speed for a given aircraft configuration or maneuver. However, if done so, caution is advised to ensure that a low AoA continues to displace the worm above the aircraft symbol wing tip, which would indicate a fast or above optimum speed condition.

Together, the LAC and speed worm display the total energy state of the aircraft. Altering the power or changing aircraft attitude moves the speed worm and the LAC in tandem and in directly proportional amounts (Fig. 18). For example, if the speed worm symbol is 0.25 in. (6.35 mm) below the wing tip—a representation of being slower than commanded speed—then placing the LAC 0.25 in. above the wing tip (by adding power or reducing pitch) will bring the aircraft up to the commanded speed and the desired velocity.

Sometimes alternative symbology is used in lieu of the LAC and speed worm. In addition to the different mechanizations of the speed worm, it is not uncommon

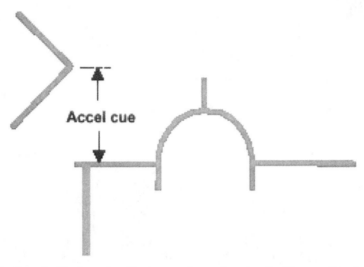

Fig. 18 Longitudinal acceleration cue and speed worm. In this case the aircraft is below commanded speed (worm below the wing), but accelerating (accelerating symbol above the wing tip). Because the displacement distance of the acceleration cue is the same as the length of the speed worm, current pitch and power settings will eventually result in neutral acceleration. The symbols can also be used to indicate the relative state of desired angle of attack (AOA). In that case, the worm would indicate deviation from reference AOA.

to find it replaced altogether by an AoA error bracket symbol. The AoA bracket is similarly presented in relation to the aircraft reference symbol.

With the increased efficiency of the cross-check that has stemmed from use of the longitudinal acceleration cue and speed worm (or AoA error bracket) on HUDs, it is reasonable to expect these concepts to eventually be widely incorporated into HDDs, as well. The correlated elements essentially reduce the several aspects of the control performance concept of flight to manipulating only two or three symbols— aircraft reference and AoA error bracket, or aircraft reference, LAC, and speed worm—all located within only millimeters of each other. Additionally, because the response of these symbols is normally quite rapid, pilots sometimes tend to make flight control and power inputs by moving *them* instead of the tachometers and/or attitude symbology. Such use of multifactorial elements of a display further confounds the distinction between classic control and performance instrumentation—a blending that is becoming more prevalent as technology advances.

    g. Flight-path vector and climb–dive marker. The flight-path vector (FPV) symbol is another carryover from the HUD (see Fig. 19). It is discussed in more detail in Chapter 10; however, its function and application to the HDD is quite relevant to this chapter. The FPV represents the aircraft's actual flight path vector, that is, the direction the aircraft is moving in three-dimensional space. It is important to realize that where the aircraft is pointed (both vertically and horizontally) and where it is actually going can be completely different (see Chapter 1). For example, the aircraft might be in a 5-deg nose-up attitude and still be descending on a 3-deg glide path. Displaying the aircraft's descent on that 3-deg dive angle

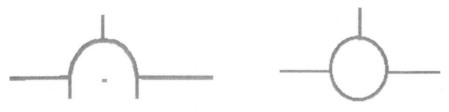

Climb Dive Marker   Flight Path Marker/Velocity Vector

Fig. 19   Flight-path vector symbology. The climb–dive marker (CDM) indicates the vertical component of the aircraft velocity vector and is limited to vertical motion only on the display. The flight-path marker (FPV) is sometimes called the velocity vector and represents the direction of the total velocity of the aircraft. It moves vertically and horizontally on the display. Neither of these symbols represents aircraft pitch.

directly on the AI reduces the pilot's workload by eliminating his or her need to calculate the resultant angle by using a combination of pitch attitude, vertical-velocity, and ground-speed information. If the pilot has a need to know the angle of descent and the FPV is not present, such calculation is required. Consequently, when establishing and maintaining an instrument or visual glide path the flight-path vector is especially useful in determining whether or not the aircraft is on the proper descent path. Not only is it easier, but also it is more accurate to set and maintain the precise, required descent angle with the FPV than to approximate it with pitch attitude constantly adjusted for changing groundspeed.

The FPV is another example of the blurring between control and performance instruments brought about by newer technology. It can serve as a control instrument in establishing a desired flight path (as long as the aircraft is not in a flight regime where power required exceeds power available), but it can also act as a performance instrument. For example, it provides an intuitive display of altitude change (climb or descent) and saves the pilot from having to look at the vertical velocity indicator, unless an exact rate of change is needed. In the horizontal plane the FPV can be used for alerting the pilot of lateral movement without his or her having to look at a yaw indicator or geographic orientation display. In one such use lateral displacement of the symbol gives immediate indication of the direction and gross magnitude of a crosswind.

Whereas display of the lateral component is especially useful on the HUD, on HDDs the FPV symbol typically presents only the vertical component of the flight-path vector, so as to maintain constant reference to the pitch ladder. (In a laterally limited mechanization the FPV is more appropriately termed the climb/dive marker, but for simplicity will not be referred to as such here.) A fully functioning FPV, utilizing the lateral component, becomes much more important if climb/dive information is presented on a sensor or virtual display of the outside scene. In that case the value of pitch-ladder referencing must then be weighed.

The benefit of the FPV to precision flying is obvious, but its significance in countering SD is not as clear. No research was found that proves a distinct advantage from incorporating the symbol on the HDD attitude indicator. However, it does satisfy Fitts' principles of quick perception, precision, completeness, and simplicity. Its use on the HUD is critical to both precision flying and spatial orientation by easing the pilot's workload. That advantage is possibly transferred to HDDs, as well, but more study is needed to confirm the benefit. Perhaps when integrated with a sensor display that replaces the traditional HDD attitude indicator, the FPV symbol will be found to have more direct use for maintaining spatial orientation.

B. Airspeed and Altitude

Unlike attitude, airspeed and altitude are only accurately depicted when looking at the displays (see Chapter 7). Most would agree that obtaining awareness of these two components of spatial orientation requires the use of an instrument display. They are grouped together in this section for several reasons—they are, as previously established, the two most critical performance instruments; they are scanned about the same amount of time during the instrument crosscheck,[34] and they are generally studied together when evaluating displays to counter SD.

Although no research was found to support the idea that the airspeed indicator and altimeter should look alike and behave in the same way, both of these displays are often found matched in format and function on the newer MFDs (see Fig. 20). Although this design likeness seems to oppose Fitts' fifth principle that states that different displays and controls should be easily distinguishable, it is possible that physical separation and conventional location on the instrument panel might sufficiently distinguish the two displays. In addition, continuity of design can actually lead to a decreased cognitive workload that could otherwise increase from assimilating different formats. However, this want for visual balance must be blended with the displays' movement attributes. Maybe the balanced approach is as good as any, but it does cause one to wonder if some kind of mixture of formats, or a completely new design for either or both parameters, might prove superior. Little work has been done to determine a preferred motif.

1. Movement

The movement dynamics of the airspeed indicator and altimeter are not nearly as controversial as with the AI. The authors speculate this contentment is because of the familiarity of these rather conventional displays. Most pilots are generally acquainted with knobs and dials and are adept at interpreting gauges in other walks of life. However, there are some axioms of mechanizing moving indicators that should be considered when developing airspeed and altitude presentations. Sanders and McCormick[4] discuss such movement in their text. A few of their pertinent concepts are listed here:

1) A pointer moving against a fixed scale is generally preferred.
2) If numerical increase is typically related to some other natural interpretation (e.g., up or down), it is easier to interpret a thermometer scale with a moving pointer.
3) Do not normally mix types of pointer-scale (moving-element) indicators when they are used for related functions—to avoid reversal errors.
4) If manual control over the moving element is expected, there is less ambiguity between the motion of the control and the display if the control moves the pointer rather than the scale.

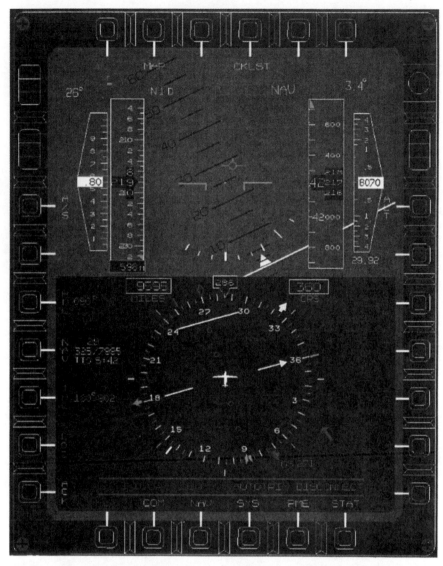

Fig. 20 Typical MFD integrating many of the traditional flight instruments onto one display surface. The display can take advantage of color, size, and density of information. Note that the airspeed tape (second from the outside on the left) is similar in form and function to the altitude tape (second from the outside on the right). (Courtesy of Gateway and Kaiser Electronics.)

5) If slight, variable movements or changes in quantity are important to the observer, these will be more apparent if a moving pointer is used.

With few exceptions, such as purely digital or numerical displays, the display format of airspeed and altitude movement has come down to two designs—circular (fixed scale with moving pointer) and vertical (moving scale with fixed pointer). The driving factor in selecting one or the other seems to be economy of space on the instrument panel and on the display itself. There are several versions of both designs that incorporate combinations of numerical readouts (counters), no counters, moving and fixed scales, and moving and fixed pointers. Regardless of the arrangement, iterations are generally classified as either counterpointer (informally termed round dial) or vertical tape.

The counterpointer format is a fixed circular scale with a moving distal pointer, and the vertical tape is a moving, vertical linear scale with a fixed pointer. In the case of the latter design, the exact quantity is usually digitally displayed in a small window within the confines of the fixed pointer. The same design technique is often used in the circular format, with the precise value digitally displayed in the center of the circular scale. The counterpointer format is shown as an altimeter in Fig. 21. Associating this design concept with the control element of the aircraft,

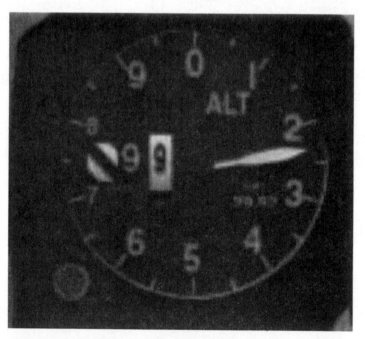

Fig. 21   Counterpointer altimeter. This altimeter illustrates the concept of clockwise and counterclockwise movement to indicate increasing and decreasing values, respectively, using a moving pointer with a fixed scale. Some counterpointer altimeters use multiple pointers. The digital value is displayed in the window to the left of center. (Courtesy of General Dynamics Advanced Information Systems.)

the movement of the altimeter pointer would correspond to the movement of the stick or yoke (e.g., stick comes back, altimeter displays an increasing value).

Although airspeed and altitude displays can be of the same basic design (circular or vertical), their scaling might or might not be the same. The objective for both, as with the AI, is to present as much range as possible to provide an overall, global view that will intuitively provide trend information while preserving enough fidelity for precision maneuvers. The physical space of the aircraft cockpit often determines how much scale can be displayed. The display of altitude requires a much greater range of motion than does airspeed. The typical displayed range of airspeed is from 0 to 1000 units, and the range of altitude is from 0 to 100,000 units. Because of the significantly smaller scale for airspeed, its indicator is often designed in a logarithmic format that includes the entire range of the scale as a means of achieving both the global view and precision interpretation. Accomplishing these dual purposes is more difficult for the altimeter because of its required greater range. In the mechanical vertical tape format, adding a second vertical-tape column increases the range, whereas in the circular scale design it is sometimes accomplished by adding multiple pointers of different shapes. As long as clutter is not a major concern, these additional symbols pose no problem. However, when they are superimposed over sensor, real, or virtual images, the degree of clutter must be taken into account.

It is conventional with vertical tapes for the altitude scale numbers to be oriented in ascending order, but for airspeed formats the scale has been found in either an ascending or descending arrangement—something that at first seems confusing, but persuasive human factors rationale exists for both methods. One philosophy is to have both scales move in the same direction in response to a pitch change. To envision this movement, one must first appreciate that in most flight maneuvers that require the stick to be pulled back, and no power added, altitude simultaneously increases as airspeed decreases. In such a maneuver, an opposites scale format (altitude in ascending order and airspeed descending) results in both scales moving downward in the display field of view to present a larger number for altitude and a smaller number for airspeed. Caution must be exercised, however, as in certain other maneuvers, such as an accelerating climb (takeoff) or decelerating descent (ILS glideslope, while slowing to final approach speed), the scales can actually move in opposite directions.

The other philosophy, of arranging both airspeed and altitude scales in ascending order, centers on the convention of placing larger numbers at the top of vertically oriented percepts, such as with floors in a building, and as suggested by McCormick.[68] Also, a benefit has been suggested in correlating movement of the throttle with the direction toward the desired airspeed value. For example, pushing the throttle forward, or up, would increase airspeed up, or toward the top of, the scale. However, the gain in intuition for locating the target value or determining appropriate throttle movement might be negated by the perception of the tape itself moving downward and contrary to the expected shift.

Another objection to the dual-ascending scheme lies in the potential for it to contribute directly to a visual illusion. If both scales are oriented in ascending order, a perception can occur of the tapes moving in opposite directions during the change in attitude described earlier. In that scenario, while holding a constant power setting, the airspeed tape will move upward, and the altitude tape will move downward.

That opposite motion of the two tapes has been hypothesized to elicit a roll-vection illusion and to, thus, be disorienting.[69] No studies were found to support one scheme of ordering vertical scales over the other, and both methods have been fielded on HUDs and HDDs. It is obvious an optimal solution is not trivial.

With scaling and movement issues being quite different for airspeed and altitude displays, one might reasonably question why it is so prevalent for their designs to be essentially identical. Notwithstanding the cognitive workload factor suggested earlier, the authors theorize that the matching style is based more on aesthetics than performance. The available research reveals that each of the two basic types of airspeed and altitude displays (circular and vertical) has its own positive and negative traits and that some attributes are specific to the medium used. Roscoe[70] studied the effects of a vertical scale, a circular scale, separated counters, and separated circular scales on command altitude, predicted altitude (1 min out), and current altitude. All displays were mechanical indicators. The study showed fewer errors and less interpretation time using the vertical scale. However, a more recent study suggested the use of a counterpointer design as an improvement over a HUD-like vertical tape scale.[71] The HUD-like vertical scale was not the same vertical scale as the one studied by Roscoe. That HUD version was an electrooptical image, used as a HUD display of airspeed and altitude, and did not include predicted and command altitude. It also displayed a smaller range of altitude than was available on the mechanical tape of the Roscoe study. As a matter of interest, it was one expert's opinion that vertical scales were adopted head up (and later carried head down to electrooptical media) because of their acceptance on HDD mechanical tapes (Lovering, personal communication, 1990). He warned that optimal performance while using tapes might not occur on the HUD medium because of the different characteristics of the displays; however, their use continues essentially unabated, especially in commercial HUDs and is a standard feature on commercial HDD EFIS. There are no known studies comparing EFIS vertical tapes to EFIS counterpointers.

As technology has improved in recent years to provide more space on head-down electrooptical displays, the capability to incorporate counterpointers on those media has correspondingly increased. With one of the primary concerns of transferring counterpointers to electrooptical HDDs now being removed, it leaves cause to consider an important attribute of the counterpointer that was identified by Hall et al.[64] During these researchers' work at Royal Aircraft Establishment, Bedford, United Kingdom, to establish an improved HUD format (see Chapter 10, Sec. III.A) they received comments by subject pilots that overwhelmingly supported counterpointers. These pilots considered the counterpointers as being not only a less-cluttered design, but also a powerful contributor to spatial orientation.

The subjects suggested that the rotating movement of the pointer was more readily noticed in the peripheral vision and was more easily interpreted as to the direction and gross rate of the parameter's change than the movement of vertical tapes (and certainly more salient and intuitive than changing digits in a numerical display). Presumably, the winding motion of the pointer in a familiar clockwise/counterclockwise fashion simplified its understanding. The apparently lower-level, cognitive deduction process seemed to provide a nearly constant, rapid, intuitive means of discerning changes in aircraft attitude and performance in all conditions, but especially during aggressive maneuvering. Changes in attitude could actually be deduced from counterpointer motion noticed in the peripheral visual field.

In his role as a member of the USAF Instrument Flight Center (IFC) instrumentation standardization team, one of this chapter's authors (Richard Evans) experienced an in-flight demonstration in the trial simulator and aircraft and concurred with the subject pilots' assessments. The total of these subjective data formed the basis for the IFC team's suggesting counterpointers for the standard USAF HUD. After validation from objective results of several other studies,[41, 71–73] the counterpointer format was included in MIL-STD 1787 as the preferred method of presenting airspeed and altitude (Hughes, personal communication, 2002).

A final point must be made regarding formatting of airspeed and altitude displays. In addition to the circular-vertical comparisons, it has been shown that the fixed scale with moving pointer type of display has been particularly useful when the information is continually changing, such as with altitude.[4] It follows that in certain scenarios this finding could apply to airspeed, as well, and is doubly relevant when considering small-spectrum presentations, such as those of airspeed on a single-turn indicator and radar altitude.

All the just-cited studies illustrate that, as with any display, determining the most efficient design for airspeed and altitude must take into account the specific flight task to be accomplished, as well as the general type of display medium to be used.

2. Color

There have been many studies showing the benefits of the use of color for information displays.[3, 74] However, with the exception of color being used to alert the pilot of preset airspeed and altitude values or recommended airspeed ranges, there is limited use of color in any of the current altimeters and airspeed indicators. One might presume that because color has been shown to improve performance in attitude awareness its use in airspeed indicators and altimeters might prove beneficial as well.

3. Location

Over time, the location of airspeed and altitude information appears to be pretty much standard (Fitts' 12th design principle)—airspeed on the left side of the AI and altitude on the right. Along with the attitude indicator the airspeed and altitude media are located directly in front of the pilot and define the top portion of the T instrument cross-check described earlier. Although the standard T arrangement has become convention over the years, it might also be justified by the natural distribution of visual attention.[75] That prioritization of attending first to stimuli immediately in front of oneself, followed by those upward and to the left of the visual field, then by those upward and to the right, melds perfectly with the generally accepted priority of attending to attitude, airspeed, and altitude in maintaining spatial orientation. The authors are aware of only one exception to this conventional arrangement, which is found in the RAH-66 Comanche helicopter. In that aircraft airspeed is placed on the right and altitude on the left of the AI. Thus far, no performance issues have surfaced with this exception. However, in order to preclude transfer of training problems, caution should be exercised in using inconsistent arrangements across aircraft.

4. Additional Symbology Modifications

A few additional symbology modifications have been applied to the airspeed indicator and altimeter over the years, but not nearly as many as with the AI. A few of these design alterations will be discussed in this section. One idea that will not be discussed in depth, but deserves mention is the implementation of numberless symbology for the displays of airspeed and altitude.[76–78] Since the proposal of this idea almost 20 years ago, it has never been implemented, most likely because of its dramatic departure from convention. Because of its extreme novelty, it seems unlikely that the concept will be used in aircraft cockpits in the foreseeable future.

5. Rate of Change in Altitude (Vertical Velocity/Speed)

The rate of change in altitude, termed vertical velocity or vertical speed, has long been an important piece of information for instrument flight and spatial orientation (see Sec. II.B.2.c). Until recently, vertical velocity/speed has always been presented on a separate, large, circular, display; however, the advent of multifunction, single PFR displays has encouraged designers to integrate vertical speed with the altimeter. This grouping approach follows Fitts' sixth design principle that encourages the clustering of similar kinds of information. Several approaches have been taken to provide the most efficient arrangement. The challenge has been to properly weigh the benefits and losses from changing the format and size of the traditional vertical-velocity indicator.

One design feature aimed at reducing clutter eliminates the display altogether and incorporates the digital-readout altimeter in presenting vertical velocity through the pilot's observing the rate of change of the numbers. Although no research is known that supports this position, anecdotal comments from pilots suggest this concept might be acceptable, especially for certain phases of flight. Others have expressed concern that this method does not command the pilot's attention quickly enough and it is ineffective for establishing a precise value during instrument maneuvers. Once again, as with the various attitude display movement concepts and airspeed and altitude formats, the quandary has surfaced over how to present enough global information from which to derive a trend, while also supporting precision flying.

The amount of precision displayed on the VVI has varied over the years, with no clear recommendation specifying an optimal amount. The most common VVI scales on the traditional round dial display a range of 0 to 6000 ft per minute (Fig. 6). A vertical speed beyond this limit places the needle (pointer) at the top or bottom of the scale, where the pilot can no longer extract the exact rate of climb or descent. Fortunately, or unfortunately (depending on the nature of the magnitude), for most aircraft the pilot has little need to know how much the rate exceeds 6000 ft per minute. Within the first 1000 ft per minute range, the scale typically is graduated to reflect 100 ft per minute increments for the sake of precision, but this scaling can vary depending upon the performance of the aircraft.

Along with the analog pointer and scale, some electrooptical displays provide a digital readout of vertical velocity, which depicts the actual rate at all times. In

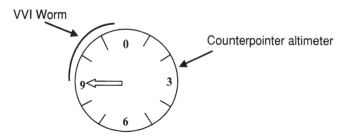

Fig. 22 Illustration of the VVI worm, showing vertical speed changes referenced to the counterpointer altimeter scale. The arc of the worm grows out of the nine o'clock position in a corresponding direction to the movement of the altimeter pointer (clockwise = climb) and approximates the magnitude of the vertical speed by reference to a value assigned to the altimeter tic marks.

an effort to reduce clutter, some of those designs present digital readout alone. These numerical counters offer ultimate precision and are unrestricted as to the maximum rate that can be displayed; however, without the analog element they are difficult formats with which to interpret trend. Consequently, for certain maneuvers a combination of an analog presentation and a digital readout might be best. At other times the mere representation of a climb or a descent by a pictorial portrayal might be sufficient to alert the pilot of an unwanted aircraft condition or to simply confirm an acceptable, general rate of change. A pictorial presentation might also adequately support the objective to reduce clutter.

One method that successfully combines these scaling and graphic attributes on electronic displays is the use of an expanding and contracting arc, sometimes called "the worm" (not to be confused with the speed worm). The worm VVI grows around the perimeter of the counterpointer altimeter and changes length based upon the magnitude of the climb or descent.[3] It is referenced to the altimeter scale markings to indicate magnitude of vertical velocity. This design feature (see Fig. 22) was developed to provide intuitive trend information and reduce clutter in spite of the symbology being in close proximity to the altitude information. It has shown improved performance and is accepted as the standard display of vertical speed on the MIL-STD HUD and it is incorporated on a few HDDs as well.

C. Integration

To this point in the chapter, each parameter of spatial-orientation information has been addressed as a separate entity. That approach is useful when describing specific attributes of displays and modification efforts, but it fails to give the full perspective needed to understand the integrated function of primary flight displays. In the dynamic and fluid environment of flight, any one spatial-orientation component can be crucial at a particular time, and each of the components takes on relevance only in conjunction with the others. Consequently, if pilots are to maintain spatial orientation, then they must obtain an integrated awareness of all spatial orientation parameters. Providing that awareness from information on instrument displays is a significant challenge for the display designer, since until relatively recently totally integrated formats have been virtually nonexistent.[79]

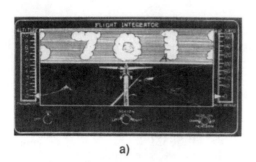

a)

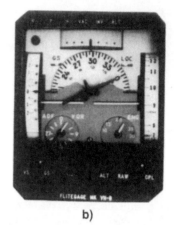

b)

Fig. 23   Early attempts to integrate flight information into one display. (Courtesy of Pam Crane.)
a) The Flight Integrator (from Ocker and Crane). Note the symbolism of clouds and terrain.
b) The FliteGage, test flown by many pilots, including one of the authors (William Ercoline), and patented by Carl Crane. The advent of computers and electro-optical displays has made this once complex mechanical integration a simple programming effort.

Actually, Ocker and Crane[9] introduced the concept of integrating spatial-orientation information in the cockpit by incorporating several of the basic flight parameters into one display, which they called the FliteGage (see Fig. 23). This apparatus presented pitch, bank, airspeed, and altitude all on one mechanical format, but for unknown reasons was never adopted for wholesale use. (Crane and his heirs maintained the patent to this design concept until 17 years after his death when it expired in 1999, but they were never able to spur enough interest to place the idea into production.) Perhaps the advent of the flight director eliminated the need for improved precision of the aircraft during approaches and landings.

The philosophy of independent displays continued until the early 1970s when the head-up display rose to prominence. [The Society of Automotive Engineers (SAE) approved standard for many years was a cluster of six separate displays that indicated airspeed, altitude, attitude, vertical speed, heading, and course guidance.] The advent of the HUD technology led to a true integration of fundamental spatial-orientation displays. At this point designers were motivated to present attitude, airspeed, and altitude information on one medium in a compact format that overlaid the outside scene. Their scheme not only met the primary objective of enabling pilots to direct their attention outside the windscreen but also had an additional beneficial effect by economizing the pilot's cross-check. Pilots appreciated having all of the crucial information readily available, immediately before their eyes, and began to use the integrated HUD information as the primary source of flight data in certain scenarios. Consequent to its great acceptance, this novel amalgamation concept was soon transferred to the head-down environment as cathode ray tubes (CRT) and flat-panel displays rapidly replaced the economically infeasible mechanical indicators.

The new technological capabilities of computer-driven media dramatically expanded the options available for providing the pilot with a holistic approach to obtaining spatial-orientation information. The major challenge became how to balance the temptation to simply duplicate conformal HUD symbology on HDDs with the obligation to provide the most effective presentation. A few problems have been mentioned that are inherent to direct replication of HUD symbology on a HDD, such as with the airspeed and altitude tapes and the conformal pitch ladder and flight-path symbol. In addition to those concerns, the effect of clutter must be taken into account. As a general rule, the less clutter the better, especially when symbology is superimposed on sensor imagery, as long as global perspective or completeness of information is not sacrificed for the sake of reducing clutter. The same dilemma occurs in weighing the importance of compatibility between head-up and head-down formats. Total compatibility is obtainable through strict duplication of the HUD symbology on the HDD (Fig. 24); however, doing so can exact too high a price by denying or degrading trend and intuitive information. It is incumbent upon the designer and the operator communities to determine the necessary degree of replication for each application. Although compatibility is extremely important to enable ease of transition and prevent negative transfer of

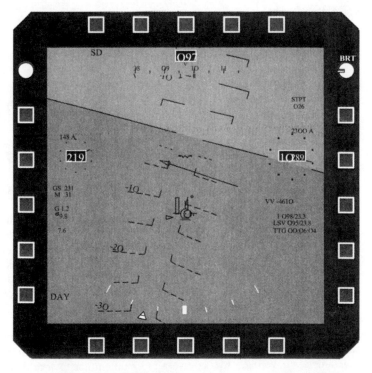

Fig. 24   An example of replicating the HUD format on an HDD medium.

training, it does not necessarily equate to duplication. As the tendency for integrating elements of SO increases, a word must be said regarding standardization. In short, it is strongly encouraged whenever possible. If information is not standardized, negative transfer of training is likely to occur—especially under high workload conditions—and pilots' time will be wasted in training programs as they unnecessarily learn new formats. Certainly it would not be practical or wise to completely standardize all cockpits—at a minimum each type aircraft's unique flight tasks would prevent such action—but it makes good sense to standardize the primary spatial orientation array.

The appeal for standardization having been made, the authors recognize and encourage development of innovative improvements that will enable the pilot to be constantly spatially oriented—mainly because there remains too many SD-related accidents. Improvements must be made. At some point, perhaps once we solve the SD problem, steps toward an improved standard will be taken. However, for the time being the frontier of totally integrated displays is replete with opportunities to build a better standard, especially in the area of combining SO and mission information. Following are some of the more noted integration concepts that arrange all of the spatial-orientation parameters on one display in conjunction with geographic (navigation) and tactical awareness information.

1.   Global Displays

The term global has been used before to denote an overall perspective when discussing specific flight parameters. In this section the term is used to designate a type of integrated display. In general, these displays incorporate all spatial, geographic, and tactical information in a pictorial representation (see Fig. 25). The concept requires either a large, single, MFD or a tight, seamless grouping of MFDs that appear as one. Global displays have shown improved performance in tasks associated with situation awareness and tracking.[80,81] As technology continues to advance, cockpits might eventually contain one large, continuous, graphical display surface for all instrument information.

2.   Highway in the Sky

This concept (also known as pathway in the sky) has been researched for several years and shown to benefit the pilot's primary spatial orientation.[82] This concept is similar to a flight director system in providing lateral course and climb and descent path guidance for a desired three-dimensional track. [The authors recommend reviewing "Display Technology (1990)"[3] for a more detailed explanation of command steering displays.] The highway in the sky (HITS) is different from a flight director in that it uses a symbolic path or roadway to represent the desired vertical and horizontal trajectory relative to the Earth's surface as opposed to command steering bars or a single command steering cue. It appears more like the real world than current flight director systems and has received many subjective accolades from novice and experienced pilots alike.[81] The primary shortfall of HITS is its difficulty in guiding the pilot back to centerline once the relatively restrictive parameters have been exceeded—a problem similar to what is experienced with the flight director when it reaches its limits of operation. This problem

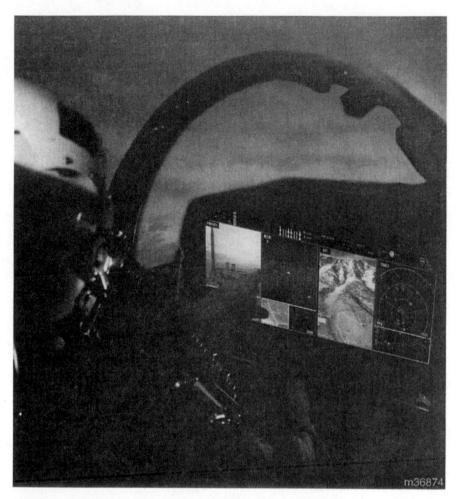

Fig. 25   Global display. Information of the many traditional head-down displays is integrated into only a few. As efficiency and effectiveness of tactical and other situation awareness displays is increased, designers and pilots hope this integration results in a more complete and intuitive depiction of the aircraft's spatial orientation as well. (Courtesy of Gateway and Kaiser Electronics.)

can be solved with a type of director arrow pointing to the correct path. The HITS concept is being studied as a potential PFR for future general aviation aircraft.[2] It is also being analyzed for use on the HUD,[83] as well as for HDDs during ground taxiing. An example of the HITS is shown in Fig. 26.

3.   Novel Flight Instrument Display

Another interesting display concept was designed and developed by the British researchers Braithwaite and Durnford while they were stationed on exchange duty at the U.S. Army Aeromedical Research Laboratory in Ft. Rucker, Alabama.[77]

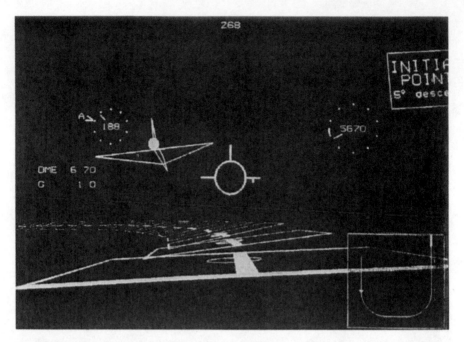

Fig. 26 Highway in the sky (HITS) display. HITS is a digitized version of an imaginary airplane as it flies through the virtual world of a highway. This example incorporates counterpointer display of airspeed and altitude. The concept has recently shown promise for high-workload, special operations military missions. (Courtesy of Dr. Mike Snow, USAF Research Laboratory, Wright-Patterson Air Force Base, Ohio.)

This display, which they termed the Novel Flight Instrument Display, presents the primary spatial orientation components in a comprehensive, purely symbolic (nonpictorial) format and integrates attitude, altitude, airspeed, heading, and vertical speed. The pilot has the option of selecting specific limits for each spatial orientation element and then performs a tracking task to maintain desired flight parameters (see Fig. 27). The presentation also allows the pilot to recognize and recover from an unusual attitude. Flight performance with this display has indicated a reduction in pilot workload.

4. OZ

The OZ display[78] is the latest and most intuitive integrated design found by the authors. The display breaks from tradition in virtually eliminating all alphanumeric characters and scales (except for heading) and replaces them with discrete symbols, colors, and shapes. The information is distributed throughout the entire display screen and contains a much larger compressed, visual field. The pilot does not need to cross-check any of the other flight instruments in order to maintain precise aircraft control (and does not have to turn his/her head to see out the side). Power symbology is provided implicit with the other control, performance, and navigation symbology (see Fig. 28). Still and Temme[78] report that novice pilots quickly grasp

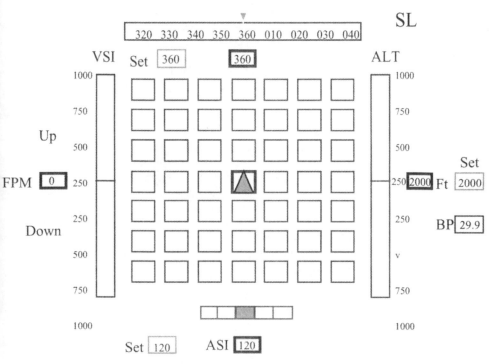

Fig. 27 Novel Flight Instrument Display. Primary spatial orientation components are presented in a comprehensive, purely symbolic (nonpictorial) format. (Courtesy of Braithwaite and Durnford; see Ref. 77 to fully appreciate the symbology and design philosophy used in this device.)

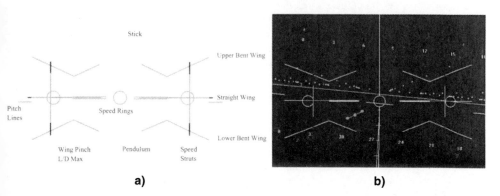

Fig. 28 OZ display: a) aircraft metaphor explained; b) computer screen shot of all symbology. (See Ref. 78 to fully appreciate the design and detail of the symbology, especially color attributes; illustrations courtesy of Drs. David Still and Leonard Temme.)

the meaning of the unique symbology and can maintain a safe level of spatial-orientation and navigation parameters with very little training. Most impressively, novice and experienced subject pilots performed exceptionally better with OZ during multiple tasking and adverse flight conditions than with a traditional display. Several of Fitts' design principles are implemented into the strategy of this futuristic display.

D. Performance Measurement

To ensure the efficacy of any improvement to SO displays while continuing to preserve the valuable lessons of the past, a new design should always produce an improvement in performance. There are several subjective means of measuring a pilot's performance using primary flight displays, and several of these have been optimized for specific flight tasks.[84] The reader is highly encouraged to appropriately apply those methods, but no further discussion of them will be included here. Accordingly, the focus of this section will be on three popular objective measures. These metrics were developed during the USAF HUD standardization effort in order to evaluate flight performance directly related to the pilot's spatial orientation (see Appendix C of this chapter). They include an unusual attitude recovery task, precision instrument control task, and an instrument landing system approach. The metrics have been used to compare HUD and HDD symbology and are easily used for evaluating any HDD.[73]

1. Unusual Attitude Recognition and Recovery Task

An UA is defined as any aircraft attitude that the pilot has not intentionally set or expected. By this definition the entrance into a UA necessarily occurs with Type I (unrecognized) SD. Encountering a UA can lead to a situation ranging from merely annoying to deadly, depending upon the setting in which it occurs (VMC, IMC, day, night, clear, weather, formation, low altitude, etc). Because of the potential for catastrophe to occur as a result of the pilot's encountering a UA, the designer must ensure that every primary flight reference enables adequate performance in the face of any unusual attitude. Fortunately, there are some performance standards available with which to assess that capability.

MIL-STD-1787C, in its specifications for a PFR, addresses the capacity of a display to inform the pilot of the aircraft's orientation and to afford him or her the ability to effectively correct an undesirable attitude. Specifically, it first requires the PFR to provide sufficient cues to enable the pilot to maintain full-time attitude awareness and minimize potential for spatial disorientation. The standard then mandates that all PFRs provide an immediately discernable attitude recognition capability that fosters a safe and effective unusual attitude recovery. In addition, acceptable performance of the display is defined as supporting the initiation of recovery from unusual attitudes within 1 s and producing a minimum correct response rate of 95% (Ref. 42, para. 4.1.1.1). Evaluating recognition of and recovery from an unusual attitude has been a method employed many times when studying the effectiveness of a spatial-orientation display.[83]

The first step is to gain awareness that an unusual attitude condition exists. This action is traditionally accomplished by interpreting a source of pitch and bank, such as the primary or secondary attitude indicators, to determine that the attitude is different than expected. Performance instruments like the airspeed indicator and altimeter should also be used to verify the situation and help rule out instrument malfunction. With flight-path-oriented displays the airspeed indicator and altimeter must always be referenced to properly respond to the attitude condition. If outside visual cues are available, they should be used as well. Regardless of how the unusual attitude is recognized, the condition should be confirmed before beginning the recovery procedure. The easier it is to recognize the spatial-orientation parameters, the sooner the pilot can commence the recovery procedure. If not done soon enough, or if the attitude is incorrectly interpreted, the resulting recovery maneuver could lead to an excessive loss of altitude at best, or a controlled flight into the terrain at worst.

The second step is to perform the recovery. The purpose of all unusual attitude recoveries is to return the aircraft to a known spatial orientation (ideally, wings level with a slight climb) with minimum loss of altitude. For purposes of measurement, this ideal attitude is often established to be ±10-deg pitch and ±5-deg bank, both held for 3 to 5 s. The recovery procedure varies depending upon whether the aircraft is in a dive or a climb. If diving, the pilot rolls to a wings level, upright attitude, and then corrects to level flight while adjusting power (and, possibly, drag devices) as deemed necessary. The pilot should not add backpressure on the stick until achieving less than 90 deg of bank. If backpressure is applied too soon, the aircraft will lose more altitude than desired.

If an UA is recognized as a climb, then the pilot is to use power as required and bank as necessary to assist pitch control and to avoid negative G forces. The vagueness in the preceding procedure implies that the pilot has multiple options. Depending upon aircraft performance capabilities, the pilot could either roll the aircraft inverted and pull the nose toward the horizon or maintain, slightly increase, or decrease toward 90 deg the present bank and allow the nose to fall toward the horizon. (The latter would be the technique for aircraft not designed for inverted flight.) As the aircraft reference symbol on the display approaches the artificial horizon, the pilot should adjust pitch, bank and power to complete the recovery and establish the desired aircraft attitude—once again, wings level with a slight climb, or for study purposes, ±10-deg pitch and ±5-deg bank held for 3 to 5 s.

The varied options for rolling the aircraft from an inverted climb condition present the researcher with a significant challenge in assessing whether or not a correct response was made to the UA. Consequently, in order to achieve standardization for recovering from all UA conditions and reduce ambiguity when evaluating the intuitiveness of a display, researchers often instruct and train subjects to always roll toward the horizon when confronted with a climb and attain inverted flight if necessary to ensure positive nose tracking toward the horizon. The authors note that it is generally considered poor practice to either achieve or continue inverted flight in IMC; however, using this single recovery technique for research purposes will aid in properly assessing roll-reversal inputs and time to recover (should the latter be considered an important parameter to measure). This technique allows collapsing of data across all UA conditions. As a means of countering subject bias against inverted maneuvering in IMC, two of the authors (Ercoline and DeVilbiss) have successfully employed the technique of training the subjects to a 70% accuracy rate before initiating trial runs. Suggested setup

Table 6   Performance metric for the unusual-attitude
recognition-and-recovery task

Maneuver	Event, deg[a]	Rating elements—each event
Unusual-attitude recognition and recovery	0 pitch 60 bank 0 pitch	Pilot initiates recovery toward correct horizon and altitude within 1 s
	135 bank +30 pitch	Minimal loss of altitude and airspeed (subjective)
	30 bank	Full time horizon reference
	−30 pitch 150 bank	Full time attitude (pitch and bank) reference
	+50 pitch 45 bank	No more than 10% errors in roll reversals
	−50 pitch −120 bank	

[a]Pitch and bank can vary with aircraft type.

parameters for the unusual attitude recognition and recovery metric are specified in Table 6.

2. Precision Instrument Control Tasks

A precision instrument control task (PICT) addresses basic aircraft control maneuvering that is common to virtually all instrument flying. It can be any basic instrument flight maneuver, but a commonly used, broadly encompassing PICT is a selected variation on the vertical S series of maneuvers. The vertical S series is used in many flying training programs to improve a pilot's instrument cross-check and control inputs and consists of four similar maneuvers labeled "alpha" (A), "bravo" (B), "charlie" (C), and "delta" (D) (Fig. 29).[86]

The baseline maneuver is the vertical S A, which is a continuous series of climbs and descents flown at a constant rate and airspeed while maintaining a constant heading. The amount of altitude change at which the vertical direction is reversed and the rate at which the maneuver is flown should be compatible with the specific aircraft involved—typically a 1000-ft (305-m) change at a 1000 ft per minute (fpm) rate. Usually the altitude reversal point is selected to be on a 1000 ft interval or 500 ft interval on the altimeter for ease of reference. The maneuver requires an efficient cross-check throughout and constantly changing control inputs during the reversals. Such maneuvering is typical of descents on final approach and climbs on a missed approach.

The other vertical S maneuvers build upon one another and become incrementally more difficult. The B adds a constant bank angle, that is, 30 deg; the C reverses the bank in the opposite direction as each descent is begun; and the D reverses the bank at each change in vertical direction. The intent is to make all transitions smooth and coordinated so as to achieve wings level and zero pitch at precisely the zenith and/or nadir of the climb/dive, respectively, while continuing without

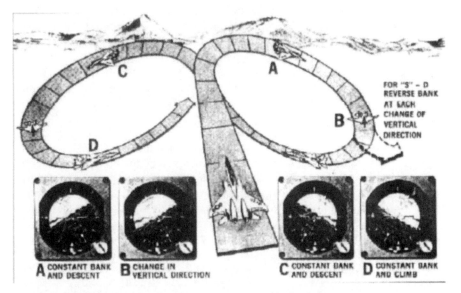

FOR "S" - D
REVERSE BANK
AT EACH
CHANGE OF
VERTICAL
DIRECTION

A CONSTANT BANK AND DESCENT   B CHANGE IN VERTICAL DIRECTION   C CONSTANT BANK AND DESCENT   D CONSTANT BANK AND CLIMB

Fig. 29   Variations of vertical SD maneuver, sometimes known as precision instrument control task. Refer to Ref. 24 for more complete description of the other three vertical S maneuvers. (Courtesy of the AF Flight Standards Agency.)

hesitation into the next attitude. Meeting this goal requires precise lead-point calculation and forces a continuous cross-check and interpretation of all parameters. The HUD standardization effort utilized a PICT consisting of vertical S A and D and analyzed the root-mean-square (RMS) error that resulted from deviations from the predetermined conditions. Some researchers have added a random perturbation function (a series of sine functions with different phases) to the task to make these routine maneuvers even more difficult.

3.   Instrument Landing System Task

The ILS approach is used to evaluate practical application of new symbology. It is a specific task performed in the final phase of flying under instrument conditions. A brief description of the navigation system, approach design, and a typical instrument display follows.

An ILS is provided at an airport to enable pilots to descend in instrument conditions along precise horizontal and vertical paths and arrive at a point from which they are able to visually acquire the runway environment and then to land. It basically consists of two separate transmitters located near the landing runway that emit radio energy of two different frequencies on opposite sides of the optimum path.[86]

One transmitter is calibrated to align with the runway centerline and the other to a normal glide path, usually at approximately 3 deg from horizontal. Standard nomenclature for the horizontal and vertical paths is localizer course (or simply localizer) and glide slope, respectively. Three other radio transmitters of single frequencies, called marker beacons, are used to highlight progress toward the runway and are placed along the localizer course. The localizer and glide-slope paths meet at the decision point, where the pilot must decide to continue the descent to landing or execute a missed approach.

Receivers on the aircraft measure frequency strength on either side of the course and glide slope. Cockpit displays interpret the relative magnitude of each and indicate deviation from center. Those displays are termed the course-deviation indicator (CDI) and glide-slope indicator (GSI). The CDI is usually placed on a horizontal navigation display that includes heading information, and the GSI normally is on the attitude indicator. Often the GSI is included on the navigation display, and sometimes CDI-like information is added to the AI. Flight directors are commonly incorporated with the AI symbology suite to command correction toward the appropriate course. In that case the AI becomes an attitude director indicator, or ADI. The directing symbols are normally vertical and horizontal lines termed bank steering and pitch steering bars, respectively, or a single wedge-shaped device toward which the aircraft symbol is flown. Sometimes single or multiple crosses or boxes (in conjunction with a flight-path vector symbol) are used in lieu of the traditional steering bars or wedges. An expanding (rising) runway symbol is also often included for precise course guidance and gross perspective of glide slope and vertical speed. Pros and cons exist for each steering bar design.

The basic challenge of an ILS approach is to keep the course deviation and glide-slope indicators centered. Sometimes an additional element is added in which the pilot must intercept the course from an oblique angle and, likewise, the glide slope from below. The pilot must then continue the approach to the decision point. The researcher can readily measure roll-and-pitch direction and amplitude during the interception, as well as deviation from course and glide slope once they are intercepted.

Thorough testing of a candidate symbol or symbology suite can be accomplished by using the unusual attitude recognition and recovery task, PICT, and ILS approach metrics. These tools adeptly evaluate utility and effectiveness of critical aircraft control and performance displays for both basic maneuvering and instrument approach environments. A flight display's usefulness during these three tasks can be reasonably interpolated to almost every instrument-flying event. In addition, it is prudent to collect subjective comments from the pilot subjects regardless of the metric used for analysis.

IV. Conclusion

This chapter establishes the foundation of the pilot's abilities to maintain SO and counter SD as a correct perception of the three flight parameters that define the meaning of SO—attitude, airspeed and altitude. An HDD PFR must provide an intuitive, efficient presentation of these parameters, and, indeed, every cockpit display should be designed with foremost consideration given to preserving that capability. Nonetheless, enabling the pilot to be aware of these three fundamental flight parameters does not necessarily eliminate the risk of SD. Even while scanning the PFR, the pilot is susceptible to experiencing Type II and Type III SD. The important concept to realize is that the proper display of fundamental spatial orientation information will lessen the likelihood of Type I SD and will enable the pilot to more effectively deal with a Type II or Type III SD event.

Great emphasis is placed on the lessons of the past. The primacy of SO information was established when the first blind sortie was flown, and the design of each instrument should be approached with the same fervor and thoughtfulness used by the display pioneers that brought that milestone about. This should not discourage endeavors to introduce unorthodox displays, but rather encourage new approaches that continue to uphold established tenets. Some examples of integrated displays are included in the discussion to illustrate how new thoughts can build upon established concepts. It is the authors' contention that even the most unorthodox design can and should hold to the basic principles established by Crane, Ocker, Doolittle, and Fitts (to name a few design pioneers). It is also important to consider the impact of new ideas like the OKCR and its potential effect on display design.

Just as fresh ideas can build upon old models, a new approach could simply be nothing more than the modified reintroduction of an old one. As the saying goes: seldom are there new ideas, only forgotten ones. Several good design features that were studied over the years and implemented, and then several others that were not implemented, were presented. Perhaps resurrecting some of these forgotten ideas, and using the improved technology now available to employ them, can breathe new life into the pursuit of preventing display-related mishaps. Or maybe a better approach would be to start from scratch and design with a better understanding of what we know of today.

Perhaps the time will come when the pilot will be less of a factor in preventing SD, and visual display design will be moot. Automation or other technology might very well solve the problem. As aircraft become more expensive and new flight regimes present increased risks from allowing the pilot to maintain constant control, there is a distinct possibility that aircraft will incorporate an artificial intelligence capable of automatically preventing controlled flight into terrain (see Chapter 11).

V. Summary

This chapter presents a basic discussion of the head-down flight instruments and flight symbology required for a pilot to maintain spatial orientation. Piloting Topics, the first major section, discusses the various displays, the way in which a pilot learns to organize the information, how the information is used to prevent spatial disorientation, and some of the terminology needed to better understand the use of the cockpit instruments. In the second major section, Design Topics, is offered a more focused approach towards the symbology design issues that enable the pilot to better interpret the information presented on the flight instruments. Basic concepts are introduced with details provided regarding the many methods of using these time-honored guidelines. The chapter also touches lightly upon some of the newer concepts that are rapidly replacing the cockpit displays almost universally found merely a generation ago. The reader is then encouraged to seek additional references for more details on the mechanization and integrated concepts already on the market and to investigate the impact of new research findings on instrument display design. Lastly, three appendices are provided to assist the reader with a deeper appreciation for terms and conditions commonly used by the flying community when applying the art of instrument flight for the prevention of SD.

Appendix A: Perceiving Horizon Position and Movement

The importance of perceiving the "correct" position and movement of the horizon from an SO display cannot be overstated. As described in Chapters 3 and 7, the horizon is the basis from which the pilot determines spatial orientation, i.e., aircraft positioning and motion relative to the Earth's surface (definition of SO Ref. 38). To adequately maintain SO, the pilot must remain constantly aware of the horizon's position, and the pilot's interpretation of that position is the foundation upon which all maneuvering is built. Correctly or incorrectly, the pilot determines fundamental aircraft positioning and motion by referencing the movement in the windscreen of whatever visual feature he or she associates with the horizon. These discernments can be equally powerful when produced from either dedicated concentration on the visual scene or from just a fleeting reference to the scene in the "corner of the eye" while attending to other tasks within the cockpit.

Visual illusions notwithstanding, the most significant problems in spatial orientation arise when horizon motion (or, more accurately, the aircraft's movement relative to the horizon) cannot be detected from an outside-the-cockpit scene and must be determined from its depiction on a display, requiring corroboration with the pilot's perception. In other words, without a visual horizon, the pilot must *decide* what the orientation of the aircraft is vs simply *sensing* its orientation from a visual horizon reference. Presenting a compelling horizon reference on an HDD with which to make a sound decision is a formidable challenge, and the success of the attempt depends upon the mental process the pilot applies in interpreting it.

While there are certainly innumerable, individual iterations of the method of mentally developing a perception of orientation—that is, there can be more than one "correct" strategy for determining SO—there can be only one "correct" presentation of the horizon on a display. That correct representation indicates the true relationship of the actual aircraft to the actual horizon. As has already been established in this text, the pilot may not perceive, or possibly accept, the accuracy of a display in replicating the real world—a misperception or reluctance attributable to his or her possessing a faulty mental image of what the display *should* indicate based upon expectancy and physiological stimuli. Therefore, in order for the pilot to attain a factual perception of horizon position and motion when the outside scene is not visible, he or she must use a spatial strategy, or mental model that takes into account conflicts between reality and the mental "image." In other words, the strategy or model must allow for correcting a flawed visualization.

Several authors have established that a mental model is developed from a pilot's training and experience. For example, a pilot learns early in his or her flying career that in a conventional aircraft, with all other variables being constant, airspeed will decrease and altitude will increase when raising the nose of the aircraft. Similarly, he or she will learn to expect the nose to "fall" after introducing a roll, as lift on the wings is lost in the bank. In the context of horizon movement in the latter example, the horizon will shift upwards in the windscreen, and the movement will become associated with the effects of rolling the aircraft. These correlations become "natural" and are inserted into the mental model. The pilot then uses the model to either produce an expected result from a given control input (confirmed by reference to the outside scene or the instrument display) or create a presumed state of orientation developed from the last perceived physiological stimulus (*hopefully*, also confirmed or corrected by reference to the instrument display).

If the pilot is distracted or experiences an illusion that masks or alters the learned, correlated factors, he or she may not insert the appropriate information into the SO model. For example, if the aircraft were rolled at a sub-threshold rate, the unnoticed, lowered pitch attitude that resulted would not be taken into account in building the mental image of present attitude. Consequently, the created mental "picture" of aircraft attitude would not match with the displayed attitude—a conflict that may prove very difficult to overcome. Overriding a false expectancy will require significant power in the display characteristics. Specifically, if the horizon reference is not sufficiently salient and intuitive, it will not overrule the expected orientation that the pilot's mental model yielded. In the case of a sub-threshold roll, the pilot's perception of being "straight and level" will be more powerful than the angled bank reference on the display. Therefore, the strength of the display is proportional to the ease with which the pilot manipulates the mental model to arrive at an acceptance of the true, correct horizon position and movement. Which model is chosen may be the determining factor as to whether or not the pilot safely controls the aircraft.

Each pilot formulates his or her own habit patterns and techniques for gaining overall spatial orientation. However, there are only two prevalent mental models with which to derive an appropriate response to displayed horizon position. These models have been termed "inside out" and "outside in." The "inside-out" approach considers the display as a window looking out toward the real world. In this model, the horizon reference will move in the display FOV in the same manner in which the real horizon would "move" in the cockpit windscreen, i.e., down as the nose is raised; up when it is lowered. On the "outside-in" display the horizon reference remains in a constant position in the display FOV, and the aircraft reference symbol moves relative to it. The perspective is as if looking at the aircraft from afar, or "outside," as the Earth remains in its stable position, and various angles of perspective from the aircraft symbol can be presented.

There is some indication that while "inside out" is the natural model for functioning in the visual scene environment, "outside in" may be more effective when no visual scene is present. This dichotomy could be attributable to the relatively less compelling visual stimulation of the horizon line on an "inside-out" display. To date, no HDD "inside-out" horizon reference extends the full width of the cockpit, as does the true horizon. The pilot must project himself or herself "into" the small FOV "window" of the "inside-out" attitude indicator and respond to the horizon reference as it moves within that restricted "window." Consequently, the position and motion of the horizon reference on a conventional, "inside-out" AI may not be nearly as strong a visual stimulant as the centrally located, moving aircraft reference symbol of the "outside-in" display. The OKCR study[36] just described in Sec. II.C of this chapter suggests this correlation to be true, because pilots had difficulty transitioning between the visual and nonvisual environments using "inside-out" attitude references. Further research is needed to validate that theory.

Based upon the potency of the OKCR and the known superior strength of influence of visual characteristics in the "natural" outside environment, the authors postulate that to be most effective, the horizon reference on an HDD should provide strong stimulation to the intrinsic, subconscious sensory systems, such as ambient vision. In the absence of such stimulation, or if it is inadequate, alerting features must be used to draw the pilot's attention to the salient characteristics of the horizon reference.

Appendix B: Visibility Definitions

1) *Visual flight rules (VFR)*: The use of this term means the aircraft is being flown under the regulatory guidance of those rules that govern flight in visual conditions. For example, in most of U.S. airspace, a pilot operating under VFR must remain 500 ft (152 m) below or 1000 ft (305 m) above and 2000 ft (610 m) horizontally away from a cloud when in controlled airspace below 10,000 ft (3050 m) MSL and must ensure the in-flight visibility is at least 3 statute miles. VFR is also used in the United States to indicate weather conditions that are equal to or greater than the minimum VFR requirements specified in federal aviation regulations (FARs). For example, one would refer to 3-mile visibility as "VFR weather" when relating to the respective operations. Notice there is no mention as to whether or not the horizon is discernible when referring to VFR. Finally, pilots and controllers use the term VFR to indicate the type of flight plan filed in the air-traffic-control (ATC) system, but that usage is not germane to this text.

2) *Visual meteorological conditions (VMC)*: The precise use of this term, per the FARs and *Aeronautical Information Manual* (AIM), relates to conditions equal to or better than minimum VFR requirements. A pilot must be operating in VMC in order to be in compliance with VFR. For example, in an airport traffic area the conditions must be at least 3 miles visibility and a 1000-ft (305-m) ceiling to enable a pilot to operate under VFR. Again, notice no mention is made of the pilot's being able to see the horizon. The preceding describes the precise, correct use of the term VMC but does not allow for pilot convention. Pilots often state they are VMC to mean they are clear of clouds, but not far enough away from them, and/or not able to see far enough ahead, to comply with VFR. Although the pilot's declaration of being VMC is not correct in those conditions, one should assume that he is at least able to incorporate some visual reference outside the aircraft—an ability that could be either helpful or detrimental depending upon the situation.

3) *Instrument flight rules (IFR)*: Here the pilot must be under the guidance of an air traffic controller and follow specific procedures specified by air regulations. Most of the time the procedures are quite restrictive as to aircraft maneuvering, but sometimes the procedures include nonspecific maneuvering freedom within general airspace or time parameters. Per FAR/AIM operating under IFR has nothing to do with visibility. The visibility could be zero or it could be clear. However, in the International Civil Aeronautical Organization (ICAO) application, IFR always refers to operating in less than VMC and, of course, still requires compliance with specific air traffic control procedures. As with the term VMC, pilots often misuse

the term IFR to mean they are in the weather. In that case, rather than stating they are IFR, they should more precisely declare they are IMC.

4) *Instrument meteorological conditions (IMC)*: These conditions are any that do not meet the minima specified for VMC. Technically, the pilot could actually be clear of cloud, see the ground and horizon, and still be in IMC, for example, distance from cloud and visibility values would be below VFR requirements (see conventional misuse of VMC just discussed). However, as just stated, if a pilot describes his state as IMC it is normally assumed that he or she is in the weather and cannot see much outside the aircraft.

Although each of these terms is important to safe and orderly flight, they can easily be a source of confusion to the display designer. Each means something specific to the pilots and might or might not be used in a technically correct manner, especially when relating to visibility. Additionally, none of the terms guarantees the presence or absence of the horizon. Because both visual contact with the Earth's surface—and especially awareness of the horizon—are critical elements in determining a pilot's spatial orientation, some practicality must be introduced into this discussion. For that reason it is suggested that the terms VMC and IMC be used when addressing a display's utility. In other words, the display designer who is considering the use of an instrument should be concerned with the visual conditions present, that is, flight visibility and the discernibleness of the horizon, not necessarily whether or not the pilot is operating under VFR or IFR.

Appendix C: Performance Standards[42]

Table C1   Basic flight performance parameters

Maneuver	Event	Rating
Takeoff/departure	Fly X radial, @ X DME turn heading X, altitude X, airspeed X	Airspeed ± 10 KIAS Altitude ± 200 ft
Navigation	Enter holding, altitude, airspeed	Heading ± 5 deg
Instrument approach	Arc from holding, partial configuration on arc, altitude (step down), airspeed Intercept final approach course (precision and non- precision), step down altitude, airspeed @ FAF, final configuration to MAP	Precision Course ± 1 dot GS ± 1 dot Airspeed ± 5 KIAS Nonprecision/radar Course ± 5o Airspeed ± KIAS Altitude ± 100 ft
Missed approach	Follow missed approach procedure, altitude, airspeed, clean configuration	Airspeed ± 10 KIAS Altitude ± 100 ft Heading ± 5 deg
Landing	Transition to land, airspeed (evaluate clutter)	Safe position to land from FAF, MAP; land visually

Table C2   Unusual attitude recognition and recovery performance
parameters

Maneuver	Event	Rating
Unusual attitude recognition and recovery	0-deg pitch[a] 60-deg bank	——
	0-deg pitch 135-deg bank	Pilot initiates recovery toward correct horizon and altitude within 1 s.
	+30-deg pitch 30-deg bank	Minimal loss of altitude and airspeed (subjective)
	−30-deg pitch 150-deg bank	Full time horizon reference
	+50-deg pitch 45-deg bank	Full time attitude (pitch and bank) reference
	−50-deg pitch −120-deg bank	No more than 10% errors in roll reversals

[a]Pitch and bank can vary with aircraft type.

Table C3   Dynamic maneuvering performance parameters

Maneuver	Event	Rating
Vertical SB	Climb: 1000 ft; 1000 fpm 30-deg bank then Descend: 1000 ft; 1000 fpm; 30-deg bank in the same direction Recover to original altitude and airspeed	Airspeed ± 10 KIAS Bank ± 5 deg
Vertical SD	Climb: 1000 ft; 1000 fpm 45-deg bank then Descend: 1000 ft; 1000 fpm; 45-deg bank in the opposite direction Recover to original altitude and airspeed	VVI ± 200 fpm (once established) Altitude ± 100 ft

References

[1]Stokes, A. F., and Wickens, C. D., "Aviation Displays," *Human Factors in Aviation*, edited by E. L. Wiener, and D. C. Nagel, Academic Press, San Diego, CA, 1988, Chap. 8.

[2]Foxworth, T. G., and Newman, R. L., "A Pilot's Look at Aircraft Instrumentation," AIAA Paper 71-787, July 1971.

[3]Stokes, A. F., Wickens, C. D., and Kite, K., "Display Technology," *Human Factors Concepts*, Society of Automotive Engineers, Inc., Warrendale, PA, 1990.

[4]Sanders, M. S., and McCormick, E. J., "Human Factors in Engineering and Design," 7th ed., McGraw–Hill, New York, 1993, p. 135.

[5]Wiener, E. L., and Nagel, D. C., *Human Factors in Aviation*, Academic Press, San Diego, CA, 1988.

[6]Gibson, J. J., *The Perception of the Visual World*, Houghton Mifflin, Boston, 1950.

[7]Pfeiffer, M. G., Clark, W. C., and Danaher, J. W., "The Pilot's Visual Task: a Study of Visual Display Requirements," U.S. Naval Training Device Center, Technical Report NAVTRADEVCEN 783-1, Port Washington, NY, 1963.

[8]O'Reilly, B., and Mackechnie, W. G., "Aerial Equilibrium and Orientation," *The Canadian Medical Monthly*, Vol. 5, No. 8, 1920, pp. 316–332.

[9]Ocker, W. C., and Crane, C. J., *Blind Flight in Theory and Practice*, Naylor, San Antonio, TX, 1932.

[10]Amalberti, R., Paries, J., Valot, C., and Wibaux, F., *Aviation Psychology: a Science and a Profession*, edited by K. Goeters, Ashgate Publishing, Limited, Brookfield, VT, 1998, pp. 19–41.

[11]Davenport, C. E., "USAF Spatial Disorientation Experience: Air Force Safety Center Statistical Review," *Proceedings of Recent Trends in Spatial Disorientation Research*, 2000.

[12]Ercoline, W. R., DeVilbiss, C. A., and Lyons, T. J., "Trends in USAF Spatial Orientation Accidents—1958–1992," *Helmret and Head-Mounted Displays and Symbology Design Requirements Conference*, edited by R. J. Lewandowski, W. Stephens, and L. A. Haworth, Society of Photo-Optical Instrumentation Engineers, Bellingham, WA, 1994.

[13]Veronneau, S. J. H., "Civilian Spatial Disorientation Mishap Experience," *Proceedings of Recent Trends in Spatial Disorientation Research*, 2000.

[14]"Definitions of Aircraft Heading and Angles," ASCC, AIRSTD 70/17, Change 3, 13 June 2001.

[15]Alkov, R. A., "The Human Factors History of Cockpit Displays," *Flying Safety*, Vol. 50, No. 9, 1994, pp. 4–8.

[16]von Wulften Palthe, P. M., "Function of the Deeper Sensibility and of the Vestibular Organs in Flying," *Acta Otolaryngologica*, Vol. 4, 1922, pp. 415–448.

[17]Doolittle, J. H., "Early Experiments in Instrument Flying," *Annual Report of the Smithsonian Institution*, The third Lester Gardner lecture, Massachusetts Inst. of Technology, Cambridge, MA, 1961, pp. 337–355.

[18]Roscoe, S. N., and Williges, R. C., "Motion Relationships in Aircraft Attitude and Guidance Displays: a Flight Experiment," *Human Factors*, Vol. 17, No. 4, 1975, pp. 374–387.

[19]Lentz, J. M., and Guedry, F. E., Jr., "Apparent Instrument Horizon Deflection During and Immediately Following Rolling Maneuvers," Naval Aerospace Medical Research Lab., NAMRL-1278, Pensacola, Florida, 1981.

[20]Roscoe, S. N., "Horizon Control Reversals and the Graveyard Spiral," *Cseriac Gateway*, Vol. 7, 1997, pp. 1–4.

[21]Perrone, J. A., "Visual Slant Misperception and the 'Black-Hole' Landing Situation," *Aviation, Space, and Environmental Medicine*, Vol. 55, 1984, pp. 1020–1025.

[22]Spady, A. A., and Harris, R. L., "How a Pilot Looks at Altitude" NASA TM 81967, 1981.

[23]Arnegard, R. J., "Operator Strategies Under Varying Conditions of Workload," NASA CR 4385, GRANT NGT-504-05, July 1991.

[24]AFM 11-217, Vol. 1, U.S. Air Force Flight Standards Agency.

[25]Dick, A. O., "Instrument Scanning and Controlling: Using Eye Movement Data To Understand Pilot Behavior and Strategies," NASA CR-3306, 1980.

[26]Barfield, W., Rosenberg, C., and Furness, T. A., "Situation Awareness as a Function of Frame of Reference, Computer-Graphics Eyepoint Elevation, and Geometric Field of View," *The International Journal of Aviation Psychology*, Vol. 5, No. 3, 1995, pp. 233–256.

[27]Wickens, C. D., *Engineering Psychology and Human Performance* 2nd ed., Harper Collins, New York, 1992.

[28]Marshak, W. P., Kuperman, G., Ramsey, E. G., and Wilson, D., "The Effect of Perspective Geometry on Judged Direction in Map Displays," *Proceedings of the Human Factors Society 31st Annual Meeting*, 1987, pp. 533–535.

[29]Ocker, W. C., and Crane, C. J., "Blind Flying and Its Teachings," *First presentation at the National Aeronautic Meeting of The American Society of Mechnical Engineers*, 1931.

[30]Sarter, N. B., and Woods, D. D., "Situation Awareness: A Critical But Ill-Defined Phenomena," *The International Journal of Aviation Psychology*, Vol. 1, 1991, pp. 45–47.

[31]Endsley, M. R., "Toward a Theory of Situation Awareness in Dynamic Systems," *Human Factors*, Vol. 37, 1995, pp. 32–64.

[32]"FAA Instrument Flyina Handbook," Federal Aviation Administration, AC 61-27C, 1 Jan. 1980.

[33]Giggin, W. C., and Rockwell, T. H., "Computer-Aided Testing of Pilot Response to Critical In-Flight Events," *Human Factors*, Vol. 26, No. 5, 1984, pp. 573–581.

[34]Wetzel, P. A., Poprik, C., and Bascom, P., "An Eye Tracking System for Analysis of Pilots' Scan Paths," *Interservice/Industry Training Systems and Education Conference Proceedings*, 1996, pp. 518–526.

[35]Bellenkes, A. H., Wickens, C. D., and Kramer, A. F., "Visual Scanning and Pilot Expertise: Their Role of Attentional Flexibility and Mental Model Development," *Aviation, Space, and Environmental Medicine*, Vol. 68, No. 7, 1997, pp. 569–579.

[36]Patterson, F., "Aviation Spatial Orientation Strategies," *Proceedings of Recent Trends in Spatial Disorientation Research*, 2000.

[37]Gillingham, K. K., "The Spatial Disorientation Problem in the United States Air Force," *Journal of Vestibular Research*, Vol. 2, 1992, pp. 297–306.

[38]Benson, A. J., "Special Senses, Work and Sleep," *Aviation Medicine, Physiology and Human Factors*, 1st ed., edited by J. Ernsting, William Clowes and Sons, Limited, London, 1978, pp. 405–467.

[39]Bryan, L. A., Stonecepher, J. W., and Aron, K., "180-Degree Turn Experiment," *University of Illinois Bulletin*, Vol. 52, No. 11, 1954.

[40]North, D. M., "A New Vision of Cockpit Displays," Editorial, *Aviation Week and Space Technology*, 8 March, 1999, p. 66.

[41]Weinstein, L. F., Gillingham, K. K., and Ercoline, W. R., "United States Air Force Head-up Display Control and Performance Symbology Evaluations," *Aviation, Space, and Environmental Medicine*, Vol. 65, 1994, pp. A20–A30.

[42]"Aircraft Display Symbology," U.S. Dept. of Defense Interface Standard, ASC/ENOI, MIL-STD-1787C, Wright-Patterson AFB, OH, 5 Jan. 2001.

[43]Boff, K. R., and Lincoln, J. E., "Engineering Data Compendium, Human Perception and Performance," Wright-Patterson Air Force Base, OH, 1988.

[44]Fitts, P. M., "Psychological Requirements in Aviation Equipment Design," *Aviation Medicine*, Vol. 17, 1947, pp. 270–275.

[45]Johnson, S. L., and Roscoe, S. N., "What Moves, the Airplane or the World?," *Human Factors*, Vol. 14, 1972, pp. 107–129.

[46]Previc, F. H., and Ercoline, W. R., "The Outside-In Attitude Display Concept Revisited," *International Journal of Aviation Psychology*, Vol. 9, 1999, pp. 377–401.

[47]Beringer, D. B., Williges, R. C., and Roscoe, S. N., "The Transition of Experienced

Pilots to a Frequency-Separated Aircraft Attitude Display," *Human Factors*, Vol. 17, 1975, pp. 401–414.

[48]Ercoline, W. R., "The Attitude Component of the Primary Flight Reference," *Proceedings of Recent Trends in Spatial Disorientation Research*, 2000.

[49]Ponomarenko, V. A., Lapa, V. V., and Lemeshchenko, N. A., "Psychological Foundation of Aircraft's Spatial Attitude Indication Design," *Psykhologicheskiy Zhurnal*, Vol. 11, 1990, pp. 37–46.

[50]Ponomarenko, V. A., "Psychophysiological Substantiation of the Mode of Piloted Aircraft's Spatial Attitude Information Presentation on a Helmet-Mounted Display in Complex Aircraft's Spatial Altitude Identification and Its Leveling," F61708-97-W0031, EOARD, London, 1998, pp. 22–36.

[51]Ponomarenko, V. A., Vorona, A. A., Gander, D. V., and Usov, V. M., "Computerized Teaching of Pilots to Spatial Orientation Flight Tasks," *AIAA Flight Simulation Technologies Conference*, AIAA, Washington, D.C., 1993, pp. 337–340.

[52]Ponomarenko, V. A., "Kingdom in the Sky—Earthly Fetters and Heavenly Freedoms. The Pilot's Approach to the Military Flight Environment," translated by I. Malinin, RTO-AG-338, 2000.

[53]Cohen, D., Otakeno, S., Previc, F. H., and Ercoline, W. R., "Effect of inside-out and outside-in attitude displays on off-axis tracking in pilots and nonpilots," *Aviation, Space, and Environmental Medicine*, Vol. 72, 2001, pp. 170–176.

[54]Malinin, I., "The Consequences of Adding Runway Symbology to the Head-Up Display," *Proceedings of Recent Trends in Spatial Disorientation Research*, 2000.

[55]Pongratz, H., Vaic, H., and Reinecke, M., Ercoline, W. R., and Cohen, D., "Outside-in vs. Inside-Out: Flight Problems Caused by Different Flight Attitude Indicators," *SAFE Journal*, Vol. 29, 1999, pp. 7–11.

[56]Reising, J. M., and Emerson, T. J., "Color Display Formats: a Revolution in Cockpit Design," *AGARD Conference Proceedings No. 329: Advanced Avionics and the Military Aircraft Man/Machine Interface*, 1982, pp. 6-1–6-11.

[57]Reising, J. M., Liggett, K. K., and Hartsock, D. C., "New Flight Display Formats," *Proceedings of the Eighth International Symposium on Aviation Psychology*, edited by R. S. Jensen, Dept. of Aerospace Engineering, Ohio State Univ., 1995.

[58]Christ, R. E., "Review and Analysis of Color Coding Research for Visual Displays," *Human Factors and Ergonomics Society Inc.*, Vol. 17, No. 6, 1975, 542–470.

[59]Thomas, S. R., "Laser Eye Protection Flight Test Questionnaire Meeting," Air Force Materiel Command, AL-SR-1992-0011. Brooks Air Force Base, TX, 1992.

[60]Burns, R. K., and Lovering, P. B., "F-15E EADI Evaluation: a Comparison of Three Formats," Aeronautical System Div., ASD-TR-88-5030, Wright-Patterson Air Force Base, OH, 1988.

[61]Malcolm, R., "The Malcolm Horizon—History and Future," *Proceedings Peripheral Vision Horizon Display (PVHD)*, NASA, 1983, pp. 11–39.

[62]Malcolm, R., "Pilot Disorientation and the Use of a Peripheral Vision Display," *Aviation, Space, and Environmental Medicine*, Vol. 55, 1984, pp. 231–238.

[63]Carmack, D. L., "Landing Weather Minimums Investigation," Air Force Flight Dynamics Lab., IPIS-TR-70-3, Wright-Patterson AFB, OH, 1972.

[64]Hall, J. R., Stephens, C. M., and Penwill, J. C., "A Review of the Design and Development of the RAE Fast/Jet Head-Up Display Format," Royal Aerospace Establishment, Working Paper 89/34, Bedford, England, U.K. 1989.

[65]Weinstein, L. R., and Ercoline, W. R., "Utility of a Ghost Horizon and Climb/Dive Ladder Line Tapering on a Head-Up Display," Air Force Material Command, AL-TR-1992-0168, Brooks Air Force Base, TX, 1993.

[66]Ercoline, W. R., and DeVilbiss, C. A., "C-141 Head-Down Display Unusual Attitude Recovery Study," *Proceedings of the 66th Annual Aerospace Medical Association*, 1995.

[67]Newman, R. L., "Improvement of Head-Up Display Standards," Flight Dynamics Lab., AFWAL-TR-87-3055, Wright-Patterson AFB, OH, 1987.

[68]Sanders, M. S., and McCormick, E. J., "Human Factors in Engineering and Design," 7th ed., McGraw-Hill, New York, 1993, p. 135.

[69]Weintraub, D. J., and Ensing, M., *Human Factors Issues in Head-up Display Design: The Book of HUD*, CSERIAC SOAR 92-2, Defense Logistics Agency, Cameron Station, VA, 1992, pp. 125–127.

[70]Roscoe, S. N., "Airborne Displays for Flight and Navigation," *Human Factors*, Vol. 10, No. 4, 1968, pp. 321–332.

[71]Ercoline, W. R., and Gillingham, K. K., "Effects of Variations in Head-Up Display Airspeed and Altitude Representations on Basic Flight Performance," *Proceedings of the Human Factors Society 34th Annual Meeting*, 1990, pp. 1547–1551.

[72]Hughes, T., Hassoun, J., and Barnaba, J., "A Comparison of Head-up and Head-down Formats During Instrument Flying Tasks," ASC-TR-93-5003, Wright-Patterson Air force Base, OH, 1993.

[73]Bailey, R. E., Knotts, L. H., Priest, J. E., Gawron, V. J., and Parada, L. O., "Evaluation of Proposed USAF HUD Standard, Session II," Arvin Calspan Corp., Contract No. F33615-88-C-3602, Buffalo, NY, 1992.

[74]Reising, J. M., and Emerson, T. J., "Color in Quantitative and Qualitative Display Formats: Does Color Help?" *Proceedings of the Conference on Color in Information Technology and Visual Displays*, 1985.

[75]Previc, F. H., "Towards a Physiologically Based HUD Symbology," USAF School of Aerospace Medicine, USAFSAM-TR-88.25, Brooks Air Force Base, TX, 1989.

[76]McNaughton, G. B., "The Role of Vision in Spatial Disorientation and Loss of Aircraft Attitude Awareness by Design," *Proceedings of the Attitude Awareness Workshop*, Flight Dynamics Laboratory, Wright-Patterson AFB, OH, 1985, pp. 1-3-1–1-3-53.

[77]Braithwaite, M. G., and Durnford, S. J., "A Novel Flight Instrument Display to Minimize the Risk of Spatial Disorientation," *Proceedings of the Human Factors and Ergonomics Society, 41st Annual Meeting*, Vol. 2, 1997, p. 897.

[78]Still, D. L., and Temme, L. A., "Oz: a Human-Centered Computing Cockpit Display," *Proceedings of the I/ITSEC Conference*, 2001.

[79]Emerson, T. J., and Moss R. J., "The Cockpit of the 21st Century—Will High Tech Payoff?," IEEE/AESS, 1990.

[80]Best, P. S., Schopper, A. W., and Thomas, G., "State-of-the-Art Glass Cockpits and Human Factors Related Issues," Human Engineering Div., Armstrong Lab., CSERIAC-RA-95-008, Wright-Patterson Air Force Base, OH, 1995.

[81]Stein, K. J., "Navy Evaluates Pictorial Cockpit Display," *Aviation Week and Space Technology*, 12 Sept. 1983.

[82]Snow, M. P., and Reising, J. M., "Effect of Pathway-in-the-Sky and Synthetic Terrain Imagery on Situation Awareness in a Simulated Low-Level Ingress Scenario," Air Force Material Command, ASC-99-1229, Wright-Patterson Air Force Base, OH, 1999.

[83]Fadden, S., Ververs, P. M., and Wickens, C. D., "Pathway HUDs: Are They Viable?" NASA, Technical Rept. ARL-00-13/NASA-00-3, 2000.

[84]Lehman, E. F., and Jenkins, M. L., "Handbook for Conducting Pilot-in-the-Loop Simulation for Crew Station Evaluation," Human Systems Div., Air Force Systems Command, HSD-TR-90-007, Brooks Air Force Base, Texas, 1990.

[85]Newman, R. L., Haworth, L. A., Kessler, G. K., Eksuzian, D. J., Ercoline, W. R., Evans, R. H., Hughes, T. C., and Weinstein, L. F., "TRISTAR I: Evaluation Methods for Testing Head-Up Display (HUD) Flight Symbology," NASA TM 4665, 1994.

[86]Bannach, B., "Instrument Flight Procedures," *Air Force Manual 11-217*, Vol. 1, HQ AFFSA/XOFD, Dept. of the Air Force, 2000.

Chapter 10

Flight Displays II: Head-Up and Helmet-Mounted Displays

Richard L. Newman*

Crew Systems, San Marcos, Texas

Loran A. Haworth[†]

Federal Aviation Administration, Seattle, Washington

I. Introduction

I N this chapter we will review selected head-up display (HUD) and helmet-mounted display (HMD) properties contributing to spatial orientation/disorientation and HUD and HMD research. We will then discuss what the design engineer should consider to minimize any adverse display effects on the pilot's ability to maintain spatial awareness. For more general issues related to HUDs and HMDs, the reader is referred to Weintraub and Ensing[1] or Newman.[2]

Pilot spatial disorientation (SD) has been a persistent problem since the first flight into (and probably spiral dive out of) a cloud. In the early 1980s HUDs were blamed as contributing to SD, and this reputation has persisted to the present, but this criticism is not necessarily still warranted. The HUD SD issue was first identified by Barnette[3] who surveyed U.S. Air Force (USAF) pilots flying HUD-equipped airplanes and found that approximately 30% of the pilots reported an increased tendency towards SD. Newman[4] reported similar findings. HUD-induced SD was reported to occur within one of several scenarios, the most common of which is flying in and out of clouds. Other disorienting situations included extreme maneuvers such as night pull-ups from a target, air combat maneuvering (ACM), and recoveries from unusual attitudes. These are conditions under which SD tendencies are most likely to occur *with or without a HUD*.

The preceding studies were performed shortly after the first HUDs became operational. These first HUDs were primarily intended as weapon-aiming devices with limited flight data included in the HUD symbology, as HUDs were not developed

---

This material is declared a work of the U.S. Government and is not subject to copyright protection in the United States.

*Engineer and test pilot.

[†]Member, FAA Transport Airplane Directorate Standards Staff.

as flight instruments nor were they tested as such. A later survey by Newman and Foxworth[5] found a reduced tendency to SD reported by F-18 pilots, and no Dassault *Mercure* pilot reported an increased tendency to disorientation. Newman and Foxworth[5] attributed this improvement in spatial orientation to better cockpit/HUD integration and better HUD training.

II. Basic Characteristics of HUDs and HMDs

To understand the shortcomings of existing head-up display designs, some understanding of HUD principles is needed. This section discusses the basic optics associated with HUD design. More detail can be found in Gard[6] or Newman.[2] *Optical Design*[7] is a very informative source book, but was unfortunately cancelled in 1986.

A. Types of Optical Arrangements

The cathode-ray-tube image in most HUDs is driven by a HUD computer called the symbol-generator. The symbol-generator takes input data from a mission computer or flight management computer and converts the data into symbology to convey meaningful information to the pilot. The symbology appears as a virtual image, with the HUD symbols appearing to float in space overlying the real-world view. The virtual image is created by a backwards extension of the rays impinging on the pilot's eye. The virtual image does not exist in the sense that it can be detected by a photographic plate. It appears only when viewed through another lens (such as the lens in a human eye or a camera).

1. Conventional HUDs

The traditional HUD uses a refractive optical design with a combining glass (Fig. 1) to superimpose HUD symbols on the real-world view. In a system of this type, the image of the symbology is passed through a collimating lens (or series of lenses) to produce a parallel set of rays. Often, the light rays are reflected in a "folding mirror" to allow for more room in the instrument panel. These parallel rays are reflected by the semitransparent combining glass back to the pilot's eyes. The view from the external scene passes directly through the combining glass to the pilot's eyes. In this type of HUD, the generation of the parallel rays of light takes place in the final collimating lens—the combiner contributes no optical power. Because the collimation is based on lenses using the principle of refraction, this type of HUD is often called a *refractive HUD*. This is the general arrangement of most early HUDs.

The exit aperture of the collimating lens will limit how much of the virtual image is visible at a particular pilot eye location and creates what has been termed the porthole or knothole effect.[9] Only part of the virtual image—the instantaneous field of view (FOV)—can be seen at a time. If the viewer's eye is shifted, all of the image can be seen, but only part at a time (see Fig. 1). The *instantaneous FOV* is a function of the exit aperture and the exit aperture-eye distance. The *total FOV* is the combined visual area that can be seen by the viewer by moving his or her head. Figure 2 shows the knothole effect and the difference between the instantaneous FOV and total FOV available as the pilot moves his or her head.

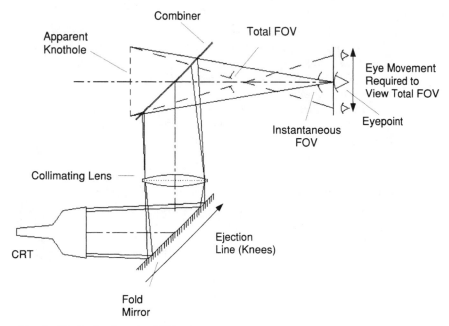

Fig. 1 Typical refractive HUD. (Reproduced with permission of Hussey; Ref. 8.)

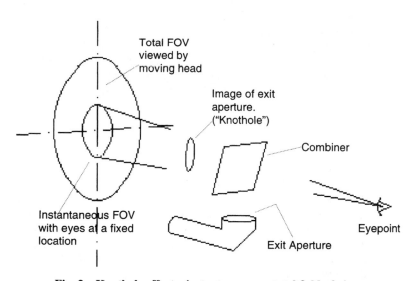

Fig. 2 Knothole effect—instantaneous vs total field of view.

2. Reflective HUDs

A second HUD optical arrangement uses a curved combiner. In such a HUD the curvature of the combiner generates the parallel rays of light.[10] It is necessary to shape both surfaces of the combiner to allow the rays from the external scene to pass through without being distorted. This type of HUD is referred to as a reflective HUD. Reflective HUDs combine the exit aperture with the total reflecting surface. As a result, the instantaneous and total FOVs are identical. There is a downside to this: the HUD symbology can suddenly disappear as the pilot moves his or her head out of the eyebox and out of the total FOV.

3. Disparity

If the incoming rays are parallel, the eyes accommodate as if the symbology image is infinitely far away. In fact, most HUDs do not quite achieve perfect collimation. Typically, the maximum disparity is about 2.5 mrad, which corresponds to an image about 25 m in front of the pilot. The larger problem with incoming rays not being parallel is that the location of the symbology can differ from one eye to the other. This binocular disparity will cause the two eyes to converge or diverge slightly and might cause eye discomfort, particularly for long-duration flights.[11]

4. Eye-Reference Point

Each HUD has an eye-reference point where the design is optimized. As the pilot's eye is moved from the *design eye-reference point*, optical performance (distortion, accuracy of symbol location, etc.) can degrade. Because the pilots constantly move their heads during flight, it is better to speak of an *"eyebox"* volume rather than a single eye point. The performance specifications should be met at any location within this eyebox, rather than at a single point.

As the pilot moves his or her head beyond the limit of the eyebox, the view of the symbology will be lost. With a conventional or refractive HUD, this will happen gradually, whereas with a reflective HUD—with its identical instantaneous and total FOVs—the symbology will vanish abruptly. Particularly in an air-to-air engagement, for example, pilots can move their heads outside the eyebox to keep the adversary in view. With a conventional, refractive HUD the symbology will usually remain visible as pilots move their heads and will thus aid in returning their gaze to the eyebox. With a reflective HUD symbology can be "lost" and require additional pilot effort to regain the symbology.

B. Primary Flight Symbols

Early HUDs presented symbology similar to head-down instruments. Generally they displayed some form of pitch reference with a background scale in addition to weapon-aiming symbols. The early HUDs were intended for use as weapon sights, and collimation was added primarily to eliminate parallax. Eventually, other flight information was added to improve performance: airspeed, altitude, heading, etc. Figure 3 shows an example of such early symbology. New symbols showing the aircraft's trajectory or flight path were added later. The display of flight-path information was a natural addition to a forward-facing display, which allowed simultaneous viewing of the external scene.

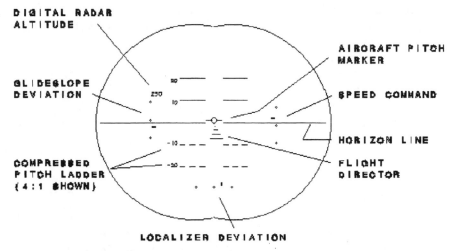

Fig. 3 Early pitch-referenced HUD symbology. (Reproduced with permission of Newman; Ref. 2.)

1. Pitch Ladder

The *pitch ladder* is the scale against which the various pitch and flight-path references are measured. In most HUDs and HMDs the pitch ladder consists of a series of lines parallel to the horizon, usually at 5-deg intervals. The pitch ladder maintains its orientation relative to the horizon and provides a stable frame of reference for instrument flight.

2. Pitch Marker

The *pitch marker* is a fixed reference on the HUD representing the extension of the fuselage reference line. Its projection against the pitch ladder is the aircraft's pitch attitude. It is sometimes called the waterline.

3. Flight-Path Marker

The *flight-path marker* (FPM) is the projection of the aircraft's flight path. When viewed through the HUD (or HMD), it shows where the airplane is going. Some pilots refer to it as the location of the "smoking hole." The FPM moves both vertically (showing the flight-path angle) and laterally (showing either drift or sideslip angle). Some HUDs allow the pilot to "cage" the FPM or constrain it to the center of the FOV. In this case it is referred to as a *climb–dive marker*. The early term for the FPM was the velocity vector. This term should be avoided to prevent confusion with the hover vector in helicopter HMDs.

Flight-path markers can be either inertial or air mass derived. Inertial FPMs show the flight path relative to the world, whereas air-mass show the flight path relative to the air through which the aircraft is flying. Each depiction has its advantages and disadvantages. Inertial FPMs show the actual trajectory and will indicate directly whether the airplane will miss a ridge or will impact it. On the other hand, air-mass flight-path information allows the pilot to directly assess the aircraft's aerodynamic performance. Further discussion is found in Sec. VII.D.

4. Ghost Horizon

If the aircraft maneuvers in such a manner that the horizon line leaves the HUD FOV, some HUDs leave a *ghost-horizon* line to indicate the direction of the horizon. Current U.S. Federal Administration Agency (FAA) policy requires a ghost horizon on all electronic flight instruments.[12]

C. Conformality

Conformality means having the same angular relationship in relation to the outside world. In HUDs or HMDs it means the pitch ladder and related symbols have the same angular relationship to each other as the real world, that is, the symbols overlie the real world objects they represent. For example, the spacing of 5-deg conformal pitch-ladder lines subtends 5 deg of the background world in which they are superimposed. Some designers use contact analog as a synonym for conformality. This is incorrect; a contact-analog display or symbol looks like the real world, but need not be the same size. A related term is *world fixed,* which refers to a symbol that retains its orientation relative to the outside visual scene.

D. Electronic Display Characteristics

1. Clutter

A visually cluttered display can prevent the pilot from interpreting the cues needed for prompt recognition and recovery from unusual attitudes. The 2.5-deg pitch line spacing on early F-16 HUDs has been criticized as distracting clutter, as has the presentation of excessive data on this and other HUD displays. In an extreme unusual attitude almost complete declutter might be desirable until the airplane has been stabilized. Clutter presents an additional problem for HUDs and HMDs in flight tasks requiring a view of the real-world cues—excessive clutter blocks the pilot's view of the real world and might prevent detection of ground-based obstacles or other aircraft.[13]

2. Digital Data and Rate Information

Some pilots have criticized the HUD's all-digital displays because they make the determination of airspeed and altitude-rate information difficult. This seems to be more of a problem with airspeed than altitude, because the flight-path marker provides altitude-rate information. Incorporating a flight-path acceleration cue, for example, could assist the pilot in airspeed control. Recent HUDs incorporate circular scales with a pointer and reference marks surrounding the digital airspeed and altitude displays.[14,15] When either airspeed or altitude change, the circular motion of the pointer provides the pilot with rate information.

3. Pitch-Ladder Precession Passing Zenith or Nadir

Many early electronic displays rolled their pitch ladders 180 deg as the airplane's pitch passed through 90 deg nose up or nose down, in what is termed precession. This was required in early mechanical attitude indicators (AI) because they were mounted on gimbal rings with axes oriented to allow free rotation. If the gimbal axes became aligned, the inner axis could lock (called *gimbal-lock*), and the display would no longer function correctly. The controlled precession prevented this, allowing the display to move freely. Early electronic displays incorporated a roll motion in their design to emulate the familiar behavior of mechanical instruments, even though it was not required.

At best, this rotation in the reference frame during precession makes controlled flight difficult during nose-up or -down attitudes; at worst, it creates disorientation. In one F-15 unusual attitude incident the negative effect of this HUD feature was apparent.[16] The pilot stated that he rolled wings level and pulled, when viewing of the videotape frame by frame shows that the airplane actually pulled through from the inverted position in a *split-S* recovery. Thus, the apparent roll was actually the display's controlled precession. Fortunately, such precession is no longer a feature in current displays.

4. Automatic Declutter

Some electronic attitude indicators remove "unneeded" information during extreme attitudes—a process designed to enhance the ability of the pilot to use the display for recovery without distraction. This removes mode awareness from the pilot and was thought to have contributed to a crash of an Airbus A-330 at Toulouse.[17] During the accident sequence, the flight controls automatically switched to a mode that removed some pitch limits. The AI symbology was automatically decluttered by excessive pitch attitude at about the same time. This declutter was intended to remove all unnecessary information during an unusual attitude. In this case, however, this declutter prevented the pilot from detecting mode information that might have prevented to the accident.*

III.   HUD Symbology and Spatial Disorientation

A.   Current HUD Limitations

HUDs and HMDs are see-through displays. Although HUDs and HMDs present collimated symbology or images superimposed on the external visual scene that will ideally lead to improved situation awareness, such see-through displays have some characteristics that can impose increased difficulty in interpreting certain orientation cues when compared to conventional AIs, as discussed in the following sections.

1. Ability to Distinguish Upright from Inverted Flight

Conventional AIs use black (or brown) and blue (or light gray) hemispheres to depict Earth and sky. These hemispheres help the pilot distinguish upright from

---

*Personal communication with H. B. Green, FAA, Seattle, WA, Aug. 1994.

inverted flight. Many AIs also provide patterns on one or both hemispheres to represent ground texture or clouds. The HUD AI, on the other hand, has been limited to monochromatic lines and by design avoids textures and patterns that might block external visual cues. This might partly explain why the percentage of roll reversals during recovery from an unusual attitude using a typical HUD is slightly higher than using a traditional AI.[18] It is unlikely that HUDs will be able to incorporate color with sufficient contrast in the foreseeable future. Regardless of technological advances, it might not be practical to use blue and brown to depict sky and ground. Blue symbols would not be clearly visible against the actual sky, and brown symbols would not sufficiently contrast with some terrain. (There is developmental work currently underway for color HUDs, but generally these programs are developing two color displays, not full color HUDs.) Consequently, a number of shape and size cues, as well as directional cues, have been incorporated into the pitch and/or climb–dive ladder of HUDs to aid in the recognition of unusual attitudes (see Sec. VII.C.).

2. Full-Scale Pitch Angles

It can be difficult to assess aircraft pitch attitude with the HUD's full-scale but limited FOV display. The conventional AIs compressed, pictorial format makes aircraft attitude interpretation easier during dynamic maneuvering (Chapter 9, Sec. III.A.4.c). The compressed pitch scales slow down the angular rates on the display, and the depiction of a wider FOV keeps the displayed horizon in view. An extended discussion of how display scaling, including pitch-compression, affects attitude recognition and recovery is included in Section VII.D.

3. Accommodation Traps

The issue of HUD accommodation traps has been raised by Roscoe[19–21] and Iavecchia.[22] They maintain, with justification, that the pilot's eyes during HUD viewing accommodate inward to near the plane of the HUD frame, in spite of the HUD symbology being collimated to optical infinity. It is asserted that as the pilot shifts between HUD symbols and real-world objects the accommodation shift will induce SD (see Sec. III of Chapter 7). HUD studies have not supported this accommodation concern, however. Randle et al.[23] used the accommodation argument to predict HUD landing approaches that are much shallower and more dispersed than non-HUD approaches, yet every study to date has indicated more precise control of approach angle and tighter touchdown dispersion using HUDs.[2] In any event the accommodation distance of the HUD would be at least as far as that of conventional instruments, and HUDs should be no worse than head-down displays in this regard. The inward shift of the pilot's attention might be more problematic for perceiving the outside world properly than the inward shift of accommodation, as discussed in Sec. III.A.5.

4. Framing

Another concern is the sense of combiner structure or, in some HUDs, by the symbology itself.[24] During the F-15 incident discussed earlier in Sec. II.D.3, the airplane was rolled 90 deg while the pilot thought he was wings level. As observed on the videotape, the 90-deg orientation of the altitude and airspeed tapes led to this sense of verticality. The edges of the pitch ladder, lining up in horizontal rows, helped to create the apparent wings-level attitude. Many of the conventional head-down AIs are round, thereby avoiding part of this problem. Many AIs also have pitch lines that lengthen as they extend further below the horizon. As a result, the edges of the pitch lines do not form parallel rows, and a false sense of horizontal does not occur when the airplane is rolled 90 deg.

5. Attentional Capture

The inability to detect outside ground and air objects using the HUD has been noted for more than a decade.[13] This tendency has been repeatedly demonstrated in laboratory and simulator studies and is believed to have resulted in several near misses in the air.[13] There are many reasons for this, including the excessive salience, clutter, and difficulty in interpreting HUD symbology along with the inward optical and attentional shift of the pilot.[13] There is also a two-dimensional attentional capture caused by the HUD, in that pilots tend to restrict their head movements and ocular scanning to the HUD rather than the rest of the cockpit and peripheral visual world.[13,25] Some solutions to this problem include making HUD symbology more intuitive, more widely spaced (by means of larger HUDs and declutter options), and even making some HUD symbology scene fixed.[26]

6. Flight Path Control—Flight Path vs Pitch

The tendency of pilots to use the HUD FPM as the primary control symbol rather than pitch attitude during unusual attitudes can lead to inappropriate control inputs for recover. Particularly at large angles of attack (AoA), applying nose-up elevator (pulling on the control stick) can result in descent, the opposite to that of normally expected flight control response. Such a "backside" condition can occur during maneuvering at extreme angles of attack or during vertical-short-takeoff-and-landing (VSTOL) operations. Klopfstein[27] developed HUD symbology to emphasize the angular pitch/flight-path/angle-of-attack relationship. Klopfstein's format was not widely accepted because it used an early symbol-generator, which could only produce a set of straight lines and intentionally showed no airspeed or altitude data. Its critics admitted, however, that a pilot could use the AoA presentation well enough to allow for precise pitch and airspeed control.[28] Klopfstein's format is shown in Fig. 4.

B. Novel Designs

Many new display designs are departing from the traditional attitude display or its cousins. Some of these displays have characteristics that can interfere with unusual attitude recognition and recovery.

1. Pathway in the Sky

The various pathway (also known as "tunnel" or "highway") formats, some of which are described in Chapter 9, Sec. III.C.2, are intended to serve as intuitive, natural displays. These displays are being proposed by a number of researchers for HUDs.[29-33] They have also been proposed for HMDs[34] and for head-down displays.[35-39]

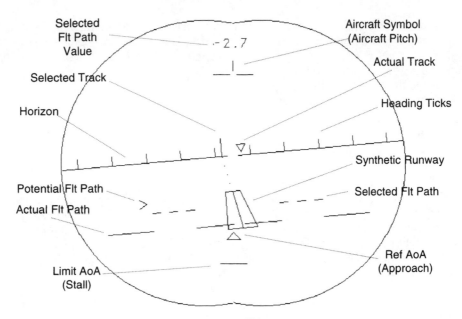

Fig. 4   Klopstein[28] symbology.

A limited number of studies have shown that the pathway displays offer many advantages in terms of maintaining a proper flight path, including altitude, airspeed, and heading performance (see Ref. 40 for a review). Nonetheless, all such displays contain a multitude of line segments, which can conflict with attitude awareness. Tunnel or pathway formats are very compelling and can overwhelm the background display of attitude information. Figure 5 shows a typical pathway format.

2.   Other Attitude References

Several global attitude awareness cues have also been proposed. These are intended to provide a small cue to enhance attitude awareness on the part of the pilot—preventing unusual attitudes, not merely helping in their recovery. The attitude cues are usually presented full time and are generally nonconformal so as to appear more intuitive to the pilot. One of the most promising of these global attitude symbologies is the *arc segmented attitude reference* (ASAR), which is also referred to as the "orange peel." The ASAR is an attitude cue surrounding the aircraft reference symbol. The ASAR has a thick circle that rotates to show roll angle and expands and contracts to show downward and upward pitch, respectively. Figure 6 shows the mechanization of this symbology. The ASAR has also been proposed as a global symbol surrounding the entire display near the edge of the HUD FOV and is known as the "grapefruit" in this case. Another global attitude symbol that has been actually flown is the French *le boule*,[41] a small attitude ball located in the lower left corner of the HMD FOV. Anecdotal reports indicate that *le boule* is a very effective orientation aid.* Global displays

---

*Personal communication with Capt. Scott Horowitz, USAF, July 1992.

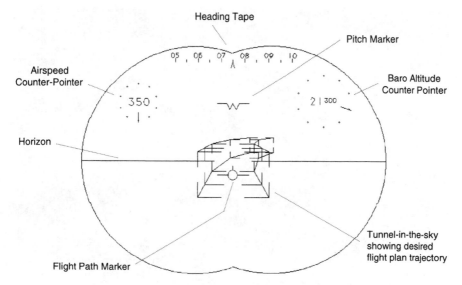

Fig. 5   Example of a pathway format

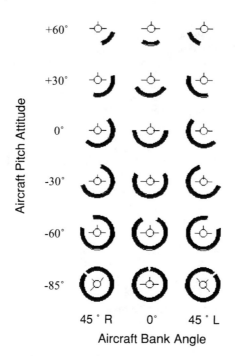

Fig. 6   Arc segmented attitude indicator, shown for different pitch-and-bank angles.

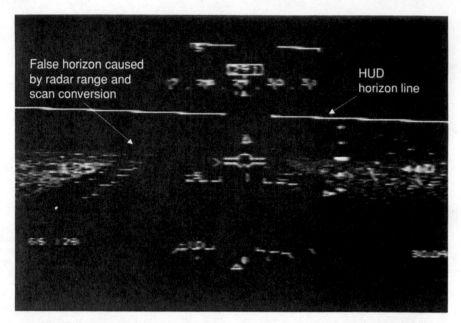

Fig. 7   Millimeter-wave radar image with superimposed HUD symbology.

such as the ASAR, *le boule*, and the theta ball[42] depict the aircraft's attitude using an inside-out, moving-horizon format, whereas others portray a moving-aircraft attitude symbol.[43] A recent modification to the ASAR that includes more distinct horizon and flight-path and bank-angle discrimination shows promise with the HMD as part of Geiselman's nondistributed flight reference (NDFR) (see Sec. VI.D.1) and the advanced NDFR being developed by Jenkins and Havig.*

3. Enhanced Vision

Enhanced vision is the presentation of sensor imagery in the primary flight display, regardless of where it is located (on a HUD, HMD, or HDD). Forward-looking infrared (FLIR) or millimeter-wavelength radar has been commonly proposed for use with HUDs and HMDs. The problems with FLIR and other night-vision devices are discussed in Chapter 7, Sec. III.C, but millimeter-wavelength radar images also provide misleading visual cues when compared to the normal out-the-window scene. The image processor converts angle/azimuth data (B-scan) data into a perspective view (C-scan). Because of the range characteristics, the image is usually confined to a band across the lower half of the display with a false horizon somewhat below the out-the-window horizon, as shown in Fig. 7. The result is a display that can challenge the pilot's ability to maintain orientation.[44]

4. Synthetic Vision

Synthetic vision is the presentation of a computer-generated picture of the external scene and, as with enhanced vision imagery, can be overlaid with flight

---

*Personal communication, March 2002.

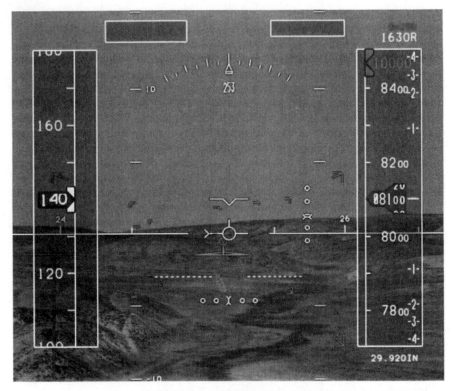

Fig. 8   Synthetic vision display with superimposed HUD symbology. (Reproduced with permission of NASA Langley Research Center.)

symbology (Fig. 8). Synthetic vision displays, which are a type of virtual display, are created from an onboard computer database in much the same fashion as is a computer-generated simulator scene. The fidelity of the image can be extremely high, approaching photographic or video quality; but, although the presentation can contribute greatly to spatial orientation, it can still contain SD-producing attributes. Although photorealistic images would seem to be intuitive, Kruk et al.[45] indicate that extreme realism seems to detract from the pilot's ability to detect ridgelines. In mountainous terrain, as with the actual out-the-window visual scene, the true horizontal might be hidden. Consequently, if the synthetic view ahead of the aircraft is used in lieu of an attitude display it must be presented such that correct attitude information is conveyed. Few studies have been performed to assess potential difficulties with synthetic displays.

IV. HMD Symbology and Spatial Disorientation

Helmet- (or head-) mounted displays share many of the same characteristics with their HUD cousins; however, HMDs are "in your face," creating a greater visual dependency on information displayed in the HMD.[46] In addition to characteristics held in common with HUDs, other HMD-unique characteristics discussed in the following sections appear to exacerbate SD.

A. HMD Characteristics

1. Conflicting Frames of Reference

Haworth and Seery[47] and Newman[48] reported pilot difficulty with the *Apache* hover symbology (a fixed, symbolic plan view) superimposed on a direct view of sensor imagery. Such a combination of coordinate systems was difficult for pilots to interpret, especially during recoveries from unintentional sideways flight. The pilots were observed primarily attending to the dynamics of the symbology rather than the sensor imagery because of the difficulty in interpreting the symbology. Walrath[49] reported similar forms of visual bias when symbology overlies dynamic video. Ercoline et al.[50] also noted greater errors in recovering from unusual attitudes when a virtual scene conflicts with the attitude depicted by the HMD symbology. However, the frame-of-reference conflict caused by head movements relative to the view depicted by the symbology is not debilitating if an outside scene is not visible.[51] And, a conflict between a fixed forward view in the symbology and a different view of the outside world might be better than attempting to produce a fully conformal HMD symbology.[52]

2. Head-Tracker Shortcomings

Key concerns for any head-tracker system are the accuracy, repeatability, and latency of the measurements. Unwanted motion of the symbology because of head-tracking deficiencies has also been reported.[53,54] Generally, the accuracy of the pointing should be commensurate with the need for image registration. Accuracy requirements at present are driven by weapon-aiming requirements, not by the need to avoid SD.

The head tracker must also follow the pilot's head without excessive lag. No specific requirements have been determined, but the responses should be fast enough to minimize display image lag if head-tracked flight symbols or head-steered images are used. Based on the normal rule of thumb of sampling at four times the observed frame time, a preliminary latency requirement of 20 ms (50 Hz) should be a first estimate. The head-tracker system should also be able to respond to head movements as high as 120–240 deg/s (2–4 rad/s) (Ref. 55).

3. Head Orientation

There are normally four dynamic degrees of freedom (DOF) for the pilots' head: three rotations (elevation, azimuth, and roll tilt) and one translation (leaning forward). Leaning forward is considered in many HUD designs that define an alert eye position somewhat forward of the design eye position. Additional DOFs might be required as well. Lateral translation might be important if the cockpit geometry requires leaning to the side to see out. Vertical translation can be significant under $+G_Z$ load.

Some head-tracking systems have ignored head tilt in roll. These systems have not usually presented symbology stabilized in either aircraft or world coordinates. As a result, there was thought to be little effect of roll head tilt, especially with the presentation of sensor images that do not align with the real world or the aircraft. When using aircraft- or world-stabilized symbology or sensor imagery, as in the virtual HUD (see Sec. IV.B), ignoring pilot head tilt can lead to visual conflicts as the pilot looks through the HMD.

Pilots are also subject to losing head-referenced orientation cues in those HMDs that prevent a direct view of the cockpit because of their optics and video overlay. Pilots have returned from flights with disturbed vertical orientation, particularly with HMDs that lack roll-tilt correction (Pat Garman, U.S. Army, personal communication, 1996). There appears to be a need for additional head-orientation symbology to assist in maintaining a normal vertical orientation. Proposals for addressing this issue include displaying virtual cockpit structure (cockpit rails) and the addition of head-tilt compensation in the head tracker.

4. HMD Symbology Location

Unlike the HUD, the HMD has an extremely large field of regard, for presenting stabilizing flight information. This poses a situation where the necessary flight information can be located outside the instantaneous FOV of the HMD. For example, if the horizon line is visually stabilized on or near the real-world horizon, the horizon line will be outside the FOV when the pilot looks away from the horizon line (up or down). When the pilot looks from side to side, the aircraft water-line symbol and FPM, normally overlaid on or near the nose of the aircraft, might again be outside the display FOV. Although this creates a situation where the information is cognitively easier to interpret because it is in the correct frame of reference, all flight information cannot always be observed at the same time.

Other HMD symbology display strategies include stabilization of all of the flight information at the same screen location (screen fixed), usually near the center of the display. The pilot then can observe all of the flight information all of the time [as in night-vison goggle (NVG) symbology], but cognitive interpretation of flight information and orientation becomes more difficult because the overlaid spatial information (symbology) must be cognitively corrected to the visual frame of reference that the pilot is observing through the sensor. This decreases the pilot's ability to remain oriented because the horizon line is not a true horizon line; directional hover information is not oriented in the direction of flight, etc. Screen-fixed symbology can also result in a cluttered display.

5. Binocular Rivalry

Some HMDs present the display to a single eye. This is desirable from a cost and weight standpoint. If the HMD is a monocular device, such as in the *Apache* helicopter, then both symbology and imagery will be shown to one eye while the other has an unaided and unobstructed view of the real world. Monocular display of symbology along with binocular intensification of outside images has also been incorporated in some NVGs.[56]

Gopher et al.[57] performed studies with pilots who performed tracking tasks with flight-control symbols presented to one eye and reference images to one eye. There was no significant degradation (compared to binocular viewing) if both symbol and reference were presented to the same eye; however, when the information was presented to different eyes, performance deteriorated. Cohen and Markoff[58] performed an experiment where a target was presented to one eye and an aiming reticle to the other. They examined simultaneous presentation and sequential presentation (hypothesized to minimize rivalry) and concluded that rivalry is negligible in HMDs. However, it must be remembered that their application was for a helmet-mounted sight. Page and Frey[53,54] evaluated a monocular HMD in an F-16 flight-test program and reported intermittent binocular rivalry issues, including eye strain and diplopia.

Binocular viewing can cause a variety of problems, including improper accommodation and misconvergence and reduced visual acuity whenever there is an inability to fuse the images from the eyes.[59] The issue of flight with dichoptic vision was raised as a possible cause of a recent accident involving a commercial MD-88 in which the pilot wore different contact lenses in his eyes, correcting for near vision in one and distant vision in the other.[60,61] These and other visual problems involving flight displays are also reviewed in Chapter 7, Sec. III.

6.   Field-of-View Limitations

The effect of HMD FOV limitations on SD are more pronounced than those reported with the HUD because the HMD is located on your face, unlike a HUD that is fixed in the cockpit like other instrument displays. No longer does the pilot have a direct and unobstructed view of the cockpit for both flight and system information and the outside world. This extreme FOV limitation decreases pilot orientation cues and negatively impacts the ability to subjectively access maneuvering performance.

7.   Parallax

Video presented on the HMD can often originate from a sensor displaced from the pilot's eye position, as in HMD-mounted FLIR imagery. This sensor can be located a half-meter or more forward and above or below the pilot. The displacement of the sensor (called parallax) creates an unusual situation where by the pilot must constantly interpret his or her physical position and orientation based on this remote viewpoint. Often, the video from a displayed eye point presents a God's-eye view from the sensor without visual reference to any airframe structure. Both conditions reduce the pilot's ability to quickly and accurately interpret vehicle orientation, especially during low-altitude, low-airspeed (nap-of-Earth) helicopter flight. (Parallax has also been reported to be an issue with fixed-wing HUDs displaying enhanced vision images.[44])

B.   Virtual HUD

The *virtual HUD* is the concept of allowing a HMD to perform the function of a forward-facing, conformal HUD. The virtual HUD is attractive to designers because it eliminates the need for a dedicated HUD in addition to the HMD. In the virtual HUD, HUD-like symbology is presented on the HMD with aircraft-stabilized positioning when the pilot looks forward from the design point of what would otherwise be an actual HUD. As the pilot turns his or her head to the side (or looks up) within the viewing angle of the HUD, the flight symbology remains superimposed on the center of the windscreen. Once the pilot's head has moved outside the normal viewing cone of the HUD, a different set of nonconformal symbology is presented that is designed to maintain the pilot's spatial orientation. Difficulties with current virtual HUDs are mainly a result of inadequacies of the head tracker. If the pilot's line of sight cannot be determined accurately enough, the virtual HUD might not provide sufficient accuracy for many tasks. From an orientation viewpoint unwanted symbol movement (jitter or "swimming") can detract from the pilot's ability to use the display. Head-tracker lags can also produce unwanted symbol movement if the pilot moves his or her head rapidly. Page and Frey[53,54] reported such unwanted symbol movement in a flight-test evaluation of a virtual HUD.

C. NVG Characteristics

Night-vision goggles can be thought of as, in most cases, a special case of an image-only HMD where the sensor is worn on the head. These have been used for several years to aid pilots in flying at night and have provided a great tactical advantage to pilots in this respect. However, many orientation problems exist with NVGs, including difficulties with judging size and distance, poor resolution, and limited FOV[62] (see also Chapter 7, Sec. III.C.1). From the standpoint of symbology and orientation information, NVGs also pose many problems such as the need to scan different types of visual information (below the NVGs for flight instrument readings and extra head scanning to increase the field of regard beyond the 40-deg FOV typical of most NVGs). One solution has been to superimpose primary flight symbology over the intensified image, which leads to a head-fixed, nonconformal attitude symbology.[63-65] The efficacy of such a symbology format has not been formally studied. Most NVG symbology evaluations have concentrated on mission performance or on subject pilot assessments.[66]

To date, NVG symbologies have not been head tracked. This should lead to conflicting frames-of-reference issues as found in the *Apache* HMD.[48,55] Other authorities have expressed concern over possible situation-awareness problems.[67,68] However, pilots in Piccione and Troxel's survey[66] report an overall improvement in situation awareness.

V. Development of HUDs and HMDs and Their Standards

It is important to review the historical development of HUD and HMD designs before discussing how to improve them. Many of the developments follow from the research described in the preceding section.

A. First Step—F-18

The F-18 HUD was the first operational HUD intended for use as a *primary flight display* and is shown in Fig. 9 (Ref. 69). No formal document is available to cite approval for the HUD as the primary flight display; however, it was (and remains) the only primary flight display installed on the airplane other than the standby attitude indicator. Prior to the F-18, HUDs were developed for specific flight tasks, usually weapon-aiming or approach-monitoring and were not designed *or tested* for use in routine flight tasks.

The F-18 HUD incorporated articulated pitch-ladder lines, also known as "bendy bars." These pitch lines are inclined at half the pitch angle forming a series of Vs pointing to the horizon; hence, the Vs are more compelling the further away they are from the horizon. The F-18 HUD also allowed the pilot to select a caged or uncaged flight-path marker. The caged flight-path marker, later known as the climb–dive marker, was constrained to the center of the FOV. When the flight-path

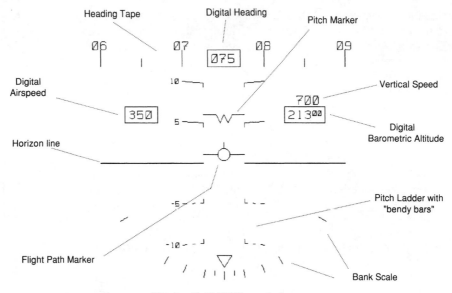

Fig. 9   F-18 HUD symbology.

marker was caged, a ghost marker was drawn to indicate where the airplane trajectory was going. The F-18 also used digital airspeed and altitude cues.

B.   Royal Aircraft Establishment FastJet

In the 1980s the Royal Aircraft Establishment (RAE) at Bedford developed the FastJet HUD symbology for the *Harrier* and *Tornado* aircraft.[70] The FastJet symbology is shown in Fig. 10. The goal of the FastJet format was to ease the pilot's task in routine and dynamic flight tasks. The major features are a tapered pitch ladder

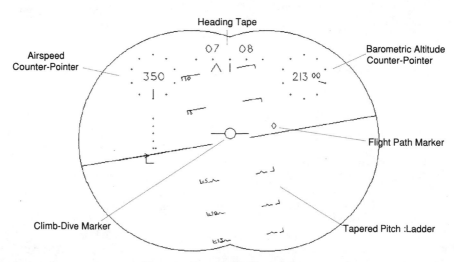

Fig. 10   FastJet HUD symbology.

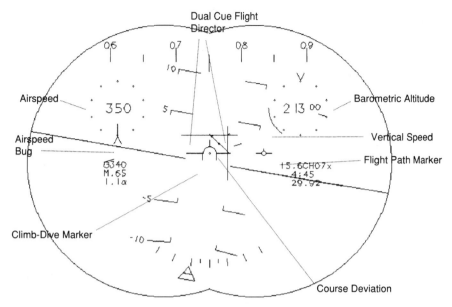

Fig. 11   MIL-STD-1787 symbology.[15]

with variable scaling, a full-time caged climb–dive marker, pitch-rate quickening for the climb–dive marker, and counterpointer scales as well as digital readouts for airspeed and altitude.

The pitch ladder incorporated scaling that ranged from 1:1 when the climb–dive marker is within 5 deg of the horizon and varied linearly to 4.4:1 at the zenith and nadir of the pitch-ladder. (The value of 4.4 was an accident of the field of view of the *Harrier* HUD. Early on, a decision had been made to use 5-deg pitch spacing up to 30 deg, and 10-deg spacing thereafter. A second, independent decision was made to set the scaling to ensure that three lines were present in the HUD FOV at any time. These two decisions, when matched with the 15-deg field of view of the *Harrier*, led to 2:1 scaling at an angle of 30 deg. This extrapolates to 4.4:1 at the zenith and nadir.*) The FastJet pitch-ladder tapers as the angle from the horizon increases to give a sense of attitude awareness. The pitch ladder was scaled around the climb–dive marker. Thus the climb–dive marker overlay the point of impact exactly in spite of the pitch scale compression. (The flight dynamics HUD, on the other hand, compresses around the waterline. As a result, its FPM does not overlay the "point of impact when operating with a compressed pitch scale."[71])

The FastJet flight symbol is a caged climb–dive marker with no option to uncage. A flight-path marker (a small diamond) shows the trajectory, but this is not intended to be an aircraft control symbol. No pitch marker is shown. Because of the elimination of the pitch reference, the climb–dive marker incorporates pitch-rate quickening based on *Harrier* flight characteristics.

In the 1980s the U.S. Air Force inaugurated a program to develop a standardized HUD symbology. The result, shown in Fig. 11, was heavily influenced by the RAE FastJet symbology, with the addition of some navigation and guidance cues.[15]

---

*Personal communication with John Hall, RAE, Bedford, England, April 1991.

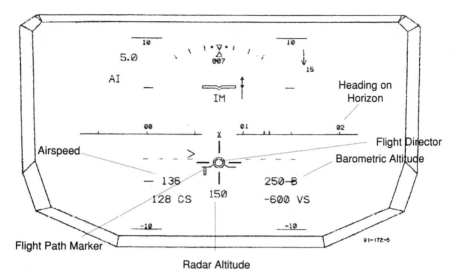

Fig. 12   Flight Dynamics HUD symbology. (Reproduced with permission of Rockwell-Collins/Flight Dynamics.)

In the recommendations of the MIL STD 1787, the pitch ladder was changed from tapered (as in the FastJet) to an asymmetric format—articulated (angled) below the horizon and tapered above. The climb–dive marker and flight-path-marker symbols were changed and a traditional course deviation indicator symbol overlaid on the climb–dive marker for lateral deviation. A conventional glide-slope indicator and split-axis flight director cues were added, as were a number of digital readouts for acceleration, ground speed, and vertical velocity. Quickening of the climb–dive marker was retained, and the initial standard mandated the *Harrier* algorithm for this feature. [Quickening refers to the addition of integrated predictor terms to a control display to provide the operator with immediate knowledge of the results of his own actions.[72] Quickening eliminates the need for the operator (i.e., pilot) to integrate the displayed values and eases the task load.] Recent airplanes that can reach extremely large AoAs have had to modify the quickening to prevent the presentation of misleading data at the extreme values.*

C. Civil HUD Development

In the 1980s, Flight Dynamics[71] developed a HUD intended for manually flying Category IIIa ILS approaches. The symbology, shown in Fig. 12, was developed from the NASA HUD studies of the 1970s (Ref. 72). Alaska Airlines was the launch customer, flying the display in their B-727 aircraft.[73] This HUD was intended for use only during instrument-landing-system (ILS) approaches, although there is no proscription against its use during other flight regimes.

The Flight Dynamics pitch ladder is oriented around the pitch marker, not the flight-path marker normally used in military HUDs. The airspeed, altitude, and

---

*Personal communication with Kevin Greeley, Lockheed Martin, April–Aug. 2001.

vertical speed cues are digital readouts arranged around the FPM, and heading is shown on the horizon. The pitch ladder is quite understated when compared with military HUDs. The pitch scaling is 1:1 until the horizon leaves the HUD FOV. As pitch is increased, the scaling is adjusted to retain the horizon line within the FOV. Additional discussion of the unusual-attitude mode of the Flight Dynamics HUD can be found in Section VII.C.

D. Military Transport HUD Development

The C-130J HUD (Ref. 74) was developed using features from the FastJet, MIL-STD-1787 (Ref. 15), and Flight Dynamics[71] symbologies. The pitch ladder was kept at 1:1 during normal operations, with no tapering or articulation. (None of these distinctive unusual-attitude features would be discernible during C-130 operations.) A climb–dive marker referenced format was intended to be the usual mode for operation because of the general lack of directional stability of the C-130. (The C-130 exhibits a significant degree of directional instability because of lateral oscillations in sideslip, which make instrument flight with an uncaged FPM difficult.) Because of initial concerns about Federal Aviation Administration (FAA) certification, the original design allowed logic switching between a flight-path marker and a climb–dive marker (a laterally caged FPM). The pitch ladder rotated around the climb–dive marker or FPM as appropriate. Following development and certification testing, the climb–dive marker was accepted by the FAA Atlanta Aircraft Certification Office and adopted as the standard for the C-130J. Figure 13 shows the C-130J HUD symbology.

The C-130J HUD switches automatically to an unusual-attitude mode when pitch or bank exceeds trigger values. This mode is pitch based, with the pitch

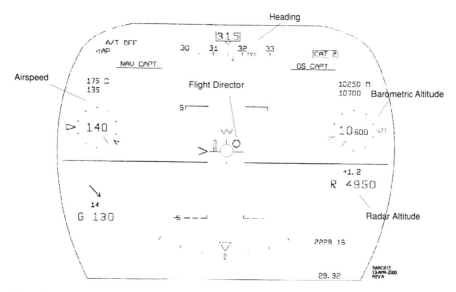

Fig. 13   C-130J HUD symbology. (Reproduced with permission of Rockwell-Collins/ Flight Dynamics.)

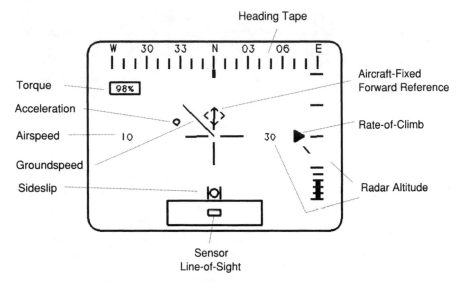

Fig. 14   MIL-STD-1295A hover symbology.[75]

ladder rotating around the pitch marker. During nose-low unusual attitudes, an *Augie Arrow* is drawn at the pitch marker. During nose-high unusual attitudes, the Augie Arrow is omitted, but extra cues are added to the pitch ladder emphasizing the recovery. The C-130J unusual-attitude mode is discussed further in Sec. VII.C.

E.   Military HMD Standard

The only HMD standard that has been published is MIL-STD-1295 (Ref. 75), describing the AH-64, *Apache* helicopter HMD system. Almost all Apache HMD symbols are *screen fixed* and are not adjusted for head movements. However, MIL-STD-1295A does show one aircraft-fixed symbol representing the forward direction to help orient the pilot. Two modes, hover and cruise, are shown in Figs. 14 and 15. The third mode, transition, has a symbology similar to the hover mode, differing only in scaling.

This HMD appears to have been adapted from what would have been presented on a fixed display. Altitude is shown both digitally and with a thermometer scale. Vertical speed is shown as a moving caret. All altitude information is on the right. Airspeed is shown digitally on the left. Aircraft heading is shown as a conventional tape and lubber line at the top of the display. Sideslip information is shown in a ball-bank format at the bottom of the display. The hover symbology depicts a screen-fixed plan (God's eye) view of the scene. The hover-velocity vector (hereafter termed the hover vector) is shown emanating from a reticle. There is also an aiding cue (a small circle) showing acceleration. The hover vector is scaled such that full length corresponds to 6 kn (11.1 km/h) ground speed. The transition-mode symbology is similar to the hover symbology, except for scaling of the hover vector and the addition of a screen-fixed horizon line. The scaling of the hover vector is 10 times the hover scaling [i.e., full length equals 60 kn (111 km/h ground speed] in this mode.

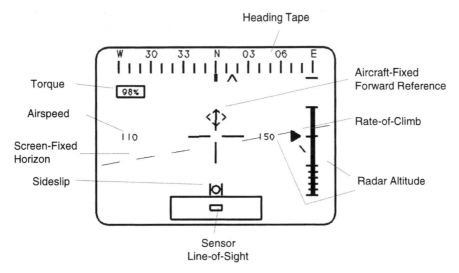

Fig. 15   MIL-STD-1295A cruise symbology.[75]

VI.   Spatial Disorientation Research Related to HUDs and HMDs

Most in-flight and simulator evaluations of effects of displays on SD have concentrated on the speed and accuracy of recovery from unusual attitudes (see also Chapter 9, Sec. III.D.1). The typical scenario involves placing a pilot (known as the evaluation pilot) in an unusual attitude and measuring the reaction time to the first correct control input and the number of reversals during the recovery. Some researchers measure the full recovery time, but this seems to be more a function of the initial conditions than of the recovery itself.[76] By necessity, the evaluation pilot is expecting the unusual attitude; as a result, unusual-attitude-recovery tasks do little to measure directly the ability of a flight display to prevent SD.

By comparison, there have been fewer studies of the entry into SD. Bryan et al.[77] studied the entry of noninstrument-rated pilots into simulated instrument conditions. They removed external visual cues from the evaluation pilot's view and monitored the entry. The average time to loss of control was 178 s after loss of visual cues. Newman and Quam[78] introduced unexpected attitude-indicator failures in a light airplane, forcing pilots to revert to the standby turn-and-slip indicators. Eight of nine evaluation pilots maintained control, defined in the experiment as a deviation of less than 300 ft (91.5 m) in altitude. The ability to maintain a proper flight path—including the ability to maintain airspeed and altitude, two important components of spatial orientation—has been investigated in numerous studies related to flight displays and symbology (e.g., Ref. 40).

Several experiments have been reported in which military pilots were forced to switch from a formation task in visual conditions to an instrument task (lost wingman). In the first study[79] the evaluation pilot flew as wingman in the rear seat of an F-100F and had the instrument hood lowered without warning. Upon losing reference, the evaluation pilot was to turn 30 deg away from the lead aircraft's heading. The time to perform this task ranged from 19 to 36 s (Ref. 79). Recently, Patterson et al.[80] and Smith et al.[81] studied the *optokinetic-cervical reflex* (OKCR) and its relation to head position and attitude interpretation in fixed-wing pilots. This reflex causes pilots to tilt their heads in an apparent attempt to align their eyes with the horizon. Their studies indicate that pilots maintain orientation with reference to the aircraft during flight in *instrument meteorological conditions* (IMC), but tend to align their heads more to the real-world horizon during flight in *visual meteorological conditions* (VMC). The observation was made that the OKCR could be a cause of SD during the transition from instrument to visual conditions. Two studies of potential difficulties during the entry into instrument flight were carried out in simulators.[80,81] Merryman and Cacioppo[82] concluded that this effect could be conducive to SD as a pilot moves his or her head during flight and that this effect must be taken into account during the design of attitude displays for HMDs. Findings from these studies should be considered when making flight symbology modifications.

A. HUD Studies

A comparison of unusual-attitude recoveries with HUD and HDD attitude displays was reported by Kinsley et al.[83] Both a static format and a fixed-base simulation of F-18 airframe dynamics were used for the evaluations. Their results show that use of the HDD AI ball resulted in faster reaction times and faster overall recovery times than with the HUD format. They found that the visual background interfered with recoveries using the HUD. Guttman[84] compared the F-18 HUD with an electronic AI during unusual attitudes in a fixed-base generic simulator. His results also showed that an electronic head-down attitude indicator produces superior recoveries than does a HUD.

Recovery from unusual attitudes was studied by Newman[16,76] using an F-14 simulator at Patuxent River Naval Air Station (NAS). (Although this study was conducted at Patuxent River NAS, it was sponsored by the Flight Dynamics Laboratory at Wright-Patterson Air Force Base, Ohio.) A number of variations on a modified F-18 HUD symbology were studied separately. Several modifications were recommended to enhance spatial awareness or to ease of recovery from unusual attitudes, including 1) pitch scale compression (2:1), 2) automatic change from 1:1 to compressed pitch (2:1) during unusual attitudes, 3) adding an arrow (Augie Arrow) to indicate the recovery direction, and 4) F-18-style slanted pitch lines (bendy bars).

Some modifications offered slight improvements, but not significant enough to warrant recommending their inclusion: 1) six-to-one pitch scale compression (both full time and changing automatically on unusual attitude entry), and 2) vertical asymmetry in the pitch ladder (different line arrangement above and below the horizon).

Various styles of bank scales (sky pointers or ground pointers) were evaluated. No effect was noted. Laterally asymmetric pitch ladders were tried ("rungs" on one side only), but proved to be extremely disorienting.

Deaton et al.[85] examined the effect of various HUD pitch ladders on unusual-attitude recovery and on the ability of the pilot to detect outside visual targets. They proposed an enhanced pitch ladder with slanted pitch lines and sharks teeth at extreme nose-low angles. A subsequent study[86] also examined the effect of orientation cues embedded in the HUD symbology. They found the Augie Arrow developed earlier[76] to be effective in aiding the pilot during recoveries from unusual attitudes. Chandra[87] and Chandra and Weintraub[88] found similar results.

In 1989, researchers at the USAF School of Aerospace Medicine reported the results of static evaluations of various pitch-ladder formats on orientation recognition. Ercoline et al.[89] compared articulated bars vs a combination of bendy bars below the horizon and straight lines above. The combined format was presented in three versions: all lines of equal length, lines becoming shorter as the angle from the horizon increased (tapering), and lines becoming thicker at extreme negative pitch angles. The results for pitch recognition favored bendy bars and increasing the thickness of the pitch lines as the angle from the horizon increases.

For bank orientation,[89] the conclusion was drawn that lateral asymmetry favored bank recognition. This result differed from that of the earlier Patuxent River study, which found that lateral asymmetry promoted disorientation.[16,76] The difference was one of degree of asymmetry. Newman used a pitch ladder drawn on one side only, which was described by the evaluation pilots as lopsided and promoted a tendency to bank the airplane. Ercoline et al.[89] used a subtler lateral asymmetry.

Later studies, however, concluded that articulated pitch-ladder lines created problems with bank recognition during unusual attitudes. In 1990, the United Kingdom studied alternative pitch-ladder formats for the multinational European Fighter Aircraft. This HUD was to have used F-18 style pitch-ladders, which Penwill and Hall[90] evaluated with the tapered pitch lines of the FastJet. The simulation was conducted on a simulator that had large-amplitude motion cues and an inflatable seat cushion to simulate G forces. The results showed a clear subjective and objective preference for tapered pitch ladders over the articulated pitch ladders. Several pilots made 180-deg errors in judging bank with the articulated lines and rolled the wrong way during recoveries. This observation was supported by a USAF-sponsored study by Weinstein et al.[18] They noted that control errors during unusual-attitude recoveries were about twice as likely with articulated vs tapered lines in the bottom of the display. Weinstein et al.[91] also evaluated airspeed and altitude scales, comparing conventional tapes with various formats. The task was maintenance of airspeed and altitude in the presence of disturbances. The results indicate that digits plus counterpointers are preferred. Vertical tapes tended to promote more incorrect responses than counterpointers.

The primary flight display on HUDs in civilian aircraft must be shown to display the correct attitude throughout 360 deg of pitch and roll by orienting the attitude gyro on a tilt table prior to flight tests.[92] There is no formal requirement for unusual-attitude recovery studies to be performed for HUDs on fixed-wing civilian aircraft, although most HUD development projects do evaluate unusual attitude recoveries.[12] To be approved for IFR flight, primary flight symbology on rotary-wing aircraft is required to undergo an unusual-attitude recovery evaluation.[93,94] Normally, the most cluttered navigation format should be used during unusual-attitude recoveries. Automatic declutter of navigation data during unusual-attitude recoveries has been incorporated in some HUDs to avoid a cluttered format.[95]

B. HMD Studies

1. Fixed Wing

There have been a limited number of studies dealing with a variety of HMD SD issues. Experiments have compared the use of HMD symbology to no symbology, the use of Earth-fixed symbology to nonconformal symbologies, and the advantage of specific attitude and other primary flight displays.

Jones et al.[52] had pilots fly simulated air-to-air missions with two different types of HMD primary flight symbology formats. There were more attitude judgment errors with an Earth-fixed (conformal) symbology rather than one that always depicted the horizon movement from a forward view of the aircraft. Pilots also preferred the forward-view symbology by a margin of 7:1.

Osgood et al.[96] and Geiselman and Osgood[42,97−99] developed a symbology (theta format) to aid in unusual-attitude encounters. Osgood et al.[96] compared using a HUD with a combination of HUD and HMD for attitude control and concluded that the combination of a HUD and HMD was superior. Geiselman and Osgood[89] studied several fixed-wing symbologies designed to convey aircraft orientation while the pilot was looking off axis. They determined that ownship attitude information enhanced the ability of the pilot to spend more time looking off axis (and presumably looking for targets). Geiselman and Osgood[42] found that the theta ball (a miniature version of a virtual world with a climb–dive marker in the middle of it) and the orange peel (ASAR) version both proved superior to the traditional climb–dive ladder in maintenance of spatial orientation and avoidance of ground collisions when pilots were subjected to turbulence. Geiselman[100] followed this line and developed the NDFR, which used the ASAR. Geiselman's symbology is flight-path based to better present aircraft energy state to the pilot.

DeVilbiss et al.[101] addressed the effect of off-axis targeting and unusual-attitude recovery. In their experiment the pilot was required to acquire a target and then recover from an unusual attitude. They found that when pilots were looking off axis with no flight instrumentation in their view recoveries from unusual attitudes were delayed by about 0.5 s—the time necessary to look at the HUD to begin recovery. They found that by displaying (screen-fixed) information on the HMD recoveries could begin sooner. This study did not evaluate the usefulness of screen-fixed symbology on mission performance, only on unusual attitude recovery.

2. Rotary Wing

Haworth and Seery[47] examined several improvements on AH-64 (*Apache*) helicopter symbols. Their test results indicate that pilots perform significantly better when using *Earth-fixed* symbology over the standard *Apache* screen-fixed symbol set. Haworth and Seery noted that both the standard and modified symbology caused incorrect cyclic inputs during hover tasks while looking off axis. They recommended further improvements in hover symbology

Haworth et al.[102] studied the effect of different stabilizations based on AH-64 symbols. The performance improved with *Earth-fixed* flight path marker and horizon line combined with screen-fixed nonspatial data (airspeed, etc.). The best symbol set appeared to be that of the *Longbow Apache* but with an uncompressed pitch ladder, compass rose, and ownship symbol with the horizon *Earth-fixed* and visible off axis.

C. Pathway Displays

Nontraditional symbologies, such as pathway in the sky, are being developed for use in HUDs, HMDs, and head-down displays (HDD) (see Chapter 9, Sec. III.C.2). The use of both sensor images and database terrain imagery are also being proposed for inclusion into flight displays. Several studies have evaluated the effectiveness of these displays on spatial awareness and unusual-attitude recovery.

Reising et al.[30] compared unusual-attitude recoveries using two traditional HUD symbology formats and a pathway format. In this experiment the pathway display commanded the recovery in accordance with standard USAF procedures. Nevertheless, the average reaction time was significantly slower (by about 100 ms) with the pathway than with either HUD symbology. Following the experiment, the pilots were given five days of practice with the pathway and were able to reduce their reaction times. The conclusion seems to be that the intuitive pathway still requires training or practice to meet the unusual-attitude recovery performance of standard HUD symbology.

On a HUD, Fadden et al.[40] reported superior lateral and vertical tracking performance with a pathway compared with conventional ILS formats. This advantage was presumably caused by the predictive flight information provided by a three-dimensional view of the intended trajectory. Fadden et al.[40] found little cost in detection of airplane-related events, although there was some evidence of attentional tunneling with the pathway format. Fadden et al.[40] also demonstrated the optimal use of a pathway display is on a HUD as opposed to a HDD panel.

VII. Unusual-Attitude-Recovery Techniques

An overall reassessment of unusual-attitude (UA)-recovery techniques is essential at this point in time, particularly with HUD- and HMD-equipped airplanes. In a critical UA the airplane is likely to be in an extreme nose-high or nose-low attitude, and the rotation about one of more or its axes can be quite high. In this situation immediate recovery is imperative. Fortunately, the typical unusual attitude is not critical. Most UAs are noticed when the airplane has just begun to depart from level, unaccelerated flight. Recovery from these mild unusual attitudes can be accomplished using normal instrument techniques. Most instrument flight manuals direct their UA recovery techniques to these mild excursions. If an UA is allowed to develop, the recovery technique must be rapid and instinctively clear to the pilot, who might be confused, disoriented, and possibly incapacitated by G forces.

A basic issue concerning HUD symbology design has been whether its primary objective should be to keep the pilot oriented or to facilitate recovery from an unusual attitude. Although maintenance of spatial orientation is clearly a priority, pilots will occasionally enter extreme UAs attitudes regardless of the symbology, in which case rapid recovery is then paramount. A slightly nonoptimum symbology in terms of orientation maintenance might be a small price to pay for faster reaction time during a critical UA. With HUD displays, particularly those with 1:1 or near

1:1 pitch scaling, the lines and symbols might be moving too fast for a pilot to assess aircraft attitude easily. In the midst of a UA, the pilot should not have to decide whether the aircraft is nose high or nose low, upright or inverted—the display in use should clearly indicate the recovery. Judicious declutter of data not needed for recovery should be considered, although FAA regulations do not support this. However, important information, such as type of symbology set (mode annunciation), should remain available. (This can be an argument against excessive mode annunciations on the primary flight display.)

A. Tactical-Aircraft Recoveries

The UA recovery technique practiced with traditional gyroscopic artificial horizons on tactical (e.g., fighter and attack aircraft) remains the basis for unusual-attitude recoveries with all monochrome electronic displays (HUDs and HMDs) (see also Chapter 9, Sec. III.D.1). This technique calls on the pilot to roll to the horizon and does not require a decision about whether the airplane is upright or inverted. In adapting this UA recovery technique for a HUD-equipped airplane, the pilot would roll the aircraft to wings level, position the horizon at the top of the display, and then pull the aircraft's nose to the horizon. In the more critical, nose-low situation the effect of this recovery will be to roll upright and then pull to the horizon. In the nose-high situation the initial roll will lead into an inverted, nose-high position and a subsequent pull down to the horizon, leaving the aircraft in an inverted attitude. Such a stabilized inverted attitude is not considered to be a problem in a tactical or trainer aircraft.

A compressed pitch ladder, tapering of pitch lines, and an Augie Arrow all provide valuable information for attitude recovery. During an unusual attitude, the pilot need only roll toward the arrow and then pull to the horizon. Although the pitch ladder might be moving too fast to read during the roll, once the airplane is wings level, its motion should be slow enough for the pilot to assess the attitude and assist in the pull to the horizon. Bendy bars on the pitch ladder should also help in recovery, although the rapid display motion during the initial recovery probably prevents full use of this cue.

B. Transport Recoveries

The UA recovery technique just described might not be suitable for transports or helicopters. Alternative techniques that do not lead to inverted recoveries from nose-high unusual attitudes should be considered for transports. Appropriate recovery techniques will depend on the pilot recognizing the difference between a nose-high and a nose-low unusual attitude. Obviously, interpretation of the display to make this nose-high/nose-low determination will slightly delay the start of the recovery. For a transport the HUD should display the Augie Arrow only for nose-low unusual attitudes, as is done in the C-130J.

One of two nose-high recovery techniques should be followed, probably dependent on the type of aircraft: 1) roll to a near-90-deg bank, with a slice back to a near-level pitch attitude and a subsequent recovery to a wings-level upright position; or 2) roll to a wings-level, nose-high attitude followed by an easing back to a level pitch attitude. The nose-low recovery technique should be the same for transports as for tactical aircraft, with a roll to upright followed by a pull to the horizon.

C. HUD Symbology Features Relevant to Unusual-Attitude Recognition

There are a number of symbology features that can assist a pilot in recognizing and recovering from an unusual attitude. The pitch ladder and its reference are the most common symbology components that are used in spatial orientation. Both articulated pitch lines and tapered lines have been used. Most HUDs use a flight-path symbol, either in the form of a FPM or a climb–dive marker. Since the mid-1980s, military standards used climb–dive markers and pivoted the pitch ladder around the climb–dive marker. Civil transport HUDs, on the other hand, pivot the ladder around the aircraft pitch symbol. This is based on the requirements of the civil airworthiness requirements requiring aircraft pitch as the primary flight reference.[103]

The original HUD for the B-727 (Ref. 71) did not have an unusual-attitude mode as such. It did provide pitch scale compression based on keeping the horizon line within the FOV. Figure 16 shows the unusual-attitude-recovery format for the Flight Dynamics' most recent design, the HGS-4000 (Ref. 104). This format mimics the standard head-down AI familiar to all pilots, thereby taking advantage of pilots' previous head-down experience. No heading, sideslip, or flight-path information is shown.

Another civil transport HUD, the BAE Systems Visual Guidance System (VGS) HUD, enlarges the pitch marker during unusual attitudes. This HUD also changes its pitch-ladder format during unusual-attitude recoveries. The bottom portion pitch ladder mimics a ground plane to emphasize the difference between above-horizon and below-horizon attitudes, as shown in Fig. 17. It retains the heading scale (on the horizon) as well as flight-path information.

The C130J HUD uses a commercial off-the-shelf design that also complies with the FAA's pitch-centered attitude requirements. During normal attitudes, its HUD shows a pitch ladder pivoting around the climb–dive marker. During extreme attitudes, however, the HUD automatically reverts to the unusual-attitude mode (Fig. 18), in which the HUD uses a fully pitch-referenced ladder. In addition,

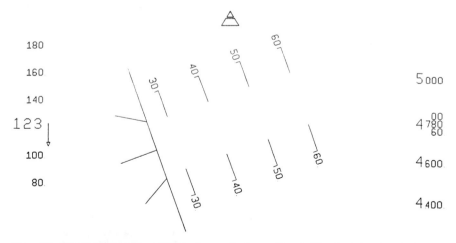

Fig. 16 HGS-4000 unusual-attitude symbology. (Reproduced with permission of Rockwell-Collins/Flight Dynamics.)

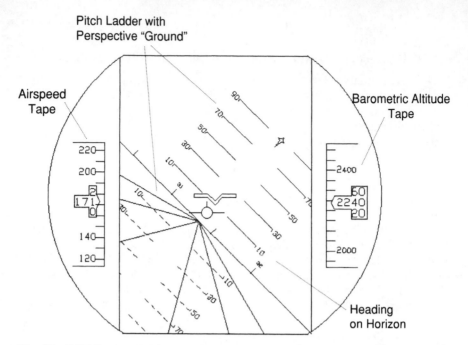

Fig. 17 BAE Systems VGS unusual-attitude symbology. (Reproduced with permission of BAE Systems.)

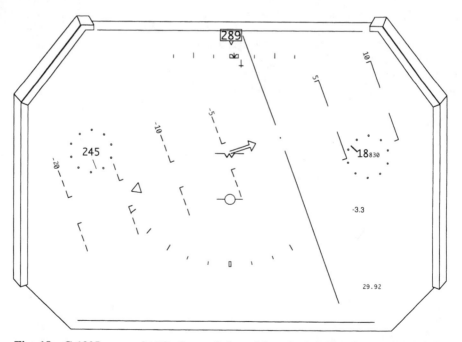

Fig. 18 C-130J unusual-attitude symbology. Note the roll-recovery arrow (Augie Arrow) at the pitch reference symbol. (Reproduced with permission of Rockwell-Collins/Flight Dynamics.)

the pitch ladder becomes enhanced to improve attitude awareness and, during nose-low recoveries, a roll-recovery arrow (Augie Arrow) directs the pilot's actions.

Table 1 gives a summary of the features of HUDs applicable to unusual-attitude recognition and recovery.

D. Display Scaling and Unusual-Attitude Recovery

Scaling (or compression) is the apparent size of the display. There are three aspects of scaling: gain, FOV, and registration. Gain is the amplitude of the display motion relative to airplane motion. Indirectly, it is the amplitude of display motion for a given control input. The predominant effect of gain determines the ease with which the pilot can close the loop and control the airplane. The primary effect of FOV is situation awareness; large FOVs generally favor improved situation awareness. This is primarily because of the presentation of a more global picture.

Registration means the HUD symbol overlays the out-the-window scene. These parameters are all intertwined; for example, variations in the FOV are directly related to changes in gain for a given display, and perfect registration automatically implies a 1:1 gain in pitch movement of the display relative to the outside world.

Display gain affects the ability of the pilot to control the aircraft through the display. Generally 1:1 (unity) scaling has been used for precise tasks, with more compression used for dynamic tasks, such as UA recovery.[14,70,76,105] Walters[106] reported improved instrument tracking with gains of the order of 1.5:1 or 2:1. This is in contrast to Roscoe et al.[107] who found that improved performance was found with display gains less than unity. Recently, Comstock et al.[108] showed no significant performance effects for various scalings on head-down image-based displays. They did show a pilot preference for unity or near-unity gains for several display sizes.

Many HUD designers have insisted on conformality, so that all symbol icons representing the real world exactly overlie the out-the-window scene. The definition of conformal means that angular representations in the out-the-window scene and in the display are identical, meaning that conformality is always associated with 1:1 pitch scaling. If matching the out-the-window scene is not essential, then there is no particular reason to insist on 1:1 scaling. There have been many HUDs designed without conformal symbology. Newman[2] describes these as pitch-referenced nonconformal HUDs. Other HUDs have used compressed scaling for specific flight regimes, usually during acrobatic maneuvers or UA recovery and involving non-ground-referenced symbols. Although no unconventional nonconformal symbologies have been used on the HUD such as the theta ball or ASAR, they have been tried with some success on HMDs, where conformality is less desirable.[52]

If a ground-referenced symbol is required for a compressed display, such a symbol can be displayed overlying its out-the-window counterpart. This will require that the compression be made about that symbol. This is the case in the RAF FastJet symbology[14] and in the MIL-STD-1787 symbology,[15] in which the compression center is the climb–dive or flight-path marker. Thus, the aircraft trajectory will over fly the projected flight path as seen out of the windshield. Civil HUDs usually program the compression about the aircraft's fuselage reference line (the water-line) and adjust the compression to keep the displayed horizon line just within the

Table 1 Unusual-attitude features of HUD standards

Format	UA mode	Pitch ladder	Scaling	Pivot	Aircraft symbol	Other cue	Scales
F-18	No	Bendy bars	1:1	Pitch marker	CDM or FPM[a]	—	Digital
FastJet	No	Tapered	Variable	CDM	CDM	—	CP[b]
MS-1787	No	Tapered above Bendy below	1:1	CDM	CDM	Ghost horizon	CP
B-727	No	Straight	Variable	Pitch marker	FPM	—	Digital
HGS-4000	Yes	Straight	Variable	Pitch marker	FPM	—	Tapes
C-130J	Yes	Straight	1:1	Pitch	Pitch marker	Augie Arrow	CP

[a]CDM-climb–dive marker and FPM-flight-path marker.
[b]CP-counterpointers.

display's FOV. Unfortunately, this virtually guarantees that no symbol will register over its out-the-window counterpart.

E.   Air-Mass Flight-Path Data

If the flight-path cue is based on motion relative to the air mass instead of motion relative to the world, the angular difference between pitch and flight path is equal to the AoA.

Although most modern HUDs use inertial flight-path cues, air mass cues have significant benefits in terms of maintenance of airspeed and AoA awareness. In the mid-1960s, Klopfstein[27] proposed the air-mass-derived HUD symbology shown in Fig. 4. He reported superior airspeed and attitude-tracking during flight tests, even with nonpilots. Figure 19 shows modified Klopfstein[27] symbology with a dashed line showing air-mass flight path (denoted γ). The figure shows how the pilot can compare the air-mass flight path with the desired approach AoA (α_{REF}, shown by the Δ symbol). Figure 19 also shows a fast approach with the AoA less than α_{REF}—the flight-path line is above the Δ. Figure 20 shows an on-speed AoA condition with the flight-path line just touching the Δ. Figure 21 shows the airplane at a stall position with the flight-path line touching the stall limit (shown as an area of slanted lines). The *Mercure* HUD symbology uses a pitch reference depressed at the desired AoA for a landing approach. This approach was developed from Klopfstein's original HUD symbology. Although the resultant scale is a "fly-from" index, it appears to promote AoA awareness. If airspeed is slow, the AoA becomes too great, and the index appears below the flight-path symbol. Anecdotal reports suggested that airspeed and flight-path control are very precise with Klopfstein's and related formats, but unfortunately no hard data are available to substantiate

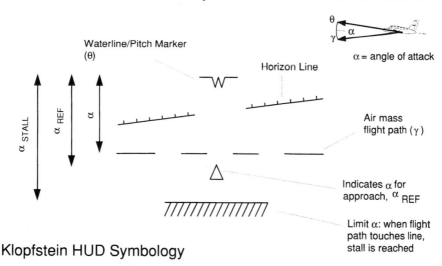

Klopfstein HUD Symbology

Fig. 19   Relationship between pitch, air-mass flight-path angle, and angle of attack. In this example airspeed is faster than approach speed ($\alpha < \alpha_{REF}$). That is, distance between $\overline{\text{W}}$ (θ) and horizontal dashed line (γ) is less than distance between $\overline{\text{W}}$ and top of $\triangle$.

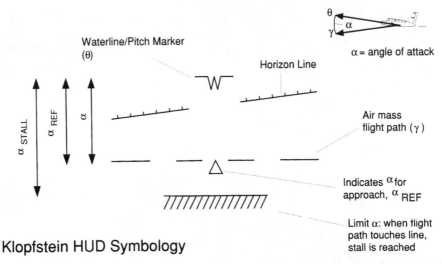

Klopfstein HUD Symbology

Fig. 20   Airspeed equal to approach speed ($\alpha = \alpha_{REF}$). That is, distance between ⌐W¬ (θ) and horizontal dashed line (γ) equals distance between ⌐W¬ and top of △.

these claims. A similar index was used in the A-7 HUD and led to the backwards AoA scale on that airplane.*

Newman et al.[109] proposed a HUD symbology for general aviation emphasizing air-mass data for airspeed awareness. Their approach changed the airspeed counterpointer from a multiple-revolution dial with a central digital airspeed to a

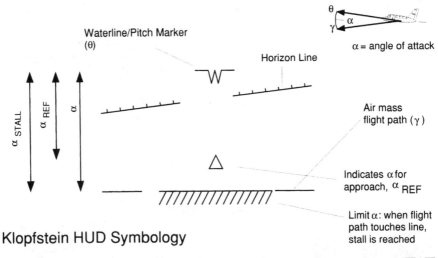

Klopfstein HUD Symbology

Fig. 21   Airspeed equal to stall speed ($\alpha = \alpha_{STALL}$). That is, distance between ⌐W¬ (θ) and horizontal dashed line (γ) equals distance between ⌐W¬ and top of slanted lines.

---

*Personal communication with Norm Driscoll, LTV, Oct. 1973.

single-revolution dial, still with the digital readout. The scaling is such that the pointer is at the half past one o'clock position at 1-G stall speed, at the three o'clock position at approach reference speed, and directly upward at the red line.

VIII. Conclusions and Recommendations

A. Display Issues

Head-up displays do not, by themselves, cause SD. They do have some features that can be improved to provide pilots with more help during UA recoveries. Overall, the advantages of HUDs far outweigh any disadvantages, and several decades of HUD research have produced a number of benefits, notably improved symbology, improved attitude-recovery standardization and pilot training, as well as the inclusion of unusual attitude recoveries as part of certification testing.

Unfortunately, the net advantage of HUDs cannot be ascribed to HMDs *at this time*. The current level of HMD technology development is about where HUDs were in the mid-1980s. Some questions need to be answered:

1) Does the HMD promote SD? There is some evidence that conflicts between out-the-window and display orientation cues, as well as head-tracker limitations, contribute to the onset of SD.

2) Is there a clear understanding of the best techniques to use to recover from an unusual attitude using a HMD?

3) What primary flight symbology should be used in HMDs?

Despite the promise shown by novel displays such as pathway displays and synthetic vision displays that are being proposed for all three display instruments (HUD, HMD, and HDD), SD and unusual-attitude issues must be addressed with the same care that was taken with HUD evaluations in recent years. Several questions must be addressed:

1) Does the use of a realistic scene help or hinder spatial awareness?

2) Do the geographical awareness benefits of a terrain- based background, with possible false horizons, outweigh the potential for SD?

3) Do the many lines associated with the pathway in the sky interfere with spatial orientation?

The NASA synthetic vision program is currently investigating general aviation applications with a heavy emphasis on inadvertent loss of control in IMC. Simulator experiments have been completed and should be reported in the near future.[110]

B. Design Recommendations

Display designers must consider the likelihood that pilots will encounter SD and must therefore incorporate cues to enhance recognition of, and recovery from, unusual attitudes.

Although flight-path data surely enhance tracking performance and general situation awareness, loss of attitude awareness can lead to SD. Including a pitch reference in the basic HUD symbology should maximize attitude awareness. Although there are reasons for omitting the pitch marker, such omission should be done with care, as the flight-path marker can provide misleading recovery cues once in an unusual attitude. It is recommended that an enhanced pitch reference, similar to that on the HGS-4000 or the C-130J HUD, be displayed at least during an unusual attitude.

Conformality carries some advantages, but a unity pitch gain during air combat maneuvers, acrobatics, or unusual attitudes can be disorienting. The HUD designer should consider the use of pitch scale compression during such phases of flight. Certainly, pitch compression is appropriate for an unusual-attitude mode and might even generally improve performance on instrument tasks.[106]

Directed recovery cues, such as the Augie Arrow, can enhance the recognition of, and recovery from, unusual attitudes. Unusual-attitude-recovery cues are generally mechanized to appear when the horizon disappears from the display's FOV. Directed recovery cues should be oriented to point to the sky, which will allow their use as a simple roll-to-and-pull attitude-recovery cue. Because of this, a horizon pointer is preferred to a pointer mechanized to point to the sky. For many aircraft, such as transports and helicopters, this means that the Augie Arrow should only be displayed during nose-low unusual attitudes. Because unusual attitudes can be associated with unreliable flight-path information, reversion to a pitch reference will be likely. For this reason the directed recovery cue should be designed to work well with the pitch marker.

C. Research and Evaluation Issues

Research into the mechanism of aircraft control during the transition between visual flight and instrument flight is needed to supplement unusual-attitude-recovery studies currently employed for display evaluation. Peripheral cues are likely to be important. They will affect both the visual flight prior to entering instrument conditions and the transition from visual to instrument flight. Good peripheral cues should be provided during visual flight conditions, at least during follow-on experiments. It is especially important to record pilot-fixation points and to document the presence or absence of the OKCR and the role of the OKCR on symbology development. Finally, it is important to consider aircraft dynamics, particularly spiral divergence. Aircraft dynamics must be realistic and representative of the aircraft being considered.

Any design of a new display or display symbology must include testing for its effect on SD and other elements of situation awareness. This normally means an evaluation of the display's effect on unusual-attitude recoveries. These tests should be conducted using the most cluttered formats available for display. Newman and Greeley[111] outline the procedures for conducting these tests and are summarized in Appendix A (see also Chapter 9, Sec. III.D). (Test methods are covered in detail in Appendix A.)

Appendix A: Flight-Test Techniques

There are several so-called standard flight and simulator techniques used in spatial-disorientation evaluations. These are unusual-attitude recoveries, attitude awareness evaluations, and studies of entry into loss of control. Of these, the unusual-attitude recovery is the most common test.

Following some general considerations for the selection of evaluation pilots and data recording issues, we will outline test procedures for unusual attitude recovery studies, failure detection, and attitude awareness evaluations. Further details can be found in Newman and Greeley.[111]

A. Choice of Pilots

A significant issue is what type of pilots should be used to perform the display evaluations: test pilots or operational pilots? The chief advantage of using operational pilots is their recent mission experience. A second advantage is the ability to obtain a range of experience levels from recent pilot training graduates to experienced pilots.

One problem with using operational pilots is that each pilot is often overtrained on a particular display and might be predisposed to that display—F-16 pilots prefer F-16 symbology, F-18 pilots prefer F-18 symbology, etc. Ideally, one should use operational pilots with no symbology background. Unfortunately, this is not possible. To avoid this problem, the experimenter must ensure that no particular symbology is overrepresented and that the subjective data are used with care.

Arguments favoring test pilots include having trained evaluators. Test pilots are used to rate airplane handling and should be familiar with rating scales such as the Cooper–Harper-type of walk-through ratings. Test pilots are also skilled at communicating with engineers and can provide insight into display or control problems. The specific choice between operational and test pilots should be based on the particular test issues.

The choice of numbers of evaluation pilots is driven by the desire for a large statistical sample and the cost/schedule constraints of flight test. Generally, simulator evaluations using a fairly large number (10–25) of pilots are used to provide a statistical sample. Flight testing is then performed to validate the simulator results. For most *flight* evaluations of displays, six evaluation pilots is a reasonable compromise between a sufficient statistical sample and the typical cost and time constraints associated with a display evaluation program.

B. Data Consideration

1. Objective Data

Table A.1 shows typical data that should be recorded as functions of time. Sampling rates should be frequent enough to ensure that the bandwidth of interest is recorded. The basic rule of thumb is to sample at 2–4 times the highest frequency present in the data. As a matter of practice, however, sampling will be driven by the data bus rates. Digital data will be sampled from the data bus at the bus rate (or its submultiple).

Sampling at too great a rate can lead to storage problems and excessive posttest processing requirements. Sampling at too small a rate can lead to loss of high-frequency data. The flight-test engineer must ensure that neither occurs. Table A1 shows typical data sampling rates. Specific aircraft and system issues might require greater sampling rates.

2. Subjective Data

Pilot ratings are an integral part of these evaluations. Both preference-based scales[112] and subjective ratings Cooper–Harper[113] ratings have been used.

Table A.1   Typical data sampling

Type of data	Normal sampling rate, Hz
Indicated airspeed	4
Pitch	20–40
Heading	20
Bank	20–40
Elevator control position	20–40
Aileron control position	20–40
Rudder control position	20
Radar altitude	4
Display image	30
Event marker indicating start	10

Preference ratings must be used with caution.[114] Haworth and Newman[115] developed display ratings based on the Cooper–Harper scales. Their display readability and display flyability ratings measure both the ease of reading the display and the ease of controlling the aircraft. Additional details can be found in Newman and Greeley.[111] Normally, subjective ratings are hand-recorded. Voice recording can be used to indicate the start of the maneuver and to supplement the hand-recorded data.

There are two aspects of flight displays that must be considered: 1) can the pilot determine the value of a specific parameter, such as airspeed? and 2) can the display be used to control that parameter? These two questions must be answered in the context of a specific task scenario.

Because of the widespread acceptance of the handling qualities rating scale[113] in the flight-test community, Haworth and Newman[115] constructed two flowcharts to rate the readability and the controllability of displays. Like the handling qualities rating, these display evaluation ratings are flight task dependent and require the evaluator to rate his or her ability to determine parameter values with desired/adequate accuracy or control the aircraft in the context of the flight task being performed.

a.   Display readability rating.   The display readability rating (DRR) is a subjective assessment of how well the pilot can determine the values of parameters shown on the display in question. The display readability chart is shown in Fig. A.1. It requires the evaluator to rate his or her ability to determine parameter values with desired/adequate accuracy in the context of the flight task being performed. The DRR can also be applied to the ease of overall maintenance of situation awareness (SA). However, such ratings are only a subjective assessment of SA.

Display readability ratings are normally expressed on a 1 (=good) to 10 (=bad) scale are often divided into several levels:

1) Level 1 (DRR = 1–3):   Satisfactory without improvement
2) Level 2 (DRR = 4–6):   Acceptable, deficiencies warrant, but do not require improvement
3) Level 3 (DRR = 7–8):   Unacceptable, deficiencies require improvement
4) Level 4 (DRR = 9–10): Unacceptable, display cannot be interpreted

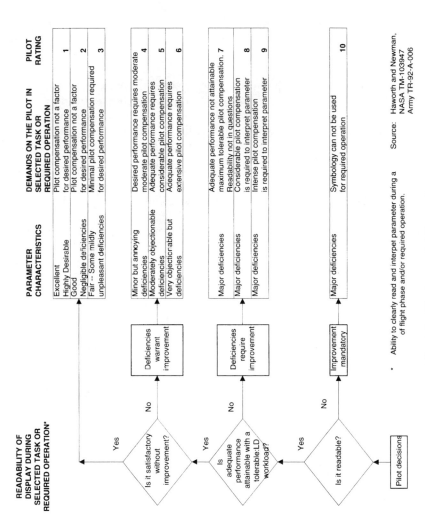

Fig. A.1 Display readability rating.

b. Display flyability rating. The display flyability rating (DFR) is a subjective assessment of how well the pilot can control specific parameters using on the display in question. The display flyability ratings follow the Cooper and Harper[113] original handling qualities rating decision tree closely. The difference between the display flyability rating and a handling qualities rating is the requirement that the evaluation pilot consider aircraft control using the display for information. The flowchart is shown in Fig. A.2.

The DFR is essentially a handling qualities rating of the airplane handling qualities in series with the display control laws. This rating will be expected to vary from aircraft to aircraft for a given symbology. Like the handling qualities rating, the DFRs are flight task dependent. Careful attention must be paid to ensuring that the flight tasks are appropriate and that proper performance criteria are established. The DFRs require the evaluator to rate his or her ability to achieve desired/adequate performance goals and the amount of compensation required to correct for deficiencies in the context of the flight task being performed.

The ratings are normally expressed on a 1 (=good) to 10 (=bad) scale and are often divided into several levels:

1) Level 1 (DFR = 1–3):   Satisfactory without improvement
2) Level 2 (DFR = 4–6):   Acceptable, deficiencies warrant, but do not
                                         require improvement
3) Level 3 (DFR = 7–9):   Unacceptable, deficiencies require improvement
4) Level 4 (DFR = 9–10):   Unacceptable, control cannot be maintained

c. Display data cards. We have already stated that a deficiency in these ratings is the amount of time it takes for an untrained evaluator to learn to use the scales. This is a minor concern for flying qualities or handling qualities evaluations because the evaluators are trained test pilots. It can be a significant concern for display evaluations because of the large number of issues being evaluated and, perhaps more important, because of the need to use operational pilots.

For this latter reason, programs in the past (such as Ref. 116) have broken the logic diagrams down and constructed data cards that asked the questions for the various choices in the Cooper–Harper logic trees and indicated the desirable and acceptable performance criteria. These data cards have, for example, constructed the DFR from the two questions shown here:

Could you read airspeed to an accuracy of

(_) 2 kn (desirable?)
(_) 5 kn (acceptable?)
(_) __ kn
(_) couldn't read airspeed at all

How much compensation or effort was required to read the airspeed?

(_) none
(_) minimal
(_) moderate
(_) considerable
(_) intense

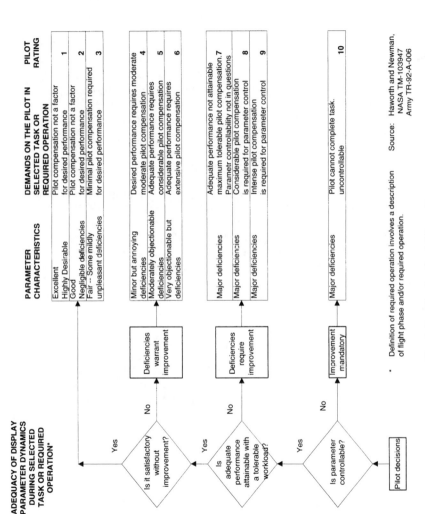

Fig. A.2 Display flyability rating.

From these questions the actual DRR can be constructed after the flight without requiring the evaluation pilot to memorize the logic chart or constantly refer to it. The safety pilot or flight-test engineer can ask these questions and mark the answers on a data card. For example, if the evaluation pilot checked the first block on question 1 (2 kn) and the third block on question 2 (moderate), the DRR would be 4. A second advantage is that it requires the evaluation pilot to state his or her achieved performance explicitly. This will become useful later in the situation awareness testing.

It has been suggested that stating the acceptable and desired performance goals creates a bias on the part of the evaluation pilot. This might be true, but it is important for the pilot flying a particular task to know his or her performance objectives. It is difficult to conceive of an operational pilot not trying to maintain a target level (i.e., performance not achieved, but workload very low). For this reason the preceding questionnaire states the performance goals. Newman and Greeley[111] present sample data cards.

3. Performance Criteria

Cooper–Harper and Haworth–Newman ratings both require that the evaluator compare actual performance with desired and acceptable standards. It is important that the performance criteria be explicitly stated as part of the experimental briefings for the evaluation pilots standards. The main function of performance criteria is to provide the evaluation pilot with performance targets. However, they also serve to aid in pass/fail decisions. For display evaluations intended for aircraft or display certification, the performance criteria will normally be established by the certification authority. The normal pass/fail threshold is 95% of test points meeting acceptable performance. In many cases the evaluation might be intended to compare several display concepts. The researcher might wish to modify these criteria to aid in this evaluation. Recommended criteria from Newman and Greeley[111] are given for each test described in Secs. A.3.9.4, A.3.9.5, and 4.6.

Criteria should reflect the intended operational use of the aircraft or display. A good source for performance criteria is the training syllabus for the aircraft in question (or for a related aircraft). The pass/fail standards for trainees should be used for the adequate performance criteria. Desired performance criteria should be one-half to two-thirds better than the pass/fail standards.

C. Unusual-Attitude Recovery

Unusual-attitude recovery is the most common test used for determining the effectiveness of a display in providing orientation cues to the pilot. In these evaluations the aircraft is placed in an extreme UA, and the evaluation pilot is asked to recover to straight and level. Recoveries should be evaluated in simulators and in flight. The simulator evaluation should encompass all unusual attitudes (including the more extreme attitudes), followed by enough aircraft unusual attitudes to ensure a valid statistical sample. Unusual attitudes should go beyond 90 deg of bank in all aircraft (at least in simulated flight).

There are usually one or both of the following objectives for this test: 1) to check the adequacy of the attitude display; and 2) to determine the utility of the display to allow the pilot to recognize and recover from unusual attitudes.

1. Conduct of the Test

Unusual-attitude recovery tests require a fully functioning display and a means to prevent the evaluation pilot from viewing the external visual scene. It is important during display evaluations that the complete range of display declutter options be investigated—from the basic, fully decluttered format through the complete display with all navigation and auxiliary scales present. Some early HUD unusual-attitude studies did not allow for declutter, and redesign was required following testing.[114] Difficulties with cluttered displays have led to the use of automatic declutter during UAs.

A predetermined number (eight is typical) of pitch-and-bank attitudes should be established covering the range of unusual attitudes to be flown. These will vary depending on the type of aircraft. Fighter aircraft and general aviation airplanes should cover attitudes through 180 deg of roll and at least 45 deg of pitch (30 deg for light airplanes). Transport airplanes and helicopters should include banks beyond 90 deg and pitch angles of 30 deg. A number of replications are usually performed.

With the aircraft in straight-and-level flight, the evaluation display should be blanked. The safety pilot flies the aircraft into a predetermined UA at which point the display is restored and the flight controls are given back to the evaluation pilot for recovery. Recent flight-test programs have programmed unusual-attitude entries into the autopilot.[54,117] This program makes the entries much more consistent but is probably only available for variable-stability fly-by-wire aircraft.

During simulator evaluations, the operator normally simply resets the simulator to the desired unusual-attitude entry conditions. An alternative simulator entry has the pilot fly in trail to a lead aircraft, which then performs a series of maneuvers covering the desired envelope of attitudes. At an unexpected time the lead aircraft is removed from the simulator scene, and the pilot recovers to straight and level. This approach was used by Gallimore et al.[118] This entry technique should be more realistic than the conventional reset initialization.

Regardless of the entry procedure, once the desired attitude has been reached, the evaluation pilot recovers to straight and level using standard procedures (see Refs. 119 and 120).

2. Choice of Pilots

A combination of test pilots and operational pilots should be used for unusual-attitude-recovery evaluation. Test pilots bridge the gap between handling qualities testing, which might be important if the display or aircraft dynamics are in question. Operational pilots bring mission experience and provide a spectrum of experience. The operational pilot experience should include diversity of experience, which is important for operational display issues.

3. Data

The following aircraft performance data should be recorded as a function of time: 1) airspeed, 2) barometric altitude, 3) heading, 4) pitch attitude, 5) bank angle, 6) sideslip, 7) bank control input, 8) pitch control input, 9) yaw control input, and 10) throttle input. Also, subjective pilot ratings should be obtained for each replication.

4. Performance Criteria

Typical performance criteria are listed here. The criteria for desired performance are reaction time to initial correct control input <0.7 s, no initial control reversals, initial control input in accordance with published standards, and no overshoots on recovery. (Published standards include instrument flight manuals[119-121] or aircraft flight manuals.) The criteria for adequate performance are reaction time to initial correct control input <1.2 s, single initial control reversal, initial control input in accordance with published standards, and single overshoot on recovery. Some experiments have used total time to recovery, altitude lost, or altitude gained as performance measures. These have generally been more sensitive to the entry conditions than to the display characteristics.

5. Safety Considerations During Flight Tests

These flight tests involve a hooded evaluation pilot. Adequate scan of the external visual scene by the safety pilot is essential. Care must be taken to ensure that the vision restriction for the evaluation pilot does not impair the vision of the safety pilot. The unusual attitudes flown in flight must be within the safe capability of the aircraft. More extreme attitudes should be performed in the simulator.

D. Attitude Awareness

Attitude awareness testing complements the standard unusual-attitude recovery where the pilot is placed in an unusual attitude and tasked to recover. This test is designed to evaluate the ability of the display symbology to convey spatial-orientation awareness to the pilot. The objectives are to evaluate the ability of the display and symbology to convey spatial-orientation awareness pilot and to evaluate the display's cues that allow pilots to recognize and recover from inadvertent unusual attitudes.

1. Conduct of the Test

The attitude awareness test should be flown in ground-based simulators in appropriate aircraft configurations. It should be performed in all display modes, including decluttered. The evaluation pilot should be tasked to follow another aircraft in trail formation. The lead aircraft or symbol will fly a series of maneuvers within the capability of the aircraft under evaluation similar to the method of Gallimore et al.[118]

The evaluation pilot will be instructed to follow the aircraft but not to exceed normal limitations in bank and pitch angle, minimum and maximum airspeed, and minimum altitude. These values should be clearly defined. The lead aircraft will, during the course of the test, approach these limits and periodically exceed them. When any limit is exceeded, the pilot will be instructed to make a verbal call and recover to straight-and-level flight using standard procedures from instrument flight manuals or other published standard. Following recovery, the pilot should complete the subject display ratings. If the evaluation pilot fails to note penetration of the envelope limits, the lead aircraft will be removed from the scene after 2 s, forcing the pilot to initiate an unusual-attitude recovery. Several replications of these flight envelope limit test points will be required.

2. Choice of Pilots

Pilots used in these evaluations should be current in the mission or a similar mission. These tests are embedded in mission scenarios, and it is important that operational crews be used. Normally, test pilots would not be appropriate for these evaluations. It is important that there is a diversity of experience among the evaluation pilots.

3. Data

The following aircraft performance data should be recorded as a function of time: 1) airspeed, 2) barometric altitude, 3) heading, 4) pitch attitude, 5) bank angle, 6) sideslip, 7) bank control input, 8) pitch control input, 9) yaw control input, and 10) throttle input. Also, subjective pilot ratings should be obtained for each replication.

Pilot estimates of bearing should be obtained from his or her initial course decisions. Once established on the new course, the safety pilot/simulator operator should ask for estimates of distances and course line aspect.

4. Performance Criteria

Performance criteria for attitude awareness are similar to those used in unusual-attitude recoveries. The criteria for desired performance are as follows: abandoned pursuit at aircraft limitations [±5 kn (9.5 km/h), ±10-deg bank tolerance], abandoned pursuit at altitude floor [±100-ft (30.5-m) tolerance], reaction time to initial correct control input <1.5 s, no initial control reversals, initial control input in accordance with published standards, and no overshoot on recovery. [These reaction times are somewhat longer that those for the simple unusual-attitude recovery (see Sec. C.4). This reflects the difference between an expected unusual attitude and an unexpected one (as in this test).] The criteria for adequate performance are as follows: abandoned pursuit at aircraft limitations [±10 kn (18.5 km/h), ±20-deg bank tolerance], abandoned pursuit at altitude floor [±500-ft (151.5-m) tolerance], reaction time to initial correct control input <2.0 s, single initial control reversal, initial control input in accordance with published standards, and single overshoot on recovery.

5. Safety Considerations During Flight Tests

These tests are flown in the simulator because of the hazards involved with aggressive formation flight in instrument conditions.

E. Failure Detection

Failure-detection tests are intended to measure situation awareness during display evaluation. They are means of introducing unusual attitudes in a more realistic fashion than the traditional UA recovery. The tests shown here are based on the presumption that the best measure of SA is the effect on pilot performance.

These tests are designed to verify that the pilot can recognize critical failures and take appropriate corrective action while maintaining aircraft control. They should be flown in conjunction with other evaluations, particularly the mission task testing. Navigation, sensor, and display system failures should be introduced during mission-related tasks to determine the reaction time and responses of the pilot. Appropriate procedures for operating the aircraft following these failures should be established prior to conducting these tests.

1. Conduct of the Test

Typical failures (and representative simulation means) include 1) navigation failure (pull circuit breaker); 2) attitude gyro failure (software simulation of both hardover and slow failures); 3) flight director failure (software simulation of both hardover and slow failures); 4) compass failure (pull circuit breaker or software simulation); 5) airspeed or altitude transducer (pull circuit breaker or equivalent); or 5) head tracker failure (pull circuit breaker or software simulation).

A special software version might be required to allow the flight-test engineer to introduce some system failures such as simulating attitude gyro failures. If such software versions are used, the response of the system to the simulated failure should be verified prior to conducting these tests. For tests involving operations in instrument conditions, the evaluation pilot should be hooded or otherwise prevented from using outside visual cues. System failures should be introduced during operations at unexpected times by the safety pilot or flight-test engineer.

Upon recognition of the failure, the evaluation pilot should take appropriate action as described in the aircraft/system-operating procedures. The evaluation pilot will be briefed to make a verbal call upon recognition of all system failures as a means of determining detection time. Following recovery, the evaluation pilot should complete display ratings.

2. Choice of Pilots

Pilots used in these evaluations should be current in the mission or a similar mission. These tests are embedded in mission scenarios, and it is important that operational crews be used. Normally, test pilots would not be appropriate for these evaluations. A wide range of pilot experience should be used.

For flight evaluations test pilots will normally serve as safety pilots and have in-flight responsibility for ensuring that test conditions are met. For multicrew airplanes the test pilot can serve as the copilot. For simulator evaluations only operational crewmembers should be used.

3. Data

Aircraft performance data should be recorded as functions of time: 1) airspeed, 2) barometric altitude, 3) radar altitude, 4) heading, 5) course deviation, 6) glide-slope deviation, 7) geographical position, 8) signal indicating start of failure, and 9) system parameters as appropriate. Also, subjective pilot ratings should be obtained for each failure introduced.

4. Performance Criteria

Generally, the criteria depend on the type of failure introduced. Examples for attitude failures and heading failures are shown in Table A.2. The pilot should

Table A.2   Performance criteria for failure detection testing

Failure detection performance	Attitude failures	Heading failures
	Desired performance	
Failure detection time	Less than 1 s	Less than 2 s
Maintain altitude	Within ±200 ft (61 m)	Within ±100 ft (30.5 m)
Maintain airspeed	Within ±10 kn (18 km/h)	Within ±5 kn (9.25 km/h)
Maintain heading	Within ±10 deg	Within ±10 deg
Pilot actions	In accordance with published standards	In accordance with published standards
	Adequate performance	
Failure detection time	Less than 2 s	Less than 5 s
Maintain altitude	Within ±500 ft (152.5 m)	Within ±200 ft (61 m)
Maintain airspeed	Within ±20 kn (37 km/h)	Within ±10 kn (18.5 km/h)
Maintain heading	Within ±20 deg	Within ±20 deg
Pilot actions	In accordance with published standards	In accordance with published standards

detect an attitude failure faster than a heading failure, although he or she will likely have larger excursions while coping with the failure. Slowly developing failures, such as autopilot softovers might require more time to detect. In such cases it is better to describe performance in terms of flight-path deviations rather than time.

5.   Safety Considerations During Flight Tests

For flight tests suitable precautions must ensure that the safety pilot's systems are not affected by these simulated failures for the evaluation pilot. The safety pilot must also ensure that air-traffic clearances are not jeopardized.

F.   Geographic Awareness

Geographic awareness tests evaluate scenarios duplicating situations encountered during normal flight operations, where the pilot must maintain geographical orientation. Typical scenarios include 1) a deviation from a planned flight plan caused by intentional deviations around weather, obstacles, or threats, followed by a return to the original flight plan; 2) a deviation from a planned flight plan caused by intentional deviations around weather, obstacles, or threats, followed by a modification to the flight plan (such as bypassing the next waypoint); 3) changing the flight-plan route; 4) changing to another, unplanned instrument approach; or 5) diverting to an alternate.

These tests are intended to determine if the navigation display permits the maintenance of geographical awareness. At the same time other parallel evaluations should be conducted to ensure that the navigation display is suitable and the pilot can enter the necessary data to generate a new flight plan during those tests which involve flight-plan modification. Geographic evaluations should be flown in conjunction with other evaluations, particularly full mission simulations.

1. Conduct of the Test

The pilot should be given a typical mission profile to fly. During the course of flying this profile, he or she will be given diversion instructions by the safety pilot. The diversions should be representative of normal operations. The evaluation pilot should be hooded or otherwise prevented from using outside visual cues. Examples of such instructions might include the follwoing:

1) The first example is a series of heading instructions around a hypothetical weather buildup, an obstacle, or a threat. The evaluation pilot will then be told to return to the original flight-plan route.

2) The second example is a series of heading instructions around a hypothetical weather buildup, an obstacle, or a threat. The evaluation pilot will then be told to fly directly to a waypoint on the original flight plan. This need not be the next sequential waypoint; some evaluations should involve flying to another waypoint. These instructions should include terminal area navigation simulating air-traffic radar vectoring followed by a clearance to join the published instrument approach procedure, either a planned procedure or an alternate procedure.

3) The third example is an instruction to fly directly to a subsequent waypoint, bypassing the active waypoint.

4) The last example is an instruction to divert to an alternate destination.

2. Choice of Pilots

Pilots used in these evaluations should be current in the mission or a similar mission. These tests are embedded in mission scenarios, and it is important that operational crews be used. Normally, test pilots would not be appropriate for these evaluations. A wide range of pilot experience should be used.

For flight evaluations test pilots will normally serve as safety pilots and have in-flight responsibility for ensuring that test conditions are met. For multicrew airplanes the test pilot can serve as the copilot. For simulator evaluations only operational crewmembers should be used.

3. Data

Aircraft performance data should be recorded as functions of time: 1) airspeed, 2) barometric altitude, 3) radar altitude, 4) heading, 5) geographical position, 6) course deviation, and 7) glide-slope deviation. Also, subjective pilot ratings should be obtained for each replication. It is important to ensure, for the purposes of evaluating the display, that the evaluators rate the display and not the ease of data entry (although such data-entry ratings are important to the overall evaluation of the cockpit). Pilot estimates of bearing should be obtained from his or her initial course decisions. Once established on the new course, the safety pilot/simulator operator should ask for estimates of distances and course-line aspect.

4. Performance Criteria

Generally, the criteria depend on the type of failure introduced and on the operational precision required (see Table A.3). For example, a failure during an

Table A.3 Performance criteria for geographic awareness testing

Maintain geographical awareness	En route	Instrument approach	Ingress to target	Nap of the Earth
		Desired performance		
Bearing to waypoint	± 5 deg	±2 deg	±2 deg	±5 deg
Distance to waypoint	±0.5 n mile (0.93 kn)	±0.1 n mile (0.19 kn)	±0.2 n mile (0.37 kn)	±600 ft (183.5 m)
Distance to course line	±0.2 n mile (0.37 kn)	±0.1 n mile (0.19 kn)	±0.1 n mile (0.19 kn)	±300 ft (91.5 m)
Course-line aspect	±10 deg	±2 deg	±5 deg	±10 deg
		Adequate performance		
Bearing to waypoint	±10 deg	±5 deg	±5 deg	±10 deg
Distance to waypoint	±1.0 n mile (1.85 kn)	±0.5 n mile (0.93 kn)	±0.5 n mile (0.93 kn)	±1200 ft (366 m)
Distance to course line	±0.5 n mile (0.93 kn)	±0.2 n mile (0.37 kn)	±0.2 n mile (0.37 kn)	±600 ft (183 m)
Course-line aspect	±30 deg	±5 deg	±10 deg	± 30 deg

instrument landing system (ILS) approach should have tighter tolerances than failures during high-altitude cruise.

5. Safety Considerations During Flight Tests

These tests have no particular hazard other than the high workload for the safety pilot. Standard precautions for instrument training flights should be observed.

References

[1]Weintraub, D. J., and Ensing, M., "Human Factors Issues in Head-up Display Design: The book of HUD," Crew System Ergonomics Information Analysis Center, Wright-Patterson AFB, OH, 1992.

[2]Newman, R. L., *Head-up Displays: Designing the Way Ahead*, Ashgate Publishing, Aldershot, England, U.K., 1995.

[3]Barnette, J. F., "Role of Head-up Display in Instrument Flight," Air Force Instrument Flight Center, AFIFC LR-76-2, Randolph Air Force Base, TX, 1976.

[4]Newman, R. L., "Operational Problems Associated with Head-up Displays During Instrument Flight," Air Force Aeromedical Research Lab., AFAMRL TR-80-116, Wright-Patterson AFB, OH, 1980.

[5]Newman, R. L., and Foxworth, T. G., "A Review of Head-up Display Specifications," Crew Systems, TR-84-04, San Marcos, TX, 1984.

[6]Gard, J. H., *HUDs in Tactical Cockpits. A Basic Guidebook*, Kaiser Electronics, San Jose, CA, 1989.

[7]"Military Handbook: Optical Design," Naval Publications and Forms Center, MIL-HDBK-141, Philadelphia, PA, 1962.

[8]Hussey, D. W., "Wide Angle Head-up Display Design and Application to Future Single Seat Fighters," *Impact of Advanced Avionics Technology on Ground Attack Weapon Systems*, AGARD, 1981.

[9]Sleight, G. R., and Lewis, C. J. G., "Practical Experience with Electronic Head-up Displays in Transport Aircraft," Elliott, Rept. 29/11/2/BO5, Rochester, England, U.K., 1969.

[10]"System Specification: Visual Approach Monitor for the B-737 Aircraft System No. 960-2008," Sundstrand Data Control, Rept. 060-1624, Redmond, WA, 1977.

[11]Gold, T., and Hyman, A., *Visual Requirements Study for Head-up Displays*, JANAIR 680712, Sperry Rand, Great Neck, NY, 1970.

[12]"Transport Category Airplane Head-up Display (HUD) Systems," Society of Automotive Engineers, SAE ARP-5288, Warrendale, PA, 2001.

[13]Stuart, G. W., McInally, K. I., and Meehan., J. W., "Head-up Displays and Visual Attention: Integrating data and Theory and Data," *Human Factors and Aerospace Safety*, Vol. 1, 2001, pp. 103–124.

[14]Henson, J. M., "A Review of the Development of the FASTJET Head-up Display Drive Laws and Symbology Suite," Royal Aircraft Establishment, RAE TM-FS(F)-657, Bedford, England, U.K., 1987.

[15]"Military Standard, Aircraft Display Symbology," Joint Cockpit Office, MIL-STD-1787B, Wright-Patterson, AFB, OH, 1996.

[16]Newman, R. L., "The HUD in Spatial Disorientation," *Proceedings of the 20th European Symposium*, Society of Experimental Test Pilots, 1988.

[17]"A330 Crashed on CAT 3 Test Flight," *Aviation Week and Space Technology*, 3 April, 1995, pp. 72, 73; 10 April, 1995, p. 60; 17 April, 1995, pp. 44, 45; 15 May, 1995, pp. 58, 59; 22 May, 1995, pp. 54–56; 29 May, 1995, pp. 69, 70.

[18]Weinstein, L. F., Gillingham, K. K., and Ercoline, W. R., "United States Air Force Head-up Display Control and Performance Symbology Evaluations," *Aviation, Space, and Environmental Medicine*, Vol. 65, 1994, pp. A20–30.

[19]Roscoe, S. N., "Designed for Disaster," *Human Factors Society Bulletin*, Vol. 29, No. 6, 1986, pp. 1, 2.

[20]Roscoe, S. N., "Spatial Misorientation Exacerbated by Collimated Virtual Flight Display," *Information Display*, Vol. 9, 1986, pp. 27, 28.

[21]Roscoe, S. N., "The Trouble with HUDs and HMDs," *Human Factors Society Bulletin*, Vol. 30, No. 7, 1987, pp. 1, 2.

[22]Iavecchia, J. H., "The Potential for Depth Perception Errors in Piloting the F-18 and A-6 Night Attack Aircraft," Naval Air Development Center, NADC-87037-20, Warminster, PA, 1987.

[23]Randle, R. J., Roscoe, S. N., and Petit, J. C., "Effects of Magnification and Visual Accommodation on Aimpoint Estimation in Simulated Landing Tasks with Real and Virtual Imaging Displays," NASA TP-1635, 1980.

[24]Norton, P. A., Dickens, P. G., Hardy, G. H., Miller, A. D., Newman, R. L., Snyder, R. G., and Tucker, C. V., "Findings and Recommendations of the Cockpit Design Subcommittee," *Proceedings of the 1981 Test Pilot's Aviation Safety Workshop*, AIAA, New York, and Society of Experimental Test Pilots, Lancaster, CA, 1981, pp. 19–47.

[25]Way, T. C., Hornsby, M. E., Gilmour, J. D., Edwards, R. E., and Hobbs, R. E., "Pictorial Format Display Evaluation," Flight Dynamics Lab., AFWAL-TR-84-3036, Wright-Patterson Air Force Base, OH, 1984.

[26]Levy, J. L., Foyle, D. C., and McCann, R. S., "Performance Benefits with Scene-Linked HUD Symbology: An Attentional Phenomenon?," *Proceedings of the 42nd Human Factors and Ergonomics Society Annual Meeting*, Human Factors and Ergonomics Society, Santa Monica, CA, 1998.

[27]Klopfstein, G., "Rational Study of Aircraft Piloting," *INTRADOS*, (reprint), Thomson-CSF, Villacoublay, France, 1966.

[28]McCloskey, St. J., "Flying the TC-121: A Visit to Bretigny to Fly the Thomson-CSF Head-up Display," International Federation of Air Line Pilots Associations, Rept. 74c95, Egham, England, U.K., 1973.

[29]Dorr, D. W., Moralez, E., and Merrick, V. K., "Simulation and Flight Test Evaluation of Head-up Display Guidance for Harrier Approach Transitions," AIAA Paper 92-4233, 1992.

[30]Reising, J., Barthelemy, K., and Hartsock, D., "Unusual Attitude Recoveries Using a Pathway-in-the-Sky," *Proceedings Flight Simulation Technologies Conference*, AIAA, Washington, D.C., 1991, pp. 131–138.

[31]Reising, J. M., Liggett, K. K., Solz, T. J., and Hartsock, D. C., "Comparison of Two Head-up Display Formats Used to Fly Curved Instrument Approaches," *Proceedings of the 39th Human Factors and Ergonomics Society Annual Meeting*, Human Factors and Ergonomics Society, Santa Monica, CA, 1995, pp. 1–5.

[32]Snow, M. P., Reising, J. M., Liggett, K. K., and Barry, T. P., "Flying Complex Approaches Using a Head-up Display: Effects of Visibility and Display Type," Air Force Research Lab., AFRL-HE-WP-TR-2000-0011, Wright-Patterson Air Force Base, OH, 1999.

[33]Ververs, P. M., and Wickens, C. D., "Designing Head-up Displays (HUDs) to Support Flight Path Guidance While Minimizing Effects of Cognitive Tunneling," *Proceedings of the IEA2000/HFES2000 Congress*, 2000.

[34]Rogers, S. P., and Asbury, C. N., "Evaluation of Intelligently-Moded HMD Symbology for Rotorcraft," *Proceedings of the Fourth Helmet and Head-Mounted Displays Conference*, Vol. 3689, International Society for Optical Engineers, Bellingham, WA, 1999.

[35]Adams, J. J., "Simulator Study of a Pictorial Display for General Aviation," NASA TP-1963, 1982.

[36]Brown, M. A., "An Integrated Three-Dimensional Terrain and Primary Flight Display for Terrain Awareness and Alerting," National Aerospace Lab., Rept. NAL-TR-13911, Tokyo, Japan, 1999.

[37]Ethrington, T. J., Vogl, T. L., Lapis, M. B., and Razo, J. B., "Synthetic Vision Information Systems," *Proceedings 19th Digital Avionics Systems Conference*, Inst. of Electrical and Electronic Engineers, New York, 2000.

[38]Theunissen, E., *Integrated Design of a Man-Machine Interface for 4D Navigation*, Delft Univ. Press, Delft, the Netherlands, 1997.

[39]Theunissen, E., and Rademaker, R. M., "Spatially Integrated Depiction of Dynamic Trajectories," Society of Automotive Engineers, Paper 2001-01-2960, Warrendale, PA, 2001.

[40]Fadden, S., Ververs, P. M., and Wickens, C. D., "Pathway HUDs: Are They Viable," Univ. of Illinois Inst. of Aviation, Rept., ARL-00-13/NASA-00-3, Savoy, IL, 2000.

[41]"Mirage 2000 Flight Manual," Avions Marcel Dassault-Breguet Aviation, 1F-M2000-1-1, Vaucresson, France, 1990.

[42]Geiselman, E. E., and Osgood, R. K., "Helmet-Mounted Display Attitude Symbology: An Evaluation of Compression Ratio," *International Journal of Industrial Ergonomics*, Vol. 15, 1995, pp. 111–121.

[43]Previc, F. H., and Ercoline, W. R., "The 'Outside-in' Attitude Display Concept Revisited,"*International Journal of Aviation Psychology*, Vol. 9, 1999, pp. 377–401.

[44]Burgess, M. A., Chang, T., Dunford, D. E., Hoh, R. H., Horne, W. F., Tucker, R. F., Hudson, R. H., and Zak, J. A., "Synthetic Vision Technology Demonstration," Federal Aviation Administration, FAA/RD-93/40, Washington, D.C., 1993.

[45]Kruk, R., Link, N., Reid, L., and Jennings, S., "Enhanced/Synthetic Vision for Search and Rescue Operations," Society of Automotive Engineers, SAE 1999-01-5659, Warrendale, PA, 1999.

[46]Garman, P. J., and Trang, J. A., "In Your Face! The Pilot's/Tester's Perspective on Helmet-Mounted Display (HMD) Symbology," *Proceedings of the Helmet- and Head-Mounted Displays and Symbology Requirements Symposium*, Vol. 2218, International Society for Optical Engineers, Bellingham, WA, 1994, pp. 274–280.

[47]Haworth, L. A., and Seery, R. E., "Rotorcraft Helmet Mounted Display Symbology Research," Society of Automotive Engineers, SAE 921977, Warrendale, PA, 1992.

[48]Newman, R. L., "Helmet-Mounted Display Symbology and Stabilization Concepts," U.S. Army Aeroflightdynamics Directorate, USAATCOM TR-94-A-021, Moffett Field, CA, 1994.

[49]Walrath, J. D., "Visual and Cognitive Issues In the Design of Displays," Army Research Lab., ARL-TR-1116, Aberdeen Proving Ground, MD, 1996.

[50]Ercoline, W. R., Self, B. P., Mathews, R. S. J., and Orzech, M. A., "The Effects of Three Helment-Mounted Display Attitude Symbology Sets on Unusual Attitude Recognition and Recovery," *Aerospace Medical Association*, 2000.

[51]Cohen, D., Otakeno, S., Previc, F. H., and Ercoline, W. R., "Effect of 'Inside-Out' and 'Outside-In' Attitude Displays on Off-Axis Tracking in Pilots and Nonpilots," *Aviation, Space, and Environmental Medicine*, Vol. 72, 2001, pp. 170–176.

[52]Jones, D. R., Abbott, T. S., and Burley, J. R., "Evaluation of Conformal and Body-Axis Attitude Information for Spatial Awareness," *Proceedings of the Third Helmet Mounted Displays Symposium*, Vol. 1695, International Society for Optical Engineers, Bellingham, WA, 1992, pp. 146–153.

[53]Frey, T. W., and Page, H. J., "Virtual HUD Using an HMD," *Proceedings of the Sixth Helmet- and Head-Mounted Displays Symposium*, Vol. 4361, International Society of Optical Engineers, Bellingham, WA, 2001.

[54]Page, J., and Frey, T., "Virtual HUD Flight Test," Lockheed-Martin Aeronautical Co. and BAE Systems, Fort Worth, TX, 2000.

[55]Newman, R. L., and Greeley, K. W., "Helmet-Mounted Displays Design Guide," U.S. Army Aeroflightdynamics Directorate, AFDD TR-98-A-006, Moffett Field, CA, 1997.

[56]Troxel, D., and Chappell, A., "ANVIS/HUD. An Operational and Safety Enhancement for Nap-of-the-Earth Night Flight," *US Army Aviation Digest*, March/April 1993, pp. 53–57.

[57]Gopher, D., Kimchi, R., Seagull, F. J., Catz, I., and Trainin, O., "Flying with Dichoptic Displays: The Interplay Between Display Characteristics and Attention Control," *Proceedings of the 36th Human Factors Society Annual Meeting*, Human Factors Society, Santa Monica, CA, 1992, pp. 1469–1473.

[58]Cohen, B. J., and Markoff, J. I., "Minimization of Binocular Rivalry with a See-Through Helmet Mounted Sight and Display," *Proceedings of the Symposium on Visually Coupled Systems*, School of Aviation Medicine, Brooks Air Force Base, TX, 1972, pp. 159–173.

[59]Levelt, W. J. M., *On Binocular Rivalry*, Mouton, The Hague, Netherlands, 1968.

[60]McKenna, J. T., "Pilot's Vision Studied in MD-88 Crash Probe," *Aviation Week and Space Technology*, 26 May, 1997, pp. 42–47.

[61]"Aircraft Accident Report: Descent Below Glidepath and Collision with Terrain, Delta Air Lines Flight 554, McDonnell-Douglas MD-88, LaGuardia, New York, October 19, 1996," National Transportation Safety Board, NTSB AAR-97-03, Washington, D.C., 1997.

[62]Sampson, W. T., Simpson, G. B., and Green, D. L., "Night Vision Goggles in Emergency Medical Service (EMS) Helicopters," Federal Aviation Administration, FAA RD-94/21, Washington, D.C., 1994.

[63]Clarkson, G. J. N., "Symbology Night Vision Goggles for Combat Aircraft," *Proceedings Helmet- and Head-Mounted Displays and Symbology Design Requirements Symposium*, Vol. 2218, International Society for Optical Engineers, Bellingham, WA, 1994, pp. 316–327.

[64]Lahaszow, A. J., "Aviator's Night Vision Imaging System Head-up Display (ANVIS/HUD) Assessment and Symbology Rationale," *Proceedings of the Helmet- and Head-Mounted Displays and Symbology Design Requirements Symposium*, Vol. 2218, International Society for Optical Engineers, Bellingham, WA, 1994, pp. 316–327.

[65]Nicholson, R., and Troxel, D., "Update of the AN/AVS-7 Head-up Display Program," *Proceedings of the Head-Mounted Displays Symposium*, Vol. 2735, International Society for Optical Engineers, Bellingham, WA, 1996, pp. 215–220.

[66]Piccione, D., and Troxel, D., "ANVIS/HUD. User and Maintainer Survey," DCS Corp., Alexandria, VA, 1996.

[67]Hart, S. G., "Helicopter Human Factors," *Human Factors in Aviation*, edited by E. L. Weiner and D. C. Nagel, Academic Press, New York, 1988, pp. 591–638.

[68]Ruffner, J. W., Grubb, M. G., and Hamilton, D. B., "Selective Factors Affecting Rotary-Wing Aviator Performance with Symbology Superimposed on Night Vision Goggles," U.S. Army Inst. for Behavioral and Social Sciences, ARI Research Rept. 1622, Alexandria, VA, 1992.

[69]"F-18 Flight Manual," Naval Air Systems Command, Flight Manual NAVAIR-A1-F18AC-NFM-000, Washington, D.C., 1996.

[70]Hall, J. R., Stephens, C. M., and Penwill, J. C., "A Review of the Design and Development of the RAE Fast-Jet Head-up Display Format," Royal Aircraft Establishment, RAE FM-WP(89)034, Bedford, England, U.K., 1989.

[71]"Flight Dynamics Model 1000 Head-up Display System Specification," Rockwell-Collins/Flight Dynamics, Document 404-0249, Portland, OR, 1989.

[72]Bray, R. S., *A Head-up Display Format for Application to Transport Aircraft Approach and Landing*, NASA TM-81199, 1980.

[72]Birmingham, H. P., and Taylor, F. V., "A Design Philosophy for Man-Maching Control Systems," *Selected Papers on Human Factors in the Design and Use of Control Systems*, edited by H. W. Sinaiko, Dover, New York, 1961, pp. 67–87.

[73]Johnson, T., "Alaska Airlines Experience with the HGS-1000 Head-up Guidance System," Society of Automotive Engineers, SAE 901828, Warrendale, PA, 1990.

[74]"Historical Overview of the Development of the Two-Person Flight Station on the 382J, Lockheed Aeronautical Systems Co., Rept. J11E02A510, Marietta, GA, 1995.

[75]"Military Standard, Human Factors Engineering Design Criteria for Helicopter Electro-Optical Display Symbology," Naval Publications and Forms Center, MIL-STD-1295A, Philadelphia, PA, 1984.

[76]Newman, R. L., "Evaluation of Head-up Displays to Enhance Unusual Attitude Recovery," Air Force Wright Aeronautical Lab., AFWAL TR-87-3055, Vol. II, Wright-Patterson AFB, OH, 1987.

[77]Bryan, L. A., Stonecipher, J. W., and Aron, K., "180 Degree Turn Experiment," *University of Illinois Aeronautical Bulletin*, Vol. 12, 1954, pp. 1–60.

[78]Newman, R. L., and Quam, D. L., "Pilot Reaction to Attitude Gyro Failure," *Canadian Aeronautics and Space Journal*, Vol. 28, 1982, pp. 303–310.

[79]Kraus, R. N., "Disorientation: An Evaluation of the Etiologic Factors," School of Aviation Medicine, Rept. 59–90, Brooks Air Force Base, TX, 1959.

[80]Patterson, F. R., Cacioppo, A. J., Gallimore, J. J., Hinman, G. E., and Nalepka, J. P., "Aviation Spatial Orientation in Relationship to Head Position and Attitude Interpretation," *Aviation, Space, and Environmental Medicine*, Vol. 68, 1997, pp. 463–471.

[81]Smith, D. R., Cacioppo, A. J., and Hinman, G. E., "Aviation Spatial Orientation in Relationship to Head Position, Attitude Interpretation, and Control," *Aviation, Space, and Environmental Medicine*, Vol. 68, 1997, pp. 472–478.

[82]Merryman, R. K. F., and Cacioppo, A. J., "The Optokinetic Cervical Reflex in Pilots of High Performance Aircraft," *Aviation, Space, and Environmental Medicine*, Vol. 68, 1997, pp. 479–487.

[83]Kinsley, S. A., Warner, N. W., and Gleisner, D. P., "A Comparison of Two Pitch Ladder Formats and an ADI Ball for Recovery from Unusual Attitudes," Naval Air Development Center, NADC 86012-60, Warminster, PA, 1986.

[84]Guttman, J., "Evaluation of the F/A-18 Head-up Display for Recovery from Unusual Attitudes," Naval Air Development Center, NADC 86157-60, Warminster, PA, 1986.

[85]Deaton, J. E., Barnes, M. J., Lindsey, N. J., and Greene, J. L., "The Effect of Windscreen Bows and HUD Pitch Ladder Format on Pilot Performance During Simulated Flight," Naval Air Development Center, NADC 89084-60, Warminster, PA, 1989.

[86]Deaton, J. E., Barnes, M. J., Kern, J., and Wright, D., "Evaluation of the Augie Arrow HUD Symbology as an Aid to Recovery from Unusual Attitudes," *Proceedings of the 34th Annual Meeting of the Human Factors Society*, Human Factors Society, Santa Monica, CA, 1990, pp. 31–35.

[87]Chandra, D., "Design of Head-up Display Symbology for Recovery from Unusual Attitudes," Ph.D. Dissertation, Univ. of Michigan, Ann Arbor, MI, 1993.

[88]Chandra, D., and Weintraub, D. J., "Design of Head-up Display Symbology for Recovery from Unusual Attitudes," *Proceedings of the Seventh International Symposium on Aviation Psychology*, Ohio State Univ., Columbus, OH, 1993.

[89]Ercoline, W. R., Gillingham, K. K., Greene, F. A., and Previc, F. H., "Effects of Variations in Head-up Display Pitch-Ladder Representations on Orientation Recognition," *Proceedings of the 33rd Human Factors Society Annual Meeting*, Human Factors Society, Santa Monica, CA, 1989, pp. 1401–1405.

[90]Penwill, J. C., and Hall, J. R., "A Comparative Evaluation of Two HUD Formats by All Four Nations to Determine the Preferred Pitch Ladder Design for EFA," Royal Aircraft Establishment, RAE FM-WP(90)021, Bedford, England, U.K., 1990.

[91]Weinstein, L. F., Ercoline, W. R., Evans, R. H., and Bitton, D. F., "Head-up Display (HUD) Symbology Standardization and the Utility of Analog Vertical Velocity Information During Instrument Flight," *International Journal of Aviation Psychology*, Vol. 2, 1992, pp. 245–260.

[92]"Transport Category Airplane Electronic Display Systems," Federal Aviation Administration, FAA AC-25-11, Washington, D.C., 1987.

[93]"Certification of Normal Category Rotorcraft," Federal Aviation Administration, FAA AC-27-1B, Fort Worth, TX, 1999.

[94]"Certification of Transport Category Rotorcraft," Federal Aviation Administration, FAA AC-29-2C, Fort Worth, TX, 1999.

[95]Newman, R. L., "Flight Test Report. Flight Visions FV-2000/KA HUD Installed in a Beechcraft BE-A100," Crew Systems, TR-93-09, San Marcos, TX, 1993.

[96]Osgood, R. K., Geiselman, E. E., and Calhoun, G. C., "Attitude Maintenance Using an Off-Boresight Helmet-Mounted Virtual Display," *NATO/AGARD Symposium on Helmet-Mounted Displays and Night Vision Goggles*, AGARD, 1991.

[97]Geiselman, E. E., and Osgood, R. K., "A Comparison of Three Attitude Display Symbology Structures During an Attitude Maintenance Task," *Proceedings of the 36th Human Factors Society Annual Meeting*, Human Factors Society, Santa Monica, CA, 1992, pp. 1450–1454.

[98]Geiselman, E. E., and Osgood, R. K., "Toward an Empirically Based Helmet-Mounted Symbology Set," *Proceedings of the 37th Human Factors and Ergonomics Society Annual Meeting*, Human Factors and Ergonomics Society, Santa Monica, CA, 1993.

[99]Geiselman, E. E., and Osgood, R. K., "Utility of Off-Boresight Helmet-Mounted Symbology During a High Angle Airborne Target Acquisition Task," *Proceedings of the Helmet- and Head-Mounted Displays and Symbology Design Requirements Symposium*, Vol. 2218, International Society for Optical Engineers, Bellingham, WA, 1994, pp. 328–338.

[100]Geiselman, E. E., "Development of a Non-Distributed Flight Reference Symbology for Helmet-Mounted Display Use During Off-Boresight Viewing," *Proceedings of the 4th*

Annual Symposium on Situational Awareness in the Tactical Air Environment, June 1999, pp. 118–127.

[101]DeVilbiss, C. A., Ercoline, W. R., and Sipes, W. E., "Effect of Arc Segmented Attitude Reference Symbology on a Helmet-Mounted Display During an Unusual Attitude Recovery Task," *Proceedings Helmet- and Head-Mounted Displays and Symbology Design Requirements,* Vol. 2465, International Society for Optical Engineers, Bellingham, WA, 1995, pp. 255–262.

[102]Haworth, L. A., Sharkey, T. J., and Lee, A., "TRISTAR III: Helmet-Mounted Display Symbology," *Proceedings of the Helmet- and Head-Mounted Displays and Symbology Design Requirements,* Vol. 2465, International Society for Optical Engineers, Bellingham, WA, 1995, pp. 235–245.

[103]"Airworthiness Requirements: Transport Category Airplanes," Federal Aviation Administration, Federal Aviation Regulations Part 25, Amendment 25-105, Washington, D.C., 2001.

[104]"HGS®Pilot Guide, Boeing 737 NG," Rockwell-Collins/Flight Dynamics, Document 9701-1071, Portland, OR, 2000.

[105]Hall, J. R., "The Design and Development of the New RAF Standard HUD Format," *Combat Automation for Airborne Weapon Systems: Man/Machine Interface Trends and Technologies,* AGARD, Neuilly-sur-Seine, France, 1992.

[106]Walters, D. J., "The Electronic Display for Primary Flight Data," *Problems of the Cockpit Environment,* AGARD, 1968.

[107]Roscoe, S. N., Hasler, S. G., and Dougherty, D. J., "Flight by Periscope: Making Take-offs and Landings; the Influence of Image Magnification, Practice, and Various Conditions of Flight," *Human Factors,* Vol. 8, 1966, pp. 13–40.

[108]Comstock, J. R., Glaab, L. J., Prinzel, L. J., and Elliott, D. M., "Can Effective Synthetic Vision Systems Displays be Implemented on Limited Size Display Spaces?," *Proceedings of the Eleventh International Symposium on Aviation Psychology,* Ohio State Univ., Columbus, OH, 2001.

[109]Newman, R. L., Greeley, K. W., Schwartz, R. J., and Ellis, D. R., "A Head-up Display for General Aviation," Society of Automotive Engineers, SAE 2000-01-1697, Warrendale, PA, 2000.

[110]Bogart, E. H., Doyle, T. M., Glaab, L. J., Hughes, M. F., McGee, F. G., Newman, R. L., Takallu, M. A., and Wong, D. T., "Detection of the Onset of Low Visibility Loss-of-Control in Low-Hour General Aviation Pilots," *2001 World Aviation Congress,* 2001.

[111]Newman, R. L., and Greeley, K. W., *Cockpit Displays: Test and Evaluation,* Ashgate Publishing, Aldershot, England, U.K., 2001.

[112]Murphy, and Likert, 1938.

[113]Cooper, G. E., and Harper, R. P., "The Use of Pilot Rating in the Evaluation of Aircraft Handling Qualities," NASA TN-D-5153, 1969.

[114]Newman, R. L., and Anderson, M. W., "HUD Flight Testing: Lessons Learned," *Southeast Section SETP Symposium, Stone Mountain, Georgia,* Society of Experimental Test Pilots, Lancaster, CA, 1994.

[115]Haworth, L. A., and Newman, R. L., "Techniques for Evaluating Flight Displays," NASA TM-103947, 1993.

[116]Anderson, M. R., French, D. D., Newman, R. L., and Phillips, M. R., "Flight Testing a General Aviation Head-up Display," *Journal of Aircraft,* Vol. 33, 1996, pp. 235–238.

[117]Bailey, R. E., and Knotts, L. H., "Flight and Ground Simulation Evaluation of the Proposed USAF Head-up Display Standard," AIAA Paper 93–3605, 1993.

[118]Gallimore, J. J., Brannon, N. G., Patterson, F. R., and Nalepka, J. P., "Effects of FOV and Aircraft Bank on Pilot Head Movement and Reversal Errors During Simulated Flight," *Aviation, Space, and Environmental Medicine*, Vol. 70, 1999, pp. 1152–1160.

[119]"All-Weather Flight Manual," U.S. Navy Bureau of Aeronautics, NAVAER 80-80T-60, Washington, D.C., 1957.

[120]"Instrument Flight Handbook," Federal Aviation Administration, FAA AC-61-27C, Washington, D.C., 1979.

[121]"Instrument Flying," U.S. Air Force Flight Standards Agency, AFI 21-216; formerly AFM-51-37, Andrews Air Force Base, MD.

Chapter 11

Spatial Disorientation Countermeasures—Advanced Problems and Concepts

Willem Bles*
TNO Human Factors, Soesterberg, The Netherlands

I. Introduction

WITH the introduction of the next generation of fighter aircraft and helicopters, maneuverability is increased considerably. This is particularly true
of the poststall regime, in which flight directions are not as closely coupled to the
longitudinal axis of the aircraft because of thrust vectoring. Because these maneuvers have their impact on the pilot's spatial orientation, they are dealt with in some
detail in this chapter. In flying those modern aircraft, pilots prefer a head-out concept. This requires innovative technologies for weapon and aircraft information
displays and controls. In this chapter display technologies like three-dimensional
audio and TSAS (tactile situation-awareness system) will be discussed in some detail because of the implications of these systems for improved situational awareness
and spatial disorientation (SD) preventive capabilities. Automated systems like
ground-proximity warning system (GPWS) or traffic-alert and collision-avoidance
system (TCAS) and automated ground-collision-avoidance systems (auto-GCAS)
will find their application in the cockpit and likely affect the number of SD accidents. Finally, because SD is not restricted to the pilot in the cockpit the chapter
concludes with spatial orientation problems when flying unmanned aerial vehicles
(UAV).

Over the last decade SD has been a major cause of flight accidents (see Chapter
5). Better insight into the causes of SD and better SD training have not always
resulted in a decrease in the number of SD accidents. Reasons for the apparent
ineffectiveness of pilot SD training are that the increased understanding of SD
over the years and the development of appropriate human–machine interfaces do
not fully compensate for the ever-increasing maneuverability of the aircraft, the
increase of the pilot's workload to almost unacceptable levels, and the increase

This material is declared a work of the U.S. Government and is not subject to copyright protection
in the United States.
*Senior Scientist.

in the demands of the flight conditions. Some examples include flying day and night, flying more head down in the cockpit, flying formation, flying low level, etc. It is therefore rather unfair to blame the SD community for not being able to significantly reduce the risk of SD. Based on a review of advanced SD problems and concepts, it is hard to predict whether the balance will turn in favor of a decrease in the number of SD accidents or whether SD will become an increasing threat in the near future.

The bad news (from an SD point of view) is the development of supermaneuverable aircraft. This development adds new dimensions to the spatial-orientation task because of the increasing number of degrees of freedom (DOF) of the flight path. The more extensive use of all six DOFs, will therefore make the task more demanding and introduce new illusions to the flight environment, as will be discussed in Sec. III.

The good news is that some new nontraditional display tools are being developed especially to counter SD, such as the TSAS, to be discussed in Sec. IV.B.2. Although additional features of these tactile devices, such as a directionally sensitive threat warning system, might eventually become the primary reason for acceptance of the device by the pilots, their SD countermeasure potential would be a valuable byproduct. Similarly, three-dimensional auditory displays are being developed to enhance situational awareness and indirectly counter SD by diminishing the burden of reading visual displays (Sec. IV.B.1). Together with head-mounted devices with head tracking (HMD/T), which are being developed to extend the capabilities of the head-up display (HUD) (Chapter 10), these displays are meant to improve situation awareness.

Another development is the expansion of automation in the cockpit. Examples, with respect to SD, are the systems introduced to prevent midair collisions or controlled flight into terrain (CFIT). These systems are receiving more attention and are discussed in Sec. IV.A. Although in the present versions of these systems the pilot is still in command, methods to circumvent the pilot by taking over command automatically are under consideration such as auto-GCAS. In the future cockpit (Sec. IV), most of the preceding display and automation improvements will be introduced, along with large graphic displays with synthetic vision. Despite the development of alternative controls (Sec. IV.C), automation will ultimately expand to an empty cockpit instead of the aircraft taking over command automatically from the pilot. The pilot/operator of a UAV can be positioned in command as a supervisor outside the aircraft.[1] With these unmanned aerial vehicles, spatial orientation will remain an issue, as discussed in Sec. V.

Given the fact that operational considerations will require a continuous extension of the flight envelope, a desirable approach would be to involve human-factor SD specialists at an early stage to analyze the consequences of these extensions for spatial orientation and to give adequate feedback to the engineers during the development of flight envelope and human–machine interfaces. This approach is preferred over establishing SD shortcomings after the implementation of a new technology. However, this requires a common language for all disciplines involved: the operational strategists, the aircraft-design team, and human-factor specialists. Serious steps in this direction have been made, such as the publication of the *Engineering Data Compendium on Human Perception and Performance*, edited by Boff and Lincoln.[2] The next step for the SD community requires simulation of the pilot in the loop, taking into account the interactions among the different sensory systems under realistic flight conditions.[3] In Sec. II a framework will be defined to facilitate the discussion of the provocativeness of future developments in regards to SD.

II.   Modeling Spatial Orientation for Advanced Technologies

All of the illusions described in preceding chapters are, in fact, the normal reaction of the human spatial-orientation system to an unusual environment. This implies that if the human spatial-orientation system could be modeled then (new) maneuvers with the proposed aircraft design could be evaluated to determine the likelihood of SD problems in advance. In modeling spatial orientation, models on motion sickness have proven to be very useful. This is no surprise because in both cases there were problems relating the sensed orientation and that of the real environment. Just as with motion sickness, SD only makes its appearance if the equilibrium system is stimulated outside its normal operational envelope.[3–6] Many researchers have been active in modeling spatial orientation and motion sickness qualitatively and quantitatively (for reviews see Refs. 7–10). One such model, a flowchart representing the process of spatial orientation and motion sickness, is summarized in Fig. 1 (Ref. 11). This model describes the control of body motion, and the control variable is the state of the body, attitude, and motion. This state is the combination of linear and angular position, velocity and acceleration, where the linear acceleration is composed of accelerations caused by motion *and* by gravity; the resultant of the latter is also called the specific force or gravitoinertial force. Thus, a desired body state results in the preparation phase in motor commands that subsequently drive the muscles in our body to adhere to the desired state. Together with external perturbations (e.g., motion of aircraft), this results in the actual body state. This state is sensed by the sensory systems such as the visual and vestibular systems and to some degree also by the auditory system, all of which would be included in the "sensors" block of Fig. 1. After some central nervous system (CNS) processing and delay, this results in signals that can only estimate the state of the body. Parallel to this primary path of signal flow, corollary signals are supposed to be generated by a copy of the primary path, together called an internal model or neural store, which is supposed to be created by previous experiences. The input of this internal model is a copy of the motor commands (called an efference copy). Here the basic output of the internal model should be a better estimate of the body state as compared to the output of the primary path, and it is this estimate that is compared with the desired state to generate the error signal that actually drives the controller. Optimally, the output of the internal model should be equal to that of the primary path. The difference or conflict can then give rise to an additional weighted feedback signal and can be used by the internal model to drive the difference towards zero. In terms of Kalman filtering, this conflict is also called innovation.

Despite the fact that a complete quantitative model as such is not yet available, analysis with the present model (limited in DOFs) corresponds quite well with experimental data sets.[12] From the model we see that SD occurs if the motion input does not match the motion percept. For details concerning the various sensory systems in the model, see Chapters 2 and 3. According to the model in Fig. 1, the

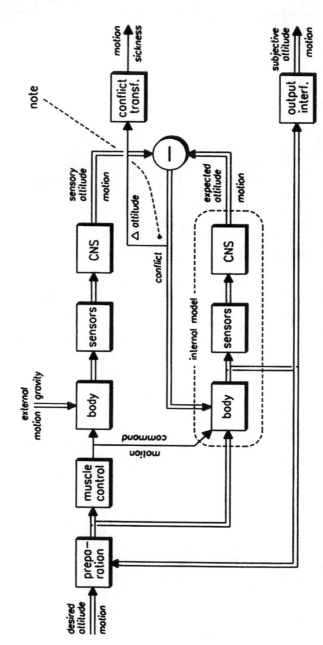

Fig. 1 Flow diagram showing the main characteristics of the spatial orientation and motion-sickness model according to Ref. 11.

sensed orientation and motion signals are matched with the outcome of an internal model (e.g., expectation),[3,8] which is especially important when the pilot is in the loop. The internal model depends highly on previous experience and training (see Chapter 4). One current motion-sickness model is based on the concept that the main conflict causing motion sickness is a difference between the vertical determined from the sensory inputs and the vertical determined on the basis of previous motion information, as is also shown in Fig. 1 (Ref. 5).

Unfortunately, the model as depicted in Fig. 1 is not sufficient to describe the process of flying. One must realize that when the pilot is in the loop, that is, there is a human–machine interface with the aircraft. Accounting for this interface results in a model describing the visual-vestibular contribution to a pilot's control output as shown in Fig. 2, which should be combined with the model of Fig. 1 (Refs. 13 and 14).

With this approach, in which the human equilibrium system is incorporated to the process of controlling the aircraft and perceiving the aircraft's movement in its environment, it is also possible to determine the necessary motion cueing algorithm for a (flight) simulator to avoid negative learning effects caused by discrepancies between real and simulated flight.[15]

Figures 1 and 2 can be useful tools for operational strategists, engineers, and human-factor SD specialists in evaluating new technologies, even before these technologies are realized. Although this is not easy to realize for the various new developments as discussed in the subsequent sections, the models displayed in Fig. 1 and 2 are helpful for qualitative judgments.

III.   Supermaneuverability

A.   Introduction

A prominent development in the operational environment occurred with the introduction of the so-called superagile aircraft like the Sukhoi-27. Superagility involves the ability to execute maneuvers in the poststall regime, with controlled sideslip and with an angle of attack (AoA) beyond maximum lift. In discussing SD consequences, this supermaneuverability of the aircraft is the most relevant. The motion of supermaneuverable flight is different from conventional aircraft in that the pilot is confronted with motion along the x (longitudinal or chest-to-back), y (lateral or side-to-side), and z (vertical or head-to-toe) axes.[16] Slightly lower $+G_z$ levels, shorter $+G_z$ duration, very high G-onset rates, high angular rates, and multiple-axis G stress as compared to the conventional fighter environment also characterize the high-agility flight environment. Only a few jet aircraft are currently capable of this type of flight. Those aircraft that are equipped with thrust-vectoring jet engines (MiG 29, SU-27, SU-37, Harrier, X-31, F-22, and F-35) are capable of directing thrust in a direction other than along the longitudinal axis of the aircraft. By directing the thrust up and down, the aircraft becomes agile in the pitch axis. When the thrust is directed laterally, the aircraft has the capability to yaw while traversing along a longitudinal velocity vector.

In terms of maneuverability, the differences between these agile jets and modern reconnaissance and attack helicopters like the RAH-66 Comanche become smaller and smaller, restricting the messages of the following paragraphs not only to fixed-wing aircraft but also to modern helicopters. Insight into the flight profiles

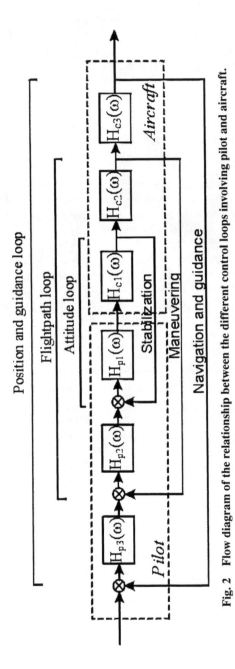

Fig. 2 Flow diagram of the relationship between the different control loops involving pilot and aircraft.

of these aircraft is required in order to estimate the possible consequences for maintaining spatial orientation when flying these aircraft.

B. Flight Profiles

Albery[16] discusses typical superagile flight profiles. They include the Cobra and the Herbst maneuvers.

The Cobra maneuver is characterized by flight in the plane of symmetry of the aircraft by pitching up of the aircraft more than 90 deg, while maintaining approximate altitude and the aircraft's original velocity vector direction. During this maneuver, $+G_z$ is experienced because of pitch and drag. After a while, the nose is pitched down again towards its original orientation (striking like a cobra). In this phase $-G_z$ will be experienced, which will vary with the distance of the pilot from the center of the pitch rotation. The Cobra maneuver can be used to slow the aircraft abruptly or to gain a lock on an adversary flying above the aircraft. The maneuver typically generates only $+4$ G_z and some negative G_z.

The Herbst maneuver is a poststall maneuver, which requires lateral thrust vectoring. The aircraft is pitched up into a stall; the thrust is laterally vectored as the aircraft slows at the top of the maneuver. The lateral force rotates the aircraft about its yaw axis over approximately 180 deg, and the aircraft is directed back along its original flight path but in the opposite direction. The Herbst maneuver eliminates the need for a long turning maneuver of a conventional fighter aircraft attempting to reverse directions. The maneuver involves G_x, G_y, and G_z exposures in combination with pitch-and-yaw motion.

Complex maneuvers like the Herbst and Cobra maneuvers are combinations of basic linear and angular motions. In most cases the maneuvers consist of a complex flight path (with all of the necessary accelerations to accomplish this path) and superimposed attitude changes (nose pointing) of the aircraft, also providing additional accelerations to the pilot. The worst-case range of the human complex stress envelope in supermaneuverable flight, as derived from several data sources, is shown in Table 1.

Table 1   Maximum (changes in) G load and maximum angular velocities and accelerations to be encountered in agile aircraft for the different body directions (from Ref. 17)

Movement Properties	Range
G_x	$+6.5/-6.5$ G
G_y	$+4/-4$ G
G_z	$+9.5/-2$ G
ω_{yaw}	$+90/-90$ deg/s
ω_{pitch}	$+180/-170$ deg/s
ω_{roll}	$+90/-150$ deg/s
dG_x/dt (G/s)	$+5/-5$ G/s
dG_y/dt (G/s)	$+2/-2$ G/s
dG_z/dt (G/s)	$+5/-5$ G/s
α_{yaw}	$+68/-68$ deg/s^2
α_{pitch}	$+289/-253$ deg/s^2
α_{roll}	$+289/-253$ deg/s^2

According to Welch et al.,[18] it is expected that superagile flight will lead to both a hyper-G environment, (i.e., $+G_z$ values of 9 to 15 G), as well as high $-G_z$ loading (-3 to -6 G for routine missions, even up to a momentary -10 G_z in avoidance maneuvers). The amount of $+G_y$ and $-G_y$ experienced is the consequence of the yaw rate and depends on the distance of the pilot in front of the center of gravity. For angular motion the situation is more complicated: The roll rate of the X-31 is about 240 deg/s up to 10-deg AoA, 150 deg/s at 20-deg AoA, and 45 deg/s up to 70-deg AoA. For the pilot this means that he will experience primarily eccentric yaw instead of roll motion at high AoA. According to Le Blaye,[19] the pitch agility should be about 20 deg/s for the F-22 vs 5 deg/s for the F-16, which is substantially lower than that estimated by Repperger.[17]

Exact values are apparently difficult to define, but for the discussion of the SD consequences I will adhere to the values provided by Repperger,[17] with the expectation that the Welch values remain futuristic.[20]

C. Spatial Orientation

The magnitudes of the angular accelerations shown in Table 1 are not beyond the normal working range of the semicircular canals, and so there are no direct consequences of supermaneuvering for the semicircular canals. It is likely that the canal stimuli during the Cobra, Herbst, or the other maneuvers performed by agile aircraft will result in percepts that accurately reflect the actual angular motion because of the fast rotations over a limited angle of displacement. The nystagmus response will be adequate as well during most poststall maneuvering, based on data from a 1-G environment. Although the magnitude of the force vector will be varying, it will usually be much higher than 1 G, perhaps 3–4 G during poststall maneuvering. At this G level the gain of the canal response in terms of nystagmus or motion perception might be different from the optimal response at 1 G, based on available evidence from parabolic flight experiments.[21] It is also unclear whether suppression of the canal-induced nystagmus by visual fixation occurs normally during these higher G loads. On the other hand, poststall maneuvers do not last very long, which might help regaining adequate vision shortly after the maneuver.

According to Table 1, the G loads encountered in supermaneuvers should not impair the otolith system, as they are smaller than the G loads pulled in conventional high-performance aircraft. Sustained G_z loads ≥ 3 G will generate up-beating nystagmus (L nystagmus), which is not appropriate for maintaining spatial orientation.[22,23] There is very little known about the horizontal nystagmus following sustained stimulation along the G_y axis because of the unpleasant experimentation for subjects in conditions of $G_y > 2$ G. Even less is known about the capability to suppress the L nystagmus by visual fixation. Wientjes and Marcus[24] observed a decrease in visual search tasks during 3-G_z stimulation, especially during vertical eye movements, which they attributed to the latent presence of L nystagmus. They indicated that this phenomenon could be potentially hazardous during high-performance flight because of the much higher G loads involved. Cheung and Hofer[25] found a degradation of visual pursuit during 3 G_z, which they assume to be caused by central hypoxia and to changed visual-vestibular integration in the vestibular nuclei caused by the increased G loading. Cheung et al.[26] found some horizontal G_y nystagmus during counter-rotation experiments. G_x nystagmus has never been observed. The G loads in supermaneuvering aircraft are likely to be different from those in conventional aircraft in that they will affect the pilot from all possible directions. Changes between the $+G_z$ and $-G_z$ component are especially prevalent (push–pull effect). These direction-changing G loads combined with angular motion challenge the perception of gravity (i.e., the subjective vertical), which can easily provoke SD.

D. Subjective Vertical and Spatial Orientation

The central vestibular system has problems in accurately interpreting the otolith input during a sustained G load[27,28] (see also Chapter 6, Sec. III). Current motion perception theories proposed low-pass filtering of the otolith output to signal gravity, while the canal response is also involved in the internal reconstruction of the subjective vertical.[3,29,30] In view of the increased G load and its changing directions with respect to the pilot during supermaneuvering, it is obvious even without a detailed analysis that this will easily result in a subjective vertical that does not correspond to the gravity vector.

It can be assumed that the movement of the aircraft is more provocative for the vestibular system when the head is fixed to the head rest during air-to-air combat maneuvering than when pilots try to keep their gaze (and consequently as much as possible their head) fixed on the adversary. In the latter case the angular motion of the head is much more natural than the motion of the aircraft and therefore probably more easily and accurately interpretable. It would be of interest to investigate the consequences of the head movements for spatial orientation during supermaneuvering by comparing the output of the model of Fig. 1 with the aircraft motion as input vs the output of the model with the pilot's head motion as input.

Nevertheless, whatever head motion takes place, the vestibular system by itself will fail to indicate the flight path during supermaneuvering because of the G loads involved. To maintain spatial orientation (SO) correctly, the orientation system must therefore rely on visual information (provided no other technology is used to supplement the required SO information).

E. Vision

According to present models on visual-vestibular interactions, the poststall maneuvering should not pose insolvable problems for the data processing of the various sensory systems involved in maintaining spatial orientation. However, this is only true as long as there is ample visual position and motion information available. One might expect that especially maneuvering with a high AoA might cause problems, but test pilots did not report any problems in this respect (see also Sec. III.F). However, test flights have been flown primarily under good visual conditions with good visible horizons, and so generalization is difficult. Deployment, for instance, in a cloudy European combat theater is a completely different situation for out-the-window handling/maneuvering.

For flying these supermaneuvers under closed-cockpit conditions, intuitive instrument feedback about the flight path of the aircraft is essential to prevent SD, whereas for navigational purposes additional HMD information with navigation forward-looking infrared (FLIR) and synthetic terrain imagery is necessary. These requirements pose additional technical problems (see Chapter 10). Wider HUDs, canopy projection, or a head-mounted virtual reality system might also be required.[31]

Off-boresight targeting can pose problems in terms of a second visual frame of reference, which will affect the situational awareness of the pilot. Because this depends also on the visual information, off-boresight targeting can easily lead to SD. Whether specific symbology in the HUD or HMD will enable the pilot to remain fully aware of his or her spatial orientation during such tasks remains to be investigated (see also Chapter 10).

F. Pilot Reports

No additional human factors/physiological limitations were encountered while flying the X-31 aircraft after flying F-16 or F-18 aircraft. Maneuvering was experienced to be very comfortable because the X-31 flight-control system was set up to provide poststall maneuvering with zero sideslip, resulting in only a little G_y.

Spatial disorientation was not encountered. However, all maneuvering was in daylight, (visual meteorological conditions or VMC) in the southwestern United States, with good horizons present. One single episode, spiraling down into and through a cloud layer, suggested that in intermittent instrument meteorological conditions (IMC) with a poor horizon, transitioning to head-down conditions could pose problems. Pilots preferred out-the-window handling/maneuvering, which is important in all fighter aircraft. Such maneuvering allows full attention to the adversary and the tactical situation, without the need to monitor whether one's own aircraft might depart its own control envelope. The reports of the pilots were encouraging in view of the predicted problems caused by the complex sensory stimulation. However, it appears that clear visibility is a prerequisite for achieving superagile flight without SD.[32]

G. SD Countermeasures

In general, one could state that the SD threat in supermaneuverable flight is a threat similar to the threat in conventional aircraft. Just as in normal aircraft, SD in superagile aircraft is a threat because it can occur unexpectedly. During supermaneuvering, Type I SD is unlikely to occur, but Type II SD can occur easily in bad viewing conditions. Although it is recognized easily, it might be difficult to recover from because of the dissociation between the velocity vector of the aircraft and the aircraft's attitude. It is obvious that both normal procedural training as well as additional skills training involving recovery from Type II SD is required. Several of the items just discussed are presently under investigation. A survey of the relevant items to be studied for supermaneuverable aircraft handling would be useful, as would be joint research because in-flight research tools are expensive and scarce.

Closely related to SD is motion sickness, as indicated already in Sec. II. During supermaneuvering, it is unlikely that the internal representation[33] of a passive observer can keep up with the sensory side, giving sufficient conflict to provoke motion sickness. Because expectancy plays a large role in motion perception and the pilot is in control of the maneuvers, this will enable the internal model of the pilot to better keep up with the sensory side. Moreover, as indicated by pilot reports, the sorties flown so far have been in good visual conditions, thereby allowing the visual system to correct for the vestibular insufficiencies in determining the vertical. These two factors should reduce the chance of motion sickness considerably. Reports* that pilots do not appreciate the maneuvering anymore when they are out of the control loop (e.g., gun tracking) are in agreement with the preceding statements. Clearly pilots should avoid conflicting frames of reference, for instance, symbology on the HMD should be consistent with the out-the-window view during head movements. In general, dissociations among the reference frames of the head, display, and airframe should be avoided. Additional three-dimensional audio (Sec. IV.B.1) and tactile (Sec. IV.B.2) cueing could be helpful tools in maintaining spatial orientation during supermaneuvering and might consequently help to prevent motion sickness.

Although motion sickness might be encountered in conventional fighter aircraft, supermaneuvering is expected to be much more provocative in this respect. Extensive training with these types of maneuvers should be considered using SD trainers, advanced centrifuges, inversion demonstrations, and with aerobatic aircraft. Until more ground-based research is done on the effects of superagile maneuvering on motion-sickness provocativeness, conversion to superagile aircraft should be restricted to those pilots who have a history free of motion sickness. Demonstrations and training of supermaneuvers in ground-based devices are useful, as long as those devices give responses representative of what is encountered in the air[34] (see also Chapter 8). Otherwise, an internal representation that does not correspond to the real situation will be built up. Because the real conditions can cause motion sickness as well, one should carefully differentiate between motion sickness and simulator sickness in ground-based devices.

IV. Future Cockpit

Calhoun[35] concludes from an analysis of the agile aircraft that they have the potential to provide enhanced speed, range, flexibility, and lethality. To be able to exploit all of these abilities of agile aircraft, crew stations must enhance the interaction between situational awareness, the maneuverability envelope, and the cockpit information and control system. She anticipates that supermaneuvers go so fast that conventional symbology in the cockpit is not adequate anymore. Decisions are expected to be made in what she calls microtime. For her, the challenge of the cockpit design is to provide the right information at the right time. Because fighter pilots, including those flying agile aircraft, prefer out-the-window maneuvering and handling, information could be provided by head-up display and head-up control systems. The hands-on-throttle-and-stick (HOTAS) concept facilitates head-up control, by adding switches to the flight controls enabling selection of sensor systems, weapon systems, and navigation systems without the necessary redirection of the pilot's gaze point. This encouraged the design of head-up display and control systems. Some of these systems are rather futuristic (Sec. IV.C), but some others like head-mounted tracking systems, three-dimensional audio, and vibro-tactile displays will be introduced in the new cockpits. On top of these developments, there is also a push towards automated cockpit systems, which

---

*Personal communication with Dr. J. Linder, April 1999.

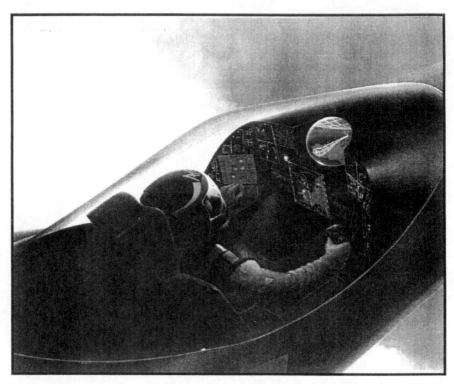

Fig. 3   Impression of a future fighter cockpit. The Boeing Advanced Technology Crew Station. (Reproduced with permission of David Snyder.)

are increasingly finding their place in the cockpits of airliners, small aircraft, and military aircraft, depending on the envisioned applications of those aircraft (Sec. IV.A). There is also a push to go to synthetic vision displays, which can potentially ease the workload of pilots in civil airliners when flying at night or in bad weather. In military aircraft, a need for flying closed cockpit is also observed because of the threat of directed-energy weapons. This might demand even a complete new design of the cockpit.[36] Some ideas about these developments are covered in Sec. IV.D. A depiction of a future fighter cockpit is illustrated in Fig. 3.

A.   Cockpit Automation

In modern airliners systems that make them safer in terms of averting midair collisions and CFIT were installed. The TCAS is a system in which neighboring aircraft computers monitor each other to prevent a midair collision. A device in one jet's cockpit warns with an automatic voice "traffic" and then commands the jet to climb, while the other jet is given a similar warning and commanded to descend. Because of these systems, several near accidents ended safely.[37] In Sec. IV.B.1 several experiments are mentioned in which three-dimensional audio shortened the time to detect the intruding aircraft. Application of three-dimensional audio requires continuous wearing of a headset, which is common in the military environment, but not in civil aviation.

A second automated warning system is the GPWS. In its newest version GPWS uses terrain databases to show the pilot on the computer screen where dangerous mountain peaks ahead are located if it senses that the plane comes too close to the ground. Jets do have GPWS setups, but in nap-on-the-Earth flying they are useless. The problem is that these systems contain a warning some seconds early in an attempt to account for the pilot's reaction time in recognizing the problem and correcting it. It is this reaction time that causes the system, in many instances, to issue a warning when the aircraft is not in danger. These early warnings are nuisances to the pilot, and therefore the warnings are either ignored or turned off.[38] To circumvent this problem, Swihart and Barfield designed an auto-GCAS, which eliminates the pilot reaction time. It is always in the background, allowing the pilot to maneuver to all attitudes and altitudes without causing a recovery action unless the aircraft is in danger of striking the ground. These authors determined the points where pilots normally react to avoid ground collisions and designed the system to activate after this moment. Auto-GCAS utilizes a digital terrain system with a terrain-referenced navigation algorithm to locate the aircraft spatially with respect to the terrain. The terrain database around the aircraft is scanned, and a terrain profile is created. An aircraft response model is used to continuously predict the aircraft's future recovery trajectory, and a recovery is automatically initiated whenever the trajectory penetrates a preset distance from the terrain profile. The flight-test results showed the benefits of such an automated system. It showed that nuisance warnings were almost zero and that interference to the pilot was nonexistent, leading the authors to believe that pilot acceptance will be much better than in the past.[28] It is obvious that all of these systems have a strong potential to prevent CFIT SD accidents, and, as such, they deserve to be deployed within all aircraft. According to Albery,* an updated GCAS is under development for the SAAB Gripen fighter aircraft. It is ready for flight testing in test aircraft and will later be operationally installed. The Gripen GCAS function warns for impending ground collision, and if no pilot recovery maneuvering occurs an automatic fly-up is initiated at the last possible moment. In line with these developments in which the flight performance is monitored to prevent an impact, techniques are being developed that monitor some vital parameters of the pilot in order to see whether he or she is still actively engaged in controlling the aircraft (smart suit). An example of this is the monitoring of breathing rhythm and head movements in Russian pilots on their long-distance flights across Siberia. If certain physiological signals indicate that the pilot is falling asleep, the pilot state monitor might decide to switch the control to an autopilot.[39]

Additional developments that might enhance situational awareness concern the introduction of an intelligent user interface for cockpit information management, such as the U.S. Army's Rotorcraft Pilot's Associate for the future attack/scout helicopter. These developments will not be discussed in detail here and the reader is referred to Miller and Hannen[40] and Svenmarck.[41] It is obvious that reduction in workload will allow more time for the real pilot's task, (i.e., flying the aircraft), thereby reducing the chance of SD.

---

*Personal communication with Dr. Bill Albery, April 1999.

B. Nontraditional Displays

Spatial-orientation functions of traditional displays are discussed in Chapters 9 and 10. In view of the ever-increasing burden of the visual displays, researchers have addressed alternative sensory systems such as the auditory and the tactile ones. The auditory system already plays an important role in the cockpit for communication and warning information, but with the development of three-dimensional auditory displays a new set of applications are feasible and being explored to determine whether this technique is advantageous in the modern cockpit (see Sec. IV.B.1). A similar approach with tactile sensors attempts to provide the pilot with three-dimensional directional information. This approach was primarily initiated to address the problems of SD, but this technology development might also show itself to be useful as a directional threat indicator, as discussed in Sec. IV.B.2.

1. Three-Dimensional Auditory Display

a. General description. A three-dimensional auditory display presents sound from arbitrary directions spanning a sphere around the listener. Such displays have become feasible through the development of techniques for creating virtual sound sources using headphone presentation.[42,43] The principle is shown in Fig. 4.

Advantages of such displays in the cockpit, in addition to the information contained in the signal itself, are that relevant directional information can be conveyed using the natural sound localization ability of humans. Because it is common in high-workload tasks to present information primarily through the visual channel, use of the auditory channel can reduce pilot workload and shorten reaction times.[44,45] Another advantage is that spatial separation of signals and noise sources lowers the threshold at which signals can be detected and discriminated, thereby improving the effective signal-to-noise ratio.[46,47] This is also important for simultaneous discrimination of multiple signals. Thus, three-dimensional audio has the potential to improve overall situational awareness in the cockpit.

Virtual sound sources are created with headphone sounds simulating the acoustic effects of the listener's shoulders, head, and external ears by linear head-related transfer functions (HRTF). Because of interindividual differences, these HRTFs

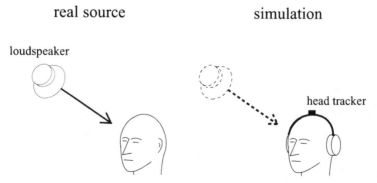

Fig. 4 **Directional hearing of a real sound source (loudspeaker) and of a virtual sound source (earphones with corresponding HRTFs).**

are optimal if they are determined for each individual. To determine such HRTFs requires recording of test signals from known directions with small probe microphones placed in the ear canals of that individual. Creating a virtual sound source with a fixed direction, relative to the listener's head, is accomplished by loading the digital filters with the individual's HRTFs for that specific angle. Creating a space-stable virtual sound source requires recording the head position and orientation with a tracking device to update the filters in real time with the HRTF corresponding to that particular position of the sound source in space.

  b. *Experimental evidence.* Wightman and Kistler[48] found that localization acuity of virtual and real sound sources in subjects with immobilized heads was equally good (about 10 deg), when using the individual's own HRTFs for the virtual sounds. They used trains of noise bursts as stimuli. Confusions, which are the refractions of the source position about the horizontal or vertical plane passing through the listener's ears,[49] were about twice as high for the virtual sounds (10.9%) compared with the real sounds (5.6%), however. In an identical setup with nonindividualized HRTFs, these confusion percentages were much higher: 23.5% vs 6.0% for the real sounds conditions, if only those seven subjects were considered with confusion percentages similar to those for the real sound conditions of the just-mentioned Wightman and Kistler study.[50] This shows the importance of individualized HRTFs. With speech stimuli instead of noise bursts, Begault and Wenzel[51] obtained similar results. They also observed that stimuli were heard inside the head about 50% of the time, depending on the source position. Bronkhorst[52] found that if head movements were allowed and signals were of long duration localization acuity as well as confusion percentages were the same for both real and virtual sound sources. Given the flight envelope for fighter aircraft, auditory localization accuracy under varying levels of sustained $+G_z$ acceleration is of interest as well. Nelson et al.[53] showed that localization error did not significantly increase between 1 and 5.6 $+G_z$, although errors increased significantly at 7.0 $+G_z$.

  Several flight simulator studies have investigated the use of three-dimensional audio for the TCAS that is installed in most commercial aircraft. (References 100–103 are suggested for further reading) An example of a laboratory setup for such experiments is shown in Fig. 5.

  These studies used a three-dimensional auditory display for the aural TCAS warning to convey the spatial location of an intruding aircraft to the pilots. All studies showed that out-the-window visual search time for the intruding aircraft was reduced with three-dimensional audio, compared to monaural warnings (reductions ranged from 8 to 47%)

  In a study that compared different methods of directing attention to peripheral targets, target acquisition time with three-dimensional tones was less than with other auditory signals (coded aural tone, speech cue, and three-dimensional speech cue).[54] Information from the auditory channel reduced search latencies about 100–200 ms.

  This advantage increased as the eccentricity of the target increased beyond the limit of the central visual field.[55] Subjects were able to detect targets with less overall head motion and reduced head velocity,[56] which might not only be helpful in high-acceleration environments to reduce the risk of neck and shoulder fatigue and injury, but also to prevent unnecessary vestibular stimulation. In actual

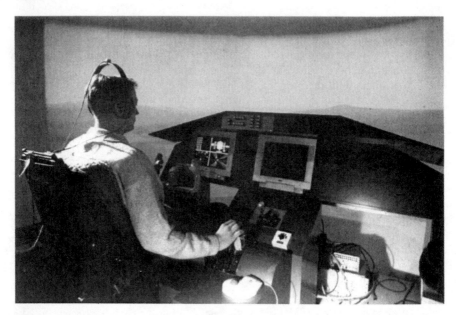

Fig. 5   Laboratory setup for experiments on three-dimensional audio in the cockpit. Note the head tracker on the headphones.

Harrier flight tests, a three-dimensional audio system was particularly effective for azimuth cueings. Aviators were able to discern targets separated by 12–20 deg (Ref. 57).

In a series of simulator studies, Bronkhorst and Veltman performed three experiments on three-dimensional audio in the military cockpit.[42,58–60] In their studies subjects used individualized HRTFs and head trackers to register head position. All experiments included an intercept task, but the visual radar information was different. A small plan-view or two-dimensional radar display in the head-down display (HDD) was used in the first experiment.[42] The authors found that performance of the intercept task improved when the subjects were supported by three-dimensional audio along with visual information. These findings were replicated in the second experiment,[59] but intercept performance with an advanced three-dimensional visual radar[61] display was almost optimal, and, therefore, no further improvement could be obtained with three-dimensional audio. Performance on a head-up display task was improved in the second experiment with both types of radar displays, indicating that the subjects had scanned the radar display less often and, therefore, had more time to check the HUD when they were supported by three-dimensional audio. In a third experiment, Veltman and Oving[60] gathered eye movement data concerning the actual scan behavior of the subjects. Subjects made about 50% fewer downward eye movements to scan the HDD when they were supported by three-dimensional audio, which might be helpful in close combat situations. In some conditions of this experiment, the positions of two independent targets were presented by three-dimensional audio. Pilots were able to discriminate these targets adequately. Furthermore, extra information was added to the sounds to reduce confusion. Pitch was used to reduce front-back confusion. (Higher frequencies were used for targets in front of their own jet.) Update frequency was used to reduce the above-below confusion. (Faster update rates were used for targets above the pilot's own jet). No confusion was reported in this experiment. In sum, all three experiments showed positive effects on primary and/or secondary task performance when three-dimensional audio was presented. Similar effects were found for three-dimensional audio added to a HMD.[56]

Speech intelligibility and discrimination are also improved by localizing speech inputs. Small angular separation of messages (45 deg) is found to greatly improve speech intelligibility. Using three-dimensional communication separation, the speech intelligibility levels were maximized.[46,57,62] A three-dimensional communication separation system also worked well in Harrier flight tests, aiding dual message traffic.[57]

Calhoun[35] proposed spatialized auditory cues to code system status information. For example, to aid the pilot in understanding a critical situation and add redundancy to the message a left engine auditory fire-alert message could be displayed, so that it appears to emanate from the left. The auditory space can also be used to indicate the level of urgency of an auditory warning. The most urgent warnings would be presented so they are perceived inside the head, whereas less urgent warnings are perceived to the sides.[63]

In reviewing all of these three-dimensional audio experiments on situation awareness, Calhoun concludes that three-dimensional auditory signals have the potential of being detected more quickly than visual signals and, at the very least, might help to relieve the pilot's heavy visual workload.[35] According to Calhoun, possible (agile) aircraft applications of three-dimensional auditory displays include 1) alerting pilots of ground or aerial threat locations and facilitating target acquisition; 2) enhancing situational awareness during air-to-air combat by localizing voice communications; 3) segregating multiple channels of communication to improve intelligibility, discrimination, and selective attention among audio sources; 4) providing an additional cue for location of urgency of an aircraft system malfunction. Calhoun[35] concludes that before these candidate applications can be implemented further research is required to determine how best to exploit the capability to present auditory signals. Finally, she stresses the need to refine the three-dimensional audio technique in order to diminish the large number of front–back confusions whenever head movements are minimal. Until this confusion is controlled, application of three-dimensional auditory displays might best be limited to serving as a redundant cue. This conclusion is in line with the findings of Bronkhorst and Veltman.[58]

   c.   *Auditory induced self-motion and self-localization.*   In the preceding examples auditory information was used to indicate the direction of a sound source (e.g., a threat) with respect to the pilot's position. This normal reflexive ability does not require training as such. In the past few decades researchers have investigated whether the auditory surround could play a role in spatial self-orientation similar to that of the visual system. Experiments were in two directions: one was to see whether a sensation of rotation could be induced along with (audiokinetic) nystagmus, whereas the other tried to demonstrate the auditory influence on posture control. It was difficult to evoke audiokinetic circular vection or nystagmus with rotating sound sources about stationary subjects.[64–67] The auditory system plays only a minor role in spatial orientation, if compared to the other sensory systems like the vestibular and visual systems.[68] For instance, subjects rotating at constant velocity with steady sound sources in the room will continue to report rotation, despite the absence of any vestibular information. However, as soon as the chair starts to decelerate the vestibular sensation of turning into the opposite direction overrules the sustained auditory sensation. In view of the visual dominance over the vestibular system, it is clear that the auditory system is not as heavily involved in self-orientation: this makes sense in view of the fact that sound sources are in many cases not stable in space. (See also Chapter 2, Sec. XII.) Studies on postural reactions to auditory stimuli have also had negative results, because the reported postural reactions observed at high sound levels look more like shock reactions.[67] Of course, blind people process auditory position information much better, but that requires continuous attention. Similar use of auditory signals for spatial orientation can be seen with an auditory routing system to guide people to the exit in case of low visibility in evacuating a building in case of fire.[69] However, this definitely requires controlled attention from the subjects.

Auditory cues in the cockpit have long been used to support spatial orientation of the pilot, mostly in the form of single frequencies and voice communications, presented monaurally. Lyons et al.[70] investigated the effects of an acoustic orientation instrument that displayed airspeed as a sound frequency (repetition rate), vertical velocity by amplitude modulation rate (increase shown by increased pitch), and bank angle by right/left lateralization (louder signal on the side that was in the same direction as the bank). This display was presented to pilots using earphones, after processing the auditory signal to map to the actual aircraft flight data. The result showed that acoustic signals can be useful indicators of the orientation of an aircraft in the absence of visual cues, with interaural intensity differences (representing bank angle) particularly effective in this regard.

From the examples just given, it is clear that auditory orientation information has proven to be useful in the cockpit for flying the aircraft. Continuous provision of the acoustic information during flight[70] will not guarantee that the pilot will maintain a correct spatial orientation and prevent SD mishaps, although it might be that matching the auditory spatial-orientation information with the environment eventually becomes automatic for pilots. In a Type I SD episode, the mismatch between the auditory information and the pilot's natural orientation percept will then trigger the pilot to restore correct orientation. It is also feasible to provide the information if the pilot requests it, for instance, when the pilot is in a Type II SD situation. In that case, three-dimensional audio could be made to indicate the gravity vector, as is done with the tactile vest (Sec. IV.B.2). Perhaps tactile and three-dimensional audio information should be combined in these cases, although this requires more research, especially under complex vestibular maneuvering. With a head-tracker system the auditory information might remain space stable despite changes of head or body position, which is an important advantage of three-dimensional audio over tactile body displays.

In conclusion, with respect to SD, three-dimensional auditory displays can reduce the pilot's visual workload, thereby providing him or her with more time for the primary mission tasks, which might thereby reduce the chance of SD. On the other hand, more research is needed to determine if three-dimensional audio has the potential to provide direct spatial-orientation information to the pilot in the cockpit during fast maneuvering.

2. Tactile Displays

a. General description. Craig and Sherrick[71] reviewed the early work on dynamic tactile displays. Tactile cueing was developed in the 1970s to overcome visual handicaps by converting visual information to patterns for the skin.[72] A nice example in this respect is a device containing a large series of vibrating tactors on the back of blind subjects used to project the image of a video camera mounted on the head of the subject. Although blind subjects after some training could learn to interpret complex patterns, the skin is not an intuitive substitute for the eye, and the interpretation required a lot of attention. Anecdotal evidence pointed to reduce fore-aft swaying of a subject when the experimenter was zooming in and out with the camera, showing incorporation of the tactile information in postural control.[73] Also, detection of motion by stimulating subsequent tactors on the skin was shown to demand less attention.

b. Basic research. Van Erp and his colleagues, initiated a series of studies on the basic aspects of vibro-tactile stimulation of the torso with respect to the perceptual characteristics in terms of the information processing capacity of the torso.[74] In their experiments on the spatial resolution of the torso, they found that the ventral part of the torso is more sensitive than the dorsal part for vibro-tactile stimulation: the distance between two actuators needed to reach a 75% correct localization performance being on the average 0.4 and 1.7 cm, respectively, as shown in Fig. 6.

They also found that the sensitivity near the sagittal plane of the torso is about two to three times better than to the sides.[76] In another experiment Van Erp[75]

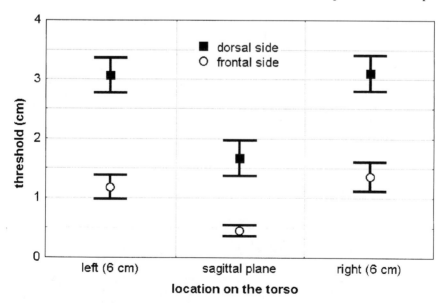

Fig. 6   Threshold for the minimum (center-to-center) distance between two actuators needed to reach a 75% correct localization performance as a measure of the torso's spatial accuracy for vibro-tactile stimuli. (Reproduced with permission of Van Erp; Ref. 75.)

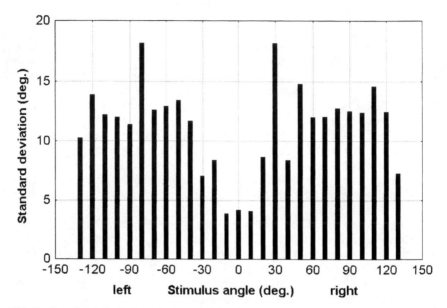

Fig. 7   Standard deviation of vibro-tactile responses as a function of stimulus angle, with 0 deg as the midsagittal plane and negative angles to the left. (Reproduced with permission of Van Erp; Ref. 75.)

investigated tactile direction discrimination of the torso. Again, several actuators were attached around the torso, and subjects had to indicate the direction of that tactile stimulus. The results showed that there was not one tactile ego-center, but instead two internal reference points: one for the left side of the torso and one for the right side. When these internal reference points are determined as a function of the body side stimulated, the left and right points are 6.2 cm apart on average across participants. Further research showed that this finding was not caused by the experimental setup, the visual system, the subjective location of the stimuli, or other anomalies.[77] The variance of the responses depends on the presented direction: performance in the front-sagittal region is very good with standard deviations between 4 and 8 deg and somewhat lower to the sides, as is shown in Fig. 7.

c. Tactile display systems for the cockpit.   Visual displays still dominate cockpit design, the interest in auditory displays is growing, but only a few groups have research programs on tactile displays. Sanneman[78] used vibrating tactors on a pilot's chest successfully to provide airspeed and glide-path information, and in the early 1990s two tactile navigation displays were developed. Gilliland and Schlegel[79] explored the use of the human head for a vibro-tactile information display to provide an egocentric view of the environment. This would allow, for instance, for direction sensitive threat warnings. The relative accuracy (how well can the subject designate the correct stimulus site) was almost 90% with 12 stimulation sites but it deteriorated with more stimulation sites.

A more interesting body locus for a tactile information display is the torso because of its large surface, its three-dimensional form, and its possible egocentric view. This approach was followed at the Naval Aerospace Medical Research

Laboratory (NAMRL) in Pensacola, Florida, where the TSAS was developed as a nonvisual tool to avoid SD.[80,81] Arrays of small pneumatically activated tactile stimulators in a vest are cued by the aircraft's inertial reference system and are designed to allow the pilot to sense the aircraft's attitude even without checking the instruments or the world outside. With the TSAS setup indicating the direction of the gravity vector, pilots recover more easily from unusual attitudes.[82] Coupled with motion feedback from the aircraft, TSAS improves pilot performance in hovering operations, by reducing drifting (which, according to accident statistics, is a very common cause for SD accidents).[83] Coupled with global-positioning-system (GPS) information, tactile cueing can also be of value in direction cueing.

   d. Flight experience with tactile display. In the first flight test in the TSAS program in 1995, a flight surgeon flew maneuvers including straight-and-level flight, standard rate turns, unusual attitude recoveries, and ground-controlled approaches as well as aileron rolls and inside loops.[81,82] He was sitting in the back seat without any instruments under the hood, to prevent viewing outside visual information, and received only limited torso stimulation located apart from auditory cues for altitude, airspeed, and G force. The TSAS provided aircraft pitch-and-roll vectors to on the pilot's torso. Stimulus frequency of a tactor increased with increasing pitch angle in discrete steps, enhancing the direction sensitivity of each tactor. With 16 tactors encoded this way for pitch and roll, the pilot in effect could determine the direction of the Earth's surface. The researchers commented that unusual-attitude recovery was possible for the TSAS-equipped pilot, unless the system was deactivated during setup maneuvering and not reactivated until the moment the subject pilot took over control.[82] This demonstrates that although TSAS might be intuitive (easy to learn) it also requires continuous attention.

   With a comparable setup a second set of flight tests was performed in a UH-60A helicopter, with similar maneuvers except for the aerobatic maneuvers. Two research pilots deprived of vision performed the maneuvers with success. In a third flight test with the same UH-60 helicopter, TSAS was used as a feedback system for controlling drift velocity in hovering operations. Here, too, application of TSAS proved to be very helpful. Pilots appreciated the increase in performance using TSAS feedback and at the same time experienced a decrease in workload.[83] As with three-dimensional audio, the question remains whether a TSAS-equipped pilot during normal operational flying could get into a Type 1 SD situation or whether the TSAS information would automatically alert the pilot to the impending danger of SD. Experiments to answer this type of questions are very difficult to set up but have to be done.

   The application of TSAS for directional threat cueing has also been proposed, similar to three-dimensional audio. Together with GPS, TSAS can also give directional way-finding information for underwater operations, which can help to prevent SD in that environment.

   e. Relevant issues. At NAMRL much effort was devoted to increasing the reliability of the tactile cueing system.[81] One of the problems of the tactors is that it is very difficult to get information on the effective stimulus when used in the cockpit environment, especially when pulling Gs. Van Veen and van Erp[74] found in psychophysical experiments in a centrifuge that the perception of vibrotactile stimulation on the torso is not substantially impaired during high G-load conditions, at least up to 6 G, which is very promising.

Van Erp stresses that just adding tactile information does not automatically enhance the human–machine interface or improve the user's performance: the results obtained so far are promising, but filling the gaps of the required knowledge is necessary before applications can be successful.[77] The nature of the interactions between the tactile and other senses is only recently being addressed.

C. Alternative Controls

There are two elements to the pilot–machine interface: getting information to the pilot through various sensory modalities and getting control commands from the pilot to the aircraft. Most research has concentrated on improving the former, but technological solutions that could improve the ease by which a pilot controls the aircraft are also needed. One advanced control technology already in use is the already mentioned HOTAS, and several other technologies that have been the subject of considerable research will be discussed here: eye-based, muscle- and brain-based, and speech-based control. Foot control, an alternative control-technology favored by Previc,[84] will not be discussed in this section.

1. Eye-Based Control

One of the candidates for alternative controls is eye-based control. In combination with the head-tracker signal, eye tracking enables control of crew station functions using the pilot's line of sight.[85,86] Calhoun prefers the direction of eye gaze to serve as a control input signal because the visual system is the primary channel for acquiring information and because eye muscles are extremely fast and respond very quickly. It is more efficient to use the pilot's gaze to aim a weapon, rather than align the head or manually slew a displayed cursor over the target. In terms of SD, eye-based control can reduce head movements, which is an advantage in terms of the provocativeness of SD during flight maneuvers.

Eye-based control can therefore increase the envelope and speed of target acquisition with a HMD/T system. Pilots were very positive as to the increased capability that could be realized with eye-based control. Moreover, eye motion is more feasible under high acceleration conditions, compared to head or hand movement. Eye-based control involves the use of a consent button, which could be located on the joystick. The system is not yet flight worthy for supermaneuverable aircraft, but it is anticipated that eye-based control will eventually be feasible for agile aircraft and will be used to designate display areas subtending approximately 17 mrad ($\sim$1 deg) of visual angle.

2. Electromyographic-Based Control

If electrodes are positioned on the surface of the skin to detect the firing of muscle fibers, these electrical signals can be used to provide electromyographic (EMG)-based control. Because these signals are very noisy, they can be used only to generate a binary control input: one control action above a reference threshold and another action below the reference level.[87] Important for implementation of EMG-based control is to choose body movements that do not interfere with the pilot's normal functions. It is questionable whether applications will be possible during supermaneuvering or when "straining" or pulling Gs.

3. Electroencephalographic-Based Control

Electrodes integrated in the pilot's headgear positioned over specific areas of the scalp can provide the necessary signals to implement electroencephalographic (EEG)-based control.[87] This type of control translates the electrical activity of the brain into a control signal. In one approach, EEG signals are brought under conscious voluntary control with training and biofeedback. Another approach harnesses naturally occurring brain responses to modulated stimuli. These brain responses (so-called evoked responses) sometimes include components that modulate at the same frequency as the evoking stimuli. Selectable items of a display are modulated at different frequencies. Detecting which frequency pattern is dominant in the visually evoked brain activity can identify the pilot's choice (gaze point) between selectable items. This method would have the advantage over the normal eye-based control in that the components of this EEG control are less expensive and obtrusive. Further refinement of the method is required, however. In terms of SD prevention, the same arguments can be made for ECG control as far as for eye-based control (Sec. IV.C.1).

4. Speech-Based Control

Speech-recognition technology allows the pilot's speech signals to be used to carry out preset activities. A prerequisite is high recognition reliability; otherwise, additional validation steps might be required. Use of speech input has the potential of rapidly accessing functions several levels down the hierarchical structure of a multifunction control. On the other hand, manual selection of a dedicated, frequently selected switch (e.g., the HOTAS concept) might be more rapid than the mental processing involved in issuing a verbal command and the time required by the voice recognizer to process the signal. The performance of speech systems is degraded by high ambient noise, vibration, stress level of the pilot, and acceleration. To compensate for these shifts in speech caused by changes in the environment, adaptation algorithms are required in the speech processing as well as noise-canceling hardware.[35,88,89]

As for SD, speech-based control enables the pilot to remain head-out and requires less head movements, thereby helping to prevent SD.

D. Virtual Cockpit

As described in preceding chapters and sections, much progress has been made in presenting the pilot with information to update his or her situation awareness. However, in most aircraft this sort of advanced avionics is not installed and will not be installed in the next couple of years. North[90] cites a report from the Flight Safety Foundation indicating that about 80% of airline fatalities resulted from controlled-flight-into-terrain and approach-and-landing accidents. The biggest reason for such accidents is pilots' failure to make critical decisions or making wrong decisions at crisis times. Lack of "geographical" awareness was the second leading cause. North[90] argues that current display technologies still have the pilot reading and interpreting letters and numbers, which they have to convert into a view of the world outside the cockpit. North pleads to invest in the virtual cockpit, a cockpit that does not rely on information displayed as letters and numbers but instead on synthetic vision displays. With the accuracy of global positioning systems and the availability of vast digital terrain databases, the pathway-in-the-sky concept (see Chapter 9, Sec. III.C and Chapter 10, Sec. III.B) could be optimized. These pathway-in-the-sky concepts have shown to be realizable in the work by Mulder.[91]

Flying closed cockpit, akin to flying under IMC, is considered by the military in order to avoid the threat of a directed-energy weapon. The HDD and HUD offer in principle enough information to allow safe flying. Fast maneuvering in military aircraft using only these displays would increase the chance of SD. Helmet-mounted displays, which display synthetic terrain imagery or FLIR imagery, all try to provide the pilot with a pictorial view from the outside world. The ultimate display as proposed by Hopper[31] is in line with this reasoning. Although such HMDs allow for a lot of what is known as "presence," they make and provoke motion sickness and SD easily.[92] Head movements must be detected before the visual image can be adjusted, which brings about an inevitable delay. Even if predictor algorithms are used, these velocity changes necessarily cause inadequacies in the visual presentation, which increases the likelihood of closed-cockpit scenes not being able to achieve visual dominance and thereby facilitating SD (see also Chapter 3, Sec. IV.D). Thus, fast head movements can cause discrepancies between the physical head motion and the visual motion, which is according to all motion sickness models provocative (see Sec. II). Therefore, technical improvements should be directed to make this delay as small as possible. Interestingly, it has been found that people adapt to these discrepancies by moving their heads more slowly after a while, which minimizes these discrepancies and diminishes the likelihood of motion sickness, but a restriction on the speed of head movement is not desirable in military aircraft.[93]

Additional problems arise if the HMD synthetic terrain is used to provide off-boresight targeting. For example, FLIR images that magnify the area surrounding a target make it more difficult for the pilot to keep track of his or her own flight path. Consequently, the chance of mismatches between the expected information and the sensed information might grow, leading to a greater risk of SD and motion sickness.

Because laser threats are not always present, one conceptualizes two solutions: retractable protection whereby the pilot flies using visual flight rules (VFR) depending on the situation and the other a full-time enclosed cockpit with no outside vision.[36]

Borah[94] summarizes the idea of the virtual cockpit as an extension of the visually coupled system to its practical limit so that it could provide an integrated and intuitive man–machine interface for all of the tasks that make up the pilot's job. Borah[94] states that to enable operations in any external visibility condition, all relevant head-out information for controlling the aircraft, navigating, finding targets, avoiding threats and maintaining tactical awareness should be superimposed directly onto the pilot's normal view of the world or, when that is unavailable, the sensor-derived and computer-generated synthetic substitute for that view. Directional sound cues (and vibro-tactile cues) could reinforce the sensory inputs. Not all technologies are at present mature enough to realize such a virtual cockpit, however.

V. Unmanned Aerial Vehicles

Another development in military aviation is the introduction of unmanned aerial vehicles (UAV), either for reconnaissance or for combat operations, in which the pilot becomes a distant operator, mostly in a ground control room. Because spatial disorientation is one of the issues of concern in operating UAVs, some attention is given to this topic as well.

It is obvious that the orientation situation for the distant operator of UAVs is not the same as for the pilot in the aircraft. In regard to the control system model displayed in Fig. 1, the basic difference is that there is no UAV motion input to mechanically stimulate the operator's orientation system. As long as the distant operator does not experience vection by the UAV camera view on a large monitor, the equilibrium system of the operator only deals with his or her orientation in the control room.

Exchange of information with the UAV is delayed, which affects control in time-critical tasks. Therefore, supervisory control[1] of the UAV is preferable for the operator, which is a rather abstract way of flying (flying between waypoints). Operating UAVs is, therefore, not a classical piloting task.

In one regard, the lack of direct motion feedback might be an advantage for the distant operator because now UAVs can operate beyond human physiological limits. On the other hand, the absence of direct motion feedback can be disadvantageous in that the distant operator might fail to experience changes in flight performance induced by some structural damage to the UAV. It is also possible that the absence of motion feedback has other consequences. The operator can manipulate the viewing direction of the camera onboard the UAV, but it is difficult for the operator to maintain a correct orientation of the flight direction and attitude of the UAV because the camera image is seen on the monitor screen straight ahead of the operator. Many UAVs have been lost because of SD of the operator with respect to the flight path of the UAV.[95] Therefore, an important issue is how the spatial awareness of the operator can be improved.

The main issue is how to display the tactical and other situational information as adequately as possible to the UAV operator on the visual display. Support of geographical orientation is possible with tunnel-in-the-sky displays, plan-view (Gods-eye) displays, maps, and compass. Several display options to provide the spatial information are possible, such as from a pilot-oriented reference frame (heading up) or from a world-oriented reference frame (north up).[96] In addition, the viewpoint from the operator in the display can be egocentric (as in pathway-in-the-sky displays[91]) or exocentric (as in maps or a plan-view display[97]). In this respect the difference between the concept of local guidance and global awareness is relevant.[96] Local guidance can, for instance, be the estimation of a target with respect to the pilot's own aircraft, whereas global awareness refers to the estimation of the relative position and distances between targets. Research has shown that egocentric information displays enhance flight performance and situational awareness primarily in local-guidance tasks. Exocentric displays providing orientational and tactical information enhance flight performance and situational awareness primarily in global awareness tasks. If the supervisory control task of the pilot requires a combination of local-guidance and global-awareness tasks, one would expect that a combined exo- and egocentric display would optimally support the pilot. However, this is not immediately evident in practice, and the optimal display depends on the tasks involved.[98,99]

In the future we can expect that the limited visual displays from the UAV cameras will be enhanced to egocentric three-dimensional visual displays in the operator station. Increasing the field of view of UAV camera images can be accomplished with computer-generated images of three-dimensional terrain databases available from satellites. By combining information from GPS and inertial navigation systems (INS), wide-base stereo displays can be created that highlight with high resolution the region of interest with variable scaling. This enhances the spatial orientation of the operator and facilitates the search for targets. Tactical information will then be superimposed on the display.

It is likely that this sort of visual display improvement will lead to a better situational awareness of the operator of the UAV. However, as a consequence of the increased visual display size and the better image quality, it is possible for the operator to become "immersed" in the task, just as if he or she were piloting an aircraft in a simulator. If so, then the visual system will provide the operator's equilibrium with some visually induced motion information. This should be no problem for the human equilibrium system as long as the motion characteristics of the UAV are modest. Some researchers have even considered supplying the UAV operator with actual motion in a motion based simulator. Because one of the aims of the UAV was to go beyond the physiological boundaries of the human equilibrium system, the discrepancy between the visually induced UAV motion and the motion of the simulator might be large, leading to simulator sickness.

Increasing the difficulty factor still further is the proposal for the navigator to operate UAVs from the cockpit. Because of the superposed movements of the navigator's own aircraft, this raises interesting SD issues. Just as is the case with the distant ground station, this operator station will probably not immerse the operator into the UAV motion. However, his or her sensory systems will detect the motion of the aircraft to create a self-motion sensation. It is an open question as to whether or not such self-motion sensations might interfere with the UAV orientation task.

VI. Summary

Because the evolution of the human equilibrium system is not fast enough to keep up with the quickly expanding motion characteristics of modern fighters and helicopters, the possibility of inducing spatial disorientation remains. Because pilots flying these aircraft prefer head-up control of the aircraft, much effort has been invested in the development of displays to enhance situational awareness. In this chapter the options of vibro-tactile (TSAS) and three-dimensional audio information displays are summarized. Based upon this review, one can expect that TSAS and three-dimensional audio will find an application in the cockpit. For specific task such as hovering, TSAS might be an ideal tool to help the pilot. TSAS and three-dimensional audio will both be able to improve situational awareness in tasks where three-dimensional spatial information has to be displayed. However, although both displays might help to maintain spatial orientation, it is not certain that using TSAS or three-dimensional audio will prevent a Type I spatial-disorientation incident.

New control concepts like gaze-based, speech-based or EMG/EEG-based controls allow for a head-out control of the aircraft. They might be of some help in enhancing situational awareness, but before application of these novel control concepts are realized a lot of dedicated research is necessary.

The development of automated systems (TCAS and auto-GCAS) that sense impending head-on collisions or a controlled flight into terrain, and consequently take over command automatically is a most promising development and might have the biggest impact on preventing SD mishaps in fixed-wing aircraft.

References

[1]Sheridan, T. B., "Supervisory Control," *Handbook of Human Factors*, edited by G. Salvandy, Wiley, New York, 1987.

[2]Boff, K. R., and Lincoln, J. E., *Engineering Data Compendium "Human Perception and Performance*," Vol. I–III, H. G. Armstrong Aerospace Medical Research Lab., Wright-Patterson Air Force Base, OH, 1988.

[3]Bos, J. E., Bles, W., and Hosman, R. J. A. W., "Modeling Spatial Orientation and Motion Perception," *AIAA Paper 01–4248*, 2001, pp. 1–9.

[4]Benson, A. J., "Spatial Disorientation—General Aspects," *Aviation Medicine*, edited by J. Ernsting and P. King, Butterworth, London, 1998, pp. 277–296.

[5]Bles, W., Bos, J. E., de Graaf, B., Groen, E., and Wertheim, A. H., "Motion Sickness: Only One Provocative Conflict?," *Brain Research Bulletin*, Vol. 47, 1998, pp. 481–487.

[6]Gillingham, K. K., and Previc, F. H., "Spatial Orientation in Flight," Armstrong Lab., AL-TR-1993-0022, Brooks Air Force Base, TX, 1993.

[7]Benson, A. J., "Motion Sickness," *Aviation Medicine*, edited by J. Ernsting and P. King, Butterworth, London, 1988, pp. 318–338.

[8]Oman, C. M., "A Heuristic Mathematical Model for the Dynamics of Sensory Conflict and Motion Sickness," *Acta Oto-Laryngologica*, Suppl. 392, 1982.

[9]Reason, J. T., and Brand, J. J., *Motion Sickness*, Academic Press, London, 1975.

[10]Wertheim, A. H., "Motion Perception During Self Motion; The Direct Versus Inferential Controversy Revisited," *Behavioral and Brain Sciences*, Vol. 17, 1994, pp. 293–355.

[11]Bles, W., Bos, J. E., en Kruit, H., "Motion Sickness," *Current Opinion in Neurology*, Vol. 13, 2000, pp. 19–25.

[12]Bos, J. E., and Bles, W., "Modelling Motion Sickness and Subjective Vertical Mismatch Detailed for Vertical Motions," *Brain Research Bulletin*, Vol. 47, 1998, pp. 537–542.

[13]Hosman, R. J. A. W., "Pilot's Perception and Control of Aircraft Motion," Ph.D. Dissertation, Delft Univ. of Technology, Delft, the Netherlands, 1996.

[14]Hosman, R. J. A. W., and Stassen, H. G., "Pilot's Perception in the Control of Aircraft Motions," *Control Engineering Practices*, Vol. 7, 1999, pp. 1421–1428.

[15]Advani, S. A., and Hosman, R. J. A. W., "Integrated Motion Cueing Algorithm and Motion-Base Design for Flight Simulation," *Conference Proceedings: "Flight Simulation — The Next Decade*," Royal Aeronautical Society, London, 2000, 24–1-9.

[16]Albery, W., "Simulation," *Human Consequences of Agile Aircraft*, RTO-TR-015 AC/323(HFM-015)TP/15, Vol. 8, 2001, pp. 111–120.

[17]Repperger, D. W., "Dynamic Scaling of One-Seventh Size F-15 Prototypes for Agile Flight Simulation," AL/CF-TR-1995-0028, 1995.

[18]Welch, H., Albery, W., and Bles, W., "Physiological Consequences: Cardiopulmonary, Vestibular and Sensory Aspects," *Human Consequences of Agile Aircraft*, RTO-TR-015 AC/323(HFM-015)TP/15, Vol. 5, 2001, pp. 49–58.

[19]Le Blaye, P., "Agility: History, Definitions and Basic Concepts," *Human Consequences of Agile Aircraft*, RTO-EN-12, Vol. 2, 2000, pp. 1–13.

[20]Banks, R. D., Lyons, T. R., and Firth, J., "Introduction," *Human Consequences of Agile Aircraft*, RTO-TR-015 AC/323(HFM-015)TP/15, Vol. 1, 2001, pp. 1–9.

[21]Lackner, J. R., and Graybiel, A., "Variations in Gravitoinertial Force Level Affect the Gain of the Vestibulo-Ocular Reflex: Implications for the Etiology of Space Motion Sickness," *Aviation, Space, and Environmental Medicine*, Vol. 52, 1981, pp. 154–158.

[22]Marcus, J. T., and van Holten, C. R., "Vestibulo-Ocular Responses in Man to $+G_z$ Hypergravity," *Aviation, Space, and Environmental Medicine*, Vol. 61, 1990, pp. 631–635.

[23]McGrath, B. J., Guedry, F. E., Oman, C. M., and Rupert, A. H., "Vestibulo-Ocular Response of Human Subjects Seated in a Pivoting Support System During 3 Gz Centrifuge Stimulation," *Journal of Vestibular Research*, Vol. 5, 1995, pp. 331–347.

[24]Wientjes, C. J. E., and Marcus, J. T., "Situational Awareness and Vestibular Stimulation (II): Influence of + Gz Load upon Visual and Memory Search," TNO Human Factors, Rep. IZF 1991 A-22, Soesterberg, the Netherlands, 1991.

[25]Cheung, B., and Hofer, K., "Degradation of Visual Pursuit During Sustained +3Gz Acceleration," *Aviation, Space, and Environmental Medicine*, Vol. 70, 1999, pp. 451–458.

[26]Cheung, B., Money, K., and Eizenman, M., "Oculomotor Response to Linear Acceleration Induced by Counter-Rotation in Supine Subjects," *Aviation, Space, and Environmental Medicine*, Vol. 69, 1998, pp. 121–128.

[27]De Graaf, B., Bos, J. E., Tielemans, W., Rameckers, F., Rupert, A. H., and Guedry, F. E., "Otolith Contribution to Ocular Torsion and Spatial Orientation During Acceleration," Naval Aerospace Medical Research Lab., Technical Rept. 96-3, Pensacola, FL, 1996.

[28]Guedry, F. E., "Psychophysics of Vestibular Sensation," *Handbook of Sensory Physiology*, Vol. VI/2, edited by H. H. Kornhuber, Springer-Verlag, Berlin, 1974, pp. 3–154.

[29]Glasauer, S., "Das Zusammenspiel von Otolithen und Bogengängen im Wirkungsgefüge der Subjectiven Vertikale," Master's Thesis, Technical Univ., Munich, Germany, 1992.

[30]Merfeld, D. M., Young, L., Oman, C., and Shelhamer, M., "A Multidimensional Model of the Effect of Gravity on the Spatial Orientation of the Monkey," *Journal of Vestibular Research*, Vol. 3, 1993, pp. 141–161.

[31]Hopper, D. G., "Hectomegapixel Aerospace Cockpit Displays," *Countering the Directed Energy Threat: Are Closed Cockpits the Ultimate Answer? RTO Meeting Proceedings*, 30/AC/323(HFM)TP/10, Vol. 11, 2000, pp. 1–13.

[32]Knox, F., and Stucky, M., "Pilot Interviews," *Human Consequences of Agile Aircraft*, RTO-TR-015 AC/323(HFM-015)TP/15, 2001, App. D, pp. 155–169.

[33]Stassen, H. G., Johannsen, G., and Moray, N., "Internal Representation, Internal Model, Human Performance Model and Mental Workload," *Proceedings of the 3rd IFAC/IFIP/IEA/IFORS Symposium On Analysis, Design and Evaluation of Man-Machine Systems*, Univ. of Oulu, Oulu, Finland, 1988, pp. 23–32.

[34]Linder, J., Tielemans, W., and Albery, W., "Selection, Training and Simulation," *Human Consequences of Agile Aircraft*, RTO-EN-12, Vol. 6, 2000, pp. 1–10.

[35]Calhoun, G. L., "Pilot-Vehicle Interface," *RTO EN-12 Human Consequences of Agile Flight*, 2000, pp. 1–20.

[36]Jarrett, D., "Alternative Crewstation Configurations for Future Combat Aircraft," *Countering the Directed Energy Threat: Are Closed Cockpits the Ultimate Answer?*, RTO-MP-30, AC/323(HFM)TP/10, Vol. 14, 2000, pp. 1–18.

[37]Carley, W. M., Fritsch, P., and Karp, J., "New Cockpit Systems Broaden the Margin of Safety for Pilots," *The Wall Street Journal*, 1 March 2000.

[38]Swihart, D., and Barfield, F., "An Advanced Automatic Ground Collision Avoidance System for Fighter Aircraft," *SAFE Assoc. Proceedings* [CD-ROM], Atlanta, GA, 1999.

[39]Voyevodin, V. S., Kapustin, A. V., Dorafeev, Y. L., Dvornikov, M. V., and Soukholitko, V. A., "Flight Safety Ensuring in Case of Pilot's Temporary Loss," *5th Biannual International Symposium on Aeronautical Sciences*, TsAGI, Shukovsky, Russia, 1999.

[40]Miller, C. A., and Hannen, M. D., "The Rotorcraft Pilot's Associate: Design and Evaluation of an Intelligent User Interface for Cockpit Information Management," *Knowledge-Based Systems*, Vol. 12, 1999, pp. 443–456.

[41]Svenmarck, P., "Decision Support in a Fighter Aircraft: From Expert Systems to Cognitive Modeling," Swedish Centre for Human Factors in Aviation, HFA Rep. 1998-04, Linkoping, Sweden, 1998.

[42]Bronkhorst, A. W., Veltman, J. A., and van Breda, L., "Application of a Three-Dimensional Auditory Display in a Flight Task," *Human Factors*, Vol. 38, 1996, pp. 23–33.

[43]Wightman, F. L., and Kistler, D. J., "Headphone Simulation of Free Field Listening: I. Stimulus Synthesis," *Journal of the Acoustical Society of America*, Vol. 85, 1989, pp. 858–867.

[44]Perrot, D. R., "Auditory Psychomotor Coordination," *Proceedings of the Human Factors Society 32nd Annual Meeting*, Human Factors and Ergonomic Society, Santa Monica, CA, 1988, pp. 81–85.

[45]Wickens, C. D., "Processing Resources Inattention," *Varieties of Attention*, edited by R. Parasuraman and D. R. Davies, Academic Press, Orlando, FL, 1984, pp. 63–102.

[46]Bronkhorst, A. W., and Plomp, R., "The Effect of Head-Induced Interaural Time and Level Differences on Speech Intelligibility in Noise," *Journal of the Acoustic Society of America*, Vol. 83, 1988, pp. 1508–1516.

[47]Ricard, G. L., and Meirs, S. L., "Intelligibility and Localization of Speech from Virtual Directions," *Human Factors*, Vol. 36, 1994, pp. 120–128.

[48]Wightman, F. L., and Kistler, D. J., "Headphone Simulation of Free Field Listening: II. Psychophysical Validation," *Journal of the Acoustical Society of America*, Vol. 85, 1989, pp. 868–878.

[49]Mills, W., "Auditory Localization," *Foundations of Modern Auditory Theory*, Vol. 2, edited by J. V. Tobias, Academic Press, New York, 1972, pp. 301–348.

[50]Wenzel, E. M., Arruda, M., Kistler, D. J., and Wightman, F. L., "Localization Using Nonindividualized Head-Related Transfer Functions," *Journal of the Acoustical Society of America*, Vol. 94, 1993, pp. 111–123.

[51]Begault, D. R., and Wenzel, E. M., "Headphone Localization of Speech," *Human Factors*, Vol. 35, 1993, pp. 707–717.

[52]Bronkhorst, A. W., "Localization of Real and Virtual Sound Sources," *Journal of the Acoustic Society of America*, Vol. 98, 1995, pp. 2542–2553.

[53]Nelson, W. T., Bolia, R. S., McKinley, R. L., Chelette, T. L., Tripp, L. D., and Esken, R. L., "Localization of Virtual Auditory Cues in a High Gz Environment," *Proceedings of the Human Factors Society 32nd Annual Meeting*, Human Factors and Ergonomic Society, Santa Monica, CA, 1988.

[54]Calhoun, G. L., Janson, W. P., and Vanlencia, G., "Effectiveness of Three-Dimensional Auditory Directional Cues," *Proceedings of the Human Factors Society 32nd Annual Meeting*, Human Factors and Ergonomic Society, Santa Monica, CA, 1998, pp. 68–72.

[55]Perrot, D. R., Cisneros, J., McKinley, R. L., and D'Angelo, W. R., "Aurally Aided Visual Search Under Virtual and Free-Field Listening Conditions," *Human Factors*, Vol. 38, 1996, pp. 702–715.

[56]Nelson, W. T., Hettinger, L. J., Cunningham, J. A., Brickman, B. J., Haas, M. W., and McKinley, R. L., "Effects of Localized Auditory Information on Visual Target Detection Performance Using a Helmet Mounted Display," *Human Factors*, Vol. 40, 1998, pp. 452–460.

[57]Gilkey, R. H., and Anderson, T. R. (eds.), "Binaural and Spatial Hearing in Real and Virtual Environments," Lawrence Erlbaum, Mahwah, NJ, 1997, Chap. 31 and 32.

[58]Bronkhorst, A. W., and Veltman, J. A., "Evaluation of a Three-Dimensional Auditory Display in Simulated Flight," *RTO AMP Symposium on "Audio Effectiveness in Aviation,"* Vol. 5, 1996, pp. 1–6.

[59]Veltman, J. A., van Erp, J. B. F., van Breda, L., and Bronkhorst, A. W., "Visuele en Auditieve 3-D Displays als Ondersteuning bij het Opsporen van Doelvliegtuigen [Visual and Aiditive 3-D Displays as Support Finding Target Aircraft]," TNO Human Factors Rep. TM-96-A036, Soesterberg, the Netherlands, 1996.

[60]Veltman, J. A., and Oving, A. B., "3-D Sound in the Cockpit to Enhance Situation Awareness," TNO Human Factors, Rep. TM-99-A061, Soesterberg, the Netherlands, 1999.

[61]Van Breda, L., and Veltman, J. A., "Perspective Information in the Cockpit as a Target Tracking Aid," *Journal of Experimental Psychology—Applied*, Vol. 4, 1998, pp. 55–68.

[62]Drullman, R., and Bronkhorst, A. W., "Multichannel Speech Intelligibility and Talker Recognition Using Monaural, Binaural, and Three-Dimensional Auditory Presentation," *Journal of the Acoustical Society of America*, Vol. 107, 2000, pp. 2224–2235.

[63]Begault, D. R., and Wenzel, E. M., "Techniques and Applications for Binaural Sound Manipulation in Human-Machine Interfaces," *The International Journal of Aviation Psychology*, Vol. 2, 1992, pp. 1–22.

[64]Dodge, R., "Thresholds of Rotation," *Journal of Experimental Psychology*, Vol. 6, 1923, pp. 107–137.

[65]Hennebert, P. E., "Nystagmus Audiocinétique," *Acta Otolaryngologica (Stockholm)*, Vol. 51, 1960, pp. 412–415.

[66]Lackner, J. R., "Induction of Illusory Self-Rotation and Nystagmus by a Rotating Sound-Field," *Aviation, Space, and Environmental Medicine*, Vol. 48, 1977, pp. 129–131.

[67]Marme, A., and Bles, W., "Circular Vection and Human Posture II: Does the Auditory System Play a Role?," *Agressologie*, Vol. 18, 1977, pp. 329–333.

[68]Previc, F. H., "The Neuropsychology of 3-D Space," *Psychological Bulletin*, Vol. 124, 1998, pp. 123–164.

[69]Whittington, D., "Use of Directional Sound for Ship Evacuation," *Proceedings of the TIEMS 2001 Conference* [CD-ROM TIEMS2001], 1.12, 2001, pp. 1–10.

[70]Lyons, T. J., Gillingham, K. K., Teas, D. C., Ercoline, W. R., and Oakley, C., "The Effects of Acoustic Orientation Cues on Instrument Flight Performance in a Flight Simulator," *Aviation, Space, and Environmental Medicine*, 1990, pp. 699–706.

[71]Craig, J. C., and Sherrick, C. E., "Dynamic Tactile Displays," *Tactual Perception: a Sourcebook*, edited by W. Schiff and E. Foulke, Cambridge Univ. Press, Cambridge, England, U.K., 1982.

[72]Bach-Y-Rita, P., "Neurophysiological Basis of a Tactile Vision-Substitution System," *IEEE Transactions on Man-Machine Systems*, MMS-11, 1970, pp. 108, 109.

[73]Jansson, G., "Human Locomotion Guided by a Matrix of Tactile Point Stimuli," *Active Touch. The Mechanism of Recognition of Objects by Manipulation: a Multidisciplinary Approach*, edited by G. Gordon, Pergamon, Oxford, England, U.K., 1978, pp. 229–242.

[74]Van Veen, H. A. H. C., and Van Erp, J. B. F., "Tactile Information Presentation in the Cockpit," *Haptic Human-Computer Interaction*, edited by S. Brewster, and R. Murray-Smith, Springer-Verlag, Berlin, 2001, pp. 164–171.

[75]Van Erp, J. B. F., "Tactile Navigation Display," *Haptic Human-Computer Interaction*, edited by S. Brewster and R. Murray-Smith, Springer-Verlag, Berlin, 2001, pp. 155–163.

[76]Van Erp, J. B. F., and Werkhoven, P. J., "Spatial Characteristics of Vibro-Tactile Perception on the Torso," TNO Human Factors, Rep. TM-99-B007, Soesterberg, the Netherlands, 1999.

[77]Van Erp, J. B. F., "Direction Determination with Vibrotactile Stimuli Presented to the Torso: Search for the Tactile Ego-Centre," TNO Human Factors, Rep. TM-00-B012, Soesterberg, the Netherlands, 2000.

[78]Sanneman, R. A., "Tactual Display for Aircraft Control," *Office of Naval Research*, DARPA 2108, Arlington, VA, 1975.

[79]Gilliland, K., and Schlegel, R. E., "Tactile Stimulation of the Human Head for Information Display," *Human Factors*, Vol. 36, 1994, pp. 700–717.

[80]Rupert, A. H., Guedry, F. E., and Reschke, M. F., "The Use of a Tactile Interface to Convey Position and Motion Perceptions," *Virtual Interfaces: Research and Applications*, AGARD C P 541: Vol. 20, 1994, pp. 1–7.

[81]Rupert, A. H., "An Instrumentation Solution for Reducing Spatial Disorientation Mishaps," *IEEE Engineering in Medicine and Biology*, Vol. 19, 2000, pp. 71–80.

[82]Raj, A. K., McGrath, B. J., Rochlis, J. L., Newman, D. J., and Rupert, A. H., "The Application of Tactile Cues to Enhance Situation Displays," *Proceedings for the Third Annual Symposium and Exhibition on Situational Awareness in the Tactical Air Environment*, 1998, pp. 77–84.

[83]Raj, A. K., Suri, N., Perry, J. F., and Rupert, A. H., "The Tactile Situation Awareness System in Rotary Wing Aircraft: Flight Test Results," *Current Aeromedical Issues in Rotary Wing Operations, Symposium Proceedings*, RTO-MP-19, Vol. 16, 1998, pp. 1–7.

[84]Previc, F. H., "Neuropsychological Guidelines for Aircraft Control Stations," *IEEE Engineering in Medicine and Biology*, Vol. 19, No. 2, 2000, pp. 81–88.

[85]Borah, J., "Technology and Application of Gaze Based Control," *Alternative Control Strategies: Human Factors Issues*, RTO-EN-3 AC/323(HFM)TP/1, Vol. 3, 1998, pp. 1–10.

[86]Calhoun, G. L., Arbak, C. J., and Boff, K. R., "Eye-Controlled Switching for Crew Station Design," *Proceedings of the Human Factors and Ergonomics Society 28th Annual Meeting*, 1984, pp. 258–262.

[87]McMillan, G. R., "The Technology and Applications of Biopotential-Based Control," *Alternative Control Strategies: Human Factors Issues*, RTO-EN-3 AC/323(HFM)TP/1, Vol. 7, 1998, pp. 1–10.

[88]Anderson, T. R., "The Technology of Speech-Based Control," *Alternative Control Strategies: Human Factors Issues*, RTO-EN-3 AC/323(HFM)TP/1, Vol. 2, 1998, pp. 1–9.

[89]Steeneken, H. J. M., "Potential of Speech and Language Technology Systems for Military Use: an Application and Technology-Oriented Survey," RTO Technical Rep. AC/243(Panel3)TR/21, 1996.

[90]North, D. M., "A New Vision of Cockpit Displays," Editorial, *Aviation Week and Space Technology*, 8 March, 1999, p. 68.

[91]Mulder, M., *"Cybernetics of Tunnel-in-the-Sky Displays,"* Ph.D. Dissertation, Delft Univ. Press, Delft, The Netherlands, 1999.

[92]Regan, E. C., and Price, K. R., "The Frequency of Occurrence and Side-Effects of Immersion Virtual Reality," *Aviation, Space, and Environmental Medicine*, Vol. 65, 1994, pp. 527–530.

[93]Bles, W., and Wertheim, A. H., "Appropriate Use of Virtual Environments to Minimise Motion Sickness," *What Is Essential for Virtual Reality Systems to Meet Military Human Performance*, RTO-MP-058 AC/323(HFM-058)TP/30, Vol. 7, 2001, pp. 1–9.

[94]Borah, J., "Technology and Application of Head Based Control," *Alternative Control Strategies: Human Factors Issues*, RTO-EN-3 AC/323(HFM)TP/1, Vol. 6, 1998, pp. 1–12.

[95]De Vries, S. C., Van der Steen, E. M., and Krabbendam, A. J., "The Position of Un-manned Aerial Vehicles in Future Airpower: Contribution of TNO-DO," TNO Human Factors, *Rep. TM-00-A038*, Soesterberg, the Netherlands, 2000.

[96]Wickens, C. D., and Prevett, T., "Exploring the Dimensions of Egocentricity in Aircraft Navigation Displays," *Journal of Experimental Psychology: Applied*, Vol. 1, 1995, pp. 110–135.

[97]Wickens, C. D., "Situation Awareness: Impact of Automation and Display Technology," *Situation Awareness: Limitations and Enhancement in the Aviation Environment*, Vol. 2, 1996, pp. 1–13.

[98]Barfield, W., Rosenberg, C., and Furness, T. A., III, "Situation Awareness as a Function of Frame of Reference, Computer-Graphics Eyepoint Elevation, and Geometric Point of View," *International Journal of Aviation Psychology*, Vol. 5, 1995, pp. 233–256.

[99]Yeh, M., Wickens, C. D., and Seagull, F. J., "Effects of Frame of Reference and View-ing Condition on Attentional Issues with Helmet-Mounted Displays," *Proceedings of 2nd Annual FEDLAB Symposium: Advanced Displays and Interactive Displays*, 1998, pp. 107–114.

[100]Begault, D. R., "Head-up Auditory Displays for Traffic Collision Avoidance System Advisories: A Preliminary Investigation," *Human Factors*, Vol. 35, 1993, pp. 707–717.

[101]Begault, D. R., and Pittman, M. T., "Three-Dimensional Audio Versus Head-Down Traffic Alert and Collision Avoidance System Displays," *The International Journal of Avi-ation Psychology*, Vol. 6, 1996, pp. 79–93.

[102]Begault, D. R., Wenzel, E. M., and Lathrop, W. B., "Augmented TCAS Advisories Using a 3-D Audio Guidance System," *Proceedings of the Ninth International Symposium on Aviation Psychology*, Ohio State Univ., Columbus, OH, 1997, pp. 353–357.

[103]Oving, A. B., and Bronkhorst, A. W., "Application of a Three-Dimensional Auditory Display for TCAS Warnings," *Proceedings of the 10th International Symposium on Aviation Psychology*, Ohio State Univ., Columbus, OH, 1999, pp. 26–31.

Glossary

acceleration—change in velocity over time, expressed in terms of meter/second^2 for linear acceleration and degree/second^2 for angular acceleration

accommodation (optical)—change in the optical power (curvature) of the human lens for different viewing distances, accomplished by contraction of the ciliary muscles of the eye

acoustic orientation instrument (AOI)—device that presents auditory cues to spatial orientation (such as interaural intensity differences to signal bank)

action extrapersonal system—brain system, coursing ventromedially through the cerebral cortex, which is responsible for our orientation and navigation in topographical (geographical) space

Advanced Spatial Disorientation Demonstrator (ASDD)—USAF spatial-disorientation demonstrator, built by ETC, Inc., and generically known as the Gyrolab 2000, that features a four-degree-of-motion platform, flight-simulation aeromodels, a wide-FOV computer-generated scene, computer-generated re-configurable cockpit instruments, and a simulated head-up display

aerial perspective—tendency of distant scene elements to appear reduced in contrast and more bluish, as a result of atmospheric scattering

agile flight—nontraditional fixed-wing aircraft maneuvers that include flat turns, lateral motion, and high angle of attacks (Cobra and Herbst maneuvers) that are mostly a capability of vectored-thrust fixed-wing or rotary-wing aircraft (*see* **vectored thrust**)

aircraft control not maintained—category used by the U.S. National Transportation Safety Board referring to a human-factors-related aircraft mishap other than controlled flight into terrain [*see* **controlled flight into terrain (CFIT)**]

aircraft-fixed symbology—flight symbology that moves in synchrony with the aircraft so as to appear 'fixed' to the aircraft

airspeed indicator—primary flight instrument that provides information concerning the aircraft's velocity through the air (*see* **performance instruments**)

alternobaric vertigo—angular sensations accompanied by nystagmus that can occur with increased barometric pressure (as during landing), particularly when a pilot has a middle-ear infection or some other predisposing condition (also referred to as **pressure vertigo**)

altimeter—primary flight instrument that provides information concerning the aircraft's altitude above ground (radar altimeter) or altitude above sea level (barometric altimeter) (*see* **performance instruments**)

ambient attitude indicator—type of attitude display that is situated in or extends into the peripheral visual field in order to tap into ambient vision [*see* **peripheral-vision horizon display (PVHD)** and **ambient extrapersonal system**]

ambient extrapersonal system—brain system that includes primary vestibular cortex, nearby parietal-temporal visual and somatosensory areas, the dorsome-dial visual cortex, and subcortical projections extending from the vestibular nuclei; this system is involved in the control of posture and orientation in Earth-fixed (gravitational) space and is synonymous with ambient-mode vision

angle of attack (AoA)—difference between the aircraft's pitch angle and the direction of its velocity vector in space (e.g., an aircraft that is pitched up while descending has a high AoA)

arc-segmented attitude reference—attitude display designed for HUDs and HMDs that depicts aircraft attitude by means of an arc that fills upward in pitch-down attitudes and retreats downward in pitch-up attitudes and rotates clockwise or counterclockwise during aircraft bank

articulation—symbology format, usually for HUD pitch ladders, in which the negative pitch lines bend at increasing dive angles toward the artificial horizon of the attitude display

attitude—pitch or bank of an aircraft (*see* **pitch** and **bank**)

attitude indicator (AI)—instrument or symbol that depicts the attitude of an aircraft, also known as an attitude director indicator (ADI) when combined with heading and command steering information (*see* **control instruments**)

Aubert (A) effect—tendency to view a vertical line as tilted away from the direction of tilt, presumably caused by an underregistration of head tilt at large tilt angles (>90 deg); this effect is opposite to the Mueller or E effect [*see* **Mueller (E) effect**]

audiogravic illusion—illusory displacement and/or linear movement of a head-fixed sound source in consonance with a shift of the gravitoinertial vector (*see* **somatogravic illusion**)

audiogural illusion—illusory displacement and/or rotatation of a head-fixed sound source in consonance with an erroneously perceived rotation (*see* **somatogyral illusion**)

Augie Arrow—roll symbol consisting of an arrow referenced to the flight-path marker, which automatically appears during unusual attitudes and indicates the roll attitude to aid recovery; the Augie Arrow was named for the late William Augustine of the U.S. Air Force's Flight Dynamics Laboratory

autokinetic illusion—illusion that a small stationary spot in an otherwise darkened environment begins to move, usually after a period of 10 s or more of fixation on it

automated ground-collision avoidance system (auto-GCAS)—system that automatically transfers control of the aircraft to a computer whenever the aircraft is headed for an impact with the ground (*see also* **ground-proximity warning system**)

bank—angular displacement of the aircraft around its longitudinal axis, in reference to the horizon (*see* **roll**)

Barany chair—reduced-friction chair that is capable of near constant velocity turning about a vertical axis and is the most widely used round-based demonstrator for angular SD illusions

binocular disparity—depth cue relying on the offset between the right-eye and left-eye images of objects that lie in front of or behind the fixation point

black-hole approach—landing approach to a runway at night, characterized by a lower-than-perceived glide slope, when the terrain surrounding the runway is not highly visible; the low-approach tendency is enhanced when additional visual illusions caused by sloping or narrow runways or fog are present

blind flight—term used early on in aviation referring to flight without the availability of outside visual references [*see also* **instrument meteorological conditions (IMC)**]

blood alcohol concentration (BAC)—a measure of alcohol intoxication that is commonly defined as milligrams of alcohol in 100 ml of blood.

breakoff illusion—SD illusion in which the pilot feels separated from the aircraft; this illusion typically occurs at high altitude in fixed-wing aircraft and is distinct from the "flying carpet" illusion (*see* **flying carpet illusion**)

brownout—visual condition that occurs when blowing sand, dust, and other ground particulates reduces low-level flying visibility (*see also* **whiteout**)

central nervous system (CNS)—all of the structures and pathways comprising the brain and spinal cord

centrifugal force—inertial force (reaction) resulting from a centripetal acceleration (*see* **centripetal acceleration**)

centripetal acceleration—acceleration of a body rotating around an external point, such as a turning aircraft or a rotating gondola in a centrifuge, which is directed toward the center of curvature (*see* **centrifugal force** and **planetary motion**)

channelized attention—devotion of excessive amounts of mental effort toward processing one piece or set of information, such as emergency warning messages

Class A mishap—serious aircraft mishap typically involving loss of life or a major financial loss, which in the U.S. Air Force is defined as $1 million (U.S.) or greater

collimation—presentation of a visual image using a parallel projection system so that the image appears to come from distant space (optical infinity)

compression—tendency for lines that are perpendicular to the line of sight on the ground to become more closely spaced in the distance; also known as foreshortening

conformal symbology—flight symbology that moves in identical relationship to the outside world, as is the case with all Earth-fixed symbologies [*see* **Earth-fixed (world-fixed) symbology**]

control instruments—instruments that display immediate attitude and power indications and that are calibrated to permit attitude and power adjustments in definite amounts; control is determined by reference to the attitude indicators and power indicators (*see*, by contrast, **navigation instruments** and **performance instruments**)

controlled flight into terrain (CFIT)—mishap in which there is no evidence of aircraft malfunction or of any effort by the pilot to prevent the mishap (*see* **Type I spatial disorientation**)

Coriolis illusion—illusion of angular motion (usually pitch or roll) that occurs when the head is removed from the plane of rotation; this illusion is also known as cross-coupling and is frequently associated with nausea, vomiting, and other symptoms in naïve subjects

corticospinal motor system—phylogenetically recent neuromotor system that contains direct projections from the cerebral cortex to spinal motoneurons that are involved in voluntary skeletal movements, including those of the wrist and hand (*see*, by contrast, **vestibulospinal motor system**)

crater illusion—illusion of landing in a crater, caused by the reflection of a helicopter landing light off a surface beneath

crew coordination—exchange of relevant information between and among aircrew to accomplish a given task

crew resource management—integrating the skills of all aircrew to perform flying tasks and enhance flight safety

cupula—gelatinous structure in the ampulla of the semicircular canals that moves in response to the inertial lag of the endolymph during head accelerations (*see* **semicircular canals**)

cyclovergence—disjunctive movement of the eyes that occurs when we rotate our eyes in opposite directions; known as incyclovergence when we rotate our eyes inward and excyclovergence when we rotate our eyes outward

degrees of motion—number of angular and linear (translatory) motion axes in a Cartesian coordinate system, usually associated with a motion base on a flight simulator or SD demonstrator (also known as degrees of freedom)

design-eye reference point—design-eye reference is a single point designated by the aircraft designer that allows the pilot to reach all required cockpit controls and an adequate external view

didactic instruction—SD teaching that is confined mainly to the classroom and that can be supplemented by ground-based and in-flight demonstrations

dip illusion—tendency to lower one's altitude when increasing separation distance to lead as a result of the tendency to maintain a constant angular relationship relative to the lead aircraft; to maintain a constant 1 deg below lead, for example, one must lose 91 m (300 ft) for each nautical mile of separation distance

Earth-fixed space—space defined in relation to the surface of the Earth (and the gravitational vertical)

Earth-fixed (world-fixed) symbology—information on flight displays that is fixed relative to the surface of the Earth and shifts in parallel with (conformal to) the outside scene when the aircraft or pilot's head move (e.g., conformal pitch lines on a HUD or HMD) [*see* **conformal symbology**, **head-up display (HUD)**, and **helmet-mounted display (HMD)**]

edge rate—rate at which texture elements flow past a moving observer, based on a combination of optical-flow rate and texture density

elevation—angular displacement of the aircraft around its lateral axis axis, in reference to the horizon (*see* **pitch**)

elevator illusion—illusion of climbing, as in an elevator, when a pilot is exposed to a >1 G force, as occurs when leveling off from a descent when the centrifugal force from the bottom of the descent adds to the force of gravity; or adds to the illusion of falling at <1 G; or the movement of small spots in accordance with the perceived self-motion (*see* **centrifugal force**)

enhanced vision—natural but aided vision using optical devices that contain special sensors, such as FLIR or NVDs [*see* **forward-looking infrared radar (FLIR)**, **night-vision devices (NVD)**, and **night-vision goggles (NVG)**]

equivalence principle—equivalence between gravitational and inertial forces, as noted by Mach and Einstein; this equivalence explains why inertial forces resulting from sustained accelerations add to the 1 G force of gravity to produce a combined gravitoinertial force vector whose direction is confused with that of gravity (*see* **gravitoinertial force**)

Euclidean space—mathematical concept that parallel lines never converge, as first described by the Greek mathematician Euclid

eye height—distance from the ground to the eye, which is used to scale optical flow velocity (i.e., larger eye heights above ground result in smaller optical-flow velocities)

fascination—excessive fixation on an visual target or other object, either by voluntary allocation of mental resources (*see* **channelized attention**) or by a preconscious visual capture by the target (as in **target-hypnosis**)

field dependence—degree to which visual inputs are relied on to maintain one's orientation in space

field of regard—total amount of angular space that can be seen on a visual display or through aided or unaided vision when the head or sensor is free to move

field of view (FOV)—amount of angular space that is visible, either on a visual display or through aided or unaided vision

flicker vertigo—visual sensations (e.g., a false sensation or movement) and nonvisual sensations (e.g., dizziness) caused by flickering visual stimuli such as reflections from a helicopter rotor blade (*see* **vertigo**)

flight director—avionics system that shows the pilot where to fly while navigating to a certain point, such as a runway

flight path—direction of the aircraft's movement in three-dimensional space

flight-path marker (FPM)—symbol on a HUD or HMD whose position indicates the direction of the aircraft's movement in three-dimensional space relative to the ground or air mass; this symbol is also referred to as the velocity vector and when its movement is constrained laterally, as the climb–dive marker [*see* **head-up display (HUD)** and **helmet-mounted display (HMD)**]

flight simulator—device that is designed to reproduce the movements of the visual world—as well as the vestibular and other physiological sensations of flight, in the case of simulators with motion devices—by relying on a realistic model of the aerodynamic response of the aircraft to control-stick inputs; such devices range from simple visual displays to complex six-degree-of-motion systems with wide-FOV, collimated visual displays

flying-carpet illusion—sensation of flying on top of the aircraft without its frame, as is most likely to be experienced in aircraft like the F-16 with its large glass canopies and restricted views of the terrain; this is similar to but distinct from the breakoff illusion (*see* **breakoff illusion**)

focal extrapersonal system—brain system coursing dorsoventrally through the cerebral cortex that is responsible for searching for and recognizing objects and alphanumeric information (synonymous with focal-mode vision)

force—product of an object's mass (m, a scalar) and its acceleration (a, a vector), based on the formula $F = ma$

forward-looking infrared (FLIR)—thermal imaging technique for transducing scene information in the 800–1200 nm region; the FLIR camera is mounted on a pod near the front of the aircraft and is displayed on head-down, head-up, and helmet-mounted displays (*see* **synthetic vision**)

frequency-separated display—attitude display that uses the frequency of the control input to determine which symbol moves in bank, either the aircraft or the horizon; typically, the rapid initial movement is of the aircraft and the slower subsequent movement is of the artificial horizon

geographical disorientation—loss of orientation in geographical or topographical space, such as when a pilot lands perfectly but at the wrong airport or runway

G-excess illusion—illusion that occurs when a pilot moves his or her head in a >1 G environment, which leads to excessive shearing of the otolith organs and to an exaggerated sensation of head, body, or aircraft tilt

ghost horizon—attitude-display feature that allows the horizon to be seen at all times even when it is conformal to a real horizon that is not in the display space because of a large amount of aircraft pitch; in the typical ghost mode, the artificial horizon appears as a dashed line resting at the edge of the display

giant-hand illusion—illusion in which the pilot believes that the aircraft no longer responds to his or her control-stick inputs, as if a giant hand has grabbed the wings of the aircraft and is preventing the pilot from moving the control stick to level the aircraft (*see* **Type III spatial disorientation**)

graveyard spin—aircraft spin resulting in a continuing loss of lift and a descent into the ground, which can be attributed to the erroneous sense of turning caused by the inertial lag of the endolymph in the semicircular canals; in turn, the illusory turning percept leads the pilot to push the rudder in direction of the spin rather than opposite to it, as would be needed to stop the spin (*see* **inertia** and **semicircular canals**)

graveyard spiral—tendency of the pilot following a prolonged turn to place the aircraft into a greater-than-desired bank without realizing the increased bank and the subsequent need to add backpressure to compensate for the loss of lift; this tendency is believed to be caused by the combination of a decay of turning sensation during the level turn and the alignment of the gravitoinertial vector with the vertical axis of the aircraft, which allows the pilot to feel level when actually banked and rolled in the opposite direction when leveling out (*see* **centrifugal force** and **inertia**)

gravitoinertial force (GIF)—resultant force that represents of the sum of the gravitational force vector and the inertial force vector created by the acceleration of the aircraft (*see* **equivalence principle**)

ground-proximity warning system—system that senses an impending aircraft impact with the ground and provides an alerting cue to the pilot [*see* **automated ground-collision avoidance system (auto-GCAS)**]

heading—angular displacement of the aircraft trajectory in reference to the horizontal plane of the Earth's surface and the direction of true north

head-down display (HDD)—flight display that is part of the instrument panel that lies in the cockpit space beneath the windscreen

head-fixed symbology—primary flight and other symbology that moves in synchrony with the head, such as the symbols on night-vision goggles

head-up display (HUD)—flight display lying directly above the glare shield in the front of the cockpit, in which primary flight and other information is presented in collimation on a *see*-through combiner glass (*see* **collimation**)

helmet- (head-) mounted display (HMD)—flight display that is presented using fiber optics and a combiner surface to appear superimposed on the pilots visor at optical infinity (*see* **collimation**)

highway in the sky (HITS)—particular flight symbology that provides navigational and spatial orientation to the pilot by means of a three-dimensional pictorial course indicator and a moving aircraft symbol (also known as the pathway-in-the-sky) (*see* **pathway displays**)

human factors analysis and classification system—system used by mishap investigators and researchers to classify and understand the human-factor contribution to aviation mishaps; this system addresses organizational influences, unsafe supervision, preconditions for unsafe acts, and unsafe acts.

induced motion—illusion of a stationary visual object moving opposite to a moving background scene, as when the moon appears to move opposite to the clouds

inertia—tendency of objects at rest to remain at rest unless acted upon by a force or torque, as exemplified by the lack of movement (inertial lag) of the endolymph in the semicircular canals during the initial acceleration during turning of a head

in-flight spatial-disorientation sortie—special flight designed to demonstrate various SD illusions to aircrew of both fixed-wing and rotary-winged aircraft

inside-out display—attitude-display format that depicts a fixed aircraft against a moving horizon, as would be seen from inside the aircraft (*see*, by contrast, **outside-in display**)

instrument flight rules (IFR)—set of regulations governing instrument flight and the conduct of fight under instrument meteorological conditions; also, a term used by pilots and controllers to indicate the corresponding type of flight plan [*see* **instrument meteorological conditions (IMC)**]

instrument flight training—specialized training that teaches pilots to become proficient in understanding and processing the information from their flight instruments

instrument landing system (ILS)—system provided at an airport to enable pilots to descend in instrument conditions along precise horizontal (localizer course) and vertical (glide-slope) paths to a point from which they are able to visually acquire the runway; an ILS consists of two transmitters located near the runway that emit at two different radio frequencies on opposite sides of the optimum path, one of which is aligned with the runway centerline and the other to a normal glide path (usually 3 deg from horizontal)

instrument meteorological conditions (IMC)—weather conditions expressed in terms of visibility, distance from clouds, and cloud ceiling height that are less than the minima specified for visual meteorological conditions [*see* **visual metereological conditions (VMC)**]

inversion illusion—SD illusion in which pilots at least temporarily feel as though they are inverted relative to the Earth; this illusion can be caused either by gravitoinertial forces that are <1 G or by visual factors (e.g., brighter water than sky)

jerk—rate of change of acceleration, expressed in terms of G/s for linear motion

labyrinth defective (LD)—person who has a profound loss of function in both the left and right vestibular organs (labyrinths)

lean on sun—tendency of pilots to fly as if the sun were directly overhead, which can result in an unperceived bank when the sun is at low angles relative to the horizon

leans—feeling of being banked when the aircraft is actually upright and level; this illusion can be caused by both gravitoinertial forces (e.g., leveling out from a prolonged turn) or by visual factors (e.g., a sloping cloud deck)

loss of situation(al) awareness (LSA)—failure to maintain situational awareness [*see* **situation(al) awareness (SA)**]

lost wingman—procedure in which a pilot who has become disoriented or loses sight of lead temporarily removes himself or herself from the flying formation

micropsia—tendency for objects to appear smaller than they actually are because of oculomotor factors (accommodative micropsia or convergence micropsia) or neuropsychological factors

motion sickness—condition consisting of both peripheral symptoms (e.g., nausea and vomiting) and central symptoms (e.g., drowsiness) caused by certain motions or conflicts involving the vestibular system

Mueller (E) effect—tendency to view a vertical line as tilted toward the direction of tilt, presumably caused by an underregistration of head tilt at moderate angles of tilt (<30 deg); this effect is opposite to the Aubert or A effect [*see* **Aubert (A) effect**]

multifunction display (MFD)—computerized flight display, usually presented on a cathode-ray tube or liquid crystal monitor located on the head-down instrument panel, which allows the pilot to switch between types of information [*see* **head-down display (HDD)**]

nap of the Earth (NOE)—low-level flight maneuvering by rotary-winged aircraft, typically at an altitude less than 30 m (100 ft)

natural orientation—spatial-orientation percept derived from outside (ambient) visual cues or nonvisual (somatosensory and vestibular) sensory inputs (*see*, by contrast, **synthetic orientation**)

navigation instruments—instruments (or displays) that indicate the position of the aircraft in relation to a selected navigation facility or fix; these include course indicators, range indicators, glide-slope indicators, and bearing pointers (*see*, by contrast, **control instruments** and **performance instruments**)

night-vision devices (NVD)—general term given to any devices used to aid pilots in flying at night, including night-vision goggles and helmet-mounted

FLIR images [*see* **forward-looking infrared (FLIR)** and **night-vision goggles (NVG)**]

night-vision goggles (NVG)—device that uses a pair of image-intensifier tubes in the near-infrared range (600–900 nm) to aid pilot visibility at night [*see* **night-vision devices (NVD)** and **enhanced vision**]

nystagmus—involuntary reflex movement of the eyes in response to head or scene movements that helps to stabilize the visual world, consisting of both slow and fast phases (beats) [*see* **optokinetic nystagmus (OKN)**, **vestibulo-ocular reflex (VOR)**, and **vestibular-ocular disorganization**]

oculogravic illusion—illusory displacement and/or linear movement of a small, head-fixed spot of light in consonance with a shift of the gravitoinertial vector [e.g., an upward movement of a cockpit light can occur as the pilot feels pitched upward (*see* **somatogravic illusion**)]

oculogyral illusion—illusory displacement and/or rotation of a small, head-fixed spot of light, usually in consonance with an erroneously perceived rotation as during a postrotatory sensation (*see* **somatogyral illusion**)

optical flow—movement of the visual scene in response to self-motion, corresponding to the geometry of visual space

optokinetic-cervical reflex (OKCR)—tilt of the head in response to movements of the visual scene, most notably in the roll plane

optokinetic nystagmus (OKN)—reflexive movement of the eyes in response to visual scene motion, in which the slow phase is in the same direction as the visual scene and the fast phase is opposite to it (*see* **nystagmus**)

oscillopsia—inability to stabilize the retinal image during movement, usually caused by damage to the vestibular system or by abnormal vestibular stimuli during flight (*see* **vestibulo-ocular disorganization**)

otoconia—calcium-carbonate crystals that lie on the otolithic membrane and move relative to the endolymph in response to linear acceleration and head tilt relative to gravity (*see* **otoliths**)

otoliths—vestibular organs that include the maculae of the utricle and saccule, which are responsible for detecting linear acceleration and head tilts relative to gravity; the maculae of the otolith organs contain an otoconia-laden membrane and hair cells that project into it; the otoliths are also referred to as the graviceptor organs (*see* **otoconia**, **utricle**, and **saccule**)

outside-in display—attitude-display format that depicts a moving aircraft against a stationary horizon, as would be seen from outside (behind) the aircraft (*see*, by contrast, **inside-out display**)

out-the-window—reference to the visual (e.g., terrain) information available to the pilot while looking through the windscreen and to the pilot's view in that situation

parallax—perceived change in visual angle to an object with different viewpoints or distances, as when the elevation of a target or terrain feature erroneously appears to descend as distance increases

pathway displays—navigational displays that depict the desired path of the aircraft relative to the outside terrain, usually in the form of a moving set of contours, e.g., a highway or tunnel [*see* **highway in the sky (HITS)**]

performance instruments—instruments (or displays) that indicate the aircraft's actual performance, which include the altimeter, airspeed, Mach indicator, vertical-velocity indicator, heading indicator, angle-of-attack indicator, and turn-and-slip indicator (*see*, by contrast, **control instruments** and **navigation instruments**)

peripersonal system—brain system that courses dorsolaterally through the cerebral cortex and handles our visuomotor interactions within reaching space

peripheral-vision horizon display (PVHD)—attitude display presented by a laser beam that extends into the peripheral visual field overlying the cockpit instrument panel; also known as the Malcolm horizon after its inventor (*see* **ambient attitude indicator**)

perspective—geometrical tendency for parallel lines to appear to converge as they approach the horizon

pitch—angular motion around the lateral or left-right axis of the aircraft (also referred to as the interaural or *y* axis for movements of the head and body). Pitch often is used to describe the angular displacement of the aircraft around its lateral axis, in reference to the horizon, but the proper term for this is elevation (*see* **elevation**)

pitch compression—format used in the display of attitude on pitch-ladder displays, which shows a nonconformal $>1:1$ mapping between each pitch line and its out-the-window reference at large pitch angles (*see* **pitch ladder**)

pitch ladder—series of lines (usually evenly separated by a specified interval) that reflect precise amounts of aircraft pitch movement on an attitude display; this display is referred to as a climb–dive ladder when a laterally caged flight-path marker is present on the head-up or helmet-mounted display

pitch marker—aircraft reference symbol that is fixed on the head-up display; also known as the waterline [*see* **head-up display (HUD)**]

planetary motion—motion of an object around an external center of rotation, as in the case of an aircraft in a banked turn or a gondola on a centrifuge (*see* **centripetal acceleration** and **centrifugal force**)

plan view—aircraft map display that shows a two-dimensional world from above (also known as a God's-eye view); such a view can be contrasted with two-dimensional side (profile) and three-dimensional (perspective) views

positional alcohol nystagmus (PAN)—ocular movements created by the effects of alcohol ingestion on movements of the endolymph in the semicircular canals (see **semicircular canals**)

postroll effect—tendency of a pilot to continue to apply bank to an aircraft in the same direction as a previous roll once the original roll is stopped, presumably caused by the postrotatory response of the cupulae in the roll plane; this effect is also known as the Gillingham illusion (*see* **postrotatory** and **somatogyral illusion**)

postrotatory—refers to the period following the cessation of rotation, which can often be accompanied by a turning sensation opposite to the previous turning direction

poststall maneuver—maneuver (e.g., yawing) that occurs after an aircraft has reached a pitch-up (stall) attitude of 30 deg or more, facilitated in agile aircraft by vectored-thrust (*see* **agile flight** and **vectored thrust**)

primary flight reference (PFR)—display or suite of displays that contains all of the minimum required control, performance, and navigation information to permit the safe operation of the aircraft for a specific flight task

proprioception—sensory system, and receptors within that system such as muscle spindles and Golgi tendon organs, that give rise to a perception of muscle and joint movement (also known as the kinesthetic sense) (*see* **somatosensation**)

quickening—addition of integrated predictor terms to an aircraft control display to provide the pilot with immediate knowledge of the results of his or her own control inputs

rod-and-frame illusion—illusion that a small vertical rod is displaced opposite to the tilt of a larger frame, resulting in the tendency of observers to set the rod in the direction of the frame when asked to align it with the perceived vertical (*see* **field dependence** and **visual vertical**)

roll—angular motion around the aircraft's longitudinal or fore-aft axis (also referred to as naso-occipital or *x* axis for movements of the head and body) (*see* **bank**), Although bank and roll are often interchanged, the former describes position in relation to the horizon, whereas the latter describes motion referenced to the aircraft

roll-reversal error—control input by the pilot, usually caused by a misinterpretation of bank attitude, that changes the bank of the aircraft in a direction opposite to that required to level the aircraft

root-mean-square error—a measure of variability determined by calculating the deviations of points from their true position, summing up the measurements, and then taking the square root of the sum.

saccule—sac-like structure of the vestibular apparatus that contains the saccular macula, which is the less sensitive of the two otolith organs; it is oriented best for the detection of vertical and fore-aft movements and pitch tilt (*see* **otoliths**)

screen-fixed symbology—flight symbology that remains centered on the display screen during movements of the aircraft or pilot's head (as on an NVG HUD)

seat of the pants—sensations as to the direction of aircraft motion and tilt relative to gravity that are conveyed by the pressure receptors in the back and buttocks; the term "flying by the seat of one's pants" refers to flying based on natural orientational sensations rather than instruments when the pilot is deprived of external visual cues (*see also* **natural orientation** and **somatosensation**)

semicircular canals—vestibular organs responsible for detecting angular acceleration, which are composed of a elliptical canal containing endolymph fluid and a widened end known as the ampulla, in which the cupula and hair cells reside; the three canals known as the lateral, superior, and anterior canals are orthogonal to each other (*see* **cupula**)

shape constancy—tendency for objects to appear rigid in their shape so that any objective shape change is perceived as a change in distance or orientation to the object (*see* **size constancy**)

simulator sickness—symptoms that develop after pilots have flown in visual simulators for a period of time, which are mainly oculomotor but can include dizziness, headaches, and even nausea

situation(al) awareness (SA)—perception of the elements in the environment within a volume of time and space, the comprehension of their meaning, and the projection of their status in the near future [*see* **loss of situation(al) awareness (LSA)**]

size constancy—tendency for objects to appear rigid in their size so that any objective size change is perceived as a change in distance to the object (see **shape constancy**)

somatogravic illusion—false sensation of body tilt that results from perceiving the direction of a nonvertical gravitoinertial force as vertical (*see* **audiogravic illusion** and **oculogravic illusion**)

somatogyral illusion—false sensation of rotation or absence of rotation which results from misperceiving the magnitude and direction of an actual rotation (*see* **audiogural illusion, graveyard spin**, and **oculogyral illusion**)

somatosensation—sensory system comprised of mechanoreceptors such as free nerve endings, Meisner's corpuscles, Merkel's discs, and Pacinian corpuscles that convey information concerning the motion of the body in space and its tilt relative to gravity (*see* **seat of the pants**)

spatial disorientation (SD)—failure to sense correctly the position, motion, or attitude of the aircraft or the pilot within the fixed coordinate system provided by the surface of the Earth and the gravitational vertical [*see* **spatial orientation (SO)** and **Type I, Type II,** and **Type III spatial disorientation**]

spatial disorientation demonstrator/trainer—ground-based device whose motion and visual scenes combine to reproduce common SD illusions and demonstrate the limitations of the senses in flight

spatial orientation (SO)—ability to sense correctly the position, motion, or attitude of the aircraft or the pilot within the fixed coordinate system provided by the surface of the Earth and the gravitational vertical [*see* **spatial disorientation (SD)**]

split-S maneuver—maneuver consisting of a half-roll to the inverted position, followed by a half-loop to upright flight in the opposite direction; during unusual attitude recoveries, a recovery from inverted flight is made by using a half-loop rather than rolling upright [*see* **unusual-attitude recovery (UAR)**]

suddenly unfamiliar—phenomenon in which the pilots can suddenly find themselves unsure as to which mode the aircraft is in, where the aircraft is in relation to known landmarks, and with whom they might be communicating

synthetic orientation—spatial-orientation percept derived from the flight instruments, usually requiring more attentional resources than when orienting with good outside visual references (*see*, by contrast, **natural orientation**)

synthetic vision—out-the-window terrain imagery that is created by digital databases and presented on a computer-generated display

systems approach to training (SAT)—process to determine whether 1) aircrew training has achieved both its specified objectives (internal validation) and 2) the training objectives themselves reflect the operational requirements (external validation)

tactile situational awareness system (TSAS)—tactile orientation vest, developed by the U.S. Navy, that stimulates various points on the body by means of small tactors to depict lateral acceleration and other flight parameters

target hypnosis—effect of a visual target, such as lights in the distance, to mesmerize the pilot and capture his or her attention (*see* **channelized attention**)

task saturation—high-workload situation in which the pilot is overwhelmed by the amount and/or difficulty of the processing required by one or more tasks (see **workload**)

temporal distortion—erroneous perception of elapsed time, usually caused by changes in arousal

torque—rotational analogue of force, as in the torque exerted by head accelerations upon the mass of the cupula, which is defined as the product of the rotational inertia of a body (J) and its angular acceleration α, or $M = J\alpha$ (see **force**)

torsional eye movements—conjunctive rotation of the eyes that occurs in response to a lateral head tilt or visual roll motion (also known as ocular torsion)

traffic-alert and collision-avoidance system (TCAS)—automated system for alerting the pilot of other aircraft in the immediate environment and directing the pilot as to which evasive movements should be performed

trim—"neutral" control-stick setting in which pressures are minimized; proper trim reduces inadvertent aircraft drift and allows for easier control of the stick

turn-and-slip indicator (previously known as bank-and-turn indicator)—one of the earliest flight instruments developed, which depicts the turn rate of the aircraft and any deviation (i.e., slip) from the bank required to produce a coordinated (level) turn

Type I spatial disorientation—"unrecognized" SD, which is more likely to cause fatal mishaps such as CFIT [*see* **controlled flight into terrain (CFIT)**]

Type II spatial disorientation—"recognized" SD, in which the pilot might realize that some conflict exists among his or her natural spatial-orientation percept and what is being conveyed by the flight instruments or the outside world; accompanying sensations include vertigo (*see* **vertigo**)

Type III spatial disorientation—"incapacitating" SD, in which the pilot is unable to control the aircraft because of motor conflicts or uncontrollable nystagmus (*see* **giant-hand illusion** and **vestibulo-ocular disorganization**)

unmanned (uninhabited) aerial vehicle (UAV)—aircraft that is piloted or navigated by a person at a remote site, whether on the ground or in the air

unusual-attitude recovery (UAR)—process of returning the aircraft to near straight and level from an unexpected bank and/or pitch angle (typically >45-deg, although it can occur following any assumed attitude)

utricle—sac-like structure of the vestibular apparatus that contains the utricular macula, the more sensitive of the two otolith organs; it is oriented best for the detection of lateral and fore-aft movements and roll-and-pitch tilt (*see* **otoliths**)

vection—illusion of self-motion, opposite to a moving visual scene, in a stationary observer; it usually requires wide-FOV scenes and can be experienced as either translation (in which case it is termed linear vection) or rotation, in which case it is termed angular vection (or circularvection when experienced in yaw) (see **optical flow**)

vectored thrust—aircraft technology in which the thrust is movable in direction, as in vertical short takeoff and landing (VSTOL) aircraft such as the Harrier jumpjet (*see* **agile flight**)

velocity—change in position over time, whose magnitude is expressed in terms of meters/second in the case of linear velocity and degrees/second in the case of angular velocity

vergence—disjunctive movement of the eyes that occurs as fixation is changed in depth; known as convergence when we move our eyes inward to fixate on near objects and divergence when we move our eyes outward to fixate on distant objects

vertical-velocity indicator—instrument display that depicts the vertical acceleration (i.e., rate of climb or descent) of the aircraft (*see* **altimeter**)

vertigo—state in which the person and/or the outside world appear to spin or otherwise be in some sensory conflict; aviator's vertigo or pilot vertigo have historically been used to describe SD events, mainly of the Type II variety, in which the aviator might have experienced disorientation with or without vertigo (*see* **Type II spatial disorientation**)

vestibular habituation—term used to describe the diminished response of the vestibular system following exposure to sustained or repeated angular or linear motion

vestibulo-ocular disorganization—state in which the ocular nystagmic reflexes that normally help to stabilize the world on the retina become excessive or inappropriate (e.g., the nystagmus that occurs during the postrotatory period following a turn or during cross-coupled motion) and might even prevent the pilot from adequately viewing the flight instruments (*see* **nystagmus**)

vestibulo-ocular reflex (VOR)—reflexive movement of the eyes in response to motion of the head, which is controlled by a three-neuron arc from the vestibular nuclei to the oculomotor nuclei; the slow phase of the VOR moves in the opposite direction to the head and the fast-phase moves in the same direction as the head (*see* **nystagmus**)

vestibulospinal motor system—portion of the neuromotor system that is stimulated by vestibular inputs and that innervates mostly the proximal (upper arm and lower leg) and axial musculature used in postural control and whole-body locomotion (*see* **corticospinal motor system** and **giant-hand illusion**)

virtual cockpit—totally enclosed cockpit in which a computer-generated visual scene is used to represent the outside world to the pilot, usually by means of a helmet-mounted display (*see* **synthetic vision**)

virtual display—any visual display that depicts the outside world or elements within it using a computerized format

visual dominance—normal ability of an external visual scene to predominate over vestibular, somatosensory, and proprioceptive cues in the perception of spatial orientation

visual flight rules (VFR)—rules that govern the procedures for conducting flight under good visual conditions (in U.S. airspace, for example, a pilot operating under VFR must remain 500 ft below, 1000 ft above, and 2000 ft horizontally away from a cloud when in controlled airspace below 10,000 ft mean sea level and must ensure the in-flight visibility is at least 3 statute miles); a term also used in the U.S. to indicate weather conditions that are equal to or greater than minimum VFR requirements and by pilots and controllers to indicate a corresponding type of flight [*see* **visual meteorological conditions (VMC)**]

visually perceived eye level—perception of where the eyes are located in elevation as measured by setting a spot or line to the same height as the eyes

visual meteorological conditions (VMC)—visual conditions, typically associated with clear weather, that exceed the minimum VFR requirements [*see* **visual flight rules (VFR)**]

visual transition—pilot's switch from an out-the-window visual reference to a reliance on flight instruments and vice versa

visual vertical—perception of where upright lies as measured by setting a line to vertical (*see* **rod-and-frame illusion**)

whiteout—visual condition that occurs when blowing snow reduces low-level flying visibility (*see also* **brownout**)

workload—overall amount and difficulty of the tasks required to be performed at a particular moment (*see* **task saturation**)

yaw—angular motion around the aircraft's vertical axis (also referred to as dorsoventral or z axis for movements of the head or body)

Index

Acceleration, 2, 5, 23–28, 31, 33, 36, 39, 41, 42, 45–49, 51–56, 58, 59, 61–63, 66, 67, 73, 75, 77, 80, 85–89, 93, 101, 106, 107, 124, 129, 155, 157, 177, 188, 198, 227–231, 234, 243, 246–248, 250–260, 263, 264, 266, 267, 269, 274–280, 286, 290, 307, 309, 320, 341–344, 363, 364, 369, 370, 402, 417, 418, 456, 470, 472, 511, 523, 530, 531, 536
Accessory Optic System (AOS), 128
Accommodation Traps, 458
Acoustic Orientation Instrument (AOI), 79, 93
Acoustic Orientation Research, 79
Action-Extrapersonal, 98, 130
Advanced Spatial Disorientation Demonstrator (ASDD), 123, 338
Advanced Spatial Disorientation Trainer (ASDT), 337, 338
Aerial Perspective, 99, 119–121, 292, 298, 314
Aerospace Medical Association, 14, 15, 277, 326, 373, 374, 376
AGARD, 18, 35, 36, 87, 91, 94, 133, 138, 185, 187, 192–194, 240, 241, 275, 277–280, 318, 319, 321, 326, 372–376, 447, 500, 505, 506, 539
Agile Flight, 535
Aircraft Control, 4, 71, 79, 80, 82, 164, 197, 211–213, 238, 270, 273, 277, 279, 328, 329, 341, 361, 384, 387, 395, 432, 436, 438, 469, 486, 490, 539
Aircraft Displays, 379, 381, 403
Airspeed Indicator, 181, 235, 382, 388, 389, 397, 399, 420, 426, 435
Air Standardization Coordinating Committee (ASCC), 326
Alternobaric Vertigo (Pressure Vertigo), 268
Altimeter, 10, 152, 163, 169, 173, 235, 246, 252, 328, 333, 367, 382, 388–391, 397, 399, 400, 404, 410, 420, 422, 423, 426, 427, 435, 436
Ambient-Extrapersonal, 81, 97, 98, 130, 132
Ambient Vision, 18, 39, 96, 99, 100, 107, 110, 114, 123, 124, 126–133, 143, 284, 286, 288, 289, 293, 298, 314, 442
AMST, 19, 340, 344–347
Angle-of-Attack (AoA), 391
Angular Acceleration, 25, 27, 31, 42, 45–49, 56, 59, 66, 67, 85, 157, 177, 188, 246–248, 250, 259, 275, 276, 278, 280, 363

Angular Displacement, 25, 46, 405
Angular Motion, 5, 22, 23, 25–27, 29, 30, 44, 46, 57, 59, 60, 63, 77, 84, 93, 107, 110, 129, 163, 244, 247, 250, 251, 267, 271, 307, 363, 364, 516, 517
Angular Motion Perception, 46
Angular Velocity, 25, 48, 247, 261
Arc Segmented Attitude Reference, 460, 461, 506
Articulation, 412, 471
Artificial Horizon, 10, 13, 112, 126, 172, 262, 273, 328, 365, 386, 398, 405, 407, 413, 415, 435, 478
Attentional Capture, 459
Attitude, 1, 2, 9, 13, 16–18, 20, 21, 31, 33–39, 56, 79, 80, 82, 91, 112, 126, 134, 141, 151–153, 163, 169, 172, 175, 177, 179, 181–184, 205, 206, 211, 228, 231, 233–235, 237, 239, 243, 246, 251, 252, 254, 257, 259–263, 266, 275–277, 288, 325, 328, 330, 339, 341–343, 353, 354, 361–364, 366, 369–372, 382–388, 395, 397, 399, 400, 403–420, 423–426, 428, 432, 434–438, 441, 442, 444–448, 455–464, 467, 469, 471–483, 485–487, 492–497, 501–506, 511, 515, 518, 529, 533
Attitude Director Indicator (ADI), 416
Attitude Displays, 16, 18, 126, 384, 387, 408, 410, 412, 413, 447, 474, 503
Attitude Indicator (AI), 385
Aubert (A) Effect, 68, 69, 100
Auditory Orientation Information, 78, 526
Augie Arrow, 472, 474, 475, 478, 480–482, 486, 505
Autokinetic Illusion, 288, 307, 310
Automated Ground-Collision-Avoidance Systems (auto-GCAS), 509
Awe, 150, 152, 180

Bank, 2, 7, 13, 16, 21, 30, 34, 64, 69, 79, 134, 143, 153, 172, 183, 229, 243, 246, 251, 257, 259–263, 271, 276, 289, 291, 299–301, 328, 346, 362, 364, 368, 370–372, 382, 383, 385–387, 398, 399, 401, 402, 404–410, 412, 413, 416, 428, 434–436, 438, 440, 441, 444, 461, 462, 471, 472, 474, 475, 478, 488, 492–495, 507, 526
Bank and Turn Motion, 385
Barany Chair, 6, 7, 10, 197, 337, 347, 358
Barany, Robert, 6

Benson, Alan, 14, 15, 17–19, 22, 173, 179, 181, 248, 250, 291, 327, 361

Binaural, 78, 79, 538

Binocular, 97, 99, 115–117, 122, 124, 125, 134, 139, 315, 316, 454, 465, 466, 503

Binocular Disparity, 454

Binocular Rivalry, 466, 503

Black-Hole Approach, 342

Bles, Willem, 509

Blind Flight, 12, 13, 32, 373, 397, 445

Blood Pooling, 66

Braithwaite, Malcolm, 171, 175, 204, 222, 223, 225, 283, 313, 323, 325, 326, 335, 431, 433

Brooks Field, 12

Brown, Lex, 268, 323, 332, 349, 351, 367, 368, 416

Brownout, 175, 288, 291, 298, 299, 315

Cartesian Coordinate Axes, 42

Central Nervous System (CNS), 511

Centrifugal Force, 7, 26, 29, 31, 124, 252, 255, 264

Centripetal Acceleration, 26, 27, 252, 276

Cerebral Cortex, 44, 84, 129, 130, 132, 133, 143

Channelized Attention, 167, 168, 170, 172, 220, 222, 340

Civil Aviation, 145, 156, 185, 188, 208–210, 212–216, 374, 521

Class A mishap, 221

Climb–Dive Marker (CDM), 419

Clutter, 18, 423, 426, 427, 429, 443, 456, 459

Cobra Maneuver, 515

Cockpit Instrument, 112, 309, 380–382, 384

Collimated Flight Displays, 288, 312, 313

Collimated Viewing Displays, 311

Collimation, 452, 454

Compression, 118–120, 122, 254, 266, 302, 413, 414, 458, 469, 474, 479, 481, 486, 502

Conformal, 126, 409, 413, 414, 429, 456, 464, 466, 476, 481, 503

Conformality, 456, 481, 486

Constant-Radius Planetary Device, 345

Constant-Radius, Planetary Arm Devices, 343, 348

Control Instruments, 385, 395

Controlled Flight Into Terrain (CFIT), 3, 206, 510

Conventional HUDs, 452

Convergence Micropsia, 116

Coriolis Illusion, 246–248, 263, 276

Corticospinal Motor Mechanisms, 70

Corticospinal Motor Strategy, 266

Course Deviation Indicator, 438, 470

Course Indicators, 2

Cramer, Robert, 14

Crane, Carl J., 338, 384, 394, 408, 428

Crater Illusion, 288

Crew Coordination, 150, 176, 325

Crew Resource Management (CRM), 199

Cross-Coupling, 85, 249, 250, 258, 259, 271, 275, 344

Cupula, 5, 42, 44–49, 71, 83, 245, 247, 248, 261, 267

Cyclovergence, 117, 140

Degrees of Freedom (DOF), 339, 510

Design Eye-Reference point, 454

Design Recommendations, 485

DeVilbiss, Carita, 379, 416, 435

Didactic Instruction, 324, 330

Dip Illusion, 288, 301

Disorientation Stress, 21, 22, 331

Disparity, 20, 116, 117, 119, 120, 134, 139, 152, 454

Display Issues, 382

Divergence, 486

DME, 443

Doolittle, James, 10, 12, 13, 391, 393, 397, 410, 439

Dorsoventral, 42, 52, 53, 59, 72, 244, 257, 274

Drugs, 148, 154, 155, 167, 168, 171, 180, 181, 186, 188, 190, 194, 269, 363, 364

Duckworth, Joseph, 14

Earth-Fixed Space, 1, 2, 31, 95, 97, 101, 104, 125, 132, 133, 299, 310

Edge Rate, 105, 106

EEG-Based Control, 531

Elevation, 30, 80, 119–121, 134, 138, 159, 290, 297, 303, 332, 383, 397, 445, 464, 540

Elevator Illusion, 256, 263, 277, 288, 320, 342, 352

EMG-Based Control, 530, 535

Emotion, 3, 21, 148, 150, 153, 154, 185, 205, 266

Endolymph, 5, 7, 39, 42, 43, 45–49, 51, 58, 245, 247, 248, 261, 269

Equivalence Principle, 51

Ercoline, William (Bill), 1, 9, 246, 323, 337–339, 379, 407, 409, 416, 428, 435, 464, 475

Evans, Richard, 325, 379, 425

Eye-Based Control, 530, 531

Eyebox, 454

Eye-height, 103, 119

Eye-Reference Point, 454

False Horizons, 102, 285, 288–291, 319, 485

False Surface Planes, 288, 289, 291

Fascination, 152, 172, 180–182, 193, 363

Fatigue, 3, 80, 148–150, 155, 168, 171, 175, 180, 181, 186, 187, 189, 262, 272, 284, 318, 332, 363, 368, 403, 523

Fear, 80, 145, 150, 151, 155, 180, 182, 205, 409

Field Dependence, 126, 127, 141, 142

Field of Regard, 316, 317, 411, 467
Field of View (FOV), 314, 332
Filehne Illusion, 100
Fitts, Paul, 16, 403, 409, 411, 419, 420, 425, 426, 434, 439
Flicker Vertigo, 295, 363
Flight Director, 386, 402, 428, 430, 470, 496
Flight-Data Recorders (FDR), 229
Flight-Instrument Training, 237
Flight Instruments, 2, 3, 8, 9, 16, 20, 21, 64, 235, 237, 273, 328, 332, 352, 359, 399, 412, 421, 432, 439, 452
Flight-Path, 418, 419, 429, 435, 438, 454–456, 459, 462, 467, 469–471, 476, 479, 481–483, 485, 486, 497
Flight Simulator, 7, 80, 93, 190, 275, 337, 338, 342, 346–348, 357, 358, 523, 538
Flying Carpet Illusion, 182
Focal Extrapersonal System, 97
Force, 2, 6, 7, 12, 14, 16, 18–20, 22, 26–29, 31, 32, 34–36, 39, 45, 49–53, 69, 72–75, 77, 79, 81, 85, 86, 89, 92, 93, 95, 114, 123, 124, 135, 136, 140, 147, 149, 152, 171, 177, 184, 187, 190–193, 204, 220, 228, 230, 231, 237, 239, 240, 243, 244, 246, 250–258, 260–262, 264, 265, 271, 272, 275, 277–280, 285, 289, 297, 309, 317–319, 321, 323, 325, 326, 332, 337, 339, 341, 343, 345, 347–349, 351, 362, 367, 368, 372–376, 384, 398, 401, 406, 409, 432, 445–449, 451, 469, 474, 500, 501, 503, 504, 507, 511, 515, 516, 529, 535, 536
Formation Flying, 298, 299, 330
Forward-Looking Infrared (FLIR), 286, 334, 462, 518
Framing, 458
Frequency-Separated Display, 408

G-Excess Illusion, 278, 342
G-Induced Loss of Consciousness (GLOC), 65, 220
Gawron, Valerie, 145, 150
Geographical Disorientation, 2–4, 170
Geographical Orientation, 2, 170, 497, 533
Ghost Horizon, 415, 456, 482
Giant Hand Illusion, 183, 184, 194, 265, 266, 271, 279, 375
Gillingham Illusion, 34, 245, 271, 275, 342, 352
Gillingham, Kent K., 4, 14, 15, 17, 19, 22, 173, 178, 182, 208, 209, 221, 245, 250, 256, 263, 273, 283, 299, 308, 330, 342, 352
Glide Slope, 122, 302, 303, 437, 438
God's-Eye View, 466
Graveyard Spin, 72, 244, 245, 263, 271, 342
Graveyard Spiral, 261–263, 271, 278, 342, 445
Graviceptor, 63, 112
Gravitational Vertical, 1, 2, 28, 29, 50, 51, 54, 98, 113, 206, 233, 361
Gravitoinertial Force (GIF), 51, 261

Graybiel, Ashton, 14, 15, 77, 245, 255, 265, 307, 309
Green Card, 14
Grief, 150, 154, 180
Ground-Based Requirements, 341
Ground-Based Training, 6, 18, 336, 341, 346, 347, 351, 356, 357, 360
Ground Proximity Warning System (GPWS), 206
Guedry, Fred, 14, 15, 47, 54, 149, 167, 174, 175, 178, 259, 289, 291, 295, 299, 307

Haworth, Loran, 451, 464, 476, 488, 492
Head-Down Display (HDD), 174, 316, 346, 379–381, 431, 438, 448, 458, 459, 477, 524
Heading, 2, 15, 21, 30, 37, 100, 105, 134, 152, 159–162, 165, 170, 236, 257, 316, 330, 366, 368, 369, 372, 384, 385, 399, 402, 428, 432, 436, 438, 443, 445, 454, 460, 471, 472, 474, 479, 488, 493, 495–498, 533
Heading Indicator, 385, 388
Head-Mounted Display (HMD), 381, 463, 502
Head-up Display (HUD), 18, 35, 449, 451, 500, 505
Hegenberger, Albert, 12
Helmet-Mounted Display (HMD), 18, 125, 286, 346, 413, 451, 463, 532
Herbst Maneuver, 515
Highway in the Sky (HITS), 8, 18, 430, 432
Horizon, 10, 13, 18, 20, 30, 55, 59, 69, 70, 87, 97, 98, 104, 112–114, 119, 121, 126, 161, 172, 179, 228, 229, 236, 237, 245, 246, 260–265, 273, 278, 285, 288–291, 297–300, 304–306, 311, 315, 328, 332, 342, 363, 365, 367, 386, 397, 398, 403–409, 413–416, 435, 436, 440–445, 447, 448, 455, 456, 458, 459, 462, 465, 467, 469–472, 474–479, 481, 482, 486, 518
Human Factors Analysis and Classification System, 201

IERW, 357
Illusions, 4, 5, 7, 14, 16, 17, 29, 32, 64, 68, 72, 75, 77, 78, 80, 108, 111, 114, 124, 125, 127, 132, 175, 178–181, 185, 204–206, 209–211, 220, 223, 225, 227–229, 237–239, 243–245, 250–252, 254, 256, 260, 262–265, 270, 271, 274, 283–291, 293–296, 298, 300, 301, 307–311, 313, 315, 316, 318, 319, 324, 325, 327, 331, 332, 337–342, 344, 346, 347, 349, 351, 352, 356, 357, 360, 363–365, 367, 391, 411, 440, 510, 511
Induced Motion, 64, 136–138, 534
Inertia, 27, 42, 45, 251
Inertial Lag, 7, 308
Inside-Out Display, 408
Instantaneous Field of View, 452
Instrument Crosscheck, 341, 395–397, 420

Instrument Displays, 32, 39, 58, 381, 382, 384, 393, 396, 427, 466
Instrument Flight Rules (IFR), 260
Instrument Flight Training, 12, 352
Instrument Landing System (ILS), 500
Instrument Meteorological Conditions (IMC), 146, 198, 286, 289, 398, 518
Inter-aural Translational VOR, 61
Inversion Illusion, 50, 114, 254–256, 263, 277, 294, 342

Jerk, 23–25
Jones–Barany Chair, 7, 10

Kinesthetic Sense, 75

Labyrinthine-Defective (LD), 265
Lackner, James, 14, 74, 81
Lack of Discipline, 145, 147, 180
Lateral Vestibulospinal Tract (LVST), 70
Lean-on-Sun, 204, 288, 295
Leans, 21, 173, 260, 261, 263, 271, 289, 330, 338, 339, 342, 352, 356, 363, 364, 371
Linear Acceleration, 24–27, 33, 36, 39, 47, 49, 51–55, 62, 63, 66, 67, 77, 88, 89, 124, 228, 229, 243, 246, 256, 269, 276, 307, 364, 369, 511, 536
Linear Displacement, 23–25, 87
Linear Velocity, 24, 55, 246
Localizer, 165, 437, 438
Loss of Situational Awareness (LSA), 3, 167, 185, 206, 211, 220, 238, 325
Lost Wingman, 330, 331, 334, 473
Love of Flying, 145, 146, 180
Luminance Illusions, 293

Mach, Ernst, 4, 5, 251
Malcolm Horizon, 413, 447
Mechanoreceptors, 54, 74–76, 83, 92
Medial Vestibulospinal Tract (MVST), 70
Melvill-Jones, Geoffrey, 15
Mental and Physical State, 145, 148
Merkel's disks, 76
Micropsia, 116, 312
Military Aviation, 1, 18, 204, 220, 311, 313, 352, 533
Millimeter-Wavelength Radar, 462
MIL-STD 1787C, 401
Mitchel Field, 10
Motion Sickness, 38, 67, 68, 83, 85, 88, 89, 93, 127, 187, 205, 249, 270, 276, 280, 511, 518, 519, 532, 535, 536, 540
Motions in Flight, 3, 22
Multifunctional Displays (MFD), 18, 411
Myers, David, 7, 9

NAMRL, 14, 15, 194, 376, 445, 529
Nap-of-Earth (NOE), 296, 331, 466, 499, 503, 521

Naso-Occipital, 42, 52, 59–61, 68, 69, 87
Natural Orientation, 20, 21, 56, 526
Navigation Instruments, 2, 393
Newman, Richard, 451
Nighttime Landings, 122, 288, 302, 304
Night-Vision Devices (NVD), 18, 121, 175, 204, 288, 298, 313, 327, 361, 364, 462
Night-Vision Goggles (NVG), 125, 286, 313, 315, 332, 364, 465, 467
Nonplanetary Devices, 343, 344
Nonvisual, 4, 37, 38, 96, 100, 123, 126–128, 176, 225, 243, 244, 246, 262, 263, 271, 275, 283, 286, 289, 299, 318, 349, 362, 442, 529
NTSB, 4, 146, 156, 167, 169, 194, 211–216, 219, 230, 503
Nystagmus, 6, 7, 21, 48, 57–59, 62, 63, 67, 70–72, 76, 78, 84, 85, 87, 90, 91, 93, 99, 110, 138, 143, 156–158, 188, 198, 205, 206, 245, 249, 268–272, 274, 275, 280, 309, 310, 362, 364, 516, 525, 538

Occipital-Parietal Cortex, 131
Ocker, William, 9, 10
Ocular Torsion, 536
Oculogravic Illusion, 33, 93, 135, 253, 254, 256, 264, 278, 288, 309, 320
Oculogyral Illusion, 67, 124, 288, 307–310, 320, 321
Oculomotor, 7, 36, 44, 49, 55–57, 64, 82, 87, 90, 93, 98, 100, 108–111, 133, 266, 267, 536
Optical Flow, 103–106, 119, 122, 174, 284, 285, 295, 296, 319
Optokinetic-Cervical Reflex (OKCR), 69, 99, 100, 109, 112, 113, 125, 299, 397, 474
Optokinetic Nystagmus (OKN), 99
Oscillopsia, 59, 101, 271
Otoconia, 49–51, 251
Otolithic Membrane, 49, 258, 277
Otoliths, 38, 41, 49–51, 53–55, 61, 62, 65, 87, 90, 197, 229, 231, 243, 253, 267, 271, 309, 339, 369
Otolith-Spinal Modulation, 74
Outside-in Display, 407, 408
Out-the-Window, 20, 124, 286, 298, 311, 313, 346, 409, 413, 462, 463, 481, 483, 485, 517–519, 523
Overconfidence, 145, 146, 167, 180, 182, 185

Pacinian Corpuscles, 74, 76
Parallax, 99, 103, 118, 135, 292, 293, 301, 316, 454, 466
Pathway Displays, 460, 485
Pathway-in-the-Sky, 448, 532, 533
Perceptual-Motor Apparatus, 133
Performance Instruments, 370, 388, 391, 395, 396, 398, 420

Perilymph, 39, 269
Peripersonal System, 81, 97, 98
Peripheral Vision Horizontal Display (PVHD), 447
Perspective, 99, 102, 115–122, 125, 126, 133, 135, 139, 140, 172, 177, 192, 193, 201, 217, 218, 232, 284, 291, 292, 298, 302, 304, 314, 381, 382, 393, 410, 413, 414, 427, 429, 430, 438, 441, 446, 462, 502, 538
Pilot Vertigo, 2, 198
Pitch, 13, 19, 29–31, 42, 47–49, 55–57, 59, 65, 66, 79, 85, 89, 104, 110–113, 123, 127, 138, 141, 142, 157, 163, 173, 189, 225, 228, 229, 231, 232, 237, 247, 248, 250–259, 263, 266, 267, 271, 275, 276, 279, 285, 289–291, 309, 310, 320, 337, 338, 340–346, 352, 363, 369–372, 382, 383, 385–387, 399, 401, 402, 404–406, 408–419, 428, 434–436, 438, 441, 444, 454–461, 467, 469, 471, 474, 475, 477–483, 485, 486, 488, 493–495, 505, 513, 515, 516, 524, 526, 529
Pitch Compression, 486
Pitch Illusion, 228, 234, 235, 237, 291
Pitch Ladder, 21, 410, 412, 429, 455, 456, 468–472, 474, 475, 478, 479, 481, 504, 505
Pitch marker, 469, 470, 472, 482, 485, 486
Planetary Motion, 229, 342–344, 346
Plan View, 394, 464
Ponomarenko, Vladimir, 15, 408
Position, 1, 2, 7, 8, 12, 20, 30, 31, 36, 38, 39, 41, 44–46, 48–52, 54–56, 61–63, 66, 70–72, 74–77, 79, 81, 82, 85, 86, 91, 92, 95, 97–99, 101, 110, 114, 116, 127, 133, 134, 138, 157, 163, 169, 170, 172, 177, 178, 181, 183, 206, 211, 228, 231, 234–236, 243, 244, 246–248, 254, 255, 257, 258, 263–266, 270, 271, 277, 278, 283, 288, 293–295, 299, 300, 304, 309, 313, 318, 330, 331, 357, 361, 365, 372, 389, 390, 392, 393, 398, 399, 416, 426, 427, 440, 441, 443, 457, 464, 466, 474, 478, 483, 485, 488, 496, 498, 504, 511, 517, 523–526, 533, 539, 540
Positional Alcohol Nystagmus (PAN), 156, 269
Positional Vertigo, 267, 271
Postroll Effect, 352, 371
Postrotatory, 7, 57, 67, 72, 87, 245, 270, 308, 310, 363
Poststall Maneuver, 515–516
Power Displays, 396
Precision Instrument Control Task (PICT), 436
Precision Instrument Control Tasks, 436, 437
Previc, Fred, 1, 95, 283
Primary Flight Reference (PFR), 400, 401
Proprioception, 72, 75, 134
Pseudo-Coriolis, 64, 66, 88, 89
Psychic Reflection, 102
Purkinje Cells, 44

Quickening, 469, 470

Radial Acceleration, 26, 31, 255, 343
Reason's Human-Error ("Swiss Cheese") Model, 200, 201
Reflective HUD, 454
Research and Evaluation Issues, 486
Reverence, 150, 180
Rod-and-Frame Illusion, 111
Roll, 2, 16, 19, 29–31, 34, 42, 47–49, 56, 57, 59, 63, 65, 66, 69, 77, 85, 88, 89, 100, 103, 104, 107–112, 123, 126, 127, 129, 138, 141, 142, 151, 156, 163, 172, 173, 183, 192, 244–248, 250, 251, 256–258, 260, 261, 266, 267, 271, 275, 279, 285, 300, 320, 337, 338, 340, 342–345, 368, 371, 383, 385, 399, 405–409, 424, 435, 436, 438, 440, 441, 444, 457, 458, 460, 464, 465, 475, 478, 480, 481, 486, 493, 516, 529
Roll-Reversal Error, 16
Roscoe, Stanley, 16
Rotary Wing, 241, 260, 375, 377, 539
Rotorcraft, 204, 223–225, 502, 505, 521, 537
Ruggles Orientator, 7, 8, 338

Saccular Macula, 51–53
Saccules, 54
Screen-Fixed Symbology, 465, 476
SD Countermeasures, 7, 14, 17–19, 207, 218, 220, 272, 324, 325, 338, 340, 348
SD Countermeasures Trainers, 340
SD Mechanisms, 14, 17, 239
Seat-of-the-Pants, 75, 168, 272, 370, 371
Self-Tilt, 99, 110, 111, 127, 138
Semicircular Canals, 7, 40, 41, 46, 47, 49, 55–57, 63, 83–85, 128, 197, 227, 231, 243, 244, 246–248, 250, 260, 269–271, 279, 339, 343, 362, 363
Serenity, 150, 153, 180
Shape–Slant Invariance, 122
Shape-Constancy, 123
SHEL(L) Model, 199, 200
Simulator Sickness, 127, 142
Situational Awareness (SA), 3, 32, 59, 80, 148, 167–169, 206, 211, 237, 326, 332, 334–335, 346, 365, 367, 368, 393, 394, 396, 397, 430, 431, 447, 467, 481, 485, 486, 488, 492, 495, 509, 510, 518, 519, 521, 522, 525, 531, 533–535
Size Constancy, 116, 135, 172
Size–Distance Invariance, 122
Somatogravic Illusion, 5, 7, 55, 123, 124, 138, 142, 231, 232, 234, 251, 254, 264, 271, 309, 341, 347, 363, 370
Somatogyral Illusion, 9, 244, 245, 271, 308, 349, 363, 371
Somatosensation, 75

Somatosensory, 37, 38, 45, 47, 54, 62, 64, 68, 69, 72, 73, 76–78, 81, 82, 93, 95, 96, 98, 101, 112, 128, 131, 204, 209, 243, 264, 265, 269, 271, 309, 339
Somatosensory (Arthrokinetic) Nystagmus, 78
Spatial Ability, 145–147, 180, 185, 186
Spatial Disorientation Trainer, 229
Speech-Based Control, 530, 531, 539
Sperry, Elmer, 9, 405
Sperry Gyroscope Company, 9
Stress, 20–22, 80, 89, 148, 152, 154, 155, 167, 168, 171, 180, 185, 187, 188, 198, 229, 249, 266, 272, 327, 331, 513, 515, 531
Subthreshold motion, 342
Suddenly Unfamiliar, 180, 184
Synthetic Orientation, 20, 22, 56, 299
Synthetic Vision, 462, 463, 485, 502, 506, 520, 532
Systems Approach to Training (SAT), 354

T arrangement, 12, 425
T instrument cross-check, 425
Tactile Situation-Awareness System, 509
Tactile Systems, 73
Target Hypnosis, 171
Target-fixation, 182, 301, 330
Task Saturation, 3, 167, 168, 170, 172, 220, 332
Temporal Distortion, 168, 172, 180, 185
Terrain Misjudgments, 296
Three-Dimensional Space, 15, 18, 75, 95–98, 117, 118, 251, 418
Thresholds, 33, 47, 54, 64, 65, 74, 85, 86, 106, 124, 127, 128, 141, 194, 277, 320, 538
Torque, 5, 27, 71, 76, 247, 248
Torsion Pendulum Model, 51
Torsional Eye Movements, 99, 100
Traffic-Alert and Collision-Avoidance System (TCAS), 509
Training, 6, 7, 9, 12–14, 16–19, 32, 34, 35, 39, 67, 82, 83, 90, 142, 146, 147, 151, 155, 167, 171–173, 179, 181, 184, 191–193, 198, 209, 211, 212, 219, 220, 222, 229, 233, 237, 241, 272, 273, 276, 281, 292, 298, 317–319, 323–329, 331, 332, 334, 336–338, 340, 341, 343, 344, 346–361, 364–368, 371–377, 379, 384, 388, 393, 394, 396, 401, 403, 407–409, 426, 430, 434–436, 440, 445, 446, 452, 477, 485, 487, 492, 500, 509, 513, 518, 519, 525, 527, 531, 536
Trim, 155, 236, 256, 371, 372, 384, 395
Turn and Slip Indicator, 2, 388, 399, 473
Type I (Unrecognized), 20, 204, 205, 219, 222, 341, 381, 395, 400, 434
Type II (Recognized), 20, 204, 205, 219, 222, 341, 381, 398, 400
Type III (Incapacitating), 20, 204, 205, 341, 400

Unmanned Aerial Vehicles (UAV), 509, 510, 533
Unusual Attitude Recovery, 353, 434, 448, 476, 504, 506
US Army, 373, 503
USAARL, 94, 186, 187, 189, 192, 241, 319, 322, 326, 365, 367, 373–376
USAF, 2, 7, 12, 14, 15, 17, 20, 34, 35, 149, 159, 167, 171, 179, 183, 191, 192, 195, 204, 208, 209, 211, 220–223, 226, 229, 239, 240, 283, 289, 290, 292, 300, 301, 311, 313, 315, 318, 319, 321, 325, 335, 337, 338, 347, 348, 355, 356, 373, 375, 376, 400, 401, 413, 414, 416, 425, 432, 434, 445, 448, 451, 460, 475, 477, 506
USAF Advanced Instrument School, 167, 325, 347, 414
USAF Instrument Flight Center, 425
USAFSAM, 14, 16, 337, 348, 375, 448
USASAM, 326
USN, 209, 225–227
Utricles, 49, 51, 52, 69, 266
Utricluar Macula, 52

Van Wulfften Palthe, P. M., 7, 8
Variable-Radius Planetary Device, 345
Vection, 5, 45, 76, 92, 93, 100, 104–110, 112, 126, 127, 129, 131–134, 136–138, 142, 174, 288, 289, 295, 296, 299–301, 319, 424, 525, 533, 538
Vection Illusions, 108, 300
Vectored Thrust, 331
Velocity, 2, 23–27, 31, 37, 41, 45–49, 54–56, 58, 59, 62–64, 67, 74, 76, 78, 79, 84, 95, 100, 103, 104, 107, 122, 124, 129, 135, 140, 177, 246–248, 250, 258, 259, 262, 274, 299, 310, 343, 362, 385, 388, 391, 397, 399, 402, 419, 426, 455, 472, 505, 511, 513, 515, 518, 526, 529, 532
Vergence, 62, 81, 115, 116, 130, 139
Veronneau, Stephen, 445
Vertical-Speed Indicator, 235, 252, 388, 391, 397
Vertical-Velocity Indicator, 388, 397, 399
Vertical-Velocity/Speed Indicator (VVI/VSI), 391
Vestibular Habituation, 67, 80, 94
Vestibular System, 5, 7, 25, 27, 38, 40, 41, 63–65, 67, 70, 76–78, 81, 83–86, 90, 95, 96, 132, 133, 177, 206, 231, 239, 244, 269, 270, 275, 511, 517, 526
Vestibulo-Ocular Disorganization, 267
Vestibulo-Ocular Reflex (VOR), 41
Vestibulospinal Motor System, 21
Vestibulo-Spinal Reflexes, 205
VFR, 81, 174, 207, 233, 234, 236, 398, 442, 443, 532
Virtual Cockpit, 465, 532
Virtual Display, 419, 463, 505
Virtual HUD, 464, 466, 467, 503

Viscous Resistance, 46
Visual Dominance, 81, 112, 124, 125, 286, 299, 308, 532
Visually Perceived Eye Level, 111, 138
Visual Transition, 174
Visual Vertical, 69, 109, 112, 132
Visual-Vestibular Interaction, 5, 18, 35, 63, 64, 86–88, 136, 142, 143, 265, 280, 517
Visuomotor, 14
VMC, 69, 72, 174, 215, 226, 238, 239, 273, 286, 296–298, 315, 353, 362, 364, 365, 370, 398, 434, 442, 443, 474, 518
VOR, 41, 56–61, 63, 67, 70, 82, 84, 163, 198, 270

Waterline, 455, 469, 481
Whiteout, 146, 175, 206, 288, 291, 298, 299
William R. Ercoline, 1, 323, 379
Wobblies, 65, 267
Wright-Patterson AFB, 35, 446–448, 500, 504
Wyle, 340, 346, 348

Yaw, 19, 29–31, 42, 47–49, 51, 56, 58, 59, 64, 66–68, 72, 85, 104, 107, 108, 110, 132, 157, 165, 189, 219, 244, 247, 248, 250, 251, 256, 259, 264, 266, 267, 271, 279, 337, 338, 340, 342–346, 371, 384, 385, 387, 402, 419, 493, 495, 513, 515, 516
Young, Larry, 14

PROGRESS IN ASTRONAUTICS AND AERONAUTICS
SERIES VOLUMES

*1. Solid Propellant
Rocket Research (1960)
Martin Summerfield
Princeton University

*2. Liquid Rockets and
Propellants (1960)
Loren E. Bollinger
Ohio State University
Martin Goldsmith
The Rand Corp.
Alexis W. Lemmon Jr.
Battelle Memorial Institute

*3. Energy Conversion
for Space Power (1961)
Nathan W. Snyder
*Institute for Defense
Analyses*

*4. Space Power Systems
(1961)
Nathan W. Snyder
*Institute for Defense
Analyses*

*5. Electrostatic
Propulsion (1961)
David B. Langmuir
*Space Technology
Laboratories, Inc.*
Ernst Stuhlinger
*NASA George C. Marshall
Space Flight Center*
J. M. Sellen Jr.
*Space Technology
Laboratories, Inc.*

*6. Detonation and Two-
Phase Flow (1962)
S. S. Penner
*California Institute of
Technology*
F. A. Williams
Harvard University

*7. Hypersonic Flow
Research (1962)
Frederick R. Riddell
AVCO Corp.

*8. Guidance and Control
(1962)
Robert E. Roberson
Consultant
James S. Farrior
*Lockheed Missiles and
Space Co.*

*9. Electric Propulsion
Development (1963)
Ernst Stuhlinger
*NASA George C. Marshall
Space Flight Center*

*10. Technology of Lunar
Exploration (1963)
Clifford I. Cumming
Harold R. Lawrence
Jet Propulsion Laboratory

*11. Power Systems for
Space Flight (1963)
Morris A. Zipkin
Russell N. Edwards
General Electric Co.

*12. Ionization in High-
Temperature Gases (1963)
Kurt E. Shuler, Editor
*National Bureau of
Standards*
John B. Fenn,
Associate Editor
Princeton University

*13. Guidance and
Control-II (1964)
Robert C. Langford
General Precision Inc.
Charles J. Mundo
Institute of Naval Studies

*14. Celestial Mechanics
and Astrodynamics (1964)
Victor G. Szebehely
Yale University Observatory

*15. Heterogeneous
Combustion
(1964)
Hans G. Wolfhard
*Institute for Defense
Analyses*
Irvin Glassman
Princeton University
Leon Green Jr.
*Air Force Systems
Command*

*16. Space Power
Systems Engineering
(1966)
George C. Szego
*Institute for Defense
Analyses*
J. Edward Taylor
TRW Inc.

*17. Methods in
Astrodynamics and
Celestial Mechanics
(1966)
Raynor L. Duncombe
U.S. Naval Observatory
Victor G. Szebehely
*Yale University
Observatory*

*18. Thermophysics and
Temperature Control of
Spacecraft and Entry
Vehicles
(1966)
Gerhard B. Heller
*NASA George C. Marshall
Space Flight Center*

*19. Communication
Satellite Systems
Technology
(1966)
Richard B. Marsten
*Radio Corporation of
America*

*20. Thermophysics of Spacecraft and Planetary Bodies: Radiation Properties of Solids and the Electromagnetic Radiation Environment in Space (1967)
Gerhard B. Heller
NASA George C. Marshall Space Flight Center

*21. Thermal Design Principles of Spacecraft and Entry Bodies (1969)
Jerry T. Bevans
TRW Systems

*22. Stratospheric Circulation (1969)
Willis L. Webb
Atmospheric Sciences Laboratory, White Sands, and University of Texas at El Paso

*23. Thermophysics: Applications to Thermal Design of Spacecraft (1970)
Jerry T. Bevans
TRW Systems

*24. Heat Transfer and Spacecraft Thermal Control (1971)
John W. Lucas
Jet Propulsion Laboratory

*25. Communication Satellites for the 70's: Technology (1971)
Nathaniel E. Feldman
The Rand Corp.
Charles M. Kelly
The Aerospace Corp.

*26. Communication Satellites for the 70's: Systems (1971)
Nathaniel E. Feldman
The Rand Corp.
Charles M. Kelly
The Aerospace Corp.

*27. Thermospheric Circulation (1972)
Willis L. Webb
Atmospheric Sciences Laboratory, White Sands, and University of Texas at El Paso

*28. Thermal Characteristics of the Moon (1972)
John W. Lucas
Jet Propulsion Laboratory

*29. Fundamentals of Spacecraft Thermal Design (1972)
John W. Lucas
Jet Propulsion Laboratory

*30. Solar Activity Observations and Predictions (1972)
Patrick S. McIntosh
Murray Dryer
Environmental Research Laboratories, National Oceanic and Atmospheric Administration

*31. Thermal Control and Radiation (1973)
Chang-Lin Tien *University of California at Berkeley*

*32. Communications Satellite Systems (1974)
P. L. Bargellini
COMSAT Laboratories

*33. Communications Satellite Technology (1974)
P. L. Bargellini
COMSAT Laboratories

*34. Instrumentation for Airbreathing Propulsion (1974)
Allen E. Fuhs
Naval Postgraduate School
Marshall Kingery
Arnold Engineering Development Center

*35. Thermophysics and Spacecraft Thermal Control (1974)
Robert G. Hering
University of Iowa

*36. Thermal Pollution Analysis (1975)
Joseph A. Schetz
Virginia Polytechnic Institute
ISBN 0-915928-00-0

*37. Aeroacoustics: Jet and Combustion Noise; Duct Acoustics (1975)
Henry T. Nagamatsu, Editor
General Electric Research and Development Center
Jack V. O'Keefe,
Associate Editor
The Boeing Co.
Ira R. Schwartz,
Associate Editor
NASA Ames Research Center
ISBN 0-915928-01-9

*38. Aeroacoustics: Fan, STOL, and Boundary Layer Noise; Sonic Boom; Aeroacoustics Instrumentation (1975)
Henry T. Nagamatsu, Editor
General Electric Research and Development Center
Jack V. O'Keefe,
Associate Editor
The Boeing Co.
Ira R. Schwartz,
Associate Editor
NASA Ames Research Center
ISBN 0-915928-02-7

*39. Heat Transfer with Thermal Control Applications (1975)
M. Michael Yovanovich
University of Waterloo
ISBN 0-915928-03-5

*40. Aerodynamics of Base Combustion (1976)
S. N. B. Murthy, Editor
J. R. Osborn,
Associate Editor
Purdue University
A. W. Barrows
J. R. Ward,
Associate Editors
Ballistics Research Laboratories
ISBN 0-915928-04-3

---

*Out of print.

*41. Communications Satellite Developments: Systems (1976)
Gilbert E. LaVean
Defense Communications Agency
William G. Schmidt
CML Satellite Corp.
ISBN 0-915928-05-1

*42. Communications Satellite Developments: Technology (1976)
William G. Schmidt
CML Satellite Corp.
Gilbert E. LaVean
Defense Communications Agency
ISBN 0-915928-06-X

*43. Aeroacoustics: Jet Noise, Combustion and Core Engine Noise (1976) Ira R. Schwartz, Editor *NASA Ames Research Center*
Henry T. Nagamatsu, Associate Editor *General Electric Research and Development Center*
Warren C. Strahle, Associate Editor *Georgia Institute of Technology*
ISBN 0-915928-07-8

*44. Aeroacoustics: Fan Noise and Control; Duct Acoustics; Rotor Noise (1976)
Ira R. Schwartz, Editor *NASA Ames Research Center*
Henry T. Nagamatsu, Associate Editor *General Electric Research and Development Center*
Warren C. Strahle, Associate Editor *Georgia Institute of Technology*
ISBN 0-915928-08-6

*45. Aeroacoustics: STOL Noise; Airframe and Airfoil Noise (1976)
Ira R. Schwartz, Editor *NASA Ames Research Center*
Henry T. Nagamatsu, Associate Editor *General Electric Research and Development Center*
Warren C. Strahle, Associate Editor *Georgia Institute of Technology*
ISBN 0-915928-09-4

*46. Aeroacoustics: Acoustic Wave Propagation; Aircraft Noise Prediction; Aeroacoustic Instrumentation (1976)
Ira R. Schwartz, Editor *NASA Ames Research Center*
Henry T. Nagamatsu, Associate Editor *General Electric Research and Development Center*
Warren C. Strahle, Associate Editor *Georgia Institute of Technology*
ISBN 0-915928-10-8

*47. Spacecraft Charging by Magnetospheric Plasmas (1976)
Alan Rosen
TRW Inc.
ISBN 0-915928-11-6

*48. Scientific Investigations on the Skylab Satellite (1976)
Marion I. Kent
Ernst Stuhlinger
NASA George C. Marshall Space Flight Center
Shi-Tsan Wu
University of Alabama
ISBN 0-915928-12-4

*49. Radiative Transfer and Thermal Control (1976)
Allie M. Smith
ARO Inc.
ISBN 0-915928-13-2

*50. Exploration of the Outer Solar System (1976)
Eugene W. Greenstadt
TRW Inc.
Murray Dryer
National Oceanic and Atmospheric Administration
Devrie S. Intriligator
University of Southern California
ISBN 0-915928-14-0

*51. Rarefied Gas Dynamics, Parts I and II (two volumes) (1977)
J. Leith Potter
ARO Inc.
ISBN 0-915928-15-9

*52. Materials Sciences in Space with Application to Space Processing (1977)
Leo Steg
General Electric Co.
ISBN 0-915928-16-7

*53. Experimental Diagnostics in Gas Phase Combustion Systems (1977)
Ben T. Zinn, Editor *Georgia Institute of Technology*
Craig T. Bowman, Associate Editor *Stanford University*
Daniel L. Hartley, Associate Editor *Sandia Laboratories*
Edward W. Price, Associate Editor *Georgia Institute of Technology*
James G. Skifstad, Associate Editor *Purdue University*
ISBN 0-915928-18-3

*54. Satellite Communication: Future Systems (1977)
David Jarett
TRW Inc.
ISBN 0-915928-18-3

---

*Out of print.

*55. Satellite Communications: Advanced Technologies (1977)
David Jarett *TRW Inc.*
ISBN 0-915928-19-1

*56. Thermophysics of Spacecraft and Outer Planet Entry Probes (1977)
Allie M. Smith *ARO Inc.*
ISBN 0-915928-20-5

*57. Space-Based Manufacturing from Nonterrestrial Materials (1977)
Gerald K. O'Neill, Editor
Brian O'Leary, Assistant Editor
Princeton University
ISBN 0-915928-21-3

*58. Turbulent Combustion (1978)
Lawrence A. Kennedy
State University of New York at Buffalo
ISBN 0-915928-22-1

*59. Aerodynamic Heating and Thermal Protection Systems (1978)
Leroy S. Fletcher
University of Virginia
ISBN 0-915928-23-X

*60. Heat Transfer and Thermal Control Systems (1978)
Leroy S. Fletcher
University of Virginia
ISBN 0-915928-24-8

*61. Radiation Energy Conversion in Space (1978)
Kenneth W. Billman
NASA Ames Research Center
ISBN 0-915928-26-4

*62. Alternative Hydrocarbon Fuels: Combustion and Chemical Kinetics (1978)
Craig T. Bowman
Stanford University
Jorgen Birkeland
Department of Energy
ISBN 0-915928-25-6

*63. Experimental Diagnostics in Combustion of Solids (1978)
Thomas L. Boggs
Naval Weapons Center
Ben T. Zinn
Georgia Institute of Technology
ISBN 0-915928-28-0

*64. Outer Planet Entry Heating and Thermal Protection (1979)
Raymond Viskanta
Purdue University
ISBN 0-915928-29-9

*65. Thermophysics and Thermal Control (1979)
Raymond Viskanta
Purdue University
ISBN 0-915928-30-2

*66. Interior Ballistics of Guns (1979)
Herman Krier
University of Illinois at Urbana-Champaign
Martin Summerfield
New York University
ISBN 0-915928-32-9

*67. Remote Sensing of Earth from Space: Role of "Smart Sensors" (1979)
Roger A. Breckenridge
NASA Langley Research Center
ISBN 0-915928-33-7

*68. Injection and Mixing in Turbulent Flow (1980)
Joseph A. Schetz
Virginia Polytechnic Institute and State University
ISBN 0-915928-35-3

*69. Entry Heating and Thermal Protection (1980)
Walter B. Olstad
NASA Headquarters
ISBN 0-915928-38-8

*70. Heat Transfer, Thermal Control, and Heat Pipes (1980)
Walter B. Olstad
NASA Headquarters
ISBN 0-915928-39-6

*71. Space Systems and Their Interactions with Earth's Space Environment (1980)
Henry B. Garrett
Charles P. Pike
Hanscom Air Force Base
ISBN 0-915928-41-8

*72. Viscous Flow Drag Reduction (1980)
Gary R. Hough
Vought Advanced Technology Center
ISBN 0-915928-44-2

*73. Combustion Experiments in a Zero-Gravity Laboratory (1981)
Thomas H. Cochran
NASA Lewis Research Center
ISBN 0-915928-48-5

*74. Rarefied Gas Dynamics, Parts I and II (two volumes) (1981)
Sam S. Fisher
University of Virginia
ISBN 0-915928-51-5

*75. Gasdynamics of Detonations and Explosions (1981)
J. R. Bowen
University of Wisconsin at Madison
N. Manson
Universite de Poitiers
A. K. Oppenheim
University of California at Berkeley
R. I. Soloukhin
Institute of Heat and Mass Transfer, BSSR Academy of Sciences
ISBN 0-915928-46-9

*Out of print.

*76. Combustion in
Reactive Systems
(1981)
J. R. Bowen
University of Wisconsin
at Madison
N. Manson
Universite de Poitiers
A. K. Oppenheim
University of California
at Berkeley
R. I. Soloukhin
Institute of Heat and Mass
Transfer, BSSR Academy
of Sciences
ISBN 0-915928-47-7

*77. Aerothermodynamics
and Planetary Entry
(1981)
A. L. Crosbie
University of Missouri-Rolla
ISBN 0-915928-52-3

*78. Heat Transfer and
Thermal Control (1981)
A. L. Crosbie
University of Missouri-Rolla
ISBN 0-915928-53-1

*79. Electric Propulsion
and Its Applications to
Space Missions (1981)
Robert C. Finke
NASA Lewis Research
Center
ISBN 0-915928-55-8

*80. Aero-Optical
Phenomena (1982)
Keith G. Gilbert
Leonard J. Otten
Air Force Weapons
Laboratory
ISBN 0-915928-60-4

*81. Transonic
Aerodynamics (1982)
David Nixon
Nielsen Engineering &
Research, Inc.
ISBN 0-915928-65-5

*82. Thermophysics of
Atmospheric Entry (1982)
T. E. Horton
University of Mississippi
ISBN 0-915928-66-3

*83. Spacecraft Radiative
Transfer and Temperature
Control (1982)
T. E. Horton
University of Mississippi
ISBN 0-915928-67-1

*84. Liquid-Metal Flows
and Magneto-
hydrodynamics (1983)
H. Branover
Ben-Gurion University
of the Negev
P. S. Lykoudis
Purdue University
A. Yakhot
Ben-Gurion University
of the Negev
ISBN 0-915928-70-1

*85. Entry Vehicle
Heating and Thermal
Protection Systems: Space
Shuttle, Solar Starprobe,
Jupiter Galileo Probe (1983)
Paul E. Bauer
McDonnell Douglas
Astronautics Co.
Howard E. Collicott
The Boeing Co.
ISBN 0-915928-74-4

*86. Spacecraft Thermal
Control, Design, and
Operation (1983)
Howard E. Collicott
The Boeing Co.
Paul E. Bauer
McDonnell Douglas
Astronautics Co.
ISBN 0-915928-75-2

*87. Shock Waves,
Explosions, and
Detonations (1983)
J. R. Bowen
University of Washington
N. Manson
Universite de Poitiers
A. K. Oppenheim
University of California
at Berkeley
R. I. Soloukhin
Institute of Heat and Mass
Transfer, BSSR Academy
of Sciences
ISBN 0-915928-76-0

*88. Flames, Lasers, and
Reactive Systems (1983)
J. R. Bowen
University of Washington
N. Manson
Universite de Poitiers
A. K. Oppenheim
University of California
at Berkeley
R. I. Soloukhin
Institute of Heat and Mass
Transfer, BSSR Academy
of Sciences
ISBN 0-915928-77-9

*89. Orbit-Raising and
Maneuvering Propulsion:
Research Status and
Needs (1984)
Leonard H. Caveny
Air Force Office of
Scientific Research
ISBN 0-915928-82-5

*90. Fundamentals
of Solid-Propellant
Combustion (1984)
Kenneth K. Kuo
Pennsylvania State
University
Martin Summerfield
Princeton Combustion
Research Laboratories, Inc.
ISBN 0-915928-84-1

*91. Spacecraft
Contamination: Sources
and Prevention
(1984)
J. A. Roux, Editor
University of Mississippi
T. D. McCay, Editor
NASA Marshall Space
Flight Center
ISBN 0-915928-85-X

*92. Combustion
Diagnostics by
Nonintrusive Methods
(1984)
T. D. McCay, Editor
NASA Marshall Space
Flight Center
J. A. Roux, Editor
University of Mississippi
ISBN 0-915928-86-8

*Out of print.

*93. The INTELSAT
Global Satellite System
(1984)
Joel Alper
COMSAT Corp.
Joseph Pelton
INTELSAT
ISBN 0-915928-90-6

*94. Dynamics of Shock
Waves, Explosions, and
Detonations (1984)
J. R. Bowen
University of Washington
N. Manson
Universite de Poitiers
A. K. Oppenheim
University of California
at Berkeley
R. I. Soloukhin
Institute of Heat and Mass
Transfer, BSSR Academy
of Sciences
ISBN 0-915928-91-4

*95. Dynamics of Flames
and Reactive Systems
(1984)
J. R. Bowen
University of Washington
N. Manson
Universite de Poitiers
A. K. Oppenheim
University of California
at Berkeley
R. I. Soloukhin
Institute of Heat and Mass
Transfer, BSSR Academy
of Sciences
ISBN 0-915928-92-2

*96. Thermal Design of
Aeroassisted Orbital
Transfer Vehicles (1985)
H. F. Nelson, Editor
University of Missouri-Rolla
ISBN 0-915928-94-9

*97. Monitoring Earth's
Ocean, Land, and
Atmosphere from Space—
Sensors, Systems, and
Applications (1985)
Abraham Schnapf
Aerospace Systems
Engineering
ISBN 0-915928-98-1

98. Thrust and Drag: Its
Prediction and
Verification (1985)
Eugene E. Covert
Massachusetts Institute
of Technology
C. R. James
Vought Corp.
William F. Kimzey
Sverdrup Technology
AEDC Group
George K. Richey
U.S. Air Force
Eugene C. Rooney
U.S. Navy Department
of Defense
ISBN 0-930403-00-2

99. Space Stations and
Space Platforms—
Concepts, Design,
Infrastructure, and Uses
(1985)
Ivan Bekey
Daniel Herman
NASA Headquarters
ISBN 0-930403-01-0

*100. Single- and Multi-
Phase Flows in an
Electromagnetic Field:
Energy, Metallurgical, and
Solar Applications (1985)
Herman Branover, Editor
Ben-Gurion University
of the Negev
Paul S. Lykoudis, Editor
Purdue University
Michael Mond, Editor
Ben-Gurion University
of the Negev
ISBN 0-930403-04-5

*101. MHD Energy
Conversion: Physiotechnical
Problems (1986)
V. A. Kirillin, Editor
A. E. Sheyndlin, Editor
Soviet Academy of Sciences
ISBN 0-930403-05-3

*102. Numerical Methods
for Engine-Airframe
Integration (1986)
S. N. B. Murthy, Editor
Purdue University
Gerald C. Paynter, Editor
Boeing Airplane Co.
ISBN 0-930403-09-6

*103. Thermophysical
Aspects of Re-Entry
Flows (1986)
James N. Moss
NASA Langley Research
Center
Carl D. Scott
NASA Johnson Space
Center
ISBN 0-930403-10-X

*104. Tactical Missile
Aerodynamics (1986)
M. J. Hemsch, Editor
PRC Kentron, Inc.
J. N. Nielson,
Editor
NASA Ames Research
Center
ISBN 0-930403-13-4

*105. Dynamics of
Reactive Systems
Part I: Flames and
Configurations;
Part II: Modeling and
Heterogeneous
Combustion
(1986)
J. R. Bowen, Editor
University of
Washington
J.-C. Leyer, Editor
Universite de Poitiers
R. I. Soloukhin,
Editor
Institute of Heat
and Mass Transfer,
BSSR Academy of
Sciences
ISBN 0-930403-14-2

*106. Dynamics of
Explosions (1986)
J. R. Bowen, Editor
University of
Washington
J.-C. Leyer, Editor
Universite de Poitiers
R. I. Soloukhin, Editor
Institute of Heat
and Mass Transfer,
BSSR Academy
of Sciences
ISBN 0-930403-15-0

*Out of print.

***107. Spacecraft
Dielectric Material
Properties and Spacecraft
Charging (1986)**
A. R. Frederickson
*U.S. Air Force Rome Air
Development Center*
D. B. Cotts
SRI International
J. A. Wall
*U.S. Air Force Rome Air
Development Center*
F. L. Bouquet
*Jet Propulsion Laboratory,
California Institute of
Technology*
ISBN 0-930403-17-7

***108. Opportunities for
Academic Research in a
Low-Gravity Environment
(1986)**
George A. Hazelrigg
*National Science
Foundation*
Joseph M. Reynolds
Louisiana State University
ISBN 0-930403-18-5

***109. Gun Propulsion
Technology (1988)**
Ludwig Stiefel
*U.S. Army Armament
Research, Development and
Engineering Center*
ISBN 0-930403-20-7

***110. Commercial
Opportunities in Space
(1988)**
F. Shahrokhi, Editor
K. E. Harwell, Editor
*University of Tennessee
Space Institute*
C. C. Chao, Editor
*National Cheng Kung
University*
ISBN 0-930403-39-8

***111. Liquid-Metal Flows:
Magnetohydrodynamics
and Application (1988)**
Herman Branover, Editor
Michael Mond, Editor
Yeshajahu Unger, Editor
*Ben-Gurion University
of the Negev*
ISBN 0-930403-43-6

***112. Current Trends
in Turbulence Research
(1988)**
Herman Branover, Editor
Micheal Mond, Editor
Yeshajahu Unger, Editor
*Ben-Gurion University of
the Negev*
ISBN 0-930403-44-4

***113. Dynamics of Reactive
Systems Part I: Flames;
Part II:
Heterogeneous
Combustion and
Applications (1988)**
A. L. Kuhl, Editor
R&D Associates
J. R. Bowen, Editor
University of Washington
J.-C. Leyer, Editor
Universite de Poitiers
A. Borisov, Editor
USSR Academy of Sciences
ISBN 0-930403-46-0

***114. Dynamics of
Explosions (1988)**
A. L. Kuhl, Editor
R & D Associates
J. R. Bowen, Editor
University of Washington
J.-C. Leyer, Editor
Universite de Poitiers
A. Borisov, Editor
USSR Academy of Sciences
ISBN 0-930403-47-9

***115. Machine
Intelligence and Autonomy
for Aerospace (1988)**
E. Heer, *Heer Associates, Inc.*
H. Lum
NASA Ames Research Center
ISBN 0-930403-48-7

***116. Rarefied Gas
Dynamics: Space Related
Studies (1989)**
E. P. Muntz, Editor
*University of Southern
California*
D. P. Weaver, Editor
*U.S. Air Force Astronautics
Laboratory (AFSC)*
D. H. Campbell, Editor
*University of Dayton
Research Institute*
ISBN 0-930403-53-3

***117. Rarefied Gas
Dynamics: Physical
Phenomena (1989)**
E. P. Muntz, Editor
*University of Southern
California*
D. P. Weaver, Editor
*U.S. Air Force Astronautics
Laboratory (AFSC)*
D. H. Campbell, Editor
*University of Dayton
Research Institute*
ISBN 0-930403-54-1

***118. Rarefied Gas
Dynamics: Theoretical
and Computational
Techniques (1989)**
E. P. Muntz, Editor
*University of Southern
California*
D. P. Weaver, Editor
*U.S. Air Force Astronautics
Laboratory (AFSC)*
D. H. Campbell, Editor
*University of Dayton
Research Institute*
ISBN 0-930403-55-X

**119. Test and Evaluation
of the Tactical Missile (1989)**
Emil J. Eichblatt Jr., Editor
Pacific Missile Test Center
ISBN 0-930403-56-8

***120. Unsteady Transonic
Aerodynamics (1989)**
David Nixon
*Nielsen Engineering &
Research, Inc.*
ISBN 0-930403-52-5

**121. Orbital Debris from
Upper-Stage Breakup (1989)**
Joseph P. Loftus Jr.
*NASA Johnson Space
Center*
ISBN 0-930403-58-4

**122. Thermal-Hydraulics
for Space Power,
Propulsion and Thermal
Management System
Design (1990)**
William J. Krotiuk
General Electric Co.
ISBN 0-930403-64-9

---

*Out of print.

123. Viscous Drag Reduction in Boundary Layers (1990)
Dennis M. Bushnell
Jerry N. Hefner
NASA Langley Research Center
ISBN 0-930403-66-5

***124. Tactical and Strategic Missile Guidance (1990)**
Paul Zarchan
Charles Stark Draper Laboratory, Inc.
ISBN 0-930403-68-1

125. Applied Computational Aerodynamics (1990)
P. A. Henne, Editor
Douglas Aircraft Company
ISBN 0-930403-69-X

126. Space Commercialization: Launch Vehicles and Programs (1990)
F. Shahrokhi
University of Tennessee Space Institute
J. S. Greenberg
Princeton Synergetics Inc.
T. Al-Saud
Ministry of Defense and Aviation Kingdom of Saudi Arabia
ISBN 0-930403-75-4

127. Space Commercialization: Platforms and Processing (1990)
F. Shahrokhi
University of Tennessee Space Institute
G. Hazelrigg
National Science Foundation
R. Bayuzick
Vanderbilt University
ISBN 0-930403-76-2

128. Space Commercialization: Satellite Technology (1990)
F. Shahrokhi
University of Tennessee Space Institute
N. Jasentuliyana
United Nations
N. Tarabzouni
King Abulaziz City for Science and Technology
ISBN 0-930403-77-0

***129. Mechanics and Control of Large Flexible Structures (1990)**
John L. Junkins
Texas A&M University
ISBN 0-930403-73-8

130. Low-Gravity Fluid Dynamics and Transport Phenomena (1990)
Jean N. Koster
Robert L. Sani
University of Colorado at Boulder
ISBN 0-930403-74-6

131. Dynamics of Deflagrations and Reactive Systems: Flames (1991)
A. L. Kuhl
Lawrence Livermore National Laboratory
J.-C. Leyer
Universite de Poitiers
A. A. Borisov
USSR Academy of Sciences
W. A. Sirignano
University of California
ISBN 0-930403-95-9

132. Dynamics of Deflagrations and Reactive Systems: Heterogeneous Combustion (1991)
A. L. Kuhl
Lawrence Livermore National Laboratory
J.-C. Leyer
Universite de Poitiers
A. A. Borisov
USSR Academy of Sciences
W. A. Sirignano
University of California
ISBN 0-930403-96-7

133. Dynamics of Detonations and Explosions: Detonations (1991)
A. L. Kuhl
Lawrence Livermore National Laboratory
J.-C. Leyer
Universite de Poitiers
A. A. Borisov
USSR Academy of Sciences
W. A. Sirignano
University of California
ISBN 0-930403-97-5

134. Dynamics of Detonations and Explosions: Explosion Phenomena (1991)
A. L. Kuhl
Lawrence Livermore National Laboratory
J.-C. Leyer
Universite de Poitiers
A. A. Borisov
USSR Academy of Sciences
W. A. Sirignano
University of California
ISBN 0-930403-98-3

***135. Numerical Approaches to Combustion Modeling (1991)**
Elaine S. Oran
Jay P. Boris
Naval Research Laboratory
ISBN 1-56347-004-7

136. Aerospace Software Engineering (1991)
Christine Anderson, Editor
U.S. Air Force Wright Laboratory
Merlin Dorfman, Editor
Lockheed Missiles & Space Company, Inc.
ISBN 1-56347-005-5

137. High-Speed Flight Propulsion Systems (1991)
S. N. B. Murthy
Purdue University
E. T. Curran
Wright Laboratory
ISBN 1-56347-011-X

---

*Out of print.

138. Propagation of Intensive Laser Radiation in Clouds (1992)
O. A. Volkovitsky
Yu. S. Sedenov
L. P. Semenov
Institute of Experimental Meteorology
ISBN 1-56347-020-9

139. Gun Muzzle Blast and Flash (1992)
Günter Klingenberg
Fraunhofer-Institut für Kurzzeitdynamik, Ernst-Mach-Institut
Joseph M. Heimerl
U.S. Army Ballistic Research Laboratory
ISBN 1-56347-012-8

*140. Thermal Structures and Materials for High-Speed Flight (1992)
Earl. A. Thornton
University of Virginia
ISBN 1-56347-017-9

141. Tactical Missile Aerodynamics: General Topics (1992)
Michael J. Hemsch
Lockheed Engineering & Sciences Company
ISBN 1-56347-015-2

142. Tactical Missile Aerodynamics: Prediction Methodology (1992)
Michael R. Mendenhall
Nielsen Engineering & Research, Inc.
ISBN 1-56347-016-0

143. Nonsteady Burning and Combustion Stability of Solid Propellants (1992)
Luigi De Luca, Editor
Politecnico di Milano
Edward W. Price, Editor
Georgia Institute of Technology
Martin Summerfield, Editor
Princeton Combustion Research Laboratories, Inc.
ISBN 1-56347-014-4

144. Space Economics (1992)
Joel S. Greenberg, Editor
Princeton Synergetics, Inc.
Henry R. Hertzfeld, Editor
HRH Associates
ISBN 1-56347-042-X

145. Mars: Past, Present, and Future (1992)
E. Brian Pritchard
NASA Langley Research Center
ISBN 1-56347-043-8

146. Computational Nonlinear Mechanics in Aerospace Engineering (1992)
Satya N. Atluri
Georgia Institute of Technology
ISBN 1-56347-044-6

147. Modern Engineering for Design of Liquid-Propellant Rocket Engines (1992)
Dieter K. Huzel
David H. Huang
Rocketdyne Division of Rockwell International
ISBN 1-56347-013-6

148. Metallurgical Technologies, Energy Conversion, and Magneto-hydrodynamic Flows (1993)
Herman Branover
Yeshajahu Unger
Ben-Gurion University of the Negev
ISBN 1-56347-019-5

149. Advances in Turbulence Studies (1993)
Herman Branover
Yeshajahu Unger
Ben-Gurion University of the Negev
ISBN 1-56347-018-7

150. Structural Optimization: Status and Promise (1993)
Manohar P. Kamat
Georgia Institute of Technology
ISBN 1-56347-056-X

151. Dynamics of Gaseous Combustion (1993)
A. L. Kuhl,
Editor
Lawrence Livermore National Laboratory
J.-C. Leyer,
Editor
Universite de Poitiers
A. A. Borisov, Editor
USSR Academy of Sciences
W. A. Sirignano, Editor
University of California
ISBN 1-56347-060-8

152. Dynamics of Heterogeneous Gaseous Combustion and Reacting Systems (1993)
A. L. Kuhl, Editor
Lawrence Livermore National Laboratory
J.-C. Leyer,
Editor
Universite de Poitiers
A. A. Borisov, Editor
USSR Academy of Sciences
W. A. Sirignano, Editor
University of California
ISBN 1-56347-058-6

153. Dynamic Aspects of Detonations (1993)
A. L. Kuhl
Lawrence Livermore National Laboratory
J.-C. Leyer
Universite de Poitiers
A. A. Borisov
USSR Academy of Sciences
W. A. Sirignano
University of California
ISBN 1-56347-057-8

154. Dynamic Aspects of Explosion Phenomena (1993)
A. L. Kuhl
Lawrence Livermore National Laboratory
J.-C. Leyer
Universite de Poitiers
A. A. Borisov
USSR Academy of Sciences
W. A. Sirignano
University of California
ISBN 1-56347-059-4

---

*Out of print.

155. Tactical Missile Warheads (1993)
Joseph Carleone, Editor
Aerojet General Corporation
ISBN 1-56347-067-5

156. Toward a Science of Command, Control, and Communications (1993)
Carl R. Jones
Naval Postgraduate School
ISBN 1-56347-068-3

*157. Tactical and Strategic Missile Guidance Second Edition (1994)
Paul Zarchan
Charles Stark Draper Laboratory, Inc.
ISBN 1-56347-077-2

158. Rarefied Gas Dynamics: Experimental Techniques and Physical Systems (1994)
Bernie D. Shizgal, Editor
University of British Columbia
David P. Weaver, Editor
Phillips Laboratory
ISBN 1-56347-079-9

*159. Rarefied Gas Dynamics: Theory and Simulations (1994)
Bernie D. Shizgal, Editor
University of British Columbia
David P. Weaver, Editor
Phillips Laboratory
ISBN 1-56347-080-2

160. Rarefied Gas Dynamics: Space Sciences and Engineering (1994)
Bernie D. Shizgal, Editor
University of British Columbia
David P. Weaver, Editor
Phillips Laboratory
ISBN 1-56347-081-0

161. Teleoperation and Robotics in Space (1994)
Steven B. Skaar
University of Notre Dame
Carl F. Ruoff
Jet Propulsion Laboratory, California Institute of Technology
ISBN 1-56347-095-0

162. Progress in Turbulence Research (1994)
Herman Branover, Editor
Yeshajahu Unger, Editor
Ben-Gurion University of the Negev
ISBN 1-56347-099-3

163. Global Positioning System: Theory and Applications, Volume I (1996)
Bradford W. Parkinson, Editor
Stanford University
James J. Spilker Jr., Editor
Stanford Telecom
Penina Axelrad, Associate Editor
University of Colorado
Per Enge, Associate Editor
Stanford University
ISBN 1-56347-107-8

164. Global Positioning System: Theory and Applications, Volume II (1996)
Bradford W. Parkinson, Editor
Stanford University
James J. Spilker Jr., Editor
Stanford Telecom
Penina Axelrad, Associate Editor
University of Colorado
Per Enge, Associate Editor
Stanford University
ISBN 1-56347-106-X

165. Developments in High-Speed Vehicle Propulsion Systems (1996)
S. N. B. Murthy, Editor
Purdue University
E. T. Curran, Editor
Wright Laboratory
ISBN 1-56347-176-0

166. Recent Advances in Spray Combustion: Spray Atomization and Drop Burning Phenomena, Volume I (1996)
Kenneth K. Kuo
Pennsylvania State University
ISBN 1-56347-175-2

167. Fusion Energy in Space Propulsion (1995)
Terry Kammash
University of Michigan
ISBN 1-56347-184-1

168. Aerospace Thermal Structures and Materials for a New Era (1995)
Earl A. Thornton, Editor
University of Virginia
ISBN 1-56347-182-5

169. Liquid Rocket Engine Combustion Instability (1995)
Vigor Yang
William E. Anderson
Pennsylvania State University
ISBN 1-56347-183-3

170. Tactical Missile Propulsion (1996)
G. E. Jensen, Editor
United Technologies Corporation
David W. Netzer, Editor
Naval Postgraduate School
ISBN 1-56347-118-3

171. Recent Advances in Spray Combustion: Spray Combustion Measurements and Model Simulation, Volume II (1996)
Kenneth K. Kuo
Pennsylvania State University
ISBN 1-56347-181-7

172. Future Aeronautical and Space Systems (1997)
Ahmed K. Noor
NASA Langley Research Center
Samuel L. Venneri
NASA Headquarters
ISBN 1-56347-188-4

*Out of print.

173. Advances in
Combustion Science:
In Honor of Ya. B.
Zel'dovich (1997)
William A. Sirignano,
Editor
University of California
Alexander G. Merzhanov,
Editor
*Russian Academy
of Sciences*
Luigi De Luca, Editor
Politecnico di Milano
ISBN 1-56347-178-7

174. Fundamentals of
High Accuracy Inertial
Navigation (1997)
Averil B. Chatfield
ISBN 1-56347-243-0

175. Liquid Propellant
Gun Technology (1997)
Günter Klingenberg
*Fraunhofer-Institut für
Kurzzeitdynamik,
Ernst-Mach-Institut*
John D. Knapton
Walter F. Morrison
Gloria P. Wren
*U.S. Army Research
Laboratory*
ISBN 1-56347-196-5

*176. Tactical and
Strategic Missile Guidance,
Third Edition (1998)
Paul Zarchan
*Charles Stark Draper
Laboratory, Inc.*
ISBN 1-56347-254-6

177. Orbital and Celestial
Mechanics (1998)
John P. Vinti
Gim J. Der, Editor
TRW
Nino L. Bonavito, Editor
*NASA Goddard Space
Flight Center*
ISBN 1-56347-256-2

178. Some Engineering
Applications in Random
Vibrations and Random
Structures (1998)
Giora Maymon
RAFAEL
ISBN 1-56347-258-9

179. Conventional
Warhead Systems Physics
and Engineering Design
(1998)
Richard M. Lloyd
Raytheon Systems Company
ISBN 1-56347-255-4

180. Advances in Missile
Guidance Theory (1998)
Joseph Z. Ben-Asher
Isaac Yaesh
*Israel Military Industries—
Advanced Systems Division*
ISBN 1-56347-275-9

181. Satellite Thermal
Control for Systems
Engineers (1998)
Robert D. Karam
ISBN 1-56347-276-7

182. Progress in Fluid
Flow Research:
Turbulence and Applied
MHD (1998)
Yeshajahu Unger
Herman Branover
*Ben-Gurion University
of the Negev*
ISBN 1-56347-284-8

183. Aviation Weather
Surveillance Systems
(1999)
Pravas R. Mahapatra
Indian Institute of Science
ISBN 1-56347-340-2

184. Flight Control
Systems (2000)
Rodger W. Pratt, Editor
Loughborough University
ISBN 1-56347-404-2

185. Solid Propellant
Chemistry, Combustion,
and Motor Interior
Ballistics (2000)
Vigor Yang, Editor
*Pennsylvania State
University*
Thomas B. Brill, Editor
University of Delaware
Wu-Zhen Ren, Editor
China Ordnance Society
ISBN 1-56347-442-5

186. Approximate
Methods for Weapons
Aerodynamics (2000)
Frank G. Moore
ISBN 1-56347-399-2

187. Micropropulsion
for Small Spacecraft
(2000)
Michael M. Micci, Editor
Pennsylvania State University
Andrew D. Ketsdever,
Editor
*Air Force Research
Laboratory, Edwards Air
Force Base*
ISBN 1-56347-448-4

188. Structures
Technology for Future
Aerospace Systems (2000)
Ahmed K. Noor, Editor
*NASA Langley Research
Center*
ISBN 1-56347-384-4

189. Scramjet Propulsion
(2000)
E. T. Curran, Editor
Department of the Air Force
S. N. B. Murthy, Editor
Purdue University
ISBN 1-56347-322-4

190. Fundamentals of
Kalman Filtering: A
Practical Approach (2000)
Paul Zarchan
Howard Musoff
*Charles Stark Draper
Laboratory, Inc.*
ISBN 1-56347-455-7

191. Gossamer Spacecraft:
Membrane and Inflatable
Structures Technology for
Space Applications (2001)
Christopher H. M. Jenkins
Editor
South Dakota School of Mines
ISBN 1-56347-403-4

192. Theater Ballistic
Missile Defense (2001)
Ben-Zion Naveh, Editor
Azriel Lorber, Editor
Wales Ltd.
ISBN 1-56347-385-2

*Out of print.

193. Air Transportation Systems Engineering (2001)
George L. Donohue,
Editor
George Mason University
Andres Zellweger,
Editor
Embry Riddle Aeronautical University
ISBN 1-56347-474-3

194. Physics of Direct Hit and Near Miss Warhead Technology (2001)
Richard M. Lloyd
Raytheon Electronics Systems
ISBN 1-56347-473-5

195. Fixed and Flapping Wing Aerodynamics for Micro Air Vehicle Applications (2001)
Thomas J. Mueller,
Editor
University of Notre Dame
ISBN 1-56347-517-0

196. Physical and Chemical Processes in Gas Dynamics: Cross Sections and Rate Constants for Physical and Chemical Processes, Volume I (2002)
G. G. Chernyi
S. A. Losev
Moscow State University
S. O. Macharet
Princeton University
B. V. Potapkin
Kurchatov Institute
ISBN 1-56347-518-9

197. Physical and Chemical Processes in Gas Dynamics: Physical and Chemical Kinetics and Thermodynamics of Gases and Plasmas, Volume II
G. G. Chernyi
S. A. Losev
Moscow State University
S. O. Macharet
Princeton University
B. V. Potapkin
Kurchatov Institute
ISBN 1-56347-519-7

198. Advanced Hypersonic Test Facilities (2002)
Frank K. Lu,
Editor
University of Texas at Arlington
Dan E. Marren,
Editor
Arnold Engineering Development Center
ISBN 1-56347-541-3

199. Tactical and Strategic Missile Guidance, Fourth Edition (2002)
Paul Zarchan
MIT Lincoln Laboratory
ISBN 1-56347-497-2

200. Liquid Rocket Thrust Chambers: Aspects of Modeling, Analysis, and Design
Vigor Yang, Editor
Pennsylvania State University
Mohammed Habiballah,
Editor
ONERA
Michael Popp, Editor
Pratt & Whitney
James Hulka, Editor
Aerojet-General Corporation
ISBN 1-56347-223-6

201. Economic Principles Applied to Space Industry Decisions (2003)
Joel S. Greenberg
Princeton Synergetics, Inc.
ISBN 1-56347-607-X

202. Satellite Communications in the 21st Century: Trends and Technologies (2003)
Takashi Iida, Editor
Communications Research Laboratory
Joseph N. Pelton, Editor
George Washington University
Edward W. Ashford,
Editor
SES GLOBAL
ISBN 1-56347-579-0

203. Spatial Disorientation in Aviation (2004)
William R. Ercoline, Editor
General Dynamics Advanced Information Systems
Fred H. Previc, Editor
Northrop Grumman Information Technology
ISBN 1-56347-654-1

---

*Out of print.